Progress in
Cancer Research and Therapy
Volume 6

IMMUNOTHERAPY OF CANCER: PRESENT STATUS OF TRIALS IN MAN

Progress in
Cancer Research and Therapy

Progress in
Cancer Research and Therapy
Volume 6

Immunotherapy of Cancer: Present Status of Trials in Man

Edited by

William D. Terry, M.D.
Chief, Immunology Branch
Division of Cancer Biology and
  Diagnosis
National Cancer Institute
Bethesda, Maryland

Dorothy Windhorst, M.D.
Assistant Medical Director
Division of Medical Research
Hoffmann–La Roche Inc.
Nutley, New Jersey
Formerly *Medical Officer*
Immunology Branch
National Cancer Institute
National Institutes of Health
Bethesda, Maryland

Raven Press ▪ New York

Raven Press, 1140 Avenue of the Americas, New York, New York 10036

Raven Press, New York, 1978

Made in the United States of America

Library of Congress Cataloging in Publication Data
Main entry under title:

Immunotherapy of cancer.

    (Progress in cancer research and therapy; v. 6)
    Includes bibliographical references and index.
    1. Cancer—Chemotherapy. 2. Immunotherapy.
I. Terry, William D. II. Windhorst, Dorothy. III. Series. [DNLM: 1. Neoplasms—Therapy. 2. Immunotherapy W1 PR667M v. 6 / QZ267 I33]
RC271.C51543   616.9'94'061   77–83696
ISBN 0-89004-182-2

Preface

This volume reviews the present state of knowledge in the field of immuno-therapy of human cancer, based on both large clinical trials and more pre-liminary studies.

Sections of the volume are devoted to the immunotherapy of melanoma, lung cancer, osteogenic sarcoma, acute myelogenous leukemia, acute lym-phatic leukemia and lymphomas, gastrointestinal cancer and breast cancer. The natural history, standard therapy, and a description of prognostically important factors for each of these cancers are also reviewed. Discussions focus on a critical evaluation of the results of clinical immunotherapy trials, both from the perspective of immunotherapy and the perspective of clinical trial design.

Contents

Contributors

J. Adamus
Oncological Institute
Gliwice, Poland

P. Alberto
Division of Oncology
University of Geneva
Geneva, Switzerland

Peter Alexander
Institute of Cancer Research
The Royal Marsden Hospital
Sutton, Surrey, England

Willem K. Amery
Janssen Pharmaceutica
B-2340 Beerse, Belgium

J. L. Amiel
Institut de Cancérologie et d'Immuno-
génétique
INSERM
Hôpital Paul-Brousse
Villejuif, France

J. M. Andrien
Hôpital Civil de Verviers
Rue Hauzeur de Simonis
Verviers, Belgium

Gerald V. Aranha
Department of Surgery
University of Minnesota
Minneapolis, Minnesota 55455

Donald Armstrong
Memorial Sloan-Kettering Cancer
Center
New York, New York 10021

C. Aubert
Institut Paoli Calmettes
Marseille, France

Richard F. Bakemeier
University of Rochester Cancer Cen-
ter
Rochester, New York 14642

Stanley Balcerzak
Ohio State University Hospital
Columbus, Ohio 43210

Alfred A. Bartolucci
Division of Hematology and Medical
Oncology
Department of Biometry
Emory University School of Medicine
Atlanta, Georgia 30322

Raymond Belanger
Department of Surgery
University of Ottawa
Ottawa, Canada

Robert E. Bellet
Department of Medicine
Temple University School of Medi-
cine
Philadelphia, Pennsylvania 19104

D. Belpomme
Institut de Cancérologie et d'Immu-
nogénétique
INSERM
Hôpital Paul-Brousse
Villejuif, France

W. Berchtold
Department of Biometry and Popu-
lation Genetics
Swiss Federal Institute of Technology
Zurich, Switzerland

David Berd
University of Pennsylvania
School of Medicine
Philadelphia, Pennsylvania 19104

Gianni Beretta
Istituto Nazionale Tumori
20133 Milan, Italy

George J. Beski
Department of Neoplastic Diseases
Mount Sinai School of Medicine
New York, New York 10029

M. P. Beumer-Jockmans
Institut Pasteur du Brabant
Brussels, Belgium

Ronald Blum
The Sidney Farber Cancer Institute
Boston, Massachusetts 02115

G. R. Blumenschein
Departments of Developmental
Therapeutics and Medicine
The University of Texas System
Cancer Center
M.D. Anderson Hospital and Tumor
Institute
Houston, Texas 77030

Gerald P. Bodey
Department of Developmental
Therapeutics
The University of Texas System
Cancer Center
M.D. Anderson Hospital and
Tumor Institute
Houston, Texas 77030

G. Bonadonna
Istituto Nazionale Tumori
Milan, Italy

G. Brenning
Karolinska Institute
Leukemia Group of Central Sweden
Stockholm, Sweden

N. Breslow
Department of Biostatistics
University of Washington
Seattle, Washington 98105

Andrew W. Bruce
Department of Urology
Queen's University
Kingston, Ontario, Canada

Michael A. Burgess
Department of Developmental
Therapeutics
The University of Texas System
Cancer Center
M.D. Anderson Hospital and
Tumor Institute
Houston, Texas 77030

J. Bury
Hôpital de Bavière
University of Liège
Liège, Belgium

James J. Butler
Department of Pathology
University of Texas System
Cancer Center
M.D. Anderson Hospital and
Tumor Institute
Houston, Texas 77030

A. Buzdar
Departments of Developmental
Therapeutics and Medicine
The University of Texas System
Cancer Center
M.D. Anderson Hospital and
Tumor Institute
Houston, Texas 77030

Robert B. Catalano
Department of Medicine
American Oncologic Hospital
Fox Chase Cancer Center
Philadelphia, Pennsylvania 19111

A. Cattan
Institut de Cancérologie et d'Immuno-
génétique
INSERM
Hôpital Paul-Brousse
Villejuif, France

Franco Cavalli
Division of Oncology
University of Bern
Bern, Switzerland

B. Chapuis
Institute of Cancer Research
The Royal Marsden Hospital
Sutton, Surrey, England

Randolph H. Chase
Laboratory of Cellular Immunology
Children's Hospital of San Francisco
San Francisco, California 94118

Wallace H. Clark, Jr.
Temple University School of Medi-
cine
Philadelphia, Pennsylvania 19140

Bayard D. Clarkson
Memorial Sloan-Kettering Cancer
Center
New York, New York 10021

A. Cochran
University of Glasgow—Western
Infirmary
Glasgow, Scotland

Martin H. Cohen
Veterans Administration Hospital
Washington, D.C. 20010

James Conroy
Cancer Institute
Hahnemann Medical College
Philadelphia, Pennsylvania 15261

John J. Costanzi
University of Texas Medical Branch
Galveston, Texas 77550

William Costello
State University of New York at
Buffalo
Buffalo, New York 14226

Richard H. Creech
Department of Medicine
American Oncologic Hospital
Fox Chase Cancer Center
Philadelphia, Pennsylvania 19111

André Crepeau
Department of Surgery
University of Ottawa
Ottawa, Canada

Alfred F. Crook
Department of Medicine
University of Ottawa
Ottawa, Canada

D. Crowther
CRC Medical Professional Oncology
Unit
The Christie Hospital
Manchester, England

Isabelle Cunningham
Memorial Sloan-Kettering Cancer
Center
New York City, New York 10021

Thomas J. Cunningham
Albany Regional Cancer Center
Albany, New York 12208

Janet Cuttner
Division of Hematology
Mount Sinai School of Medicine
New York, New York 10029

David C. Dahlin
Department of Surgical Pathology
Mayo Clinic
Rochester, Minnesota 55901

J. L. David
Hôpital de Bavièrei
University of Liège
4000 Liège, Belgium

Robert L. DeJager
Memorial Sloan-Kettering Cancer
Center
New York, New York 10021

Jean B. deKernion
Department of Surgery
University of California at
Los Angeles
School of Medicine
Center for the Health Sciences
Los Angeles, California 90024

G. Delalieux
Hôpital St. Pierre
Free University of Brussels
Brussels, Belgium

M. J. Delbeke
Akademisch Ziekenhuis
University of Gent
Gent, Belgium

M. Delgado
Institut de Cancérologie et d'Immu-
nogénétique
INSERM
Hôpital Paul-Brousse
Villejuif, France

J. De Marsillac
Institut Nacional de Cancer
Rio de Janeiro, Brazil

R. Denolin
Hôpital St. Pierre
Free University of Brussels
Service Hematologie
1000 Brussels, Belgium

P. De Porre
Akademisch Zienkenhuis
University of Gent
de Pintelaan, 135
9000 Gent, Belgium

F. De Vassal
Institut de Cancérologie et d'Immu-
nogénétique
INSERM
Hôpital Paul-Brousse
Villejuif, France

Vincent T. DeVita
National Cancer Institute
Bethesda, Maryland 20014

Nikolay V. Dimitrov
Department of Medicine
Michigan State University
East Lansing, Michigan 48824

Monroe D. Dowling
Memorial Sloan-Kettering Cancer
Center
New York, New York 10021

J. Durand
Fondation Curie
Paris, France

Francis Edgerton
Department of Thoracic Surgery
Roswell Park Memorial Institute
Buffalo, New York 14263

David Eidinger
Department of Urology
Queen's University
Kingston, Ontario, Canada

Frederick R. Eilber
Division of Oncology
Department of Surgery
University of California Medical
School
Los Angeles, California 90024

H. Ekert
Department of Clinical Haematology
and Oncology and Research Foun-
dation
Royal Children's Hospital
Parkville, Victoria 3052, Australia

Rose Ruth Ellison
Department of Medicine
School of Medicine
State University of New York
at Buffalo
Buffalo, New York 14215

L. Engstedt
Karolinska Institute
Leukemia Group of Central Sweden
Stockholm, Sweden

Paul F. Engstrom
Department of Medicine
American Oncologic Hospital
Fox Chase Cancer Center
Philadelphia, Pennsylvania 19111

Julio N. Feierstein
Centro Oncológico de Medicina
Nuclear
Instituto de Oncología "Angel H.
Roffo"
Buenos Aires, Argentina

D. Fiere
Hôpital Edouard Herriot
Place D'Arsonval
69374 Lyon, France

Bernard Fisher
Department of Surgery
University of Pittsburgh
The School of Medicine
Pittsburgh, Pennsylvania 15261

Edwin R. Fisher
University of Pittsburgh
The School of Medicine
Pittsburgh, Pennsylvania 15261

G. Flowerdew
Institut Jules Bordet
EORTC Data Center
Rue Heger Bordet
Brussels, Belgium

Joseph G. Fortner
Memorial Sloan-Kettering Cancer
 Center
New York, New York 10021

S. Franzén
Karolinska Institute
Leukemia Group of Central Sweden
Stockholm, Sweden

Emil Frei III
The Sidney Farber Cancer Institute
Boston, Massachusetts 02115

Emil J. Freireich
Department of Developmental
 Therapeutics
The University of Texas System
 Cancer Center
M.D. Anderson Hospital
Houston, Texas 77030

S. K. Frytak
Mayo Clinic
Rochester, Minnesota 55901

G. Gahrton
Karolinska Institute
Leukemia Group of Central Sweden
Stockholm, Sweden

Timothy S. Gee
Memorial Sloan-Kettering Cancer
 Center
New York, New York 10021

Edmund A. Gehan
Department of Biomathematics
The University of Texas System
 Cancer Center
M.D. Anderson Hospital and
 Tumor Institute
Houston, Texas 77030

S. L. George
Institut Jules Bordet
EORTC Data Center
Rue Heger Burdet
Brussels, Belgium

Gerald S. Gilchrist
Section of Pediatric Oncology
Department of Pediatrics
Mayo Clinic
Rochester, Minnesota 55901

Horacio M. Glait
Centro Oncológico de Medicina
 Nuclear
Instituto de Oncología "Angel H.
 Roffo"
Buenos Aires, Argentina

Oliver Glidewell
CALGB Operations Office
Scarsdale, New York 10583

Richard G. Glogau
Department of Medicine
University of California
San Francisco, California 94143

J. P. Gmür
Division of Hematology
Department of Medicine
University of Zurich
Zurich, Switzerland

Alice S. Goldsmith
Division of Hematology and Medical
 Oncology
Emory University School of Medicine
Atlanta, Georgia 30322

Raymond L. Gonzalez
Laboratory of Cellular Immunology
Children's Hospital of San Francisco
San Francisco, California 94118

Theodor B. Grage
Department of Surgery
University of Minnesota
Minneapolis, Minnesota 55455

Robert G. Graw
National Cancer Institute
Bethesda, Maryland 20014

B. Gullbring
Karolinska Institute
Leukemia Group of Central Sweden
Stockholm, Sweden

Audolfur Gunnarsson
Geitland 6
Fossvogur
Reykjavik, Iceland

Jordan U. Gutterman
Department of Developmental
 Therapeutics
The University of Texas System
 Cancer Center

M.D. Anderson Hospital and
Tumor Institute
Houston, Texas 77030

R. G. Hahn
Mayo Clinic
Rochester, Minnesota 55901

H. Hainaut
Clinique de L'Esperance
Montignee, Belgium

D. Hammond
Children's Cancer Study Group
University of Southern California
Los Angeles, California 90007

Tin Han
Department of Thoracic Surgery
Roswell Park Memorial Institute
Buffalo, New York 14263

James T. Hanlon
University of Pittsburgh
The School of Medicine
Pittsburgh, Pennsylvania 15261

John A. Hansen
Memorial Sloan-Kettering Cancer
Center
New York, New York 10021

Jules E. Harris
Department of Medicine
University of Ottawa
Ottawa, Canada

M. Hayat
Institut de Cancérologie et
d'Immunogénétique
INSERM
Hôpital Paul-Brousse
Villejuif, France

Ingegerd Hellström
Division of Tumor Immunology
Fred Hutchinson Cancer Research
Center
Seattle, Washington 98104

Karl Erik Hellström
Division of Tumor Immunology
Fred Hutchinson Cancer Research
Center
Seattle, Washington 98104

Edward S. Henderson
National Cancer Institute
Bethesda, Maryland 20014

Evan M. Hersh
Department of Developmental Thera-
peutics
The University of Texas System
Cancer Center
The M.D. Anderson Hospital and
Tumor Institute
Houston, Texas 77030

Jeanne P. Hester
Department of Developmental
Therapeutics
The University of Texas System
Cancer Center
M.D. Anderson Hospital and Tumor
Institute
Houston, Texas 77030

James S. Hewlett
Cleveland Clinic Foundation
Cleveland, Ohio 44106

Ruth Heyn
Mott Children's Hospital
University of Michigan
Ann Arbor, Michigan 48109

Elias Y. Hilal
Memorial Sloan-Kettering Cancer
Center
New York, New York 10021

Yashar Hirshaut
Memorial Sloan-Kettering Cancer
Center
New York, New York 10021

Wolfgang E. Hirte
Department of Medicine
University of Ottawa
Ottawa, Canada

P. Höcker
Karolinska Institute
Leukemia Group of Central Sweden
Stockholm, Sweden

S. Höglund
Karolinska Institute
Leukemia Group of Central Sweden
Stockholm, Sweden

James F. Holland
Department of Neoplastic Diseases
Mount Sinai School of Medicine
New York, New York 10029

Ariel C. Hollinshead
Division of Hematology and
Oncology
Department of Medicine
George Washington University
Medical Center
Washington, D.C. 20014

G. Holm
Karolinska Institute
Leukemia Group of Central Sweden
Stockholm, Sweden

E. Carmack Holmes
Division of Oncology
Department of Surgery
University of California Medical
School
Los Angeles, California 90024

David Hooper
Department of Surgery
University of Ottawa
Ottawa, Canada

P. Hörnsten
Karolinska Institute
Leukemia Group of Central Sweden
Stockholm, Sweden

G. N. Hortobagyi
Departments of Developmental
Therapeutics and Medicine
The University of Texas System
Cancer Center
M.D. Anderson Hospital and Tumor
Institute
Houston, Texas 77030

John Horton
Albany Medical College
Albany, New York 12208

Daniel F. Hoth
Division of Medical Oncology
Vincent T. Lombardi Cancer
Research Center
Georgetown University School of
Medicine
Washington, D.C. 20007

J. Hugues
Hôpital de Bavière
University of Liège
4000 Liège, Belgium

R. L. Ikonopisov
Oncological Research Institute
Sofia, Bulgaria

John C. Ivins
Section of Orthopedic Oncology
Department of Orthopedics
Mayo Clinic
Rochester, Minnesota 55901

Norman Jaffe
The Sydney Farber Cancer Institute
Boston, Massachusetts 02115

S. Jameson
Regional Hospital
Örebro, Sweden

C. Jasmin
Institut de Cancérologie et
d'Immunogénétique
INSERM
Hôpital Paul-Brousse
Villejuif, France

Robert F. Jones
Division of Tumor Immunology
Fred Hutchinson Cancer Research
Center
Seattle, Washington 98104

Stephen E. Jones
Section of Hematology and Oncology
University of Arizona College of
Medicine
Tucson, Arizona 85724

P. A. Joo
University of Wisconsin Medical
School
Madison, Wisconsin 53706

D. G. Jose
Department of Clinical Haematology
and Oncology and Research
Foundation
Royal Children's Hospital
Parkville, Victoria, Australia

André Jubert
University of Texas System Cancer
Center

M.D. Anderson Hospital and Tumor
   Institute
Houston, Texas 77030

M. Karon
Children's Hospital of Los Angeles
Los Angeles, California 90027

Richard J. Kaufman
Memorial Sloan-Kettering Cancer
   Center
New York, New York 10021

Harvey W. Kausel
Albany Medical College
Albany, New York 12208

Humphrey E. M. Kay
Leukaemia Trials Office
The Royal Marsden Hospital
London SW3 6JJ England

Y. Kenis
Institut Jules Bordet
Free University of Brussels
Brussels, Belgium

Anne Kennedy
The University of Texas System
   Cancer Center
M.D. Anderson Hospital and Tumor
   Institute
Houston, Texas 77030

A. Killander
Karolinska Institute
Leukemia Group of Central Sweden
Stockholm, Sweden

D. Killander
Karolinska Institute
Leukemia Group of Central Sweden
Stockholm, Sweden

B. Kiss
State Institute of Oncology
Budapest, Hungary

E. Klein
Karolinska Institute
Leukemia Group of Central Sweden
Stockholm, Sweden

David J. Klaassen
Department of Medicine
University of Ottawa
Ottawa, Canada

William H. Knospe
Section of Hematology
Rush Presbyterian–St. Luke's Medical
   Center
Chicago, Illinois 60612

Irwin H. Krakoff
Memorial Sloan-Kettering Cancer
   Center
New York, New York 10021

A. Kulakowski
Oncological Institute
Cracow, Poland

B. Lantz
Karolinska Institute
Leukemia Group of Central Sweden
Stockholm, Sweden

F. Lejeune
Institut Jules Bordet
Brussels, Belgium

Brigid G. Leventhal
Pediatric Oncology Branch
National Cancer Institute
Bethesda, Maryland 20014

Christian Lindemalm
Department of Medicine
Södersjukhuset Hospital
Stockholm, Sweden

J. Lindemann
Division of Experimental Micro-
   biology
Institute of Medical Microbiology
University of Zurich
Zurich, Switzerland

James Linta
University of Pittsburgh
The School of Medicine
Pittsburgh, Pennsylvania 15261

T. A. Lister
Institute of Cancer Research
Royal Marsden Hospital
Sutton, Surrey, England

D. Lockner
Karolinska Institute
Leukemia Group of Central Sweden
Stockholm, Sweden

B. Lönnqvist
Regional Hospital
Örebro, Sweden

Edward Lustbader
Institute for Cancer Research
Fox Chase Cancer Center
Philadelphia, Pennsylvania 19140

D. Machover
Institut de Cancérologic et
  d'Immunogénétique
INSERM
Hôpital Paul-Brousse
Villejuif, France

Mary Anne Malahy
University of Texas System Cancer
  Center
M.D. Anderson Hospital and Tumor
  Institute
Houston, Texas 77030

Thomas M. Malm
Laboratory of Cellular Immunology
Children's Hospital of San Francisco
San Francisco, California 94118

J. Malpas
Institute of Cancer Research
The Royal Marsden Hospital
Sutton, Surrey, England

Ralph C. Marcove
Department of Surgery
Memorial Sloan-Kettering Cancer
  Center
New York, New York 10021

Michael J. Mastrangelo
Institute for Cancer Research
Fox Chase Cancer Center
Philadelphia, Pennsylvania 19140

R. Masure
Clinique de Pediatric War Memorial
Brussels, Belgium

Georges Mathé
Institut de Cancérologie et
  d'Immunogénétique
INSERM
Hôpital Paul-Brousse
Villejuif, France

R. N. Matthews
Department of Clinical Haematology
  and Oncology and Research
  Foundation
Royal Children's Hospital
Parkville, Victoria, Australia

R. Maurus
Hôpital St. Pierre
Free University of Brussels
Rue Harte
1000 Brussels, Belgium

Carole M. Maver
Albany Medical College
Albany, New York 12208

Giora M. Mavligit
Department of Developmental Thera-
  peutics
The University of Texas System
  Cancer Center
M.D. Anderson Hospital and Tumor
  Institute
Houston, Texas 77030

Charles M. McBride
Department of Surgery
The University of Texas System
  Cancer Center
M.D. Anderson Hospital and Tumor
  Institute
Houston, Texas 77030

Kenneth B. McCredie
Department of Developmental Thera-
  peutics
The University of Texas System
  Cancer Center
M.D. Anderson Hospital and Tumor
  Institute
Houston, Texas 77030

O. Ross McIntyre
Norris Cotton Cancer Center
Dartmouth-Hitchcock Medical
  Center
Hanover, New Hampshire 03734

Charles F. McKhann
Department of Surgery
University of Minnesota
Minneapolis, Minnesota 55455

Martin F. McKneally
Albany Medical College
Albany, New York 12208

Z. Mechl
Oncological Institute
Brno, Czechoslovakia

H. Mellstedt
Karolinska Institute
Leukemia Group of Central Sweden
Stockholm, Sweden

J. Michel
Centre Hospitalier de Tivoli
La Louvière, Belgium

Valerie Miké
Biostatistics Laboratory
Memorial Sloan-Kettering Cancer
  Center
New York, New York 10021

Donald Miller
Department of Medicine
Duke University School of Medicine
Durham, North Carolina 27710

G. W. Milton
University of Sydney
Department of Surgery
Sydney, Australia

Jun Minowada
Department of Thoracic Surgery
Roswell Park Memorial Institute
Buffalo, New York 14263

J. L. Misset
Institut de Cancérologie et
  d'Immunogénétique
INSERM
Hôpital Paul-Brousse
Villejuif, France

Charles G. Moertel
Mayo Clinic
Rochester, Minnesota 55901

Thomas E. Moon
Southwest Oncology Group
Biostatistical Office
Houston, Texas 77030

Alvaro Morales
Department of Urology
Queen's University
Kingston, Ontario, Canada

Donald L. Morton
Division of Oncology
Department of Surgery
University of California Medical
  School
Los Angeles, California 90024

M. Musset
Institut de Cancérologie et
  d'Immunogénétique
INSERM
Hôpital Paul-Brousse
Villejuif, France

Larry Nathanson
Tufts University Oncology Program
New England Medical Center
  Hospital
Boston, Massachusetts 02111

M. Nesbit
University of Minnesota
Minneapolis, Minnesota 55455

P. Obrecht
Division of Oncology
University of Basel
Basel, Switzerland

M. J. O'Connell
Mayo Clinic
Rochester, Minnesota 55901

Herbert F. Oettgen
Memorial Sloan-Kettering Cancer
  Center
New York, New York 10021

Américo J. Olivari
Centro Oncológico de Medicina
  Nuclear
Instituto de Oncología "Angel H.
  Roffo"
Buenos Aires, Argentina

T. Oliver
Institute of Cancer Research
The Royal Marsden Hospital
Sutton, Surrey, England

George A. Omura
Division of Hematology
University of Alabama School of
  Medicine
Birmingham, Alabama 35294

J. Otten
Hôpital St. Pierre
Free University of Brussels
Rue Haute
1000 Brussels, Belgium

J. Palmblad
Karolinska Institute
Leukemia Group of Central Sweden
Stockholm, Sweden

W. Bradford Patterson
University of Rochester Cancer
  Center
Strong Memorial Hospital
Rochester, New York 14642

Anthony R. Paul
Department of Medicine
American Oncologic Hospital
Fox Chase Cancer Center
Philadelphia, Pennsylvania 19111

C. Pauli
Karolinska Institute
Leukemia Group of Central Sweden
Stockholm, Sweden

M. E. Peetermans
Algemeen Ziekenhuis Middelheim
2000 Antwerp, Belgium

J. Pena-Angulo
Institut de Cancérologie et
  d'Immunogénétique
INSERM
Hôpital Paul-Brousse
Villejuif, France

H. H. Peter
Abteilung fur Klinische Immunologie
  —Medizinische Hochschule
Hannover, Federal Republic of Ger-
  many

Richard Peto
Radcliffe Infirmary
Oxford University
Oxford, England

J. L. Pico
Institut de Cancérologie et
  d'Immunogénétique
INSERM
Hôpital Paul-Brousse
Villejuif, France

Yosef H. Pilch
Department of Surgery
University of California Medical
  Center
San Diego, California 92103

Carl M. Pinsky
Memorial Sloan-Kettering Cancer
  Center
New York, New York 10021

Thomas Pomeroy
Radiation Branch
National Cancer Institute
Bethesda, Maryland 20014

David G. Poplack
Pediatric Oncology Branch
National Cancer Institute
Bethesda, Maryland 20014

P. Pouillart
Institut de Cancérologie et
  d'Immunogénétique
INSERM
Hôpital Paul-Brousse
Villejuif, France

Ray L. Powles
Institute of Cancer Research
The Royal Marsden Hospital
Sutton, Surrey, England

Ross Prentice
Division of Tumor Immunology
Fred Hutchinson Cancer Research
  Center
Seattle, Washington 98104

Cary A. Presant
Division of Hematology-Oncology
Washington University School of
  Medicine
The Jewish Hospital of St. Louis
St. Louis, Missouri 63110

J. Priario
Hospital de Clinicas "M. Quintela"
Montevideo, Uruguay

D. J. Pritchard
Section of Orthopedic Oncology
Department of Orthopedics
Mayo Clinic
Rochester, Minnesota 55901

Kanti Rai
Long Island Jewish-Hillside Medical
 Center
Division of Hematology
New Hyde Park, New York 11040

Sankaranarayanan Raman
Department of Epidemiology and
 Community Medicine
University of Ottawa
Ottawa, Canada

Kenneth P. Ramming
Department of Surgery
University of California, Los Angeles
School of Medicine
Center for the Health Sciences
Los Angeles, California 90024

Edna F. Rapp
Department of Medicine
University of Ottawa
Ottawa, Canada

Herbert J. Rapp
National Cancer Institute
Bethesda, Maryland 20014

A. Reed
Statistical Center
University of Southern California
School of Medicine
Los Angeles, California 90007

M. Reginster-Bous
Hôpital de Bavière
University of Liège
Liège, Belgium

R. J. Reitemeir
Mayo Clinic
Rochester, Minnesota 55901

Peter Reizenstein
Karolinska Institute
Leukemia Group of Central Sweden
Stockholm, Sweden

Stephen P. Richman
Department of Developmental Thera-
 peutics
The University of Texas System
 Cancer Center
M.D. Anderson Hospital and Tumor
 Institute
Houston, Texas 77030

Roy E. Ritts, Jr.
Department of Microbiology
Mayo Clinic
Rochester, Minnesota 55901

Victorio Rodriquez
Department of Developmental Thera-
 peutics
The University of Texas System
 Cancer Center
M.D. Anderson Hospital and Tumor
 Institute
Houston, Texas 77030

Alejandro F. Rojas
Centro Oncológico de Medicina
 Nuclear
Instituto de Oncología "Angel H.
 Roffo"
Buenos Aires, Argentina

Marvin Romsdahl
Department of Surgery
The University of Texas System
 Cancer Center
Houston, Texas 77011

C. Rosenfeld
Institut de Cancérologie et
 d'Immunogénétique
INSERM
Hôpital Paul-Brousse
Villejuif, France

J. Rubin
Mayo Clinic
Rochester, Minnesota 55901

P. Rumke
Het Nederlands Kankerinstitut
Amsterdam, The Netherlands

J. Russell
Institute of Cancer Research
The Royal Marsden Hospital
Sutton, Surrey, England

Richard W. Sagebiel
Department of Pathology
Children's Hospital of San Francisco
San Francisco, California 94118

Harold J. Sachs
Department of Medicine
George Washington University
 Medical Center
Washington, D.C. 20014

Sydney E. Salmon
Section of Hematology and Oncology
University of Arizona College of
Medicine
Tucson, Arizona 85724

H. Sather
Statistical Center
University of Southern California
School of Medicine
Los Angeles, California 90007

Christian Sauter
Division of Oncology
Department of Medicine
University of Zurich
Zurich, Switzerland

Philip S. Schein
Division of Medical Oncology
Vincent T. Lombardi Cancer
Research Center
Georgetown University School of
Medicine
Washington, D.C. 20007

M. Schneider
Institut de Cancérologie et
d'Immunogénétique
INSERM
Hôpital Paul-Brousse
Villejuif, France

David Schoenfeld
Statistical Center
State University of New York at
Buffalo
Amherst, New York 14226

David Schottenfeld
Memorial Sloan-Kettering Cancer
Center
New York, New York 10021

A. J. Schutt
Mayo Clinic
Rochester, Minnesota 55901

Max Schwarz
Department of Developmental Thera-
peutics
The University of Texas System
Cancer Center
M.D. Anderson Hospital and Tumor
Institute
Houston, Texas 77030

L. Schwarzenberg
Institut de Cancérologie et
d'Immunogénétique
INSERM
Hôpital Paul-Brousse
Villejuif, France

H. J. Senn
Division of Oncology
Department of Medicine
St. Gallen, Switzerland

N. Shore
Children's Hospital of Los Angeles
Los Angeles, California 90027

Richard L. Simmons
Department of Surgery
University of Minnesota
Minneapolis, Minnesota 55455

Richard Simon
National Cancer Institute
Bethesda, Maryland 20014

Trevor Singh
Department of Medicine
Michigan State University
Saginaw Cooperative Hospitals
Saginaw, Michigan 48824

K. O. Skärberg
Karolinska Institute
Leukemia Group of Central Sweden
Stockholm, Sweden

A. J. Slater
Department of Haematology
University Hospital of Wales
Heath Park
Cardiff CF4 4XW Wales

Richard V. Smalley
Department of Medicine
Temple University Health Science
Center
Philadelphia, Pennsylvania 19140

Kendall A. Smith
Dartmouth-Hitchcock Medical Center
Hanover, New Hampshire 03755

P. J. Smith
Department of Clinical Haematology
and Oncology and Research
Foundation
Royal Children's Hospital
Parkville, Victoria, Australia

T. L. Smith
Department of Biomathematics
The University of Texas System
  Cancer Center
Houston, Texas 77011

Frank C. Sparks
Division of Oncology
Department of Surgery
University of California Medical
  School
Los Angeles, California 90024

Lynn E. Spitler
Department of Medicine
University of California
San Francisco, California 94143

Thomas H. M. Stewart
Department of Medicine
University of Ottawa
Ottawa, Canada

Pierre A. Stryckmans
Institut Jules Bordet
Free University of Brussels
Rue Heger Bordet
1000 Brussels, Belgium

Leife G. Suhrland
Department of Medicine
Michigan State University
East Lansing, Michigan 48824

Wataru W. Sutow
Department of Pediatrics
The University of Texas Cancer
  Center
Houston, Texas 77011

R. Sylvester
EORTC Coordinating and Data
  Center
Brussels, Belgium

Mitsuru Takada
Department of Thoracic Surgery
Roswell Park Memorial Institute
Buffalo, New York 14263

Hiroshi Takita
Department of Thoracic Surgery
Roswell Park Memorial Institute
Buffalo, New York 14263

C. K. Tashima
Departments of Developmental Therapeutics and Medicine

The University of Texas System
  Cancer Center
M.D. Anderson Hospital and Tumor
  Institute
Houston, Texas 77030

William F. Taylor
Section of Medical Research
  Statistics
Department of Medical Statistics and
  Epidemiology
Mayo Clinic
Rochester, Minnesota 55901

William D. Terry
National Cancer Institute
Bethesda, Maryland 20014

Howard Teitlebaum
Department of Medicine
Michigan State University
Saginaw Cooperative Hospitals
Saginaw, Michigan 48824

R. Tomin
Institute of Oncology
Beograd, Yugoslavia

Courtney M. Townsend
Division of Oncology
Department of Surgery
UCLA Medical School
Los Angeles, California 90024

A-M. Udén
Karolinska Institute
Leukemia Group of Central Sweden
Stockholm, Sweden

G. Uribe-Botero
Department of Pathology
Veterans Administration Hospital
Houston, Texas 77011

Manuel Valdivieso
Department of Developmental Thera-
  peutics
The University of Texas System
  Cancer Center
M.D. Anderson Hospital and Tumor
  Institute
Houston, Texas 77030

M. Van Glabbeke
EORTC Coordinating and Data
  Center
Brussels, Belgium

W. Van Hove
Akademisch Ziekenhuis
University of Gent
Gent, Belgium

F. Vànky
Karolinska Institute
Leukemia Group of Central Sweden
Stockholm, Sweden

L. Verbist
Akademisch Ziekenhuis
University of Gent
Gent Belgium

U. Veronesi
Istituto Nazionale Tumori
Milan, Italy

W. Ralph Vogler
Division of Hematology and Medical
  Oncology
Department of Medicine
Emory University School of Medicine
Atlanta, Georgia 30322

B. Wadman
Ludwig Boltzmann Institute for
  Leukemia Research
Hanusch Hospital
Vienna, Austria

Harold J. Wanebo
Memorial Sloan-Kettering Cancer
  Center
New York, New York 10021

Glenn Warner
Tumor Institute
Swedish Hospital Medical Center
Seattle, Washington 98104

K. D. Waters
Department of Clinical Haematology
  and Oncology
Royal Children's Hospital
Parkville, Australia

J. Weiner
Statistical Center
University of Southern California
School of Medicine
Los Angeles, California 90007

A. Wennerholm
EORTC Coordinating and Data
  Center
Brussels, Belgium

J. M. A. Whitehouse
CRC Medical Professorial Oncology
  Unit
Southampton University
Southampton, England

John A. Whittaker
Department of Haematology
University Hospital of Wales
  and Heath Park
Cardiff CF4 4XW Wales

H. Williaert
Kindergasthuis Good Engels
Antwerp, Belgium

Dorothy Windhorst
Hoffmann-La Roche Inc.
Nutley, New Jersey 07110

Robert E. Wittes
Memorial Sloan-Kettering Cancer
  Center
New York, New York 10021

Janet Wolter
Section of Oncology
Department of Medicine
Rush-Presbyterian
St. Luke's Medical Center
Chicago, Illinois 60612

Peter F. Wong
Department of Medicine
University of California
San Francisco, California 94143

Peter F. Wright
Division of Tumor Immunology
Program in Epidemiology and
  Biostatistics
Fred Hutchinson Cancer Research
  Institute
Seattle, Washington 98104

Yuichi Yamamura
The Third Department of Internal
  Medicine
Osaka University Medical School
Fukushima, Osaka 553 Japan

Immunotherapy of Cancer: Present Status of Trials in Man, edited by W. D. Terry and D. Windhorst.
Raven Press, New York © 1978.

Cutaneous Malignant Melanoma: Diagnosis, Prognosis, and Conventional Medical Therapy

Michael J. Mastrangelo, Wallace H. Clark, Jr.,
Robert E. Bellet, and *David Berd

*Institute for Cancer Research, Fox Chase Cancer Center, and Temple University School of Medicine, Philadelphia, Pennsylvania 19104; and *University of Pennsylvania School of Medicine, Philadelphia, Pennsylvania 19104*

Our objective is a concise review of the diagnosis, prognostic factors, and conventional medical therapy of human cutaneous malignant melanoma. It is hoped that the data presented, particularly those relating to prognosis, will be useful in assessing the results of the many therapeutic trials currently being reported.

DIAGNOSIS

There are, perhaps, nine or 10 different biologic varieties of human malignant melanoma. However, over 95% of melanomas may be classified into four kinds: lentigo maligna melanoma (LMM) (9–12, 40), superficial spreading melanoma (SSM) (9–11, 40), nodular melanoma (NM) (9–11, 40), and acral lentigenous melanoma (ALM; volar, subungual, and mucous membrane types) (1). The proper understanding and recognition of the four dominant types of melanoma are not an exercise in nosologic compulsiveness but form the basis for clinical diagnosis at a developmental stage when the disease is curable. Present information about diagnosis and therapy of malignant melanoma should result in cure of over 85% of affected patients. The reason for this optimistic statement is that three of the four kinds of melanoma are characterized by indolent peripheral enlargement of relatively flat, complexly colored, primary lesions. This period of centrifugal growth generally lasts for several years and has been termed the *radial* growth phase of the primary lesion. While a melanoma is in the radial growth phase, it acquires little or no competence to metastasize and may, therefore, be cured by relatively simple surgical procedures. LMM, SSM, and ALM all develop through an initial radial growth phase.

The acquisition of competence to metastasize by a primary melanoma is associated with a focal change in the neoplasm, a change characterized by penetration into the deeper cutaneous tissues. This focal, deep penetration is called the *vertical* growth phase. The extent of this second growth phase is the basis for *levels* of invasion and tumor *thickness* measurements that presently are the mainstays for estimating prognosis and assignment of risk immediately following surgery of the primary tumor.

LMM constitutes 10 to 15% of cutaneous melanomas and is the most benign of the four types. LMM most commonly occurs in areas heavily exposed to the sun, such as the head, neck, and dorsum of the hands. The median age at diagnosis is about 70 years, and females are probably more frequently affected. The histology of this lesion is represented schematically in Fig. 1. There are both radial and vertical growth phases. The radial growth phase of LMM is characterized by abnormal melanocytes extending centrifugally in the epidermis with minimal invasion into the papillary dermis. When only radial growth is present, the lesion is called lentigo maligna and is not malignant melanoma (12). Radial growth precedes the development of vertical growth by decades, and it is this slow progression to vertical growth that accounts for the relative benignity of LMM. Although the radial growth phase is relatively innocuous, the vertical growth phase is associated with metastases in about 25% of the cases. Clinically, the early LMM lesions are large, flat, and tan and/or brown in color. With the development of the vertical growth phase the lesion becomes focally elevated, but the basic tan-brown pattern of the radial growth phase persists. LMM is distinguished from superficial spreading melanoma by the rarity of rose and pink colors and the minimal elevation of the radial growth phase.

SSM accounts for about 70% of all cases of cutaneous melanoma in Caucasians and is intermediate in malignancy. The tumor has its peak incidence in

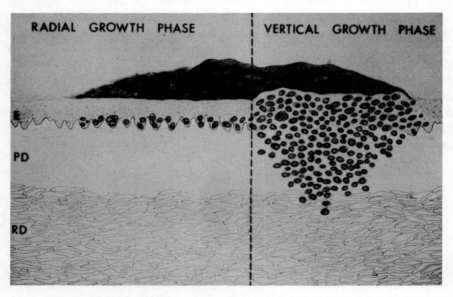

FIG. 1. LMM. E, epidermis; PD, papillary dermis; RD, reticular dermis.

the fifth decade, and the sexes are affected with equal frequency. The legs are more commonly affected in females. In males, the upper back is the predominant site. The histology of this lesion is represented in Fig. 2. As in LMM, there are both radial and vertical growth phases. The radial growth phase of SSM is characterized by melanoma cells within the epidermis (with epidermal thickening) and papillary dermis and by a host response composed of inflammatory cells, fibroplasia, and new blood vessel formation. The duration of the radial growth phase is difficult to document since the lesions are small and inconspicuous and since one-third are present on the back where they are not readily visible. It most likely ranges from 1 to as many as a dozen years. The radial growth phase of SSM is associated with recurrent or metastatic disease in less than 5% of affected patients. The vertical growth phase develops clinically rather rapidly, in a few weeks to a few months, and is heralded by the appearance of a nodule. Depending on the depth of invasion and other cellular parameters, lesions in which the vertical growth phase has supervened metastasize in 35 to 85% of cases. Early SSM lesions are a haphazard combination of tan, brown, blue, and black, and in most lesions shades of rose and pink are also present. More advanced SSM lesions have a characteristic red, white, and blue coloration. The white areas represent spontaneous regression.

NM, the most malignant of the four varieties, constitutes about 12% of all cutaneous melanomas. The median age at diagnosis is 50 years. NM occurs twice as commonly in males as in females, and this may account, at least in part, for the poorer prognosis of melanoma in males. The histology of NM is

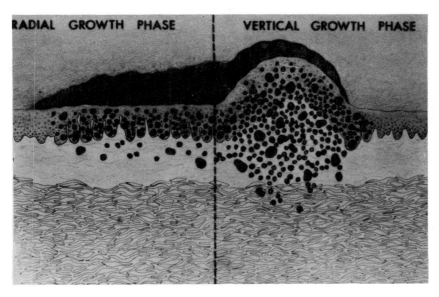

FIG. 2. SSM.

presented in Fig. 3. NM is composed exclusively of a vertical growth phase that usually shows invasion of melanoma cells into the deeper dermis. The host cellular response is variable but generally less than in other forms of melanoma. Clinically, these lesions evolve quickly over several months to a year but rarely longer. Even the earliest lesions are raised and are usually a characteristic, thundercloud gray with pinkish hues. As the lesion continues to grow, the dominant color changes to blue-black giving the tumor a blueberry like appearance. The lack of a radial growth phase makes early diagnosis difficult.

Arrington et al. (1) have documented the development and biologic characteristics of ALM. This form of melanoma occurs on the palms and soles, in subungual locations, and on mucous membranes. The developmental biology is also characterized by radial and vertical growth phases. The radial growth phase is flat, the margin nonpalpable, and the color, a mosaic of rich tans, browns, and black. In subungual locations, the radial growth phase may be a streak in the nail associated with an irregular tan-brown stain diffusing proximally from the nail bed. The radial growth phase has a duration of years, but if ignored, it will be followed by the elevated nodular areas of the vertical growth phase. The exact prognostic significance of the vertical growth phase has not been determined in a large series of cases, but once it has supervened, metastases are common.

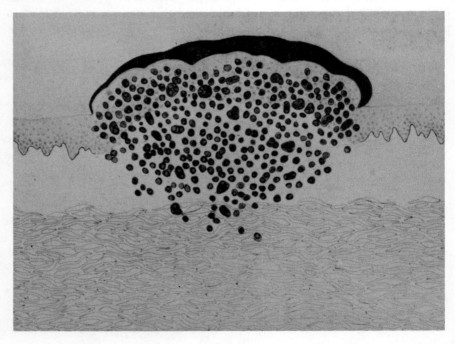

FIG. 3. NM.

PROGNOSIS

Patient Factors

Sex

Data regarding the relationship between the sex of the patient and 5-year survival are presented in Table 1. Females have a clear advantage in survival after initial diagnosis. Heise and Krementz (24) and Bodenham (5) noted an improved survival for females irrespective of whether the stage at diagnosis was local or regional. It is less clear whether females survive longer after first recurrence. Einhorn et al. (16) reported that females survived longer than males following the initiation of chemotherapy despite the lack of real difference in objective response rates. The improved survival in females may

TABLE 1. *Five-year survival as related to sex*

Study (ref. no.)	% Males	% Females
Perzik and Baum (44)	43 (33/76)	63 (45/72)
Jones et al. (26)	25 (12/48)	41 (26/63)
Shah and Goldsmith (48)	48 (368/766)	62 (445/717)
Mundth et al. (42)	35 (63/180)	54 (92/170)
Lehman et al. (29)	23 (5/22)	65 (13/20)
Nathanson et al. (43)	24 (22/92)	38 (27/72)
Cochran (13)	30 (16/54)	63 (55/88)
Totals	42 (519/1,238)	58 (703/1,202)
	$p = < 0.00001$	

be related to their hormonal milieu or to a heightened cosmetic awareness. Further, in females, the primary lesion is less frequently located in visually obscure areas of the body such as the back. The report of Jones et al. (26) that primary lesions in females are smaller in diameter than in males suggests earlier diagnosis. In summary, sex appears to be an important prognostic factor in patients with operable local or regional disease. Its importance as a stratification step in studies using more advanced cases remains a question.

Age

In reference to age at initial diagnosis, younger patients have a better 5-year survival than do older patients. Only Cochran (13) could find no difference between patients younger or older than 50 years. Three representative studies are summarized in Table 2. McLeod (37) and Heise and Krementz (24) noted that at all ages females survived longer than males. Nathanson et al. (43) failed to confirm this for the sixth and seventh decades. Again, there are few data correlating age with survival after first recurrence or dissemination.

TABLE 2. *Five-year survival as related to age at initial diagnosis*

Study (ref. no.)	>45 years	<45 years
Perzik and Baum (44)	45% (33/73)	60% (45/75)
Jones et al. (26)	27% (13/48)	40% (25/63)
Fortner et al. (17)[a]	29% (20/69)	41% (50/123)
Totals	35% (66/190)	46% (120/261)
		$p = 0.022$

[a] Trunk melanoma only.

Immunologic Studies

Delayed Hypersensitivity Responses

Melanoma patients as a group are less responsive to dinitrochlorobenzene (DNCB) than are normal controls (27). Ziegler et al. (51) and Catalona and Chretien (7) attempted to correlate DNCB reactivity with clinical stage of the disease. The data suggested that patients with less extensive disease were more responsive, but the patient populations were too small to make definite conclusions. In an effort to correlate DNCB reactivity with prognosis, Eilber and Morton (15) evaluated a series of 100 patients undergoing surgery for malignancy (18 with melanoma) preoperatively (Table 3). Ninety-two percent of patients who were operable and disease free for 6 months were positive to DNCB, whereas only 7% of those patients who were inoperable or recurred within 6 months reacted. In as much as melanoma patients constituted 18% of the total population, the overall response pattern

TABLE 3. *Relationship of immune competence to prognosis*

Study (ref. no.) Immune competence categories	Outcome of disease	
Eilber and Morton (15)[a]	Operable and/or disease free 6 mos.	Inoperable and/or recurred within 6 mos.
No. DNCB positive	50/54 (92%)	2/29 (7%) $p = 0.0005$
≥ 1 positive MAST of 6	26/47 (55%)	6/29 (20%) $p = 0.01$
Gross and Eddie-Quartey (21)[b]	No recurrence 1 year	Recurrence 1 year
Mean no. MAST positive $\pm$SD	2.27 ± 1.02	1.80 ± 1.34 $p = $ NS
Gutterman et al. (22)	Regressors	Progressors
≥ 2 positive MAST of 6	17/21 (81%)	23/35 (66%) $p = $ NS
≥ 3 positive MAST of 6	11/21 (52%)	10/35 (28%) $p = $ NS

[a] Eighteen of 100 patients with melanoma.
[b] Twelve of 26 patients with melanoma.
MAST, microbial antigen skin test; NS, p of > 0.05; SD, standard deviation.

may reflect the behavior of the melanoma patients. However, until data for the melanoma patients can be assessed separately, no firm conclusions can be drawn from this study regarding the prognostic value of DNCB skin testing in melanoma patients.

Several investigators (34,41,45) have attempted to correlate DNCB re-activity with response to intralesional Bacillus Calmette-Guérin (BCG) therapy. Pooling the data shows that reactivity to DNCB was high in both groups and that responders did not react more frequently than non-responders.

Reactivity to recall microbial antigens is depressed in melanoma patients with diffuse metastases and extensive prior treatment (47). Several investi-gators have attempted to correlate response to recall antigens with prognosis in early disease. Eilber and Morton (15) noted that 55% of patients with various malignancies who were operable and disease free for 6 months were positive to one or more microbial antigens on preoperative skin testing, whereas only 20% of those who were inoperable or recurred early reacted. These investigators concluded that DNCB reactivity more closely predicted the subsequent clinical course of the patients as only 8% of the patients who were disease free were DNCB negative, but 45% of these patients were nega-tive to all microbial antigens. Gross and Eddie-Quartey (21) evaluated re-activity to six recall microbial antigens in 26 patients (14 lung cancer, 12 melanoma) clinically free of disease and correlated these data with the sub-sequent clinical course. No significant differences (Table 3) were noted in the mean number of positive skin responses to recall antigens among controls and patients with favorable and unfavorable clinical outcomes. Again, data for melanoma patients were not presented separately.

Several investigators have attempted to correlate skin test reactivity to re-call antigens with response to therapy. Gutterman et al. (22) noted that patients experiencing objective tumor regression following dimethyl triazeno imidazole carboxamide (DTIC) + BCG therapy were more likely to be responsive than patients demonstrating tumor progression. However, Ma-strangelo et al. (34) found no difference in response to recall antigens be-tween responders and nonresponders to intralesional BCG therapy.

In summary, the carefully controlled study of Seigler et al. (47) clearly demonstrated that reactivity to recall antigens is depressed in melanoma pa-tients with diffuse metastases and extensive prior treatment. Surprisingly little conclusive data are available regarding correlation of reactivity to recall antigens and prognosis, clinical status, or response to therapy.

Lymphocytes Transformation

In a study by Seigler et al. (47) 10 of 21 melanoma patients evaluated for lymphocytes transformation (LT) to phytohemagglutinin (PHA) showed re-duced activity when compared to normal controls; none of these 10 patients had diffuse tumor involvement. Golub et al. (20) assessed the *in vitro* LT to various mitogens in 29 patients with malignant melanomas: two had no evidence of disease, 15 had regional disease, and 12 had distant metastases. The melanoma patients as a group, when compared to normal controls, had significantly decreased levels of LT to PHA, Pokeweed mitogen, and Concanavalin A. Ziegler et al. (51) were unable to demonstrate a difference in LT to PHA between patients with localized disease (8) and those with more advanced melanoma (9). A comparison with normal controls was not attempted, and an insufficient number of patients had visceral metastases to warrant separate analysis.

DeGast et al. (14) conducted a more extensive study assessing LT to PHA and antigens (diphtheria, tetanus toxoid, hemocyanin) in 61 melanoma patients (31 localized disease, 13 regional metastases, 10 distant nonvisceral metastases, seven visceral metastases). Test results were correlated with clinical stage and the course of disease over a subsequent 6-month period. The seven patients with visceral disease, all of whom experienced progression, had diminished LT to PHA when compared to normal controls and melanoma patients in all other stages. The remaining 54 melanoma patients could not be distinguished from normal controls or each other on the basis of stage of disease or clinical course over the brief 6-month observation period. LT to test antigens showed wide variation when evaluated by stage, but LT to all three was uniformly low in patients with visceral metastases. Further, a correlation between LT to test antigens and subsequent clinical course was noted: 9 of 14 (64%) patients who failed to react to all three antigens progressed as compared to 1 of 14 (3%) patients who responded to one or more of the test antigens.

These data support the prior observations of Golub et al. (20) and Seigler et al. (47) that melanoma patients with more advanced disease demonstrated decreased LT to PHA when compared with controls. These data are also in agreement with the observation of Ziegler et al. (51) who were unable to distinguish between patients with local disease and those with more advanced (not terminal) disease on the basis of LT to PHA. DeGast et al. (14) provided new data in demonstrating that patients with local or regional disease cannot be distinguished from normal controls. These results are consistent with those of Lui et al. (32) who noted that with optimal concentrations of PHA, LT was depressed only in preterminal melanoma patients. However, with threshold concentrations of PHA, impaired responses were regularly associated with disseminated disease. That a single determination of LT to PHA is not predictive of clinical course is in agreement with the observations of Gross and Eddie-Quartey (21) in a mixed group of patients (lung cancer and melanoma). A thorough assessment of the ability of LT to PHA and test antigens to indicate prognosis must await serial studies in an adequate group of surgically cured melanoma patients who are at high risk for recurrence.

Several investigators have attempted to correlate LT to PHA with the patients' response to therapy. Cheema and Hersh (8) studied LT to PHA and streptolysin "O" in 40 patients with a variety of solid tumors (18 melanoma) before and after chemotherapy and reported that a rapid recovery and overshoot of this index following chemotherapy was associated with a more favorable prognosis. Gross and Eddie-Quartey (21) noted that LT to PHA was impaired when compared to that of normal controls in patients (14 lung cancer, 12 melanoma) with both favorable and unfavorable clinical courses, and that the two groups of cancer patients could not be distinguished on the basis of a single determination. However, after 3 months of BCG therapy, patients who ultimately had a favorable clinical course demonstrated increased LT to PHA. Patients with an unfavorable clinical course did not. In these two studies, data for melanoma patients were not presented separately. Lieberman et al. (30) evaluated LT to PHA in seven patients undergoing intralesional BCG therapy. All four responders demonstrated a marked increase in LT to PHA following treatment, whereas the nonresponders did not. No effort was made to assess pretreatment values regarding their ability to predict response. Roth et al. (46) evaluated LT to PHA in 40 stage I and II melanoma patients and noted no difference between the BCG-treated group and the control group. Serial studies in individual patients were not done. Lui et al. (32) failed to note an increase in LT to PHA after BCG immunotherapy. These two groups did not attempt to correlate test results with response to therapy or clinical course.

In summary, patients with advanced visceral disease have depressed LT on exposure to PHA. Patients with more modest tumor burdens cannot be distinguished from controls. Further, a single determination of LT to PHA is not predictive of prognosis. The observation of DeGast et al. (14) that LT to a complex of antigens correlates with prognosis is encouraging and warrants further study. The data regarding the effect of therapy on this response are conflicting.

Taken as a whole, these two types of immunologic studies suggest that melanoma patients, especially those with advanced disease, are less easily sensitized to DNCB, have lower delayed hypersensitivity responses to a variety of antigens, and display impaired transformation responses to PHA and various antigens. It has not been demonstrated that any of these responses constitutes a significant independent variable in estimating the prognosis or response to treatment of melanoma patients.

Primary Lesion

Microstaging

Several workers (28,39) have clearly shown that prognosis in malignant melanoma is related to the depth of invasion of the tumor. These studies were subsequently refined by the work of Clark et al. (9–12), who defined

TABLE 4. Correlation of level of invasion of the
primary lesion with survival

Level of invasion	% Survival Clark et al. (ref. 10)	% 5-Year survival McGovern (ref. 36)
I	—	—
II	72.2	82
III	46.5	65
IV	31.6	49
V	12.0	29

five levels of microinvasion. These are as follows: level I, all tumor cells confined to the epidermis with no invasion through the basement membrane (*in situ* melanoma); level II, tumor cells penetrating through the basement membrane into the papillary dermis but not extending to the reticular dermis; level III, tumor cells filling the papillary dermis and abutting against the reticular dermis, but not invading it; level IV, extension of tumor cells between the bundles of collagen characteristic of the reticular dermis; and level V, invasion into the subcutaneous tissue. The correlation of level of invasion with survival is presented in Table 4. In our experience (*unpublished data*), level II lesions, accurately microstaged using a serial block technique, have a much better prognosis than indicated in Table 4. This variance is probably accounted for by tumor sampling errors in the older studies.

In addition to being an index of survival, microstaging has also been of assistance in predicting microscopic regional lymph node metastases in clinically negative nodes. These data are summarized in Table 5. Prophylactic lymph node dissection would seem to be indicated for patients with level IV and V primary lesions. However, it is not yet known whether this treatment favorably influences survival.

Although Clark's system of microstaging has greatly facilitated treatment planning, further refinement is required. The greatest problem is with level III lesions where prognosis is intermediate. Breslow (6) has correlated Clark's levels and the thickness of the primary lesion, as measured with an ocular micrometer, with prognosis. He has found this combination of factors of greater value in assessing prognosis than either alone. This work has been

TABLE 5. Presence of metastases in clinically negative regional
lymph nodes as related to Clark's level

Clark's level	Total patients	Tumor present	% Positive
II	19	1	5.3
III	46	2	4.3
IV	44	11	25
V	4	3	75

From Wanebo et al., ref. 50.

TABLE 6. Correlation of the diameter of the
primary melanoma with 5-year survival

Study (ref. no.)	% Surviving by diameter size	
	≥ 1.5 cm	< 1.5 cm
Perzik and Baum (44)	45.6	62.5
Shah and Goldsmith (48)	30–60	70–80
	≥ 2 cm	< 2 cm
Lehman et al. (29)	22	48
McLeod (37)	69	82
	≥ 3 cm	< 3 cm
Jones et al. (26)	9	49

extended by Hansen and McCarten (23) and Wanebo et al. (49). Both groups found an inverse relationship between depth of invasion (in mm) and survival.

Several other physical characteristics of the primary lesion have been correlated with survival. The relationship of the diameter of the primary lesion to 5-year survival is presented in Table 6. These reports are consistent in demonstrating an improved survival for patients with smaller lesions. Similarly, the relationship of ulceration in the primary melanoma with survival is summarized in Table 7. Patients with nonulcerated lesions have a better prognosis. Ulceration occurs more frequently in patients with larger primary lesions. Since the diameter of the primary is related to its depth of invasion (Clark's levels), this latter parameter alone may be adequate in assessing prognosis.

The location of the primary lesion also appears to influence survival (Table 8). Extremity lesions carry the best prognosis, head and neck primaries an intermediate prognosis, and trunk lesions the poorest prognosis. For all sites, women live longer than men (5,24,26). With the development of regional lymph node or distant metastases, it is uncertain whether the location of the primary significantly influences prognosis.

Various other aspects of the primary lesion have been studied to ascertain their relationship to prognosis. These include shape (31), mitotic activity (26,31,36), vascular invasion (5), pigmentation (5), host cellular in-

TABLE 7. Correlation of 5-year survival with the presence of
ulceration of the primary lesion

Study (ref. no.)	% Ulcerated	% Nonulcerated
Perzik and Baum (44)	46 (26/57)	75 (46/61)
Huvos et al. (25)[a]	65 (21/32)	82 (33/40)
Totals	53 (47/89)	78 (79/101)
	$p = < 0.001$	

[a] Head and neck lesions only.

TABLE 8. Correlation of 5-year survival with the location of the primary lesion

Study (ref. no.)	H & N % (A)	Arm % (B)	Leg % (C)	Trunk % (D)
Perzik and Baum (44)	53 (16/30)	71 (20/28)	53 (23/43)	57 (17/30)
Jones et al. (26)	33 (9/27)	27 (4/15)	45 (21/47)	19 (4/21)
Franklin et al. (18)	41 (21/51)	73 (22/30)	68 (59/87)	60 (47/78)
Shah and Goldsmith (48)	57 (130/228)	63 (167/265)	60 (299/498)	42 (167/397)
Mundth et al. (42)[a]	53 (60/114)	43 (20/46)	43 (38/89)	29 (26/91)
Lehman et al. (29)	45 (5/11)	50 (6/12)	66 (4/6)	0 (0/5)
McLeod (37)[b]	77	88	83	70
Totals	52 (241/461)	60 (239/396)	58 (444/770)	42 (261/622)

[a] Survival from onset symptoms.
[b] Total 342 patients.
H & N, head and neck. B vs. C, p = NS; A vs. B, p = 0.02; A vs. C, p = 0.07; D vs. A, B, or C, p < 0.001.

filtrate (6), surface contour (2), and partial regression (31). These pa-ramaters have either been of little prognostic value or are related to other more widely accepted indicators and thus are not to be considered further here.

Stage of Disease

The relationship of 5-year survival to stage of disease is summarized in Table 9. Stage I (local disease) has the best prognosis. Although stage II (regional disease) patients live longer than stage III (disseminated disease) patients, survival is poor for both groups. Survival in stage II patients has been further analyzed by the clinical status of the regional lymph nodes (Table 10). As expected, stage II patients with clinically positive lymph nodes have a poorer prognosis than stage II patients with clinically negative regional lymph nodes. These data could be used as an argument for prophylactic lymph node dissection in those patients where a high incidence of occult

TABLE 9. Correlation of 5-year survival with stage of disease

Study (ref. no.)	1 % Local[a]	2 % Regional	3 % Disseminated
Gutterman et al. (22)	—	31 (17/54)	13 (3/24)
McNeer and DasGupta (38)	71 (255/359)	19 (56/295)	—
Goldsmith et al. (19,48)	80 (256/321)	39 (178/456)	18 (43/239)
Cochran (13)	66 (67/102)	14 (5/36)	0 (0/5)
Fortner et al. (17)	55 (47/85)	19 (21/109)	—
Totals	72 (625/867)	29 (277/950)	17 (46/268)

[a] Clinical and/or histologic staging; 1 vs. 2, 2 vs. 3, p = < 0.0001.

TABLE 10. *Five-year survival of melanoma patients with histologically positive regional lymph nodes (stage II) as related to clinical status of lymph nodes*

Study (ref. no.)	Clinically positive (%)	Clinically negative (%)
Goldsmith et al. (19)	38 (154/406)	48 (24/50)
Block and Hartwell (4)	22 (6/28)	50 (1/2)
Mundth et al. (42)	16 (28/171)	57 (10/18)
Lehman et al. (29)[a]	0 (0/6)	17 (1/6)
Total	31 (188/611)	47 (36/76)
	$p = 0.005$	

[a] Five-year survival free of disease.

metastases are predicted on the basis of microstaging of the primary lesion. However, the clinically positive group includes patients who presented initially with the primary lesion plus clinically positive nodes as well as patients in whom regional nodal metastases were delayed. When comparing the results of prophylactic regional lymph node dissection with therapeutic dissection for delayed regional lymph node metastases, Goldsmith et al. (19) found no difference in 5-year survivals: 48% (24/50) versus 52% (48/83), respectively. One would anticipate that the number of nodes histologically positive would also correlate with survival, but insufficient data have been published to permit a meaningful discussion.

Stage III (disseminated disease) represents an even more heterogeneous group of patients, since melanoma has several metastatic patterns. It is generally agreed that patients with nonvisceral metastases (skin, subcutaneous, lymph node, etc.) have the best prognosis. Patients with lung lesions (with or without nonvisceral metastases) have an intermediate prognosis, whereas patients with nonpulmonary visceral metastases (e.g., liver, brain, bone, etc.) have the poorest outlook. We have found this classification useful for stratifying patients in therapy trials as well as in analysis of results.

Malignant melanoma metastases, even those in the same site, may vary widely in their growth rates and patterns. There are presently no clearly useful prospective indices for quantitating this phenomenon. The length of time from initial diagnosis to recurrence or dissemination may reflect, among other things, the growth pattern of the tumor. The validity of this procedure has not as yet been determined.

In summary, the following appear to be the important prognostic factors by stage of disease.

Stage I   * Depth of invasion of the primary
            * Clinically versus histologically negative nodes
            * Sex
            Age

The more important factors are marked (*).

Location of the primary

Stage II   * Clinical status of the regional nodes
            * Number of nodes (histologically) positive
            Sex
            Location of the primary
            Depth of invasion of the primary
            Time from initial diagnosis to regional recurrence
            Immunologic status (?)
            Age at regional recurrence (?)

Stage III   * Location of metastasis
            Immunologic status
            Time from diagnosis to dissemination
            Sex (?)
            Age at dissemination (?)

The bulk of the data reported regarding prognostic factors in patients with melanoma deals almost exclusively with survival from initial diagnosis. Little data are available regarding the pertinent prognostic indicators at the time of first recurrence or dissemination. Further, attempts to construct a system of multivariate analysis have been limited (33).

CONVENTIONAL MEDICAL THERAPY

The immunotherapy and chemotherapy of cutaneous malignant melanoma have recently been extensively reviewed (3,34,35). Presently, these modalities can be considered as conventional only in patients with surgically incurable disease. DTIC is the chemotherapeutic agent of first choice. A nitrosourea constitutes second-line treatment. We currently recommend the addition of vincristine to the nitrosoureas because of data suggesting some improvement in response rate without additive toxicity. At this report, there is no combination regimen containing an active component that has been demonstrated to be superior to the active component alone. There are no multidrug regimens containing agents of minimal individual activity that are superior to DTIC alone. For a detailed review and statistical analysis of these data, the reader is referred to Bellet et al. (3).

Immunotherapy is presently of limited value in patients with gross residual disease except for those with only dermal metastases in a nonedematous extremity. Numerous investigators have documented that BCG induces regression of injected and uninjected dermal melanoma metastases. We consider intralesional BCG conventional therapy in such patients.

ACKNOWLEDGMENT

This work was supported by U.S. Public Health Service grants no. CA-13456, CA-06927, and RR-05539 and by an appropriation from the Commonwealth of Pennsylvania.

REFERENCES

1. Arrington, J. H., III, Reed, R. J., Ichinose, H., and Krementz, E. T. (1977): Acral lentigenous melanoma: A distinctive variant of human cutaneous malignant melanoma. *J. Surg. Pathol. (In press.)*
2. Beardmore, G. L., Davis, N. C., McLeod, R., Little, J. H., Quinn, R. L., and Burry, A. F. (1969): Malignant melanoma in Queensland: A study of 219 deaths. *Aust. J. Dermatol.,* 10:158–168.
3. Bellet, R. E., Mastrangelo, M. J., Berd, D., and Lustbader, E. (1977): Chemotherapy of metastatic malignant melanoma. In: *Malignant Melanoma,* Grune & Stratton, New York. *(In press.)*
4. Block, G. E., and Hartwell, S. H., Jr. (1961): Malignant melanoma: A study of 17 cases. *Ann. Surg.,* 154:88–101.
5. Bodenham, D. C. (1972): Basic principles of surgery—malignant melanoma. In: *Melanoma and Skin Cancer,* pp. 375–383. VCN Blight, Government Printer, Sydney, Australia.
6. Breslow, A. (1970): Thickness, cross-sectional areas and depth of invasion in the prognosis of cutaneous melanoma. *Ann. Surg.,* 172:902–908.
7. Catalona, W. J., and Chretien, P. B. (1973): Abnormalities of quantitative dinitrochlorobenzene sensitization in cancer patients: Correlation with tumor stage and histology. *Cancer,* 31:353–356.
8. Cheema, A. R., and Hersh, E. M. (1971): Patient survival after chemotherapy and its relationship to *in vitro* lymphocyte blastogenesis. *Cancer,* 28:851–855.
9. Clark, W. H., Jr. (1967): A classification of malignant melanoma in man correlated with histogenesis and biologic behavior. In: *Advances in Biology of Skin and the Pigmentary System,* edited by W. Montagna and F. Hu, pp. 621–647. Pergamon Press, London.
10. Clark, W. H., Jr., Ainsworth, A. M., Bernardino, E. A., Yang, C. H., Mihm, M. C., Jr., and Reed, R. J. (1975): The developmental biology of primary human malignant melanomas. *Semin. Oncol.,* 2:83–104.
11. Clark, W. H., Jr., From, L., Bernardino, E. A., and Mihm, M. C. (1969): The histogenesis and biologic behavior of primary human malignant melanomas of the skin. *Cancer Res.,* 29:705–727.
12. Clark, W. H., Jr., and Mihm, M. C., Jr. (1969): Lentigo maligna and lentigo-maligna melanoma. *Am. J. Pathol.,* 55:39–67.
13. Cochran, A. J. (1969): Malignant melanoma: Review of 10 years' experience in Glasgow, Scotland. *Cancer,* 23:1190–1199.
14. DeGast, G. C., The, T. H., Koops, H. S., Huiges, H. A., Oldhoff, J., and Nieweg, H. O. (1975): Humoral and cell-mediated immune response in patients with malignant melanoma. *Cancer,* 36:1289–1297.
15. Eilber, F. R., and Morton, D. L. (1970): Impaired immunologic reactivity and recurrence following cancer surgery. *Cancer,* 25:362–367.
16. Einhorn, L. H., Burgess, M. A., Vallejos, C., Bodey, G. P., Sr., Gutterman, J., Mavligit, G., Hersh, E. M., Luce, J. K., Frei, E., III, Freireich, E. J., and Gottlieb, J. A. (1974): Prognostic correlations and response to treatment in advanced metastatic melanoma. *Cancer Res.,* 34:1995–2004.
17. Fortner, J. G., DasGupta, T., and McNeer, G. (1965): Primary malignant melanoma of the trunk. *Ann. Surg.,* 161:161–169.
18. Franklin, J. D., Reynolds, V. H., and Page, D. L. (1975): Cutaneous melanoma: A twenty year retrospective study with clinicopathologic correlation. *Plast. Reconstr. Surg.,* 56:277–285.
19. Goldsmith, H. S., Shah, J. P., and Kim, D. H. (1970): Prognostic significance of lymph node dissection in the treatment of malignant melanoma. *Cancer,* 26:606–609.
20. Golub, S. H., O'Connell, T. X., and Morton, D. L. (1974): Correlation of *in vivo* and *in vitro* assays of immunocompetence in cancer patients. *Cancer Res.,* 34:1833–1837.
21. Gross, N. J., and Eddie-Quartey, A. C. (1976): Monitoring of immunologic status of patients receiving BCG therapy for malignant disease. *Cancer,* 37:2183–2193.

22. Gutterman, J. U., Mavligit, G., Gottlieb, J. A., Burgess, M. A., McBride, C. E., Einhorn, L., Freireich, E. J., and Hersh, E. M. (1974): Chemoimmunotherapy of disseminated malignant melanoma with dimethyl triazeno imidazole carboxamide and Bacillus Calmette-Guerin. *N. Engl. J. Med.,* 291:592–597.
23. Hansen, M. G., and McCarten, A. B. (1974): Tumor thickness and lymphocyte infiltration in malignant melanoma of the head and neck. *Am. J. Surg.,* 128:557–561.
24. Heise, H. and Krementz, E. T. (1961): Survival experience of patients with malignant melanoma of the skin, 1950–1957. *Natl. Cancer Inst. Monogr.,* 6:69–84.
25. Huvos, A. G., Mike, V., Donnellan, M. J., Seemayer, T., and Strong, E. W. (1973): Prognostic factors in cutaneous melanoma of the head and neck. *Am. J. Pathol.,* 71:33–45.
26. Jones, W. M., Williams, W. J., Roberts, M. M., and Davies, K. (1968): Malignant melanoma of the skin: Prognostic value of clinical features and the role of treatment in 111 cases. *Br. J. Cancer,* 22:437–451.
27. Ketcham, A. S. and Chretien, P. B. (1975): Therapeutic implications of cellular immune defects in operable cancer patients revealed by dinitrochlorobenzene skin contact sensitivity. *Pan. Med.,* 17:174–178.
28. Lane, N., Lattes, R., and Malm, J. (1958): Clinicopathological correlations in a series of 117 malignant melanomas of the skin of adults. *Cancer,* 11:1025–1043.
29. Lehman, J. A., Jr., Cross, F. S., and Richey, DeW. G. (1966): A clinical study of forty-nine patients with malignant melanoma. *Cancer,* 19:611–619.
30. Lieberman, R., Wybran, J., and Epstein, W. (1975): The immunologic and histopathologic changes of BCG-mediated tumor regression in patients with malignant melanoma. *Cancer,* 35:756–777.
31. Little, J. H. (1972): Histology and prognosis in cutaneous malignant melanoma. In: *Melanoma and Skin Cancer,* pp. 109–119. VCN Blight, Government Printer, Sydney, Australia.
32. Lui, V. K., Karpuchas, J., Dent, P. B., McCulloch, P. B., and Blajchman, M. A. (1975): Cellular immunocompetence in melanoma: Effect of extent of disease and immunotherapy. *Br. J. Cancer,* 32:323–330.
33. Mackie, R. M., Carfrae, D. C., and Cochran, A. J. (1972): Assessment of prognosis in patients with malignant melanoma. *Lancet,* 2:455–456.
34. Mastrangelo, M. J., Bellet, R. E., Laucius, J. F., and Berkelhammer, J. (1970): Immunotherapy of malignant melanoma. A review. In: *Oncologic Medicine,* edited by P. F. Engstrom and A. I. Sutnick, pp. 71–93. Univ. Park Press, Baltimore, Md.
35. Mastrangelo, M. J., Berd, D., and Bellet, R. E. (1976): Critical review of previously reported clinical trials of cancer immunotherapy with nonspecific immunostimulants. *Ann. NY Acad. Sci.,* 277:94–123.
36. McGovern, V. J. (1970): The classification of melanoma and its relationship with prognosis. *Pathology,* 2:85–98.
37. McLeod, G. R. (1972): Factors influencing prognosis in malignant melanoma. In: *Melanoma and Skin Cancer,* pp. 367–373. VCN Blight, Government Printer, Sydney, Australia.
38. McNeer, G., and DasGupta, T. (1964): Prognosis in malignant melanoma. *Surgery,* 56:512–518.
39. Mehnert, J. H., and Heard, J. L. (1965): Staging of malignant melanoma by depth of invasion. *Am. J. Surg.,* 110:168–176.
40. Mihm, M. C., Jr., Fitzpatrick, T. B., Lane Brown, M. M., Raker, J. W., Malt, R. A., and Kaiser, J. S. (1973): Early detection of primary cutaneous malignant melanoma. *N. Engl. J. Med.,* 289:989–996.
41. Morton, D. L., Eilber, F. R., Malmgren, R. A., and Wood, W. C. (1970): Immunological factors which influence response to immunotherapy in malignant melanoma. *Surgery,* 68:158–164.
42. Mundth, E. D., Guralnick, E. A., and Raker, J. W. (1965): Malignant melanoma: A clinical study of 427 cases. *Ann. Surg.,* 162:15–28.
43. Nathanson, L., Hall, T. C., Vawter, G. F., and Farber, S. (1967): Melanoma as a medical problem. *Arch. Intern. Med.,* 119:479–492.
44. Perzik, S. L., and Baum, R. K. (1969): Individualization in the management of melanoma: A review of 164 consecutive cases. *Am. Surg.,* 35:177–180.

45. Pinsky, C. M., Hirshaut, Y., and Oettgen, H. F. (1973): Treatment of malignant melanoma by intratumoral injection of BCG. *Natl. Cancer Inst. Monogr.*, 39:225–228.
46. Roth, J. A., Golub, S. H., and Holmes, E. C. (1975): Effect of Bacillus Calmette-Guerin immunotherapy on tumor antigen-induced lymphocyte-stimulated protein synthesis in melanoma patients. *Surgery*, 78:66–75.
47. Seigler, H. F., Shingleton, W. W., Metzgar, R. S., Buckley, C. E., Bergoc, P. M., Miller, D. S., Fetter, B. F., and Phaup, M. B. (1972): Nonspecific and specific immunotherapy in patient with melanoma. *Surgery*, 72:162–174.
48. Shah, J. P., and Goldsmith, H. S. (1972): Prognosis of malignant melanoma in relation to clinical presentation. *Am. J. Surg.*, 123:286–288.
49. Wanebo, H. J., Fortner, J. G., Woodruff, J., MacLean, B., and Binkowski, E. (1975): Selection of the optimum surgical treatment of stage I melanoma by depth of microinvasion. *Ann. Surg.*, 182:302–315.
50. Wanebo, H. J., Woodruff, J., and Fortner, J. G. (1975): Malignant melanoma of the extremities: A clinicopathologic study using levels of invasion (microstage). *Cancer*, 35:666–676.
51. Ziegler, J. L., Lewis, M. G., Luyombya, J. B. S., and Kiryabwire, J. W. M. (1969): Immunologic studies on patients with malignant melanoma in Uganda. *Br. J. Cancer*, 23:729–734.

Immunotherapy of Cancer: Present Status of Trials in Man, edited by W. D. Terry and D. Windhorst. Raven Press, New York © 1978.

A Controlled Study of Adjuvant Therapy in Patients with Stage I and II Malignant Melanoma

Thomas J. Cunningham, *David Schoenfeld, **Larry Nathanson, ***Janet Wolter, †W. Bradford Patterson, and ††Martin H. Cohen

*Albany Regional Cancer Center, Albany, New York 12208; *Statistical Center, State University of New York at Buffalo, Amherst, New York 14226; **Tufts University Oncology Program, New England Medical Center Hospital, Boston, Massachusetts 02111; ***Section of Oncology, Department of Medicine, Rush-Presbyterian St. Luke's Medical Center, Chicago, Illinois 60612; †University of Rochester Cancer Center, Strong Memorial Hospital, Rochester, New York 14642; and ††Veterans Administration Hospital, Washington, D.C. 20010*

Immunotherapy has been suggested as an effective means for the treatment of malignant melanoma, yet its role remains to be defined. Some of the studies suggesting the effectiveness of Bacillus Calmette-Guérin (BCG) lack convincing evidence because the authors used historical control patients (3) and selected patients for treatment and control groups (2).

This study was designed to allocate randomly to control or study treatment schedules patients with malignant melanoma on the basis of similar prognostic factors. Lyophilized Tice BCG[1] given by the multiple puncture technique was chosen as the immunotherapeutic agent to facilitate group and patient participation. Initial applications were placed in the region of the lesion to maximize regional lymph node defenses.

This chapter, a preliminary report, projects the percent of patients free of melanoma at 1 year.

METHODS

Patients were eligible from all 37 member institutions of the Eastern Cooperative Oncology Group (ECOG), yet the majority came from five institutions.

Patients were considered for the study after total excision of the primary or local recurrent lesion. Patients with stage I melanoma had prophylactic node dissections at the discretion of their surgeon. A therapeutic node dissection was performed in patients with stage II disease.

Patients were placed in groups depending on stage, depth of penetration,

---

A preliminary report for the Eastern Cooperative Oncology Group
[1] Chicago Research supplied by National Cancer Institute.

and disease site (Fig. 1). Groups A and B included patients irrespective of site but were separated on the basis of Clark's levels of disease (1). Group C contained patients with stage II disease of an extremity or head and neck and those patients with melanoma of an extremity or head and neck treated only with resection who had local or regional lymph node recurrence. Patients in group D had stage II melanoma of the trunk, a localized recurrence within 5 cm of a previous trunk primary, or recurrence in adjacent lymph nodes treated only with surgical resection. Histologic slides from all patients were submitted to a referee pathologist for review.

In addition, skin reactivity to any one skin test (five units of purified protein derivative (PPD), mumps, dermatophyton, varidase), sex (premenopausal women, other), and the use of prophylactic node dissection in patients with stage I melanoma were used to stratify patients. Patients were ineligible for the study if they had received immunosuppressive or chemotherapeutic agents, if they had active tuberculosis or were on antituberculous agents, and if pregnant.

Randomization was performed through the central ECOG operations office after written informed consent was obtained. Patients in groups A, B, and C were allocated to a control group with no further therapy where they were followed every 3 months or to BCG therapy for 18 months (Fig. 2). Patients in group D were separately randomized to receive BCG alone or BCG with dimethyl triazeno imidazole carboximide (DTIC) for 18 months. Following treatment all patients entered the observation phase until tumor recurrence. The tumor-free interval was determined as the time from final surgery until

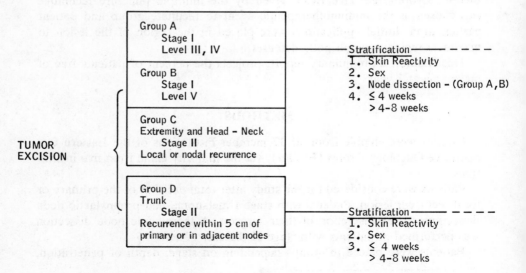

FIG. 1. Stratification factors separating patients into similar prognostic groups.

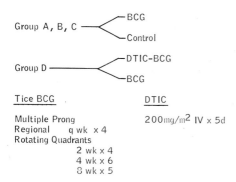

Group A, B, C
— BCG
— Control

Group D
— DTIC-BCG
— BCG

Tice BCG   DTIC

Multiple Prong $200mg/m^2$ IV x 5d
Regional   q wk x 4
Rotating Quadrants
         2 wk x 4
         4 wk x 6
         8 wk x 5

FIG. 2. Outline of the randomization to treatment schedules. DTIC, dimethyl triazeno imidazole carboximide; q, quadrant.

recurrence, and the length of survival was taken as the time from surgery until death.

Lyophilized Tice BCG was reconstituted to 0.3 ml and administered intradermally by two punctures of multiple prong discs at adjacent sites. The BCG was administered in this fashion every week times four within the regional lymph node area, i.e., adjacent to the lesion and within regional lymph node drainage areas in extremity lesions and clockwise around trunk lesions. Thereafter, other lymphatic regions were involved by rotating quadrants at each BCG administration. The frequency of administration was decreased to every 2 weeks times four, then every 4 weeks times six, and then every 8 weeks times five. Patients in group D on DTIC chemotherapy received BCG as above unless the white blood count was less than 2,000. DTIC, 200 mg/m², was given by slow i.v. push on days 1 to 5 and repeated every 4 weeks for 18 months.

RESULTS

Of 278 patients randomized to this study, 178 have been on study long enough for this preliminary evaluation.

In groups A, B, and C, 66 patients were randomized to the BCG schedule and 61 to controls. In group D, 25 patients were randomized to DTIC-BCG and 26 patients to BCG alone.

The patient characteristics were similar for each of the treatment schedules, yet there was a slight preponderance of males, nodular melanomas, and positive lymph nodes in group A, B, and C patients treated with BCG (Table 1). Full analysis of these characteristics and a pathologic review will be reported on study completion.

A positive delayed cutaneous hypersensitivity reaction to one of the biologic agents was seen on entry in greater than 80% of patients in the study, however less than 30% were reactive to five units of PPD (Table 2). Serial skin test data is available in only a few patients because of interim report

TABLE 1. *Patient characteristics*

	Groups A,B,C		Group D	
	BCG	Control	DTIC-BCG	BCG
Total patients	66	61	25	26
Age, less than 45	39	35	16	18
Male	37	28	18	18
Female, postmenopausal	15	17	3	4
premenopausal	14	16	4	4
Site				
Head-neck	9	10		
Extremity	30	29		
Trunk	22	19		
Other	5	3		
Type				
Lentigo maligna	3	2		
Superficial spreading	10	16	4	4
Nodular	37	26	9	11
Unknown, not applicable	16	17	12	10
Depth				
Level III–IV	39	39		
Level V	2	1		
Lymph nodes				
Negative	46	47		
Positive	20	14		
Inflammatory infiltrate				
Negative	13	12	6	8
Few	12	15	5	6
Moderate	21	15	5	2
Dense	2	3	1	3
Unknown	18	16	8	7

design. The conversion of negative to positive PPD skin reactions occurred in the following patients: 16 of 19 treated with BCG, three of six treated with BCG-DTIC, and zero of eight control patients.

Severe toxicity was infrequent with local reactions to BCG of increasing intensity occurring in most patients. Four patients had a severe local reaction

TABLE 2. *Initial skin testing results*

	Groups A,B,C		Group D	
	BCG	Control	DTIC-BCG	BCG
Total patients	66	61	25	26
PPD	12/62	22/59	7/25	7/26
Mumps	32/56	22/44	14/23	17/25
Dermatophyton	31/60	33/58	11/24	12/25
Varidase	26/43	27/51	6/18	10/23
% Patients positive to one test	80%	85%	80%	85%

For each treatment schedule the number of positive per number tested for each biologic antigen and the % of patients positive for at least one test are indicated.

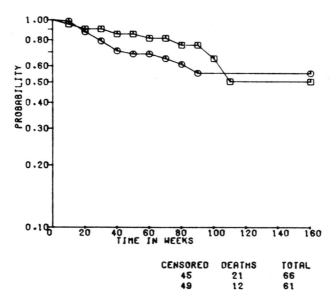

CENSORED	DEATHS	TOTAL
45	21	66
49	12	61

FIG. 3. BCG immunotherapy in early melanoma. Proportion of patients in groups A,B, and C free of tumor by treatment schedule: BCG vs. control. At 1 year p = 0.18. ①, BCG; ⊓, no therapy.

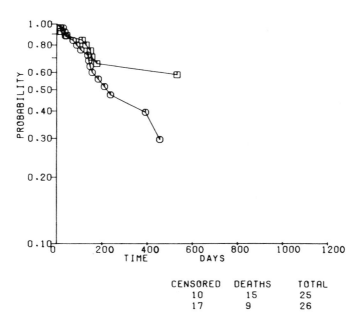

CENSORED	DEATHS	TOTAL
10	15	25
17	9	26

FIG. 4. Proportion of patients in group D free of tumor by treatment schedule: BCG-DTIC vs. BCG. At 1 year p = 0.11. ①, BCG-DTIC; ⊓, BCG.

TABLE 3. *Projected percent of patients free of tumor at 1 year*

Projected tumor	Groups A,B,C 127 of 200[a]		Group D 51 of 78[a]	
	BCG	Control	BCG	DTIC-BCG
Free 1 year	65% (p = 0.18)	86%	66% (p = 0.11)	47%
Patients relapsed	21	12	9	15
Deaths		9		13

[a] Evaluable patients.

A p value expresses the significance of the differences in treatment schedules. Deaths of relapsed patients listed.

and fever, yet no systemic BCG infections were recorded. Nausea and vomiting were seen with DTIC, whereas leukopenia was infrequent.

An actuarial estimate of the proportion of patients free of tumor at 1 year is seen in Figs. 3 and 4 and Table 3. There are more recurrences in group A, B, and C patients receiving BCG and in group D patients receiving DTIC in addition to BCG, but the differences are not significant. Deaths occurred in 27% of groups A, B, and C and 54% of group D patients who had recurred. The presence of lymph node involvement in patients in groups A, B, and C is the main factor affecting prognosis (Fig. 5). The early

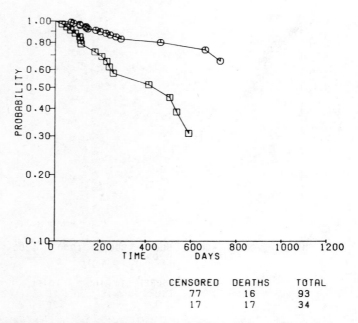

	CENSORED	DEATHS	TOTAL
	77	16	93
	17	17	34

FIG. 5. The proportion of patients in groups A,B, and C free of tumor and separated on the basis of lymph node metastasis. ①, Nodes not involved; Ⅱ, nodes involved.

data have not been analysed to relate node involvement to therapy in group A, B, and C patients.

DISCUSSION

This report establishes our design and indicates that the proportion of patients free of tumor at 1 year is statistically the same for the randomized treatments. There is a suggestion that the addition of DTIC and BCG may lead to more recurrences. Further observations may define differences and will be reported. In addition a more extensive correlation of histologic differences, serial changes in delayed cutaneous hypersensitivity reactions, and the influence of prognostic factors with the clinical response will be available. The high frequency of positive skin tests in all patients and the high incidence of positive adenopathy in patients with disease to level V have already updated our means of stratification in our new adjuvant protocol employing chemo-immunotherapy.

This preliminary report of an ongoing study indicates that ECOG can effectively undertake a program for the treatment of early cancers requiring adjuvant therapy and multidisciplinary interaction. Future successful pilot programs should be submitted to a study of this design to more quickly place the treatment in its proper perspective.

REFERENCES

1. Clark, W. H., From, L., Bernardino, E., and Mihm, M. (1969): The histogenesis and biologic behavior of primary human malignant melanomas of the skin. *Cancer Res.*, 29:705–726.
2. Eilber, F. R., Morton, D. L., Holmes, E. C., Sparks, F. C., and Ramming, K. P. (1976): Adjuvant immunotherapy with BCG in treatment of regional-lymph-node metastases from malignant melanoma. *N. Engl. J. Med.*, 294:237–240.
3. Gutterman, J. U., Mavligit, G., McBride, C., Frei, E., III, Freireich, E. J., and Hersh, E. M. (1973): Active immunotherapy with B.C.G. for recurrent malignant melanoma. *Lancet*, 1:1208–1212.

Question and Answer Session

Dr. Pinsky: What was the dose of the BCG, and what was the time of recycling of the DTIC?

Dr. Cunningham: The DTIC was repeated every four weeks. Ampules of BCG contained 10^8 viable organisms.

Dr. Rosenberg: Dr. Cunningham, what was the median follow-up of the patients that you presented? How many of the patients have actually been followed for one year?

Dr. Cunningham: About two-thirds of the patients have been followed for one year.

Question: Was the BCG given in the regional drainage of the primary tumor?

Dr. Cunningham: For an extremity lesion, such as the arm, two injections of the BCG were given on that extremity. The other two could be given in the local regional drainage area, such as in the supraclavicular region. In trunk lesions, the BCG was administered in a clockwise fashion for the first four doses. Subsequent doses were rotated between arms and thighs.

Dr. Rosenberg: Is this study still open to admission for new patients?

Dr. Cunningham: Yes, but we are changing this study, and as data become available, we will discontinue it and proceed to a different study.

Immunotherapy of Cancer: Present Status of Trials in Man, edited by W. D. Terry and D. Windhorst. Raven Press, New York © 1978.

Surgical Adjuvant Immunotherapy with BCG in Patients with Malignant Melanoma: Results of a Prospective, Randomized Trial[1]

Carl M. Pinsky, Yashar Hirshaut, Harold J. Wanebo, Elias Y. Hilal, Joseph G. Fortner, Valerie Miké, David Schottenfeld, and Herbert F. Oettgen

Memorial Sloan-Kettering Cancer Center, New York, New York 10021

Bacillus Calmette-Guérin (BCG) has been used for more than 50 years as a vaccine to prevent tuberculosis (2). For vaccination, the percutaneous route is generally recommended. Administration is by scarification, intradermal injection, or multiple tine punctures. Toxicity observed has included indolent ulceration at the vaccination site, regional lymphadenopathy, occasional chills, fever, and malaise, and, in extremely rare instances, death from disseminated BCG infection. When systemic BCG granulomatosis occurred, the clinical setting almost always suggested preexisting immunosuppression as the underlying cause (2).

Following the observation of Mathé et al. (3) that BCG administered with, or without, tumor cells was able to prolong drug-induced remissions in children with acute lymphoblastic leukemia and the report of Morton et al. (5) that BCG injected directly into melanoma nodules frequently produced regression, we began our studies of the agent in patients with melanoma. It soon became apparent that BCG given by the intralesional route led not only to regression of cutaneous nodules but also to prolonged disease-free intervals in some patients (7). This success encouraged us to try BCG vaccination, as well, in patients apparently free of disease but at high risk for recurrence.

MATERIALS AND METHODS

In 1972, a study was initiated to evaluate the effects of BCG administration by percutaneous vaccination after surgery on recurrence in patients with stage II melanoma. After regional lymph node metastases of malignant melanoma had been removed, the patients were randomized to receive either BCG

---

[1] The figures and a substantial portion of this manuscript are reprinted, by permission, from *Annals of the New York Academy of Sciences,* 277:187–194, 1976.

or no further therapy. To be eligible, the patients had to be completely free of disease and be either dinitrochlorobenzene (DNCB) or tuberculin skin test positive.

The following considerations were employed in designing the randomization scheme. According to previous studies at Memorial Hospital and elsewhere, the patients were expected to have 70% recurrence rate after 2 years. To detect a decrease of that rate to 35% with 80% probability at $p = 0.05$, it was necessary to enter 24 patients into each of the two groups. The study was initiated in the fall of 1972, and 24 patients had been entered into each of the two groups after 2 years. One of the patients in the control group could not be evaluated, because he subsequently received BCG and chemotherapy. The distribution of the prognostic factors considered to be important in patients with malignant melanoma is shown in Table 1; complete information was not available for all patients. There was no difference in sex or age distribution. It is generally believed that melanoma of the extremities has a slightly better prognosis than melanoma of the head and neck region or trunk; thus, the BCG group may have started with a slight prognostic advantage. On the other hand, there are more patients in the BCG group with Clark's level IV or V primary tumors, a distribution that would favor the control group. Also, more patients who received BCG had only one lymph node involved with tumor. In each group, three patients were DNCB negative but tuberculin positive, and no patient in either group was completely anergic by skin tests. Considering all of these factors, it is reasonable to conclude that there was no major difference in prognosis between the two groups.

TABLE 1. *Distribution of prognostic factors in control and BCG-treated groups*

	Number of patients	
Factor	Control (23)	BCG (24)
Female	7	7
Median age	48	46
Site of primary lesion[a]		
Extremity	7	11
Trunk	14	8
Head and neck	0	3
Clark's level[a]		
II or III	10	4
IV or V	7	10
Status of lymph nodes[a]		
One node	6	10
More than one node	15	10
More than one nodal area	1	3
DNCB negative	3	3
Completely anergic	0	0

[a] Information is not available for all patients.

Vaccination consisted of 4 to 6 $\times$ 10^7 viable units of BCG, supplied by the Research Foundation in Chicago, applied to the skin by means of a multiple tine technique. After the skin was cleansed and the suspension of BCG applied, a disk with 36 tines was pressed into the skin twice to produce 72 superficial punctures through which the vaccine entered the dermis. The BCG suspension was spread repeatedly over the puncture sites to ensure optimal penetration. Treatment was weekly for the first year, every other week for the second year, and every month for the third. After 3 years of treatment, BCG was stopped. The dose was increased or decreased as necessary to produce a strong but not excessive reaction at the vaccination site. In five patients initial reactivity was minimal, and the dose was increased. Nine patients continued on the same dose throughout the course of treatment. In 10 patients, local or systemic side effects became severe enough that the dose had to be decreased. BCG was applied once weekly in a rotating sequence to the extremities, with the exclusion of any extremity in which lymphadenectomy had been performed.

RESULTS AND DISCUSSION

Toxicity has been minimal. Of 24 patients treated with BCG, eight had no symptoms. Another eight patients had minor difficulties with local reactions and occasional regional lymphadenopathy, which were usually managed by decreasing the dose of BCG applied. Mild chills and low-grade fever were observed for 1 or 2 days after BCG vaccination in six patients, occasionally accompanied by mild malaise. Some but not all of these patients also had excessive local reactions, and, again, decreasing the dose of BCG generally resulted in alleviation of the symptoms. In four other patients, minor degrees of malaise only were noted that required no change in dose. Two patients complained of nausea and vomiting, but these side effects were not a major problem. Despite these side effects, the patients were quite willing to undergo weekly vaccination. After some time, when the local reaction could be predicted, many patients were trained to vaccinate themselves. Only one patient withdrew from the study.

The immunologic status of the patients was measured by serial testing for delayed cutaneous hypersensitivity to DNCB and common antigens, as described elsewhere (6). In both the BCG-treated and the control groups, two of the three initially DNCB-negative patients became DNCB positive. One of these patients in each group developed a recurrence. Also, in both groups, one patient who was previously DNCB positive became DNCB negative as he developed recurrence. Fourteen patients in the control group and 16 in the BCG-treated group had a positive tuberculin test when they entered the study. In the control group, one patient became tuberculin negative, six patients showed no change, and serial testing was not performed on the remaining 13 patients. In the BCG-treated group, 17 patients developed an increase

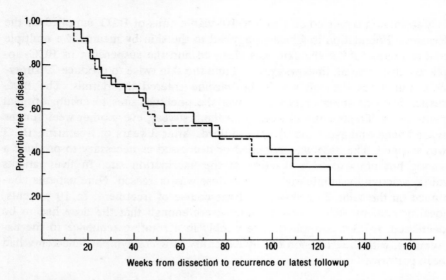

FIG. 1. The disease-free interval in the BCG-treated and control patients is depicted here. There is no apparent difference. ————, BCG, 24 patients (15 recurred, 9 no evidence of disease); ————, control, 23 patients (13 recurred, 10 no evidence of disease).

in tuberculin sensitivity, and seven patients showed no change. There were inconsistent changes in skin tests for unrelated antigens, and no difference was observed between the two groups.

At 1 year after the close of the study to patient entry, recurrence rate and survival were identical (Figs. 1 and 2) in the two groups. After 2 years of

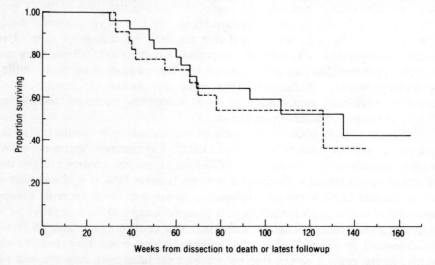

FIG. 2. The survival rate is shown here. Again, there is no difference in survival between the BCG-treated and control patients. ————, BCG, 24 patients (11 dead, 13 alive); ————, control, 23 patients (10 dead, 13 alive).

follow-up for all patients, the recurrence rate in the group treated with surgery alone is 13/23 (57%) and with surgery plus BCG is 14/24 (58%). Survival at 2 years is 15/24 (63%) for the BCG-treated group and 12/23 (53%) for the control group. Median time to recurrence is 69 and 76 weeks for the BCG-treated and control groups, respectively. Clearly, in this group of patients, BCG given by this technique is unable to positively influence the clinical course. These results are in conflict with results reported by Gutterman et al. (1) and Morton et al. (4). As discussed in this volume, several explanations are possible: (a) the types of patients seen at Memorial Hospital, M. D. Anderson, and ULCA are probably different; (b) the dose of BCG is lower in this study than in the other two; (c) BCG vaccination was omitted in limbs draining to areas of lymph node dissection only in this study; and (d) only our study is controlled by randomization. From the information available, it is not possible to decide which statement explains the difference in results. Further controlled studies will be necessary to determine whether BCG vaccination delays recurrence in patients with melanoma at high risk.

Subsequently, 31 similar patients were treated with *Corynebacterium parvum* (*C. parvum*), 4 mg i.v. per day × 5 followed by 4 mg s.c., according to the schedule for BCG. Although the study is too early for definitive evaluation, toxicity has been greater but prognosis no better than in patients treated with surgery alone or surgery plus BCG. After 2 to 3 days of daily i.v. *C. parvum* administration, nitroblue tetrazolium dye reduction of granulocytes has been markedly increased and isolated lymphocyte responsiveness to common antigens has been markedly decreased. The details of these changes will be the subject of a report that is currently in preparation.

SUMMARY

To determine if BCG administration could prevent or delay recurrence in patients with malignant melanoma, after removal of involved regional lymph nodes, a group of 47 patients was followed. By random assignment, 24 received BCG and 23 received no further therapy. Prognostic factors and delayed cutaneous hypersensitivity reactions were comparable in the two groups. In the treated group, BCG dosage was selected initially and modified, if necessary, to achieve a moderate local reaction and a minimal systemic reaction when administered percutaneously by a multiple tine technique. Toxicity was minimal. Increased reactivity to tuberculin occurred in 17 of the patients treated with BCG. There were no changes in reactivity to unrelated skin test antigens in either group. At 2 years, the recurrence rate was 14/24 (58%) and 13/23 (57%) in the BCG-treated and control groups, respectively. Median time to recurrence was 69 weeks in the patients who received BCG after surgery and 76 weeks in those who were treated with surgery alone. In conclusion, in this group of patients, BCG administration has been unable to prevent or delay recurrence of malignant melanoma.

ACKNOWLEDGMENT

This study has been supported by grants CA-05826 and CA-08748 from the National Cancer Institute.

REFERENCES

1. Gutterman, J. U., McBride, C., Freireich, E. J., Mavligit, G., Frei, E., III, and Hersh, E. M. (1973): Active immunotherapy with BCG for recurrent melanoma. *Lancet*, 1:1208–1212.
2. Mande, R. (1968): *B.C.G. Vaccination*. Dawsons, London.
3. Mathé, G., Amiel, J. L., Schwarzenberg, L., Schneider, M., Cattan, A., Schulumberger, J. R., Hayat, M., and De Vassel, F. (1969): Active immunotherapy for acute lymphoblastic leukemia. *Lancet*, 1:697–699.
4. Morton, D. L., Eilber, F. R., Holmes, E. C., Hunt, J. S., Ketcham, A. S., Silverstein, M. J., and Sparks, F. S. (1974): BCG immunotherapy of malignant melanoma: Summary of a seven year experience. *Ann. Surg.*, 180:635–643.
5. Morton, D. L., Eilber, F. R., Malmgren, R. A., and Wood, W. C. (1970): Immunological factors which influence response to immunotherapy in malignant melanoma. *Surgery*, 68:158–164.
6. Pinsky, C. M., El Domeiri, A., Caron, A. S., Knapper, W. H., and Oettgen, H. F. (1974): Delayed hypersensitivity reactions in patients with cancer. In: *Recent Results in Cancer Research*, Vol. 47, edited by G. Mathé and R. Weiner, pp. 37–41. Springer-Verlag, New York.
7. Pinsky, C. M., Hirshaut, Y., and Oettgen, H. F. (1973): Treatment of malignant melanoma by intralesional injection of BCG. *Natl. Cancer Inst. Monogr.* 39:225–228.

Question and Answer Session

Dr. Rosenberg: How do you determine dose modifications? What were you trying to achieve locally, and what were the criteria for changing the dose?

Dr. Pinsky: The dose modification was determined in order to cause the type of reaction that I illustrated in the figures. That is, at one or two weeks, inflammation should have led to pustule formation. In many of these patients there was at least some drainage. Many of these patients had some systemic reaction, but this was very minor, usually lasting a day or so, with minor chills and fever. For any patient who had more severe systemic reaction, we also decreased the dose.

Of the other 24 patients, 10 patients needed a dose reduction, nine patients had no change, and in five patients we had to increase the dose to get to this point. So there were relatively few patients in whom we did not achieve this initially and, of course, eventually we achieved it, but it took longer to get there.

Question: What was your preparation of BCG?

Dr. Pinsky: The same as that described by Dr. Cunningham. It was lyophilized TICE BCG from Chicago.

Question: Is the statistician satisfied with the number of cases in your study?

Dr. Pinsky: I don't think a statistician is ever satisfied with the number of cases, but as far as the variables were concerned, yes. I think that they felt that the randomization was quite successful even though we didn't stratify for many things. As far as coming to some sort of a final answer to whether or not this form of BCG therapy would be useful and we could translate this in a general way to a population of patients, no, it would take many more patients to be absolutely sure that this was so. I think that this is the crux of the matter.

Immunotherapy of Cancer: Present Status of
Trials in Man, edited by W. D. Terry and D. Windhorst.
Raven Press, New York © 1978.

Postoperative Immunotherapy for Recurrent Malignant Melanoma: An Updated Report

Jordan U. Gutterman, Giora M. Mavligit, *Charles M. McBride,
Stephen P. Richman, Michael A. Burgess, and Evan M. Hersh

*Departments of Developmental Therapeutics and *Surgery, The University of Texas
System Cancer Center, M. D. Anderson Hospital and Tumor Institute,
Houston, Texas 77030*

The development of adjuvant cancer immunotherapy trials has increased rapidly since the initial reports that showed that Bacillus Calmette-Guérin (BCG) could delay recurrence of metastases and prolong survival in human cancer patients with microscopic disease (32).

Immunotherapy of malignant melanoma has received intense investigation since the report of Morton and co-workers that intratumor inoculation of viable BCG organisms could induce regression of intradermal or subcutaneous metastases (38).

Based on the efficacy of BCG as an immunotherapeutic agent in experimental tumors as well as human cancer (30), in 1971, we initiated a pilot adjuvant study of systemic BCG immunotherapy in melanoma patients following surgical extirpation of recurrent metastatic disease in regional lymph nodes or in distant sites. Our initial results were encouraging; the data suggested that patients who received high doses of viable organisms of lyophilized Tice BCG had a delay in the recurrence of melanoma as well as a prolongation of survival compared to patients treated with surgery alone or with low doses of BCG (14,17). Morton and co-workers have also published their initial pilot study demonstrating similar data—BCG applied as an adjunct to surgery was associated with a delay in recurrent disease and a prolongation of survival in melanoma patients with regional or distant metastases (7,37). Other reports have also demonstrated a similar benefit of BCG immunotherapy in melanoma patients with regional metastases (3,24).

We have now followed our patients for a maximum of 5 years and report these long-term results. The following clinical data have been examined and correlated—dose and strain of BCG, anatomical location of the primary and metastatic melanoma, and amount of postsurgical residual disease as estimated by the number of positive lymph nodes.

MATERIALS AND METHODS

Between November, 1971, and July, 1973, 52 consecutive patients with regional lymph node metastases (stage IIIB disease) and 15 patients with distant metastases (stage IVA) were entered on the study. All patients had *recurrent melanoma, therapeutic* surgical resections, and were eligible for the study after they had been rendered clinically free of disease by surgery. Patients were not accepted into the study if they had been operated on more than 3 months previously.

Prior to immunotherapy patients were evaluated for residual disease with the following tests—physical examination, liver and renal function tests, chest X-ray, liver scan, electroencephalogram, and brain scan. Chest tomogram, metastatic bone survey, bone marrow biopsy, or gastrointestinal X-rays were done if specific symptoms and/or the results of other studies described above indicated they should be carried out.

Immunotherapy

Fifty-two patients with stage IIIB disease were treated. Twenty-seven were treated with a high dose of BCG (6×10^8 viable units)—20 patients were treated with lyophilized Tice strain BCG and seven with fresh liquid Pasteur BCG. Twenty-five patients received a low dose of BCG (6×10^7 viable units)—22 patients received Tice BCG and three the liquid Pasteur BCG.

Fifteen patients with stage IVA disease were treated. Nine patients were treated with high-dose BCG (eight received Tice, and one received Pasteur BCG), and six patients were treated with low-dose BCG (four received Tice, and two received Pasteur BCG).

The lyophilized Tice BCG was obtained from the Institute for Tuberculosis Research, Chicago, Illinois. The fresh liquid BCG was obtained from the Pasteur Institute, Paris, France. The Pasteur BCG was flown weekly to our Institute, stored at 4° C, and used within 14 days. BCG was administered by scarification on the upper arms and upper thighs in a rotational fashion every week for 3 months and then once a month as described previously (15,17).

Following the demonstration of a failure to maintain vigorous skin test reactivity to recall antigens during the period when the BCG was applied only once a month (18), in March, 1973, we began a maintenance schedule of every other week in all patients.

The total number of viable units administered was calculated from the number of viable units per vial as estimated by the manufacturers at the time of shipment.

The dose of BCG was not increased. The dose was decreased only if indurated lesions extending 5 cm beyond the scar were observed.

Clinical Follow-Up

Physical examination, blood chemistries, and chest X-ray were repeated every 2 months for the first 6 months of the study, and then every 3 to 4 months thereafter. Electroencephalogram and liver and brain scans were repeated whenever indicated by patients' symptoms or blood chemistry results.

Surgical Control Group

We examined the records and plotted the natural history of 260 patients with stage III disease and 121 patients with stage IVA disease who were treated at M. D. Anderson Hospital and Tumor Institute from January, 1965 to October, 1971. These patients served as the surgical control group. The natural history of these patients will be the subject of a detailed report and subsequent article.

Statistics

The statistical methods used include a generalized Wilcoxon test (12), with a one-tailed analysis, for testing differences between remission or survival curves and the methods of Kaplan and Meier for calculating and plotting remission and survival curves (27).

RESULTS

The factors known to affect prognosis for the two BCG groups and the control groups are shown in Table 1. Forty-two patients were treated with Tice BCG. Twenty received high-dose BCG (6×10^8 viable units), and 22 received low-dose BCG (6×10^7 viable units). The postoperative disease-free interval for these groups of patients is compared to that of the surgical control group in Fig. 1. Fourteen of 20 patients treated with high-dose BCG have developed recurrent disease. The median disease-free interval was 14 months. Sixteen of 22 patients treated with low-dose BCG have experienced recurrence with a median disease-free interval of 8 months. The median disease-free interval for the group of patients treated with surgery alone was 9 months. The disease-free interval for patients treated with high-dose BCG was longer than that for the surgical control group, and was statistically suggestive ($p = 0.06$). The differences between high-dose and low-dose BCG were suggestive ($p = 0.1$).

The survival for the preceding group of patients is shown in Fig. 2. Twelve of 20 patients treated with high-dose BCG have died. The median survival was 27 months. The median survival for the low-dose Tice BCG group and the surgical control group was identical (19 months). The survival of the high-dose BCG group was significantly longer than that for the surgical control group ($p = 0.01$). The low-dose BCG Tice group had a survival similar to the surgical control group.

TABLE 1. *Characteristics of surgical control and Tice BCG-treated patients with malignant melanoma*

	Control		Tice BCG (6 × 10⁸ VU)		Tice BCG (6 × 10⁷ VU)	
Male	172	(66)[a]	11	(55)	16	(73)
Female	88	(34)	9	(45)	6	(27)
Age of patient						
< 30	41	(16)	9	(45)	6	(27)
30–60	155	(60)	8	(40)	15	(68)
> 60	64	(24)	3	(15)	1	(5)
Site of primary						
Trunk	98	(37)	11	(55)	11	(50)
Extremity	88	(34)	4	(20)	5	(23)
Head and neck	52	(20)	3	(15)	4	(18)
Unknown	18	(7)	1	(5)	2	(9)
Other	4	(2)	1	(5)	0	
No. of positive lymph nodes						
1	110	(42)	5	(25)	8	(36)
2–4	64	(25)	5	(25)	5	(23)
≥ 5	61	(23)	10	(50)	9	(41)
Unknown	25	(10)	0		0	
Place of surgery						
M. D. Anderson Hospital	116	(44)	8	(40)	8	(36)
Both[b]	59	(23)	7	(35)	3	(14)
Outside	85	(33)	5	(25)	11	(50)

[a] Number of patients, with percentage in parentheses.
[b] Both means biopsy outside hospital and dissection at M. D. Anderson.
VU, viable units.

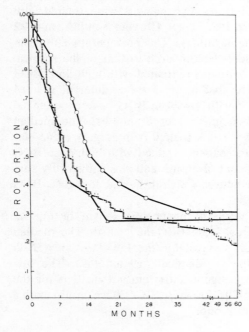

FIG. 1. Stage III melanoma. The postoperative disease-free interval for the high- and low-dose Tice BCG-treated groups (○ and △, respectively) compared to surgical control group (+). Relapses were 14/20, 16/22, and 194/260, respectively. (High-dose vs. control, $p = 0.06$; high-dose vs. low-dose, $p = 0.1$; low-dose vs. control, $p = 0.35$.)

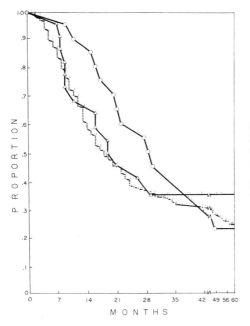

FIG. 2. Stage III melanoma. Survival of high- and low-dose Tice BCG-treated groups (O and Δ, respectively) compared to surgical control (+). Deaths were 12/20, 14/22, and 177/260, respectively. (High-dose vs. control, $p = 0.01$; high-dose vs. low-dose, $p = 0.1$; and low-dose vs. control, $p = 0.2$.)

The most notable effect of adjuvant Tice BCG occurred in the group of patients with melanoma of the trunk metastatic to regional lymph nodes. Thirteen of 21 patients with trunk melanoma treated with BCG have developed recurrent disease as shown in Fig. 3. The disease-free interval was significantly longer than the comparable group of surgical controls with trunk melanoma ($p = 0.02$).

The survival for the preceding group of trunk melanoma patients is shown in Fig. 4. Twelve of 21 patients treated with Tice BCG have died, with the median survival being 26 months. The median survival for the surgical control group was 19 months ($p = 0.009$).

Figures 5 and 6 demonstrate the results for patients with melanoma of the trunk according to the dose of BCG. In eight of the 11 patients treated with high-dose Tice and in five of the 10 treated with low-dose Tice recurrent disease has developed. The disease-free interval is longer for the high- and low-dose BCG-treated groups of patients than for the surgical controls ($p = 0.057$ and 0.07, respectively).

The survival for these patients is shown in Fig. 6. Seven of the 11 patients treated with high-dose BCG and five of the 10 treated with low-dose BCG have died. The survival for the high-dose group is significantly longer than that for the surgical control group ($p = 0.03$). The survival of the low-dose BCG group is longer than that of the surgical control group and is statistically suggestive ($p = 0.06$). The dip in the curve for the high-dose BCG group is due to the death of one patient at 45 months.

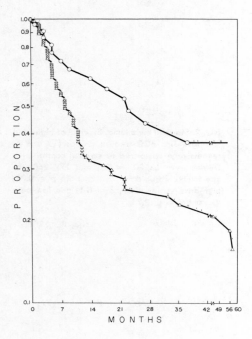

FIG. 3. Stage III melanoma of the trunk. Disease-free interval for Tice BCG-treated (○) and surgical control (△) groups. Relapses were 13/21 and 76/98, respectively. (p = 0.02.)

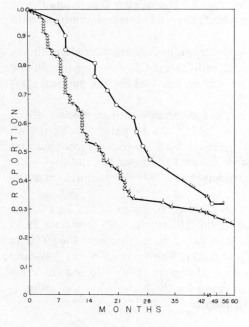

FIG. 4. Stage III melanoma of trunk. Survival of Tice BCG-treated (○) and surgical control (△) groups. Deaths were 12/21 and 68/98, respectively. (p = 0.009.)

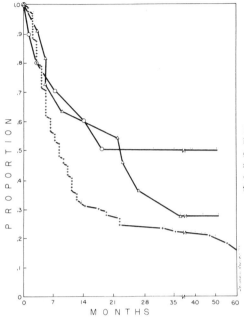

FIG. 5. Stage IIIB trunk melanoma. Disease-free interval for high- and low-dose Tice BCG-treated groups (Δ and ○, respectively) compared to surgical controls (+). Relapses were 8/11, 5/10, and 194/260, respectively. (High-dose vs. control, p = 0.057; low-dose vs. control, p = 0.07.)

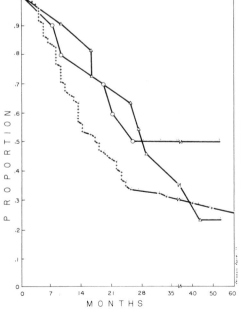

FIG. 6. Stage IIIB trunk melanoma. Survival of high- and low-dose Tice BCG-treated groups (Δ and ○, respectively) compared to surgical controls (+). Deaths were 7/11, 5/10, and 177/260, respectively. (High-dose vs. control, p = 0.03; low-dose vs. control, p = 0.06.)

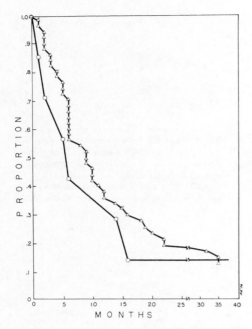

FIG. 7. Stage III melanoma of head and neck. Disease-free interval of Tice BCG-treated patients (O) compared to controls (Δ). Relapses were 6/7 and 43/52, respectively. (p = 0.25.)

In sharp contrast to the beneficial effect of Tice BCG on patients with melanoma of the trunk, there was no advantage for BCG among the group of patients with melanoma of the head and neck. Thus, in Figs. 7 and 8, it is apparent that neither the disease-free interval nor the survival was prolonged among this group of patients.

We next examined the prognosis of the groups of patients according to the number of positive nodes removed at the time of surgery. Figure 9 shows the postoperative disease-free interval for patients who had one to four positive nodes. Five of 10 patients treated with high-dose BCG and nine of 13 treated with low-dose BCG have experienced recurrence. The postoperative disease-free interval for the high-dose BCG group is statistically longer than that of the surgical control group ($p = 0.05$) and than that of the low-dose BCG group ($p = 0.04$).

The survival for these patients is shown in Fig. 10. Only three of the 10 high-dose Tice BCG patients have died compared to eight of the 13 with low-dose Tice BCG. The postoperative survival for the high-dose Tice BCG group is longer than that for the surgical control group ($p = 0.01$) and than that for the low-dose Tice BCG group ($p = 0.03$).

The prognosis for patients with five or more nodes is shown in Figs. 11 and 12. Almost all the patients treated with BCG have developed recurrent disease. However, the median disease-free interval for the high-dose Tice-treated patients was double (14 months) that of the surgical control group (7 months) ($p = 0.06$). Although there was a delay in recurrent disease for

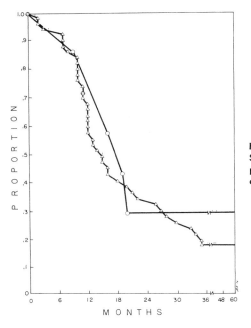

FIG. 8. Stage III melanoma of head and neck. Survival of Tice BCG-treated group (○) compared to surgical controls (Δ). Deaths were 5/7 and 40/52, respectively. (p = 0.26.)

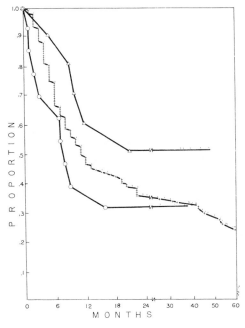

FIG. 9. Stage IIIB melanoma, one to four nodes. Disease-free interval for high- and low-dose Tice BCG-treated groups (Δ and ○, respectively) compared to surgical control (+). Relapses were 5/10, 9/13, and 116/174, respectively. (High-dose vs. control, p = 0.05; high-dose vs. low-dose, p = 0.04.)

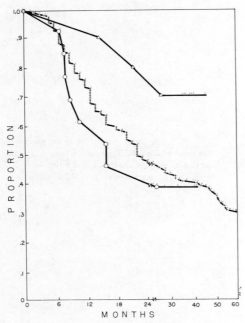

FIG. 10. Stage IIIB melanoma, one to four nodes. Survival of high- and low-dose Tice BCG-treated groups (Δ and ○, respectively) compared to surgical controls (+). Deaths were 3/10, 8/13, and 102/174, respectively. (High-dose vs. control, p = 0.01; high-dose vs. low-dose, p = 0.03.)

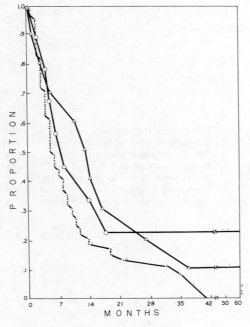

FIG. 11. Stage IIIB melanoma, five or more nodes. Disease-free interval of high- and low-dose Tice BCG-treated groups (Δ and ○, respectively) compared to surgical controls (+). Relapses were 9/10, 7/9, and 55/61, respectively. (High-dose vs. control, p = 0.06; low-dose vs. control, p = 0.14.)

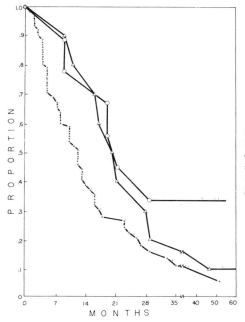

FIG. 12. Stage IIIB melanoma, five or more nodes. Survival of high- and low-dose Tice BCG-treated groups (Δ and $\bigcirc$, respectively) compared to surgical controls (+). Deaths were 9/10, 6/9, and 52/61, respectively. (High-dose vs. control, $p = 0.01$; low-dose vs. control, $p = 0.01$.)

the low-dose Tice BCG group compared to the surgical controls, this has not reached statistical significance ($p = 0.14$).

The survival for these patients is shown in Fig. 12. Although the majority of patients treated with BCG have died, there has been a significant prolongation of survival for both the high-dose and the low-dose Tice BCG group. Thus, the median survival for the surgical controls was 12 months, and the median survival for both the high-dose and the low-dose BCG groups was 21 months. Both BCG groups have lived longer than the surgical controls ($p = 0.01$ for both comparisons).

The long-term follow-up among patients treated with fresh liquid Pasteur BCG is shown in the next two figures. The disease-free interval and survival among the patients treated with high doses of Pasteur BCG were identical to the surgical control group. All three patients treated with low-dose Pasteur BCG experienced recurrence early and died (Figs. 13 and 14).

The postoperative disease-free interval for the small group of patients with stage IVA disease (patients with disseminated metastases removed by surgery) is shown in Fig. 15. Although the majority of patients treated with high-dose BCG as well as low-dose BCG has developed recurrent disease, there has been a highly significant prolongation of the disease-free interval for the group of patients treated with high-dose Tice BCG compared to surgical controls ($p = 0.001$).

The survival for the preceding group of patients is shown in Fig. 16. Five

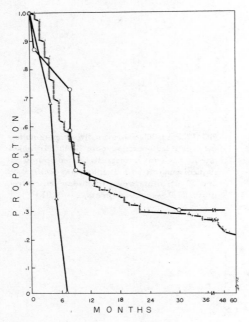

FIG. 13. Stage III melanoma. Disease-free interval for patients in high-dose (○) and low-dose (Δ) liquid Pasteur BCG compared to surgical controls (+). Relapses were 5/7, 3/3, and 194/260, respectively.

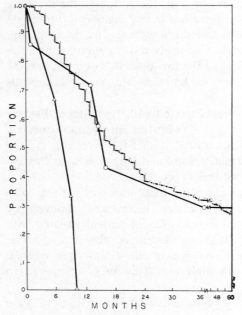

FIG. 14. Stage III melanoma. Survival of patients on high-dose (○) and low-dose (Δ) liquid Pasteur BCG compared to surgical controls (+). Deaths were 5/7, 3/3, and 177/260, respectively.

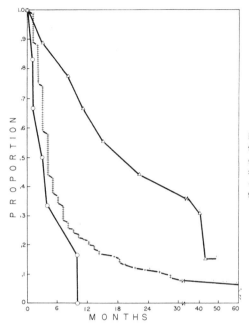

FIG. 15. Stage IVA melanoma. Disease-free interval of high- and low-dose Tice BCG-treated groups (Δ and ○, respectively) compared to surgical controls (+). Relapses were 7/9, 6/6, and 110/121, respectively. (High-dose vs. control, *p* = 0.001.)

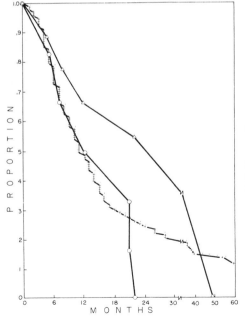

FIG. 16. Stage IVA melanoma. Survival of high- and low-dose Tice BCG-treated groups (Δ and ○, respectively) compared to surgical controls (+). Deaths were 5/9, 6/6, and 96/121, respectively. (High-dose vs. control, *p* = 0.02; high-dose vs. low-dose, *p* = 0.06.)

of the nine high-dose BCG patients have died compared to all six of the low-dose BCG patients. The survival for the high-dose BCG group is significantly longer than that for the surgical controls ($p = 0.02$).

DISCUSSION

Our initial evaluation of BCG immunotherapy was carried out in stage III patients in whom all clinical evidence of disease was removed surgically, but in whom there was a statistically high chance of residual microscopic disease recurring clinically within 6 to 12 months. We also treated a group of patients whose disease had spread beyond the regional lymphatics (stage IVA) but in whom all visible disease was removed by surgery.

The most important data derived from this study are that "adequate" doses of viable BCG organisms applied by scarification into the tumor-involved lymphatic regions significantly delayed tumor recurrence, thus prolonging the disease-free interval and survival of patients with stage IIIB disease. Similar results in small groups of patients were reported 4 years ago by Bluming and co-workers (4). In their study, high numbers of viable units of lyophilized BCG given by scarification for seven treatments after surgery were superior to low numbers of BCG organisms of intradermal Glaxo strain BCG, a strain which is weakly immunogenic (19). Morton and co-workers have recently reported results similar to those in the current study using Tice BCG multi-puncture technique in doses of 2 to 6×10^8 viable units and a schedule similar to the one outlined in this chapter (7,37). Additionally, Ikonopisov has reported prolongation of the postoperative disease-free interval and of survival in a similar group of melanoma patients with BCG or imidazole carboxamide plus BCG (24). Therefore, it seems that BCG has a definite beneficial effect in melanoma patients with minimal residual disease. In addition, there is some suggestive evidence that *Corynebacterium parvum* can delay recurrence and prolong survival in similar patients with melanoma (25). Recent confirmatory evidence on the therapeutic efficacy of BCG has been presented by Beretta (3).

The remainder of the discussion focuses on several principles that have been suggested from this study.

Dose and Strain of BCG

Dose

The published adjuvant studies in melanoma described above indicate that adequate numbers of viable BCG organisms are required to achieve a significant antitumor effect (4,7,14,17,37). It is well known that adequate numbers of viable organisms appear to be critical in curing a transplantable guinea pig hepatoma within the skin (50). Similar data have been reported by Hawrylko and Mackaness for a mouse mastocytoma model (23). It was logical to assume, therefore, that in order to control or possibly eradicate residual tumor cells in regional lymph nodes, high doses of BCG would be necessary. Our data strongly suggest that a difference of one log in numbers of viable organisms was critical for therapeutic efficacy in our patients.

The actual percentage of organisms delivered into the regional lymphatic tissue is not known. However, studies of BCG scarification in the guinea pig have demonstrated (a) increased cell-mediated immune response to sheep red blood cells (40) and (b) significant antitumor effect in animals with metastatic disease within regional lymph nodes (21). In addition, Mackaness and co-workers have recently shown that the absorption of BCG organisms after scarification in the guinea pig is greater than that delivered by the multi-puncture technique (G. B. Mackaness, *personal communication*).

The data in the current study suggest that it is imperative to design careful dose-response studies in the evaluation of various immunomodulators for human immunotherapy trials. We were not able to carry out a complete dose-response study because of the type of preparations clinically available at the time this study was initiated. Thus, we can only speculate whether a one log higher dose (6×10^9 viable units) would have further increased the therapeutic benefit. It must be stressed that excessive doses of BCG could lead to immunological incompetence or anergy (28), perhaps by increased suppressor cell activity (36) or by immunological paralysis.

In general, the prognosis of the patients treated with low doses of BCG (6×10^7 viable units) was not improved compared to the natural history of the surgical control group. An exception was the improved survival for the patients with trunk melanoma. Presumably we were able to deliver adequate doses of BCG into the regional areas to achieve a significant antitumor effect (*see below*).

Further substantiation of the clinical need for an adequate dose of viable BCG organisms in adjuvant therapy of human melanoma comes from the recent study of Pinsky et al. (41). In that adjuvant study, after surgical extirpation of regional lymph nodes, a dose of 6×10^7 viable units by the multipuncture technique was not effective in prolonging the disease-free interval or survival. We estimate that the lower applied dose and the use of the multipuncture rather than the scarification technique resulted in perhaps as much as a two-log lower effective dose. The optimal dose of BCG may also depend on other variables, including the immunocompetence of the patient (31).

Strain of BCG

In addition to the number of viable units of BCG, another important variable is the strain of BCG. BCG strains vary widely in their immunogenicity and virulence (29,45) as well as in their antitumor efficacy (10).

Both the Tice and Pasteur BCG strains used in the current study are known to be quite immunogenic and virulent (29). In addition, the Tice strain has been effective in several immunotherapy trials in both animal and human tumors (7,17,37,47,48). The numbers of patients in the current study preclude any absolute statement regarding the efficacy of fresh Pasteur BCG compared to the lyophilized Tice.

Whether the antitumor activity of a given number of organisms depends on the substrain of BCG and the method of vaccine preparation has not been firmly established in man. However, recent studies carried out by our group in collaboration with Hanna and co-workers showed that two strains, the Phipps and Pasteur, grown as a submerged culture with detergent by Mackaness and co-workers (29) permitting growth of organisms as a dispersed culture, yielded a superior result with equivalent numbers of viable organisms compared to commercially available lyophilized preparations (21). Thus, we are now studying the efficacy of a fully viable form of BCG specifically designed for cancer immunotherapy (29).

Site of Tumor

The positive therapeutic results in patients with trunk melanoma contrasted with the lack of therapeutic effect in patients with head and neck melanoma. We administered the BCG to the upper arms and upper legs, thereby presumably activating cells within lymph nodes regional to the trunk and extremity regions. BCG was not given directly into the lymphatics of the head and neck region. We suggest that the failure in head and neck melanoma patients was related to the regional effect of BCG. One of the important principles derived from some (2,5,21,22,46,50) but not all experimental studies (49) is the necessity for intimate contact between BCG (or BCG fractions) and tumor cells for maximal antitumor effect.

Further data substantiating this hypothesis come from the work of Eilber and co-workers (7). In their most recent analysis, patients with trunk and extremity as well as head and neck melanoma benefited from BCG. In contrast to our regimen, BCG was given over the site of the primary tumor, thereby delivering BCG directly in the regional lymphatics of the head and neck region as well as in the lymphatics of the trunk and extremities.

Pinsky and co-workers recently reported the failure of BCG to delay recurrence and prolong survival in melanoma (41). In addition to the use of relatively ineffective low doses of BCG, in that study the region of the lymph node metastases was not immunized, perhaps violating one of the most important principles derived from animal tumor studies.

Further, we have recently reported data suggesting that regional immunotherapy (BCG by scarification into tumor-involved lymph nodes) can potentiate the antitumor effects of chemotherapy (15).

It is now known that melanoma biopsy tissue is frequently infiltrated with a variety of cells including macrophages and lymphocytes (11). If these cells can be "activated" by regional immunotherapy, significant antitumor effects might be expected. The principles of local immunotherapy have recently been tested in other cancer trials. Ruckdeschel and co-workers observed 3 years ago that patients with operable carcinoma of the lung lived longer if they had developed postoperative empyemas (44). Therefore, a prospective trial was carried out to investigate if BCG given intrapleurally could delay recurrence and prolong survival in resectable lung carcinoma. A single dose of BCG given into the regional lymph nodes within the pleural space delayed recurrence and prolonged survival of patients with stage I lung cancer (35).

This is not to say that local or regional immunotherapy is the only effective form of adjuvant therapy. Thus, levamisole, a systemic immunopotentiator given by mouth, was effective in prolonging disease-free interval and survival in squamous lung cancer and breast cancer (1,43). Further, BCG and *C. parvum* are effective in prolonging survival in patients with disseminated cancer (13–16,25,32). Thus, local and regional as well as systemic immunotherapy seem to have a place in the management of human solid tumors.

Tumor Load—Degree of Residual Disease

It has been suggested that the immune system is generally not capable of rejecting more than a small load of tumor cells (20,30,39). Adjuvant BCG in the current study had a greater antitumor effect in the group of patients with less than five positive nodes than it did in those patients with five or more positive nodes. In particular the survival of patients with less than five positive nodes has been most significantly improved with adjuvant BCG. The survival of patients with five or more nodes was only marginally benefited by BCG. These data therefore confirm that active immunotherapy probably has more therapeutic benefit for patients with small amounts of residual tumor (33).

It should be emphasized, however, that immunotherapy did achieve a therapeutic effect even in patients with distant metastases removed by surgery (stage IVA). Similar benefit was reported by Morton and co-workers (37).

Patients with less than five nodes treated with low doses of BCG not only failed to benefit from treatment but also may have had a slight acceleration of recurrent disease and shorter survival compared to the surgical control group. This was particularly true for patients with one positive node treated with low doses of BCG (14). The possibility that patients with small amounts of residual tumor treated with low doses of BCG (? low degree of immune stimulation) may experience acceleration of tumor growth must be kept in mind. Prehn has recently hypothesized that the immune system serves a dual role in its relationship to oncogenesis or development of neoplastic cells (42). A low degree of immune stimulation in the context of a low tumor load may actually lead to stimulation of tumor growth. In Prehn's study, this seemed to be associated with cell-mediated mechanisms. Although the exact mechanism for this phenomena is not proved, it could be that low degrees of immune stimulation activates suppressor T cells that in turn suppress significant anti-tumor response. Other possible immunological mechanisms may be responsible for this phenomenon (9). Similar observations have been made in the B16 melanoma model in the mouse (6).

Additional Comments

In general, the results of this study suggest that BCG achieved cytostatis rather than cytolysis of tumor cells. Most of the patients developed evidence of recurrent disease, but BCG clearly delayed the clinical reappearance of tumor. The most marked effect of BCG was prolonged survival. In general, the major therapeutic benefit described for BCG and other forms of immuno-therapy currently in clinical use has been in survival rather than remission or disease-free interval.

Conclusion

In conclusion, BCG immunotherapy has been associated with an improved prognosis in malignant melanoma patients with limited metastatic disease. It is clear that BCG immunotherapy for the patients described in this and other studies is not optimal therapy. Further research on purification of the active components of the BCG organisms as well as the identification of additional active immunotherapy reagents (26) should continue to lead to improvement in the prognosis of such patients. Further understanding of the host–tumor relationship and the concept of shared antigens between melanoma cells and microbial organisms should add to the therapeutic results (34). Treatment of melanoma patients with primary tumors seems indicated (8). In addition combination of chemotherapy with immunotherapy should be applied in the postoperative adjuvant situation (15).

Finally, it is important to stress the limitations and variabilities of BCG (19). Thus, improved chemotherapy, immunotherapy, and immunodiagnosis are needed to further improve the treatment of patients with malignant mela-noma.

ACKNOWLEDGMENTS

This work has been supported by contract NO1-CB-33888 and grants 05830 and 11520 from the National Cancer Institute, Bethesda, Mary-land 20014. Drs. Gutterman and Mavligit are the recipients of career de-velopment awards (CA 71007–03 and CA 00130–02, respectively) also from the National Cancer Institute.

REFERENCES

1. Amery, W. (1976): Double-blind trial with levamisole in resectable lung cancer. *Ann. NY Acad. Sci.,* 277:260–268.
2. Baldwin, R. W., and Pimm, M. V. (1973): BCG immunotherapy of rat tumors of defined immunogenicity. *Natl. Cancer Inst. Monogr.,* 39:11–17.
3. Beretta, A. (1978): Controlled study for prolonged chemotherapy, immunotherapy, and chemotherapy plus immunotherapy as adjuvant to surgery. (*This volume.*)
4. Bluming, A. Z., Vogel, C. L., and Ziegler, J. L. (1972): Immunological effects of BCG in malignant melanoma: Two modes of administration compared. *Ann. Intern. Med.,* 76:405–411.
5. Carr, I., and McGinty, F. (1974): Lymphatic metastasis and its inhibition. An experimental model. *J. Pathol.,* 113:85–95.
6. Chee, D. O., and Bodurtha, A. J. (1974): Facilitation and inhibition of B16 melanoma by BCG in vivo and by lymphoid cells from BCG-treated mice in vitro. *Int. J. Cancer,* 14:137–143.
7. Eilber, F. R., Morton, D. L., Holmes, E. C., Sparks, F. C., and Ramming, K. P. (1976): Adjuvant immunotherapy with BCG in treatment of regional lymph node metastases from malignant melanoma. *N. Engl. J. Med.,* 294:237–240.
8. Everall, J. D., O'Doherty, C. J., Wand, J., and Dowd, P. M. (1975): Treatment of primary melanoma by intralesional vaccinia before excision. *Lancet,* 2:583–586.
9. Fidler, I. J. (1974): Immune stimulation-inhibition of experimental cancer metastases. *Cancer Res.,* 34:491–498.
10. Fortner, S. W., Hanna, M. G., and Coggin, J. H., Jr. (1974): Differential effects of two strains of BCG on transplantation immunity to SV40-induced tumors in hamsters. *Proc. Soc. Exp. Biol. Med.,* 147:62–67.
11. Gauci, C. L., and Alexander, P. (1975): The macrophage content of some human tumors. *Cancer Lett.,* 1:29–32.
12. Gehan, E. A. (1965): A generalized Wilcoxon test for comparing arbitrarily singly-censored samples. *Biometrika,* 52:203–223.
13. Gutterman, J. U., Hersh, E. M., Rodriguez, V., Mavligit, G. M., Burgess, M. A., Gehn, E. Hersh, E. M., McCredie, K. B., Reed, R., Smith, T., Bodey, G. P., and Freireich, E. J. (1974): Chemoimmunotherapy of adult acute leukemia prolongation of remission in myeloblastic leukemia with BCG. *Lancet,* 2:1405–1409.
14. Gutterman, J. U., Mavligit, G. M., Burgess, M. A., Cardinos, J. D., Blumenschein, G. R., Gottlieb, J. A., McBride, C. M. and McCredie, K. B., Bodey, G. P., Rodriquez, V., Freireich, E. J., and Hersh, E. M. (1976): Immunotherapy of human solid tumors and acute leukemia with BCG: Prolongation of disease free interval and survival. *Cancer Immunol. Immunother.,* 1:99–107.
15. Gutterman, J. U., Mavligit, G., Gottlieb, J. A., Burgess, M. A., McBride, C. E., Einhorn, L., Freireich, E. J. and Hersh, E. M.(1974): Chemoimmunotherapy of disseminated malignant melanoma with dimethyl triazeno imidazole carboxamide and Bacillus Calmette-Guerin. *N. Engl. J. Med.,* 291:592–597.
16. Gutterman, J. U., Mavligit, G. M., Hersh, E. M., Burgess, M. A., McBride, C. M., and Hersh, E. M. (1976): Chemoimmunotherapy of colorectal cancer, breast carcinoma, and malignant melanoma with BCG: Prolongation of disease free interval and survival. *N.Y. Acad. Sci.,* 277:135–159.
17. Gutterman, J. U., Mavligit, G. M., McBride, C. M., Frei E., Freireich, E. J., and Hersh, E. M. (1973): Active immunotherapy with BCG for recurrent malignant melanoma. *Lancet,* 1:1208–1212.
18. Gutterman, J. U., Mavligit, G. M., McBride, C. M., Frei, E., III, and Hersh, E. M. (1973): BCG stimulation of immune responsiveness in patients with malignant melanoma. *Cancer,* 32:321–327.
19. Gutterman, J. U., Mavligit, G. M., Reed, R. C., Richman, S. P., McBride, C. M., and Hersh, E. M. (1975): Immunology and immunotherapy of human malignant melanoma: Historic review and perspectives for the future. *Semin. Oncol.,* 2:155–174.
20. Halpern, B. N., Biozzi, G., Stiffel, G., and Mouton, D. (1966): Inhibitor of tumor

growth by administration of killed Corynebacterium parvum. *Nature,* 212:853–854.
21. Hanna, M. G., Jr., Peters, L. C., Gutterman, J. U., and Hersh, E. M. (1976): An evaluation of BCG administration by scarification of immunotherapy of metastatic hematomcarcinoma in the guinea pig. *J. Natl. Cancer Inst.,* 56:1013–1018.
22. Hanna, M. G., Jr., Snodgrass, M. J., Zbar, B., and Rapp, N. J. (1973): Histologic and ultrastructural studies of tumor regression in inbred guinea pigs after intralesional injection of mycobacterium bovis (BCG). *Natl. Cancer Inst. Monogr.,* 39:71–85.
23. Hawrylko, E., and Mackaness, G. B. (1973): Immunopotentiation with BCG III. Modulation of the response to a tumor specific antigen. J. Natl. Cancer Inst. 51:1677–1682.
24. Ikonopisov, R. L. (1975): The international symposium on immunological reactions to melanoma antigens. *Behring Inst. Mitt.,* 56:235–250.
25. Israel, L., and Edelstein, R. (1975): Nonspecific immunostimulation with Corynebacterium parvum in human cancer. In: *Immunological Aspects of Neoplasia,* pp. 485–504. Williams & Wilkins, Baltimore.
26. Israel, L., Edelstein, R., Depierre, A., and Simitrov, N. (1975): Brief communication: Daily intravenous infusions with C. parvum in 20 patients with disseminated cancer: A preliminary report of clinical and biological findings. *J. Natl. Cancer Inst.,* 55:29–33.
27. Kaplan, E. L., and Meier, P. (1958): Nonparametric estimation from incomplete observations. *J. Am. Stat. Assoc.,* 53:457–481.
28. Lamoureux, G., and Poisson, R. (1974): BCG and immunological anergy. *Lancet,* 2:989–990.
29. Mackaness, G. B., Auclari, D. J., and Lagrange, P. H. (1973): Immunopotentiation with BCG. I. Immune response to different strains and preparations. *J. Natl. Cancer Inst.,* 51:1655–1667.
30. Mathe, G. (1971): Active immunotherapy. *Adv. Cancer Res.,* 14:1–36.
31. Mathe, G. (1976): Surviving in company of BCG. *Cancer Immunol. Immunother.,* 1:3–5.
32. Mathe, G., Amiel, J. L., Schwarzenberg, L., Schneider, L., Cattan, A., Schlumberger, J. R., Hazart, M., and De Vassal, F. (1969): Active immunotherapy for acute lymphoblastic leukemia. *Lancet,* 1:697–699.
33. Mavligit, G. M., Gutterman, J. U., Burgess, M. A., Khankhenian, N., Seibert, G. B., Speer, J. F., Jubert, A. V., Martin, R. C., McBride, C. M., Copeland, E. M., Gehan, E. A., and Hersh, E. M. (1976): Prolongation of post-operative disease free interval and survival in human colorectal cancer by Bacillus Calmette Guerin (BCG) or BCG plus 5-fluorouracil. *Lancet,* 1:871–875.
34. Minden, P., Gutterman, J. U., Hersh, E. M., Jarrett, C., and McClatchy, J. K. (1976): Antibodies to melanoma cell and BCG antigens in sera from tumor free individuals and from melanoma patients. *Nature,* 263:774–777.
35. McKneally, M. F., Maver, C., and Kausel, H. W. (1976): Regional immunotherapy of lung cancer with intrapleural BCG. *Lancet,* 1:377–379.
36. Mitchell, M. S., Kirkpatrick, D., Mokyr, M. B., et al. (1973): On the mode of action of BCG. *Nature [New Biol.],* 243:216–217.
37. Morton, D. L., Eilber, F. R., Holmes, E. C., Hunt, J. S., Ketcham, A. S., Silverstein, M. J., and Sparks, F. C. (1974): BCG immunotherapy of malignant melanoma: Summary of a seven year experience. *Ann. Surg.,* 180:635–643.
38. Morton, D. L., Eilber, F. R., and Malmgren, R. A. and Wood, W. C. (1970): Immunological factors which influence response to immunotherapy in malignant melanoma. *Surgery,* 68:158–164.
39. Old, L. J., Clarke, D. A., and Benacerraf, S. (1959): Effect of Bacillus Calmette-Guerin infection of transplanted tumors in the mouse. *Nature,* 18:291–292.
40. Peters, L. C., Hanna, M. G., Jr., Gutterman, J. U., Mavligit, G. M., and Hersh, E. M. (1974): Modulation of the immune response of guinea pigs by repeated BCG scarification. *Proc. Soc. Exp. Biol. Med.,* 147:344–349.
41. Pinsky, C. M., Hirshaut, Y., Wanebo, H. J., Fortner, J. G., Mike, V., Schottenfeld, D., and Oettgen, H. F. (1976): Randomized trial of Bacillus Calmette-Guerin

(percutaneous administration) as surgical adjuvant immunotherapy for patients with stage-II melanoma. *Ann. NY Acad. Sci.,* 277:187–194.

42. Prehn, R. T. (1972): The immune reaction as a stimulator of tumor growth. *Science,* 176:170–171.
43. Rojas, A. F., Feierstein, J. N., Mickiewicz, E., and Glait, H. (1976): Levamisole in advanced human breast cancer. *Lancet,* 1:211–215.
44. Ruckdeschel, J. C., Codish, S. D., and Stranahan, A. (1972): Postoperative empyema improves survival in lung cancer: Documentation and analysis of a natural experiment. *N. Engl. J. Med.,* 287:1013–1017.
45. Sher, N. A., Chaparas, S. D., Pearson, and Chirigos, M. (1973): Virulence of six strains of Mycobacterium bovis (BCG) in mice. *Infect. Immun.,* 8:736–742.
46. Smith, H. G., Bast, R. C., Jr. Zbar, B., and Rapp, H. J. (1975): Eradication of microscopic lymph node metastastes after infection of living BCG adjacent to the primary tumor. *J. Natl. Cancer Inst.,* 55:1345–1352.
47. Sokal, J. E., Aungst, C. W., and Snyderman, M. (1974): Delay in progression of malignant lymphoma after BCG vaccination. *N. Engl. J. Med.,* 291:1226–1230.
48. Vogler, W. R., and Chan, Y-K. (1974): Prolongation remission in myeloblastic leukemia by Tice-strain Bacillus Calmette-Guerin. *Lancet,* 2:128–131.
49. Yron, I., Weiss, D. W., Robinson, E., Cohen, D., Adelberg, M. G., Mekory, T., and Haber, M. (1973): Immunotherapeutic studies in mice with the methanol extraction residue (MER) fraction of BCG: Solid tumors. *Natl. Cancer Inst. Monogr.,* 39:33–54.
50. Zbar, B., Bernstein, I. D., and Rapp, H. J. (1971): Suppression of tumor growth at site of infection with living Bacillus Calmette Guerin. *J. Natl. Cancer Inst.,* 46: 831–839.

Question and Answer Session

Dr. Rosenberg: I might add a clarifying point here. Most of the authors use a staging system in which patients that are Stage I are patients with local disease only, not yet disseminated to regional lymph nodes; patients with Stage II disease are patients with disease to draining lymph nodes; and patients with Stage III disease are patients with disseminated disease.

This, however, is not the convention used at the M. D. Anderson Hospital by Dr. Hersh. In Dr. Hersh's classification Stage III patients are those with positive lymph nodes; and Stage IV patients are those with disseminated disease. Stage IVA patients have disseminated disease but could be made disease-free by surgical extirpation.

One other point of clarification. As I understand the result of your first study, the group that did better with BCG treatment—represented by 20 patients who received the high dose of the BCG compared to the historical controls—did better statistically both in terms of disease-free interval and survival. Is that correct? What was the disease-free interval, and what was the survival of patients who received the high dose of BCG?

Dr. Hersh: The control disease-free interval was nine months. For the 20 patients on BCG, it was 14 months. The control median survival was 19 months and the therapeutic survival median was 27 months.

Question: What toxicity have you seen due to BCG at high doses?

Dr. Hersh: The majority of our patients do experience what I would consider evidence of systemic release of BCG organisms at the time of scarification or within the first 24 hr. That is, most of the patients have some fever, some flu-like syndrome, including backache, muscle aches, etc.

We feel that this is quite important and that the complete lack of systemic symptoms indicates that the organisms are probably staying either at the regional site or certainly are not disseminating beyond the regional lymph nodes.

We do not avoid the regional drainage areas; in fact, as time has gone along, we tended to also place the BCG around the primary site. The frequency was weekly for three months, or 12 doses approximately, and then every other week. The other side-effects which are characteristic are flaring of old lesions.

Immunotherapy of Cancer: Present Status of
Trials in Man, edited by W. D. Terry and D. Windhorst.
Raven Press, New York © 1978.

Adjuvant Immunotherapy of Malignant Melanoma: Preliminary Results of a Randomized Trial in Patients with Lymph Node Metastases

Donald L. Morton, E. Carmack Holmes, Frederick R. Eilber,
Frank C. Sparks, and Kenneth P. Ramming

*Division of Oncology, Department of Surgery, University of California Medical School,
Los Angeles, California 90024; and Surgical Service, Veterans Administration Hospital,
Sepulveda, California 91343*

Malignant melanoma is curable by operation alone in a high proportion of patients with primary stage I disease. In contrast, those with metastases to regional lymph nodes have a high rate of treatment failure despite lymphadenectomy. Treatment failure in these patients is seldom the result of uncontrolled primary or regional disease but usually of distant metastases. Since approximately 70% of these metastases become apparent within 2 years after the initial surgical treatment, it is very probable that clinically silent metastases were present in these patients at the time of their initial evaluation and operation. Therefore, in order to improve overall results, additional adjuvant therapy with systemic antitumor activity must be initiated to overcome these distant subclinical metastases. The selection of anticancer therapy for otherwise healthy patients with suspected subclinical disease presents several therapeutic and ethical problems not encountered in the treatment of known malignancy. In such circumstances, the ideal adjuvant should be relatively nontoxic, have proven results from prior investigation in animal tumor systems, and have known effectiveness in the treatment of clinically evident disease in man.

IMMUNOTHERAPY WITH BCG

Immunotherapy with Bacillus Calmette-Guérin (BCG) fulfills many of these criteria. There are many reports summarizing the effectiveness of BCG in animal tumor systems (1,2). In addition, BCG has been shown to have significant activity in patients with disseminated intracutaneous metastatic disease. We found that 90% of intracutaneous metastases from melanoma regressed when directly injected with BCG in patients who were immunologically competent, as judged by their ability to be sensitized to dinitrochlorobenzene (DNCB), or to respond to tuberculin vaccine following BCG therapy. In addition, a systemic effect was suggested when melanoma nodules at sites distant from the BCG inoculation also regressed in 15 to 20% of these immunologically competent patients. Many of these patients have remained free of disease for periods of up to 8 years (4,5). Subsequently, the early results of a simultaneously controlled but nonrandomized trial of BCG immunotherapy for patients with melanoma metastatic to regional nodes treated by surgical lymphadenectomy alone or surgery plus BCG immunotherapy suggested that this adjuvant immunotherapy was effective in lowering recurrence rates and prolonging survival (3). During this preliminary trial, we were able to evolve a technique for immunotherapy with BCG that produced minimal toxicity. Thus, we were encouraged enough to initiate a prospectively randomized trial of adjuvant immunotherapy in patients with regional lymph node metastases from melanoma.

Patients

Ninety-four patients have been entered into the study since August, 1974. All patients were seen and treated by the Division of Surgical Oncology at UCLA. Patients were evaluated by history and physical examination, chest X-ray, complete blood cell count (CBC), SMA-12 (selected blood chemistries), liver, brain, and bone scans to assess the stage or extent of disease as accurately as possible prior to therapy. All patients underwent excision of their primary melanoma site with at least a 5-cm margin in all locations except the face, along with simultaneous regional lymphadenectomy. All patients in this study had histologically proven evidence of metastasis to regional nodes and therefore were categorized as stage II malignant melanoma.

TABLE 1. *Stratification factors for randomizing stage II melanoma patients*

Factor	Control		BCG		Tumor cell + BCG	
Number	28		32		29	
Age (mean years)	42		44		40	
Sex—Male	21		23		23	
Female	7		9		6	
Site distribution						
Head & neck	21%	(6)	16%	(5)	10%	(3)
Extremity	25%	(7)	22%	(7)	20%	(6)
Trunk	43%	(12)	50%	(16)	53%	(16)
Unknown	11%	(3)	12%	(4)	17%	(4)
Lymph node status						
Clinically positive	22		21		22	
Clinically negative	6		11		7	

Patients entered through 5–1–76, data current to 10–22–76. Number of patients at each site category are given in parentheses. Percentages were derived from number of patients with disease at a given site into the total number of patients in each group.

Patients were stratified on the basis of age, sex, site of primary melanoma, and whether the nodes were thought to be involved with metastatic melanoma on clinical examination. The results of the randomization according to these stratification factors are given in Table 1.

Treatment

Systemic immunotherapy was begun 2 to 6 weeks following the operative procedure and involved the following: (a) BCG alone (Tice strain, Chicago Research Laboratories) was given at a dosage of 1 to 2×10^8 organisms by the tine technique (2 tine punctures adjacent to each axilla and groin, and circumferentially around the primary site) at weekly intervals for 12 weeks and then biweekly thereafter; (b) BCG plus allogeneic melanoma cells were given. BCG was given as described above followed by 1×10^8 allogeneic tissue-cultured melanoma cells injected intradermally into the same area at each time interval. The tumor cell vaccine was admixed with 1×10^6 organisms of Glaxo BCG during the first two inoculations, but not thereafter; and (c) control patients received no additional therapy following the initial surgical procedure. Patients were followed at monthly intervals with physical examination, CBC, SMA, and chest X-rays. None was lost to follow-up. Patients who developed recurrence continued their particular adjuvant therapy in addition to chemotherapy with dimethyltriazeno imidazole carboxamide (DTIC) combined with 1-3-bis-(2-chloroethyl)-1-nitrosourea (BCNU) or 1-(2-Chloroethyl)-3-cyclohexyl-1-nitrosourea (CCNU).

Statistical Analysis

Recurrence and survival rates were analyzed by the actuarial life table method in order to include all patients treated to date. The vertical axis on these graphs represents the proportion of patients with recurrence or alive at each point in time indicated by the horizontal axis.

RESULTS

The overall results are given in Table 2. Of the 94 patients originally entered into this study, 89 were evaluable. The remaining five patients were dropped from the study because of failure to adhere to the treatment schedule (two patients), refusal to continue in the control group (two patients), or recurrence after 1 week (one patient). Of these five, there were three recurrences, one in each treatment group.

The follow-up period of the 89 evaluable patients extends from 6 to 36 months. When the control patients are compared as a group with those receiving adjuvant immunotherapy, it can be seen that the proportion of patients in the control group who had recurrent disease is higher (50%) than in

TABLE 2. *Preliminary results of randomized trial for stage II melanoma patients*

Treatment group	Total # patients entered	Number recurred	Number expired
Control	28	14 (50%)	10 (36%)
BCG	32	13 (41%)	6 (19%)
BCG + vaccine	29	10 (34%)	7 (24%)
Combined treatment groups	61	23 (38%)	13 (21%)

Patients entered through 5–1–76, data current to 10–22–76.

either of the BCG-alone or BCG-plus-tumor-cell-vaccine group (41% and 34%, respectively). Similarly, the proportion of patients who died in the control group (36%) is higher than that in either the BCG-alone group (19%) or BCG-plus-tumor-cell-vaccine group (24%). These differences are not statistically significant at the present time, however.

When the interval from initial treatment to recurrence was plotted by the life table analysis method, those patients treated by adjuvant immunotherapy had a lower incidence of recurrence than patients treated by operation alone at all points in time. Similarly, when the survival rates of these same patients were plotted, an improvement was observed in patients who received immunotherapy (Fig. 1). However, because of the small number of patients

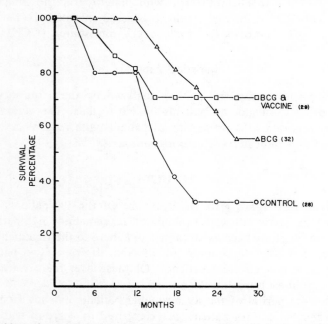

FIG. 1. Life table analysis of survival for stage II melanoma patients with involved nodes. Vertical axis represents proportion of patients who survived at each point in time. Number of patients in each treatment group is shown in parenthesis. □, BCG & vaccine (29); △, BCG (32); and ○, control (28).

available for analysis in each group, statistical analysis of the difference between the immunotherapy and nonimmunotherapy groups is not significant at the 0.05 level. Therefore, a definitive conclusion drawn from these data must await a longer follow-up period and the admission of additional patients to the study.

Side Effects of Treatment

The side effects from BCG administered by this method have been minimal and are consistent with those previously reported (6). No patient developed systemic BCG infection and/or granulomatous hepatitis secondary to BCG administration that required discontinuation of therapy. For the most part, side effects consisted of transient malaise and low-grade fever occurring on the day of immunization and local reactions at the site of BCG administration. Such complications have responded to decreased dosages of BCG.

Patients receiving BCG and melanoma cell vaccine did develop additional complications related to the vaccine itself. Seven patients contracted hepatitis B infection, presumably from the human serum in which the melanoma cells were grown. All of these patients subsequently recovered completely from the hepatitis, as evidenced by normal liver function tests and the disappearance of hepatitis B antigen from their sera.

DISCUSSION

The results from this study do not demonstrate conclusively that adjuvant immunotherapy is or is not of benefit to patients who have melanoma metastatic to regional nodes. The numbers of patients admitted to the study are too few and the period of observation too short. However, it is encouraging to note that at every point in time patients receiving adjuvant therapy appear to have fewer recurrences and longer survival than those in the control group. These results are similar to our earlier observations from the simultaneously controlled but nonprospectively randomized trial. Although these results are not statistically significant at this time, they do suggest a trend that, if it continues, should become statistically significant as larger numbers of patients are admitted to the trial.

Nevertheless, it is also clear that adjuvant immunotherapy is not the ultimate form of adjunctive treatment for patients with malignant melanoma. Recurrences continue to occur in the adjuvant immunotherapy-treated patients, despite prolonged therapy. We expect 35 to 45% of these patients to develop recurrence despite adjuvant immunotherapy by 2 years following lymphadenectomy. This prediction is based on examination of the proportion of patients free of disease at various time intervals, as predicted by life table analysis shown in Fig. 2. Thus, even if this trial does prove to be significant, it is clear that better forms of adjuvant therapy must be developed. We were

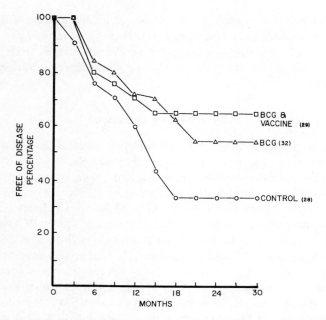

FIG. 2. Life table analysis of recurrence rate in patients with stage II melanoma with involved nodes. Vertical axis represents proportion of patients who had no evidence of recurring disease at each point in time. Number of patients in each treatment group is shown in parenthesis. ☐, BCG & vaccine (29); △, BCG (32); ○, control (28).

hopeful that the addition of specific immunization with a tumor cell vaccine would increase the specific immune response to melanoma-associated antigens over that obtained by nonspecific immunotherapy with BCG alone. At the present time, although the data suggest that immunization with the combination of BCG and tumor cell vaccine might be slightly better than BCG alone, the improvement is minimal at best. Therefore, even though adjuvant immunotherapy may be a first step in the improved treatment of malignant melanoma, it is clear that more effective adjuvant programs must be developed.

SUMMARY

This study evaluated the effect of adjuvant immunotherapy with BCG alone or combined with melanoma cell vaccine on the recurrence and survival rates of patients with melanoma metastatic to the regional lymph nodes who were treated by lymphadenectomy. Patients were prospectively randomized and stratified on the basis of age, sex, site of primary, and clinical estimate of the regional nodes. During the past 3 years, 94 patients were entered into this trial and, to date, patients receiving adjuvant immunotherapy have a slightly lower incidence of disease recurrence or death than those in the control group. However, these differences do not appear to be significant enough to advocate routine adjuvant immunotherapy in patients with melanoma metastatic to regional nodes. Therefore, this study will be continued in its present form.

ACKNOWLEDGMENTS

This study was supported by National Institutes of Health grants CA-12582 and CB-64076-TQ awarded by NIH (Department of Health, Education and Welfare), and Medical Research Services, Veterans Administration, Sepulveda, California 91343.

Computing assistance was obtained from the Health Sciences Computing Facility, UCLA, supported by NIH special research resources grant RR-3. Life table analysis was done by computer program, BMD11S, Health Sciences Computing Facility (revised 1–21–74), and two-way contingency tables were done by computer program BMDPIF, Health Sciences Computing Facility, UCLA (revised 1–3–75).

REFERENCES

1. Bast, R. C., Zbar, B., Borsos, T., and Rapp, H. J. (1974): BCG and cancer (first of two parts). *N. Engl. J. Med.*, 290:1413–1419.
2. Bast, R. C., Zbar, B., Borsos, T., and Rapp, H. J. (1974): BCG and cancer (second of two parts). *N. Engl. J. Med.*, 290:1458–1469.
3. Eilber, F. R., Morton, D. L., Holmes, E. C., Sparks, F. C., and Ramming, K. P. (1976): Adjuvant immunotherapy with BCG in treatment of regional lymph node metastases from malignant melanoma. *N. Engl. J. Med.*, 294:237–240.
4. Morton, D. L., Eilber, F. R., Holmes, E. C., Hunt, J. S., Ketcham, A. S., Silverstein, M. J., and Sparks, F. C. (1974): BCG immunotherapy of malignant melanoma: Summary of a seven-year experience. *Ann. Surg.*, 180:635–643.
5. Morton, D. L., Eilber, F. R., Malmgren, R. A., and Wood, W. C. (1970): Immunological factors which influence response to immunotherapy in malignant melanoma. *Surgery*, 68:158–164.
6. Sparks, F. C., Silverstein, M. J., Hunt, J. S., Haskell, C. M., Pilch, Y. H., and Morton, D. L. (1973): Complications of BCG immunotherapy in patients with cancer. *N. Engl. J. Med.*, 289:827–830.

Question and Answer Session

Dr. Rosenberg: I have two questions for clarification. In the historical control study that you updated for us, was there a statistically significant difference between immunotherapy and no immunotherapy?

In the randomized study, were the results for each of the two immunotherapy groups statistically significantly different from those of the control group?

Dr. Morton: If one combines the two immunotherapy arms, then there is a difference. I think there are so many prognostic factors, numbers of nodes, age, site, sex, and so many things involved here. I think when we are talking about this small number of patients, we have to be cautious at this time. Actually, looking at all the data collectively from every point in analysis, the difference is—for every way we looked at it—a p value between 0.059 and 0.09.

Immunotherapy of Cancer: Present Status of Trials in Man, edited by W. D. Terry and D. Windhorst. Raven Press, New York © 1978.

Controlled Study for Prolonged Chemotherapy, Immunotherapy, and Chemotherapy Plus Immunotherapy as an Adjuvant to Surgery in Stage I-II Malignant Melanoma: Preliminary Report[1]

G. Beretta

National Cancer Institute, 20133 Milan, Italy

The 5-year survival rate of patients with cutaneous malignant melanoma is influenced by the presence of metastatic regional nodes (N+) at the time of radical surgery. In fact, although patients with negative regional lymph nodes (N−) have an overall satisfactory prognosis when properly treated with surgery (5-year survival rate about 70%), the N+ patients show a 5-year survival of about 15% (2,11). An exception to this difference in survival rate between N− and N+ patients is malignant melanoma arising in the trunk, which is reported to bear a poor prognosis (15 to 20% 5-year survival) irrespective of the involvement of regional nodes especially when the histopathology shows a Clark's grade from 3 to 5 (7). The treatment failures after surgical procedure may present as locoregional recurrences, but very often are due to distant metastases. Since about 80% of relapses became evident at clinical observation within 2 years, it can be assumed that microscopic foci of metastatic disease are present at the time of surgical operation.

From these data it appears reasonable to approach the high-risk patients with different modalities of treatment.

Several reports summarize the rational for treatment and the actual results obtained from immunotherapeutic procedures in both animal and human neoplasms (1,5,9,10). Gutterman et al. (6) firstly and then also Eilber et al. (4) reported a significant decrease in the relapse rate in patients treated after radical surgery with long-term Bacillus Calmette-Guérin (BCG) (either with scarification or multipuncture methods), when retrospectively compared to a similar group of patients not submitted to adjuvant immunotherapy. Systemic chemotherapy as an adjuvant to surgery in experimental models produces an extension of the relapse-free period and an increased survival. Melanoma studies in humans are in progress. A preliminary report from a Central Oncology Group-controlled study failed to show any difference be-

---

[1] International Group for the Clinical Study of Melanoma, report was presented by G. Beretta. See Appendix for list of participating members.

tween surgery alone and surgery + dimethyltriazeno imidazole carboxamide (DTIC)-treated patients (8).

Since the major criticism to reported favorable results concerns the comparison between treated patients and historical controls, it is worth testing, in a large controlled series of patients, the potential usefulness of systemic chemo- and/or immunotherapy as adjuvant treatment after radical surgery.

The International Group for the Clinical Study of Melanoma planned the present controlled study in 1973 with the aim of evaluating the effect of long-term adjuvant therapy on the disease-free period in patients with radical surgery for primary or recurrent melanoma of the skin with regional node metastases (N+), as well as for primary melanoma of the trunk without regional metastases (N−) but with locally invasive tumor classified as Clark's grade 3 to 5 (7).

MATERIAL AND METHODS

Patient Admission

After radical surgery of primary melanoma and/or radical regional lymph node dissection (7), all patients with primary melanoma of the skin located in the head and neck areas, one of the four extremities, the trunk with unilateral histologically positive regional adenopathies (N+), or the trunk with histologically negative lymph nodes (N−) were eligible for the trial provided that the histologic classification in Clark's grades was from 3 to 5.

Only patients geographically accessible and providing an informed consent were accepted into the trial. Patients presenting any one of the following conditions were also excluded—previous chemotherapy or immunotherapy, fixation of lymph nodes, in transit metastases, younger than 15 or older than 75 years, concomitant neoplasia, major allergic disease, or symptomatic systemic diseases, such as cardiovascular, renal, pulmonary, or hepatic diseases (that is, patients at high-risk for surgical procedure and prolonged follow-up).

Patients were divided into two different groups: (a) untreated cases, including patients who had excisional biopsy within 6 weeks, and (b) previously treated cases, submitted to excision only of the primary melanoma in which regional node metastases were the first recurrence of the disease with or without local recurrences.

All slides of primary melanoma and of regional dissected nodes were routinely reviewed by the panel of pathologists of the group. The Clark's grade of primary melanoma (3) and the number of examined and metastatic lymph nodes had to be specified. Location of metastatic growth (intra- or extracapsular) also had to be specified.

Mechanics of Study

After surgery patients were stratified according to sex, site, and nodal involvement (head and neck, limbs N+, trunk N−, trunk N+). Then they

TABLE 1. Controlled study in operable
malignant melanoma

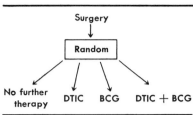

were randomized to treatments (Table 1): (a) no further therapy (control group), (b) DTIC (DIC, NSC-45388), intravenously, (c) BCG lyophilized Pasteur, percutaneously by heaf gun method, and (d) DTIC + BCG. The dose schedules and their modification according to myelosuppression or to different types of BCG reaction are reported in Tables 2 and 3. Blood counts were performed usually on day 1 of the course. Adjuvant treatment had to be started 10 to 30 days after radical surgery. Treatment was continued for 2 years or until relapse was documented.

TABLE 2. Medical treatment started 10 to 30 days from surgery

DTIC	200 mg/m² i.v. for 5 consecutive days; cycles to be repeated every 4 weeks for 24 months
BCG[a]	75 mg in 0.5-ml saline (percutaneous by heaf gun—3 shoots at 2 mm deep), weekly on 1 site of proximal region of limbs, in rotation clockwise (excluding the limb in which lymphadenectomy was performed)
DTIC + BCG	Same doses. BCG started on day 5 of the first cycle of DTIC.

[a] Lyophilized vaccine, Pasteur Institute, each vial of 37.5 mg containing 1.6 ± 0.8 × 10⁸ living units of BCG.

TABLE 3. Dose modification of adjuvant therapy

DTIC toxicity was categorized according to the drop in leukocytes (WBC) and/or platelets (PLT) count as follows:

Grade	WBC	PLT	Next dose
0	>4,000	>100,000	100%
1	3,999–2,500	99,000–75,000	50%
2	<2,500	< 75,000	No drug, wait until marrow recovering recovers

BCG reaction was red after 1 week:

Grading of reaction			Next dose	Heaf gun	Timing
0	1+	Negative	75 mg(0.5-ml saline)	4 shoots	Weekly
2+	3+	Positive	75 mg(0.5-ml saline)	4 shoots	Every 4 weeks
4+		Strongly positive	37.5 mg(0.25-ml saline)	2 shoots	Every 4 weeks

Follow-up

A physical examination and blood count were repeated every course, routine laboratory tests and chest radiogram were performed every 2 months, and liver and brain scans or other special examinations were repeated whenever indicated by the patient's symptoms or after the end of the treatment.

The endpoint of study was considered the first evidence of treatment failure, such as the appearance of tumor in local, regional, or distant sites, confirmed by biopsy or needle aspiration cytology whenever possible or by unequivocal clinical, radiologic or radioisotopic methods.

From June, 1974, 208 patients were entered into the trial from 16 participating institutions (7). After 2 years, 196 patients were adequately treated according to the protocol criteria. The main characteristics of evalu-

TABLE 4. *Main characteristics of evaluable patients (untreated/previously treated)*

	Total	Surgery alone	DTIC	BCG	DTIC + BCG
Evaluable	100/96	30/28	17/19	30/30	23/19
Sex					
M	72/50	22/16	11/9	23/15	16/10
F	28/46	8/12	6/10	7/15	7/9
Median age					
M	48/43				
F	40/49				
Site					
Limbs	26/42	7/10	10/10	3/15	6/7
Trunk N+	26/42	10/15	1/8	8/12	7/7
Trunk N−	33/2	8/1	5/0	14/1	6/0
Head + neck	15/10	5/2	1/1	5/2	4/5

able patients are reported in Table 4. Patient distribution among the four treatment groups shows no significant difference at x^2 analysis.

RESULTS

Relapses were separately considered in the two main groups of previously treated and untreated patients.

Observed relapses and first sites of relapses are reported in Table 5. From this table it appears that the number of relapses is lower in all treatment groups than in the control group treated only by surgery. The analysis of relapses for each treatment according to palpable and nonpalpable regional nodes shows no significant variations; however, currently a certain number of data on the clinical assessment of lymph nodes is not available.

TOXICITY

Treatments were well tolerated. The main symptoms due to DTIC administration were nausea and vomiting, usually presenting on day 1 of the

TABLE 5. Observed sites of first relapse in evaluable patients

	Previously untreated				Previously treated			
	Surgery	DTIC	BCG	DTIC + BCG	Surgery	DTIC	BCG	DTIC + BCG
Local	5	—	—	—	5	1	3	1
Nodes + skin	3	—	1	1	2	1	2	1
Viscera	1	—	1	—	—	—	2	—
Brain	—	4	1	—	2	1	2	—
More sites	7	1	4	4	5	6	3	5
Total with relapse[a]	16/30 (6/23)	5/17 (5/10)	6/30 (2/17)	5/23 (3/14)	14/28 (11/22)	9/19 (8/15)	12/30 (8/22)	7/19 (3/15)

[a] Patients relapsing within the first 6 months in parentheses.

course in almost all patients and with only few exceptions well controlled by phenothiazines. Myelosuppression was mild and always reversible; its incidence was less than 20% and did not significantly modify the planned treatment. BCG administration also did not provide important side effects, and only isolated hyperthermic episodes are reported. No signs of hepatic disease or spread of tubercular infection was observed in our case material.

Local reactions even more intense were kept under good local control with spontaneous regression; no deep invasion of local tissues was recorded. The association of both DTIC and BCG did not show any different toxicity than single-agent treatments until now in our case material.

COMMENT

It is too early to give useful information following the present very preliminary evaluation.

Our analysis from present data shows a slight trend in favor of immunotherapy-treated patients.

The estimated incidence of relapse actually appears to be less frequent after BCG ± DTIC in previously untreated patients and after DTIC + BCG in previously treated patients. Whether any treatment can really protect against recurrence in estimated high-risk patients is actually unknown, since only a larger number of patients would provide sufficient data for a correct statistical evaluation.

We estimate that a preliminary report on adequate case material (at least 300 evaluable patients) will become available by the end of 1977.

SUMMARY

During 2 years 208 patients with primary melanoma of the skin stage II (N+) and stage I of the trunk (Clark's level 3,4,5 only), after stratification according to previous or actual surgical treatment, sex, and site of primary melanoma, were randomized to: (a) no further therapy, (b) DTIC, 200 mg/m^2 daily × 5 every 4 weeks, (c) Pasteur BCG by heaf gun, 75 mg/ weekly (or every 4 weeks in case of positive reaction), and (d) DTIC + BCG on the same dose schedule. Very preliminary data from actuarial analysis of the recurrence rate in 196 evaluable patients seem to show a slightly longer free interval in patients receiving adequate treatment with either BCG or DTIC + BCG in previously untreated cases and with DTIC + BCG in previously treated cases, when compared with patients not submitted to adjuvant therapy. With the exception of frequent nausea and vomiting and a low number of mild myelosuppressions in DTIC-treated patients, no important side effects were observed.

APPENDIX

Dr. J. Adamus, Oncological Institute, Gliwice (Poland)

Dr. C. Aubert, Institut Paoli Calmettes, Marseille (France)

Dr. G. Beretta, Instituto Nazionale Tumori, Milan (Italy)

Dr. G. Bonadonna, Instituto Nazionale Tumori, Milan (Italy)

Dr. A. Cochran, University of Glasgow—Western Infirmary, Glasgow (United Kingdom)

Dr. J. De Marsillac, Institut Nacional de Cancer, Rio de Janeiro (Brazil)

Dr. J. Durand, Fondation Curie, Paris (France)

Dr. R. L. Ikonopisov, Oncological Research Institute, Sofia (Bulgaria)

Dr. B. Kiss, State Institute of Oncology, Budapest (Hungary)

Dr. A. Kulakowski, Oncological Institute, Cracow (Poland)

Dr. F. Lejeune, Institut Jules Bordet, Brussels (Belgium)

Dr. Z. Mechl, Oncological Institute, Brno (Czechoslovakia)

Dr. G. W. Milton, University of Sydney, Dept. of Surgery, Sydney (Australia)

Dr. H. H. Peter, Abteilung fur Klinische Immunologie-Medizinische Hochschule, Hannover (Federal Republik of Germany)

Dr. J. Priario, Hospital de Clinicas "M. Quintela," Montevideo (Uruguay)

Dr. P. Rumke, Het Nederlands Kankerinstituut, Amsterdam, (The Netherlands)

Dr. R. Tomin, Institute of Oncology, Beograd (Yugoslavia)

Dr. U. Veronesi, Instituto Tumori, Milan (Italy)

REFERENCES

1. Bast, R. C., Zbar, B., Borsos, T., and Rapp, H. J. (1974): BCG and cancer. *N. Engl. J. Med.*, 290:1413–1419, 1458–1468.
2. Cascinelli, N., Balzarini, G. P., Fontana, V., Morabito, A., and Orefice, S. (1976): Long term results of surgical treatment of melanoma of the limbs. *Tumori*, 62:233–242.
3. Clark, W. H., Jr. (1967): A classification of malignant melanoma in man correlated with histogenesis and biological behavior. In: *Advances in Biology of the Skin, Vol. 8: The Pigmentary System*, edited by W. Montagna and F. Hu, pp. 621–647. Pergamon Press, Elmsford, New York.
4. Eilber, F. R., Morton, D. L., Holmes, E. C., Sparks, F. C., and Ramming, K. P. (1976): Adjuvant immunotherapy with BCG in the treatment of regional lymph node metastases from malignant melanoma. *N. Engl. J. Med.*, 294:237–240.
5. Gutterman, J. U., Mavligit, G. M., Reed, R. C., and Hersh, E. M. (1974): Immunotherapy of human cancer. *Semin. Oncol.*, 1:409–424.
6. Gutterman, J., McBride, C., Freireich, E. J., Mavligit, G., Frei, E., III, and Hersh, E. M. (1973): Active immunotherapy with BCG for recurrent malignant melanoma. *Lancet*, 1:1208–1212.
7. International Group for the Clinical Study of Melanoma (1974): *Trial N° 6: Controlled Study for Prolonged Chemotherapy, Immunotherapy, and Chemotherapy plus Immunotherapy as an Adjuvant to Surgery.*
8. Johnson, R. O., Metter, G., Wilson, W., Hill, G., Krementz, E. (1976): Phase I evaluation of DTIC (NSC 45388) and other studies in malignant melanoma in the Central Oncology Group. *Cancer Treat. Rep.*, 60:183–187.

9. Morton, D. L. (1974): Cancer immunotherapy: An overview. *Semin. Oncol.*, 1:297–310.
10. Nathanson, L. (1974): Use of BCG in the treatment of human neoplasms: A review. *Semin. Oncol.*, 1:337–350.
11. Veronesi, U., Cascinelli, N., and Preda, F. (1971): Prognosis of malignant melanoma according to regional metastases. *Am. J. Roentgenol.*, 111:301–309.

Immunotherapy of Cancer: Present Status of
Trials in Man, edited by W. D. Terry and D. Windhorst.
Raven Press, New York © 1978.

A Randomized Double-Blind Trial of Adjuvant Therapy with Levamisole Versus Placebo in Patients with Malignant Melanoma

***Lynn E. Spitler, **Richard W. Sagebiel, ***Richard G. Glogau,
***Peter P. Wong, *Thomas M. Malm, *Randolph H. Chase,
and *Raymond L. Gonzalez

*Laboratory of Cellular Immunology and **Department of Pathology, Children's Hospital
of San Francisco, San Francisco, California 94118; and ***Department of Medicine,
University of California, San Francisco, California 94143

Levamisole, an anthelmintic, has been reported to increase cellular immune reactivity in animals (1) and man (2). Conflicting results have been reported concerning the efficacy of levamisole in the various animal tumors studied. Administration of levamisole to tumor-bearing animals resulted in inhibition of tumor growth (3), prolonged disease remission and increased survival (4), or decreased incidence of metastases (5,6). In other animal tumors, no effect was observed (5).

In our own studies of Fortner's melanotic melanoma of golden Syrian hamsters, we found that levamisole did not affect growth of the primary tumor. It did, however, impair growth of recurrent melanomas and led to cure in one-third of the animals studied, whereas this was never observed in control animals. The drug further caused a 50% reduction in the incidence of pulmonary metastases in the treated animals.

These considerations led us to conduct a randomized trial of levamisole versus placebo in patients with malignant melanoma.

MATERIALS AND METHODS

Patients

Patients included in the study are those with primary or recurrent malignant melanoma with poor prognosis. These include patients with primary malignant melanoma, levels III, IV, and V (7), with or without regional lymph node dissection. It also includes patients with regional or remote lymph node or skin recurrence of melanoma more than 90 days after excision of the primary tumor. It further includes patients with no known primary and those with mucosal or subungual lesions. The patients are divided into six groups as shown in Table 1.

TABLE 1. *Categories of patients in a randomized double-blind trial of levamisole versus placebo in malignant melanoma*

1. Primary melanoma, levels III, IV, V; no node dissection
2. Primary melanoma, levels III, IV, V; negative node dissection
3. Primary melanoma, levels III, IV, V; positive node dissection
4. Recurrent melanoma: local, in transit, regional lymph nodes (more than 90 days from primary)
5. Recurrent melanoma: remote lymph nodes or skin, completely excised
6. Mucous membrane melanoma

Patients must be 18 years of age or older. There is no upper age limit. All patients must undergo surgical excision of all known tumor and be free of tumor at the initiation of the study as determined by physical examination, chest X-ray, and liver, brain, bone, and/or gallium scans as indicated. Patients who have received prior chemotherapy or radiation therapy are not eligible. Patients receiving immunosuppressive agents such as steroids are not eligible. Patients with level II melanoma or melanoma of the eye are excluded.

Randomization and Therapy

Patients entering the study are assigned to one of the six patient groups listed in Table I on the basis of their clinical and pathologic status. They are then randomized within the group to receive levamisole or placebo. No further subrandomization is done. Each patient receives a coded vial containing either levamisole or placebo tablets that are identical in appearance. Neither the patient, the doctors, nor the technicians involved in the study know which agent the patient is receiving. Only the statistician holds the code. The patients take one tablet for 3 days in a row every 2 weeks. Each levamisole tablet contains 150 mg of the drug. They continue to take the pills for 2 years if there is no recurrence. If there is a recurrence, they continue taking the pills until they have been tumor-free for 2 years or until death. Patients are examined every 3 months, or more often if warranted.

Statistical Analysis

Data were analyzed by a modification (8) of the life table method of Cutler and Ederer (9). This is very similar to the method described by Kaplan and Meier (10). Chi square analysis was also used.

RESULTS

Patient Distribution

The age distribution of subjects in the levamisole and treatment groups was similar (Table 2). There was maldistribution between the two groups with

TABLE 2. *Age distribution of patients in randomized trial of levamisole versus placebo in patients with malignant melanoma*

Age	Levamisole	Placebo	Totals
Under 20	3		3
20–29	9	8	17
30–39	12	16	28
40–49	18	11	29
50–59	16	10	26
60–69	7	15	22
70	2	5	7
Totals	67	65	132

regard to sex. There were 31 females in the levamisole group versus only 19 females in the placebo group (Table 3). Distribution within the patient groups was similar (Table 4). Distribution according to level is reported only for patient groups 1, 2, and 3, since level was thought to be less relevant to prognosis in patients with late recurrence of tumor (groups 4 and 5) and does not apply to patients with mucosal lesions (group 6). There was maldistribution between the levamisole and placebo groups according to level of the primary tumor in that there were 15 patients with level III tumors in the treatment group and six patients with level III tumors in the placebo group (Table 5). Both female sex and level III tumors are associated with improved prognosis as opposed to male sex or level IV or V tumors. Thus, if anything,

TABLE 3. *Sex distribution of patients in randomized trial of levamisole versus placebo in patients with malignant melanoma*

Sex	Levamisole	Placebo	Totals
Male	36	46	82
Female	31	19	50
Totals	67	65	132

TABLE 4. *Distribution of patients in various groups in randomized trial of levamisole versus placebo in patients with malignant melanoma*

Patient group	Levamisole	Placebo	Totals
1	14	12	26
2	18	14	32
3	12	11	23
4	18	20	38
5	5	5	10
6	—	3	3
Totals	67	65	132

TABLE 5. *Distribution of patients by level of primary in randomized trial of levamisole versus placebo in patients with malignant melanoma*

Level of primary	Levamisole	Placebo	Totals
III	15	6	21
IV	17	17	34
V	7	12	19
Totals	39	35	74

the tendency to favorable outcome was greater in the levamisole than in the placebo group.

First Recurrence

The disease-free probability rate was similar for the levamisole and placebo groups (Fig. 1). There were no first recurrences after 16 months from initiation of the study. Chi square analysis did not reveal any significant differences between the groups.

First Visceral Recurrence

Our preliminary studies in the hamster melanoma model suggested that levamisole might not affect local recurrence but might inhibit metastatic disease. Accordingly, the probability rate of no visceral recurrence was de-

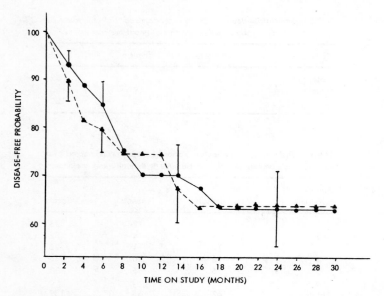

FIG. 1. Disease-free probability rate of patients with malignant melanoma randomized to levamisole or placebo. ——•——, levamisole; ——▲——, placebo.

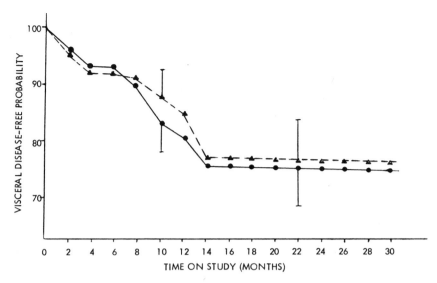

FIG. 2. Probability rate of no visceral recurrence in patients with malignant melanoma randomized to levamisole or placebo. ——●——, levamisole; ——▲——, placebo.

termined and found to be the same in the levamisole and placebo groups (Fig. 2).

Survival

The cumulative survival rate was similar in both groups (Fig. 3), and Chi square analysis did not reveal any significant differences.

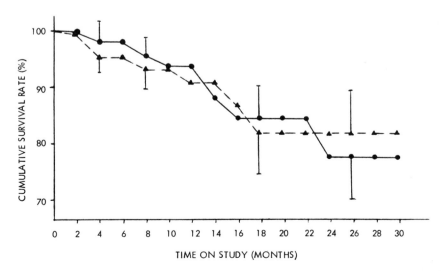

FIG. 3. Cumulative survival rate of patients with malignant melanoma randomized to levamisole or placebo groups. ——●——, levamisole; ——▲——, placebo.

DISCUSSION

We report herein the preliminary results of a randomized trial of levamisole versus placebo in patients with malignant melanoma. The results to date do not reveal any significant difference between the groups.

There are several possible explanations. One is that levamisole, in fact, does not have an effect on the outcome of this disease. Another is that the dose used was too low. In another study in which a similar dose of levamisole was used (11), clinical benefit was suggested only in subjects in low-weight categories who received a higher dose on a per kilogram basis. Another possibility is that it caused induction of enzymes causing its own degradation, and so the effective dose was lower in the patients ingesting the drug on a long-term basis.

This is a preliminary report only, and the numbers of patients followed for a prolonged time is relatively low. It is possible that levamisole may not affect early disease recurrence and early death (these patients may have had a heavy tumor burden at the initiation of therapy). Levamisole may, however, have a beneficial effect on later recurrence of tumor. In those patients, a longer period would have been permitted for its activity.

It is possible that levamisole may have a beneficial effect in one or two, but not all, of the patient groups studied. The numbers of patients within the various groups are not sufficient to permit analysis of results within the groups. Further, multivariate analysis has not been performed and might have revealed an effect not detected by our correct means.

In summary, the results of our randomized trial to date do not reveal any difference between levamisole and placebo in the therapy of patients with primary or recurrent malignant melanoma.

ACKNOWLEDGMENT

Supported by a gift from Janssen Pharmaceutica and U.S. Public Health Service grant CA-13671.

REFERENCES

1. Renoux, G., and Renoux, M. (1971): Immunostimulant effect of an imidothiazole in the immunization of mice infected with Brucella abortus. C. R. Acad. Sci. [D] (Paris), 272:349–354.
2. Tripodi, D., Parks, L. C., and Brugmans, J. (1973): Drug-induced restoration of cutaneous delayed hypersensitivity in anergic patients with cancer. N. Engl. J. Med., 289:354–357.
3. Renoux, G., and Renoux, M. (1972): Levamisole inhibits and cures a solid malignant tumour and its pulmonary metastases in mice. Nature [New Biol.,] 240: 217–218.
4. Chirigos, M. A., Pearson, J. W., and Pryor, J. (1973): Augmentation of chemotherapeutically induced remission of a murine leukemia by a chemical immunoadjuvant. Cancer Res., 33:2615–2618.
5. Potter, C. W., Carr, I., Jennings, R., Rees, R. C., McGinty, F., and Richardson, V. M. (1974): Levamisole inactive in treatment of four animal tumours. Nature, 249:567–569.

6. Sadowski, M. J., and Rapp, F. (1975): Inhibition by levamisole of metastases by cells transformed by herpes simplex virus type I (38776). *Proc. Soc. Exp. Biol. Med.,* 149:219–222.
7. Clark, W. H., Jr., From, L., Bernardino, E. A., and Mihm, M. C. (1969): The histogenesis and biologic behavior of primary human malignant melanomas of the skin. *Cancer Res.,* 29:705–727.
8. Rosenblatt, L. S., Hetherington, N. H., Goldman, M., and Bustad, L. K. (1971): Evaluation of tumor incidence following exposure to internal emitters by application of the logistic dose response surface. (Short Communication). *Health Phys.,* 21:869.
9. Cutler, S. J., and Ederer, F. (1958): Maximum utilization of the life table method in analyzing survival. *J. Chronic Dis.,* 8:699–712.
10. Kaplan, E. L., and Meier, P. (1958): Nonparametric estimation from incomplete observations. *J. Am. Statis. Assoc.,* 53:457–481.
11. Amery, W. (1975): Levamisole. (Letter to the Editor). *Lancet,* 1:389.

DISCUSSION: ADJUVANT THERAPY IN MELANOMA

Dr. Rosenberg: Six reports on the immunotherapy of malignant melanoma as an adjuvant to primary surgical treatment have been presented. Five of these reports have dealt with BCG. The reports of Drs. Cunningham and Pinsky have suggested that BCG immunotherapy is not of value in the adjuvant setting in poor-prognosis patients. Drs. Hersh, Morton, and Beretta have reported statistically significant differences with the use of immunotherapy in this type of patient. In the discussion, we should try to reconcile, as much as possible, the possible reasons for these differences in results.

To serve as a framework for the discussion, we have summarized in Table 1 various aspects of the immunotherapy used in these studies. As you can see, there is quite a difference in the way the BCG was administered in each of these studies.

Dr. Cunningham, you have reported a negative study, but I'd like to ask you a question about its experimental design. You have lumped together, in your presentation, patients having negative nodes (Clark Level III, IV, and V) with patients that have positive lymph nodes. There is no evidence that I am familiar with that the Clark level of invasion is of importance once the nodal status is positive. You have thus grouped patients that have about an 80 percent five-year survival (negative nodes) with patients that have a 20 to 30 percent five-year survival (positive nodes). In the study that you have presented and interpreted as being negative, of the 127 patients in Groups A, B and C, only 34 had positive lymph nodes and these have been divided between two groups. This number of Stage II patients is too small to bear on the question of whether poor-prognosis patients with positive nodes are helped by BCG immunotherapy.

Dr. Cunningham: Our data are very early and we have attempted to separate patients according to prognostic criteria. We did not use Clark's levels to distinguish Group C patients. Whether we will be able to distinguish between BCG or no treatment in the Group C patients I'm not sure at this time, but the study is a fairly large one and may ultimately give that information.

TABLE 1. Summary of immunotherapy methods

Investigator	Dose	Schedule	Application	Strain	Sites
Cunningham	10^8	Weekly × 4, q 2 weeks × 4, q 4 weeks × 6, then q 8 weeks × 5	Tine (2x/Rx)	Tice (Lyophilized)	Regional and then rotating quadrant.
Pinsky	$4–6 × 10^7$	Weekly × 52, q 2 weeks × 24, then q 4 weeks × 12	Tine (2x/Rx)	Tice (Lyophilized)	Extremities excluding the involved extremity.
Hersh	$6 × 10^8$	Weekly × 12, then q 2 weeks for 2 years	Scarification	Tice (Lyophilized)	One site at a time by rotation to the deltoid and thigh regions.
Morton	$2–4 × 10^8$	Weekly × 12, then q 2 weeks for 2 years	Tine (8x/Rx)	Tice (Lyophilized)	Primary site for both axillae and groins.
Beretta	75 mg $2–4 × 10^8$	Weekly × 4–6, then at ½ to 1 dose q 4 weeks for 24 months	Heaf gun (4 shots/Rx)	Pasteur (Lyophilized)	Proximal limbs except the involved limb.

I don't think I have said the BCG therapy is of no value. Rather, a better statement is that at present the tumor-free intervals do not differ.

There are some differences between our study and the others reported here: our frequency of BCG administration is much different than that of other studies; the intensity of our local reactions is greater than that noted by Dr. Morton; and we had an increasing intensity of reactions throughout treatment with BCG, as opposed to Dr. Pinsky's experience.

Dr. Rosenberg: What percent effect of BCG improvement would have been missed with only 34 patients in the positive node group? That is, what kind of difference could exist that you just wouldn't see in this study with 34 patients?

Dr. Cunningham: We have not analyzed the data for the patients in Group C alone.

Dr. Beretta: I would like to ask Dr. Cunningham if the relapses were local, regional, or distant?

Dr. Cunningham: This preliminary analysis did not include an evaluation of sites of recurrence.

Dr. Rosenberg: Dr. Pinsky, in your study of patients with positive lymph nodes you show no difference between groups receiving surgery alone or BCG as an adjuvant. Could you comment on how you reconcile your negative study with the positive studies reported by Drs. Hersh, Morton, and Beretta in patients with positive lymph nodes?

Dr. Pinsky: We do not think we have proven that BCG is of no value in the prevention of recurrence or the improvement of survival in patients with malignant melanoma. Dr. Hersh and Dr. Morton both stressed that the differences they are now seeing between control groups and treated groups are rather small. My conclusion is that we must find better therapy than that evaluated in any of the reports that we have heard today rather than to attempt to confirm or disprove these very modest therapeutic effects, which would require an enormous number of patients. Thus we have chosen not to continue this study and have gone on to other trials.

Dr. Rosenberg: I would like to ask the panel to address the differences between the trials. Clearly if some trials are positive and real, we need to understand why they are positive and why other studies are not getting the same results. Dr. Morton, could you comment on what you think are the important elements in your study that have either not been present in other studies or that you would stress be emphasized by other people who are exploring this area?

Dr. Morton: First, I would emphasize uniform criteria in admission to the study. For example, we won't admit a patient who is more than 10 weeks from the date of the diagnosis of Stage II disease. Patients that have been free of disease for six or eight months are quite a different population.

Based upon our preliminary experience with our simultaneously controlled but not prospectively randomized trial of immunotherapy in Stage II malignant melanoma, I would expect that the maximum improvement in long-term disease-free survival will be in the range of 20 to 25 percent. Although this difference is not as large as we would like, if our present randomized trial confirms this difference, the increased salvage with immunotherapy will be sufficient to justify its routine use as an adjuvant in Stage II melanoma. I would again agree with Dr. Pinsky that a 20 percent improvement is not good enough. We have to do better. But 20 percent is an important difference and can serve as a starting place for future adjuvant trials in melanoma.

Second, I believe it is important to administer the BCG in the area of the primary lesion so that the organisms drain through the same lymphatic paths as the tumor cells from the original primary melanoma.

Third, dosage is important. One has to achieve some systemic infection with BCG, because what you are trying to do is prevent not only local recurrence but systemic recurrence. From what we know from most of the human and animal data, it is important to get the BCG organism close to the tumor cells. It is clear to me, as I look at these data, that the most important differences between the studies reported here are dose of BCG and the location of the immunization sites.

Dr. LoBuglio: The figure 20 percent effect has been used by the speakers. Can you say whether you feel that this modest effect is a delay in recurrence or may be a real change in the recurrence rate?

Dr. Hersh: I think it's really too early to say. The total number of patients needs to be larger.

Dr. Rosenberg: Dr. Morton, in your randomized study, given the current data, with about 20 to 25 patients in each group, there is, as I understood it, no statistically significant difference between patients receiving BCG alone and the control group; is that correct?

Dr. Morton: Interpretation is another problem. At the point where the curves begin to separate, there are statistically significant differences. But the total curves, from the inception to the end, are not significantly different.

Dr. Rosenberg: The total curves in your *nonrandomized* study appear to be quite different and have been reported as different. What are the differences between your previous study and the current one?

Dr. Morton: The data are almost identical, but we are talking about 84 treated and 42 control patients in the non-randomized trial, compared to 28 patients in the control and 28 in the treated group in the current randomized trial. It's a matter of patient numbers and duration of follow-up. The data are remarkably consistent internally. That is, the point that the curves flatten out is within 4 percent as compared to the original trial. The 50 percent survival point in Dr. Hersh's control group is 19 months, and in ours it's 18.5 months.

Dr. Hersh: And in studies published at the turn of the century, it's exactly the same. Charles McBride has compared our data at M. D. Anderson Hospital with the data from England before 1900, and it's just about the same.

Dr. Pinsky: If the median survivals of Dr. Morton's and Dr. Hersh's control groups are the same, then something is wrong. One of the differences that hasn't been discussed yet is that for the most part the surgeons at M. D. Anderson are only operating on patients with recurrent or palpable lymph nodes, whereas Dr. Morton and we at our center are doing lymph node dissections in patients with Clark's Level III or more, whether or not the nodes are palpable. We have fewer patients who have recurrent nodal disease. The patients seen at M. D. Anderson should have a poorer prognosis from the time of lymph node dissection than the patients that Dr. Morton is treating. Despite this, if you compare our current controls and our historical controls with M.D. Anderson's, they are very similar.

Dr. Morton: As I emphasized, actually 75 to 80 percent of the patients in our trial are patients with clinically positive nodes. The number of patients with clinically negative nodes is very small.

Dr. Pinsky: Then that may be another big difference between the studies as described, and I think it should be taken into consideration. Fifty percent or less of our patients have clinically positive nodes.

Dr. Hersh: It is true that all of the patients in our study are patients who went home presumably cured after surgery for primary melanoma and then came back with recurrent nodal disease. That is a difference between our patient population and Dr. Pinsky's.

Dr. Rosenberg: Dr. Hersh, as I understand it, all of your patients have clinically positive nodes at the time they have their lymph node dissection, and that group represents a poorer prognosis group than patients that have only microscopically positive nodes. In fact, as I understood your data, the mean survival time of your control patients was 19 months compared to 23 months for that reported by Carl Pinsky. The shortened survival time of your control patients may well be a reflection of the fact that you are dealing with patients who have clinically positive nodes as opposed to microscopically positive nodes. Would you comment on why you appear to be seeing a difference between your immunotherapy series and your historical controls that is not being seen by several other workers and what might account for that difference?

Dr. Hersh: Dr. Morton covered many of these points quite well. Dose probably is the most important factor, and it relates to the truly systemic administration of BCG, as Professor Mathé says, to produce a septicemia. But when we consider dose, again I would like to raise the warning that we cannot accurately assess the doses that we are giving. We spread a certain number of organisms on the skin and introduce these systemically either by multipuncture or scarification. We really don't have a good way of evaluating the numbers of organisms that are actually delivered. The development of subcomponent fractions of BCG is extremely important, so that we can deliver an accurate dose.

Also, in regard to dose, we are really talking about viable units, and viable units are not necessarily single organisms. They may be clumps of anywhere from a few to perhaps even 100 or more organisms, and depending upon the lot and the strain and the manufacturer, this can vary a great deal. So while dose is quite important, our estimates of dose are extremely inaccurate.

Route of administration is also important, and I think that the original scarification technique does have the advantage of delivering more organisms. Dr. George Mackaness did a small study regarding this in the guinea pig in which BCG was administered by multipuncture plate or by pressure gun or by scarification. He found more organisms were introduced into the skin and more were delivered to the lymph nodes by scarification than by those other techniques.

Schedule is also important. The more frequent the schedule—weekly or every two weeks—the more likely we will be to see an immunotherapeutic benefit.

Lastly, I would like to comment on the modest therapeutic effect that we have observed. Several of the authors have put this in the proper perspective. It is the beginning of our approach to immunotherapy, and we obviously need to build on it. Historically, chemotherapy developed in a similar fashion.

Dr. Rosenberg: Dr. Beretta, in your four-arm study of patients with positive lymph nodes, you have about 20 patients in each group that are evaluable in the first two years.

We have heard from Dr. Pinsky that with 25 patients in each arm, one could expect to pick up, at a power of 0.8, 50 percent differences. You didn't give a statistical discussion of the current status of your patients with positive lymph nodes. Do you see statistically significant differences between BCG or BCG + DTIC?

Dr. Beretta: For previously untreated patients, we are seeing statistically significant differences between control groups, the BCG-treated group, and the BCG plus DTIC-treated group.

Dr. Rosenberg: Could you give us the median survival times and the disease-free intervals?

Dr. Beretta: In previously untreated patients, 50 percent of relapses are estimated to occur in patients in Group A (control) after seven months; in BCG patients, after 8.5 months; in DTIC plus BCG patients, over 12 months. This is statistically significant at the 0.05 level, but you must remember that these data are very preliminary.

We think we should have at least 100 patients in each arm, or 50 patients for untreated and 50 for previously treated patients before reasonably assessing all the data.

Dr. Pinsky: What about the medians for previously treated patients?

Dr. Beretta: For previously treated patients, the control group has a median of 6 months; DTIC group a median of 5.7 months; and the BCG group a median of 8.9 months. In DTIC plus BCG, we had a median relapse time of over 12 months.

Dr. Rosenberg: Dr. Spitler, would you like to make any comments on levamisole?

Dr. Spitler: I would like to hear the advice and comments of other people about whether this particular study should be continued or should be terminated.

Dr. Hersh: I would like to comment, if I may. I think we are beginning to know enough about some of the immunotherapy reagents to identify their activities and to classify them. Levamisole falls into the category of what I would refer to as immunorestorative agents. This agent probably is indicated in those disease categories where there is a considerable immunologic deficit.

We have also had a negative experience in melanoma with the immunorestorative agent thymosin and this probably relates to the fact that most patients with melanoma have the same level of immunocompetence as the normal population. In such a circumstance I would not actually expect immunotherapeutic benefit with levamisole whereas, in a severely immunodeficient population, it might play an important role.

Dr. Spitler: My thinking on that was quite different. When I started this study I thought levamisole acted by boosting a low level of immunologic reactivity. In melanoma the intradermal location of the tumor is ideal for stimulating cellular immune reactivity, and melanoma patients might have some reaction which hopefully could be boosted with levamisole.

Dr. Mathé: We have seen a correlation between immunotherapy effect and septicemic manifestations. I therefore don't understand why people use lyophilized instead of live BCG. Lyophilized is not as efficient in our experimental scheme. I also do not understand why you prolong treatment intervals. When the patients become more allergic, they destroy more bacteria. So when they become allergic, we give more bacteria.

I would like to ask Dr. Morton why he stops treatment after two years since he does not have a plateau in his historical trial.

Dr. Morton: We actually do continue beyond two years. Some of our first patients are actually approaching five years.

Dr. Beretta: Dr. Mathé, we decided to employ lyophilized BCG because in 1973 when we started this trial we were not able to obtain the non-lyophilized BCG. Second, we think that after obtaining a positive reaction, it is sufficient to give BCG once a month and to give it at a reduced dose in order to avoid severe local reactions.

Dr. Rosenberg: First, we have heard of some studies using BCG that have demonstrated no effect in patients in an adjuvant setting with malignant melanoma. The point has been made that before one can make a meaningful negative comment about any therapy, very large numbers of patients are needed. The negative studies presented had insufficient patients to allow a definitive negative comment. One study had 49 patients, the other had 34 patients. Dr. Pinsky has pointed out that given these numbers of patients, one can only say that 50 percent differences are not achieved by these therapies. We could be missing differences that are less than 50 percent. We need to keep in mind that the numbers of patients in the studies are small, and small differences may still exist that are due to immunotherapy.

The positive studies that have been reported differ in many details. It is very difficult to sort out, therefore—impossible in a scientific sense—whether any of these individual factors is in fact really important.

The positive immunotherapeutic effects that are being seen are modest but clinically and scientifically important. We are talking about differences of 20 to 25 percent. The numbers of patients are small and the follow-up is short. It will be very interesting and exciting to follow the data as more patients are added, and as we get more follow-up.

We can say that there are leads with the use of BCG that appear to be promising. We have to reserve any concrete conclusions, but I think you all would agree that on the basis of these results the studies are worth continuing aggressively. The hope is that we will ultimately see the firmer realization of these tentative conclusions.

Immunotherapy of Cancer: Present Status of Trials in Man, edited by W. D. Terry and D. Windhorst, Raven Press, New York © 1978.

Chemotherapy and BCG in the Treatment of Disseminated Malignant Melanoma

John J. Costanzi

University of Texas Medical Branch, Galveston, Texas 77550

The response of disseminated malignant melanoma to chemotherapy has been discouragingly low. It appears that the response rate to dimethyltriazeno imidazole carboxamide (DTIC, NSC-45388) has yielded some of the better responses, ranging from 13 to 21% (1,2). Combination chemotherapy has only minimally improved this response rate. The combination of 1,3-bis (2-chlorethyl)-1-nitrosourea (BCNU, NSC-40992), hydroxyurea, and DTIC (BHD) was reported to produce a response rate of 27% (3).

Nonspecific immunotherapy for melanoma using Bacillus Calmette-Guérin (BCG) has been extensively studied (4–6). Gutterman et al. (1) reported a superior response rate and survival in disseminated melanoma using DTIC and BCG compared to DTIC alone, particularly in patients with nodal metatases only. Since the overall response rate of 27% compared favorably to triple drug (BHD) alone (3), the present study was undertaken to determine if BCG would add significantly to the response rate and survival of patients receiving BHD. This Southwest Oncology Group (SWOG) study randomized patients with disseminated malignant melanoma to one of three treatment programs—BHD, BHD + BCG, or DTIC + BCG.

PATIENTS

The present study (SWOG 7424) was activated in October, 1974. Two hundred sixty-nine patients have been registered. Since 37 of these patients are too early for analysis, this report considers response rate and survival of 232 evaluable patients. The study was open to all members of the Southwest Oncology Group. All patients had histologically proved disseminated malignant melanoma, and they all had adequate renal and hepatic function as manifested by a blood urea nitrogen of less than 25 mg% or a serum creatinine of less than 1.5 mg% and a serum bilirubin of less than 2.5 mg%. For eligibility in the study, patients should not have been previously treated with any of the protocol agents.

Patients with brain metastases could receive corticosteroid therapy and

---

For the Southwest Oncology Group.

brain radiation (3,000 r total brain over 10 days), and those patients with massive liver involvement (span > 16 cm midclavicular line, > 12 cm anterior axillary line, and > 4 cm subxiphoid) could receive hepatic artery DTIC at 200 mg/m² daily for 5 days prior to systemic chemotherapy. These patients are analyzed with the others and separately.

All patients were randomized to receive either BHD, BHD + BCG, or DTIC + BCG. Of the 232 evaluable patients, 75 received BHD, 87 BHD + BCG, and 70 DTIC + BCG.

TREATMENT

All patients were randomized to one of three treatment arms.

1. *BHD:* BCNU, 150 mg/m², i.v., over 30 min, on day 1
   DTIC, 150 mg/m², i.v., over 30 min, daily for 5 days
   Hydroxyurea, 1,500 mg/m², orally, daily for 5 days
2. *BHD + BCG:* Same as No. 1 above plus BCG.
   BCG is administered by escarification on days 7, 14, and 21, following the beginning of chemotherapy. Each escarification was done with one vial (6×10^8 viable organism) of lyophilized Connaught strain BCG. If a patient became a responder, BCG was administered monthly (day 14) between chemotherapy treatments.
3. *DTIC + BCG:* DTIC 250 mg/m², i.v., over 30 min, daily for 5 days plus BCG per No. 2 above.

Courses are repeated every 28 days, with BCNU administered every other course. Subsequent chemotherapy doses were adjusted according to white blood count (WBC) and platelet count nadirs.

STATISTICAL ANALYSIS

Response rates were categorized as (a) *complete,* disappearance of all clinical evidence of tumor, (b) *partial,* a decrease by 50% or more in the sum of the products of two diameters of all measurable tumors, sustained for a minimum of 4 weeks, (c) *none,* an increase or decrease of less than 50% of the sum of the products of two diameters of all measurable lesions, and (d) *increasing disease,* an increase of 50% or more in the product of two diameters of any measurable tumor or the appearance of new lesions.

Toxicity was graded as *none* (WBC $> 4,000$, platelets $> 100,000$, hemoglobin > 13 g/100 ml), *mild* (WBC 3,000 to 4,000 and/or platelets 75,000 to 100,000 with hemoglobin 12 to 13 g/100 ml), *moderate* (WBC 2,000 to 3,000 and/or platelets 50,000 to 75,000 with hemoglobin 10 to 12 g/100 ml), *severe* (WBC 1,000 to 2,000 and/or platelets 25,000 to 50,000 with hemoglobin 10 g/100 ml), *life threatening* (WBC $< 1,000$ and/or platelets < 25,000), and *fatal*. This classification was also applied to nausea, vomiting, alopecia, and BCG toxicity (fever, etc.)

Statistical analyses included the Chi square test for differences in response rates, a generalized Wilcoxan test (7) to determine differences between remission or survival curves, and remission-survival curves calculated according to the method of Kaplan and Meier (8).

RESULTS

Response Rate

Seventy-five patients were randomized to BHD. Seven (9%) achieved a complete response and 14 (19%) a partial response for a total response rate of 28%. Fifty of these patients had normal brain and liver studies; their response rate was 30%. Of the eight with brain metastases receiving radiation and corticosteroids, only one (12%) responded, but of the 17 with massive liver involvement receiving intrahepatic DTIC, six (34%) responded.

Eighty-seven patients were randomized to BHD + BCG. Six (7%) had a complete response, and 19 (22%) noted a partial response for a total response rate of 29%. Fifty-eight of these patients had normal brain and liver studies, with a response rate of 31%, but of those 17 with massive liver involvement only three responded (16%). In 12 with brain metastases, three (15%) responded.

Seventy patients received DTIC + BCG. Four (5%) achieved a complete response and 10 (15%) a partial response for a total response rate of 20%. Forty-five patients had normal brain and liver studies, with a response rate of 25%. Only one (9%) of 11 with brain metastases responded, but three (21%) of 14 with massive liver metastases responded.

Therefore the addition of BCG to BHD did not increase the response rate (28 versus 29%), but either one was superior to DTIC + BCG (20%). The difference between these response rates is not statistically significant ($X^2 = 1.385$, $p = 0.25$). The addition of DTIC hepatic perfusion to those patients with massive liver involvement appears to increase their response rate (34 versus 17%) over a previous study where liver perfusion was not used (3). This response rate was achieved with chemotherapy alone with the two BCG arms noting inferior results (16 and 21%). The addition of brain radiation at the dose used (3,000 r over 10 days) did not appear to increase the response rate, although the patient numbers were small for each limb— 8, 12, and 11.

Survival

Survival curves by treatment is given in Fig. 1. The curves are similar for each treatment, and there is no evidence of a statistical difference among the

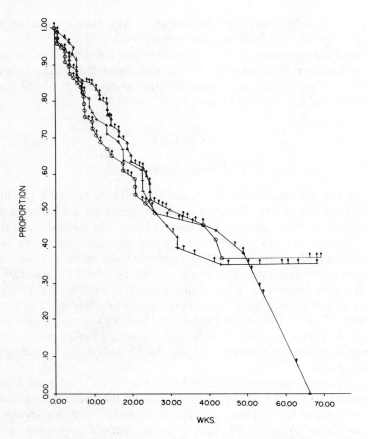

FIG. 1. Survival by treatment arm. There is no statistical difference among the curves (p > 0.28 for all paired comparisons). ○, BHD; △, BHD + BCG; +, DTIC + BCG. Arrows, individual patients.

curves (*p* > 0.28 for all paired comparisons). The median survival for patients in all treatment groups is 25 weeks, and the estimated percentage of patients surviving 1 year is about 35%.

Toxicity

The degree of toxicity is demonstrated in Table 1. The major toxicities were none, mild, and moderate. Table 2 shows the type and degree of toxicity. Dermatitis consisted of a pruritic macular-papular rash probably secondary to DTIC. The only systemic toxicity attributed to BCG was chills and fever. No instance of disseminated BCG disease was noted.

TABLE 1. Degree of toxicity by treatment

Degree of toxicity	Treatment		
	BHD	BHD + BCG	DTIC + BCG
None/mild	35 (47%)	28 (32%)	21 (31%)
Moderate	28 (38%)	44 (51%)	34 (48%)
Severe	11 (14%)	11 (13%)	13 (18%)
Life threatening	1 (1%)	4 (5%)	2 (3%)
Fatal	0	0	0
Total	75 (100%)	87 (100%)	70 (100%)

TABLE 2. Type and degree of toxicity by treatment

Type of toxicity	BHD					BHD + BCG					DTIC + BCG				
	1[a]	2	3	4	5	1	2	3	4	5	1	2	3	4	5
Leukopenia	57	11	6	1	0	69	11	6	1	0	67	1	2	0	0
Thrombocytopenia	66	3	6	0	0	78	4	1	4	0	68	1	0	1	0
Nausea/vomiting	45	5	21	4	0	48	34	5	0	0	28	34	7	1	0
Dermatitis	74	1	0	0	0	86	1	0	0	0	67	0	3	0	0
Chills/fever	75	0	0	0	0	83	3	1	0	0	67	1	2	0	0

[a] 1, None/mild; 2, moderate; 3, severe; 4, life threatening; and 5, fatal.

DISCUSSION

BCG has been reported to increase the response rate and survival when added to chemotherapy in the treatment of disseminated malignant melanoma (1), particularly in patients with only lymph node disease. The combination of BCNU, hydroxyurea, and DTIC (BHD) has been reported to produce a response rate of 27% (3), similar to the response against DTIC and BCG (1). The present study was undertaken to determine if the addition of BCG to the triple-drug regimen would increase the response rate and survival in patients with disseminated melanoma. This was not the case, and the response rate of BHD and BHD + BCG was similar (28%, 29%) but was superior to DTIC + BCG (20%), although these differences are not statistically different.

Similarly, there is no statistical difference in survival among the three treatment regimens. Since immunotherapy probably plays its greatest role in increasing survival in patients with minimal disease, those patients who have responded in this study, may demonstrate an increase in survival if they are maintained on a chemotherapy-BCG limb. Longer follow-up is necessary to determine this factor.

Toxicity in this study was very acceptable. A small number of patients noted life-threatening leukopenia with sepsis and thrombocytopenia. Toxicity to BCG was primarily systemic chills and fever, but no instance of disseminated BCG disease was recorded. Most of the toxicity was nausea and vomiting attributed to the BCNU and DTIC. In general, this was controlled by antiemetics.

In the absence of new agents specific for disseminated melanoma, immediate future efforts should be geared to more rational utilization of known effective drugs, and, probably, the major role of BCG and other immunostimulants is in maintaining patients with minimal disease.

SUMMARY

Response rate and survival were studied in disseminated malignant melanoma with a randomized effort comparing BHD with and without escarified BCG and DTIC + BCG. Seventy-five patients received the triple drug, 87 received the triple drug plus BCG, and 70 received DTIC and BCG. The triple-drug regimen produced a response rate similar to the triple drug + BCG (28 versus 29%), but the DTIC + BCG arm had a response rate of 20%. These differences are not statistically different. Survival curves, comparing the three regimens, showed no statistical differences. Although BCG may significantly prolong survival in the responder, this cannot be determined in this study at this point in time.

Toxicity was acceptable with the major types consisting of mild to moderate nausea, vomiting, leukopenia, and thrombocytopenia. Toxicity to BCG was primarily controllable chills and fever with no evidence of disseminated BCG disease.

ACKNOWLEDGMENTS

This study was supported by U.S. Public Health Service grants of the National Cancer Institute: CA-03096, CA-17701, and DHEW R R-73, J. J. Costanzi, University of Texas Medical Branch, Galveston, Texas; CA-13238, J. M. Quagliana, University of Utah Medical Center, Salt Lake City, Utah; CA-12644, B. Hoogstraten, University of Kansas Medical Center, Kansas City, Kansas; CA-03400, A. Haut, University of Arkansas Medical Center, Little Rock, Arkansas; CA-04919, J. S. Hewlett, Cleveland Clinic, Cleveland, Ohio; CA-04925, R. W. Ralley, Henry Ford Hospital, Detroit, Michigan; CA-03392, M. Lane, Baylor College of Medicine, Houston, Texas; CA-04910, H. E. Wilson, S. Balcerzak, and A. LoBuglio, Ohio State University Hospital, Columbus, Ohio; CA-12213, J. H. Saiki, University of New Mexico School of Medicine, Albuquerque, New Mexico; CA-13236, B. L. Isaacs, Northwestern University Medical School, Chicago, Illinois; CA-12014, T. Moon, Ph.D., M. D. Anderson Hospital, Houston, Texas; CA-10187, J. D. Bonnett and B. W. Amaral, Scott and White Clinic, Temple, Texas.

The following institutions also registered evaluable patients in this study: Wayne State University School of Medicine, Detroit, Michigan; Wilford Hall Medical Center, Lackland AFB, Texas; University of Virginia Medical Center, Charlottesville, Virginia; University of Arizona School of Medicine, Tucson, Arizona; VA Research Hospital, Chicago, Illinois; University of Oklahoma Medical Center, Oklahoma City, Oklahoma; VA Hospital, Little Rock, Arkansas; VA Hospital, Salt Lake City, Utah; Swedish Hospital and Tumor Institute, Seattle, Washington.

REFERENCES

1. Gutterman, J. U., Mavligit, G., Gottlieb, J. A., Burgess, M. A., McBride, C. E., Einhorn, L., Freirich, E. J., and Hersh, E. M. (1974): Chemoimmunotherapy of disseminated malignant melanoma with DTIC and BCG. *N. Engl. J. Med.,* 291: 592–597.
2. Luce, J. K. (1972): Chemotherapy of malignant melanoma. *Cancer,* 30:1604–1615.
3. Costanzi, J. J., Vaitkevicius, V. K., Quagliana, J. M., Hoogstraten, B., Cottman, C. A., and Delaney, F. C. (1975): Combination chemotherapy for disseminated malignant melanoma. *Cancer,* 35:342–346.
4. Morton, D. L., Eilber, F. T., Malmgren, R. A., and Wood, W. C. (1970): Immunologic factors which influence response to immunotherapy in malignant melanoma. *Surgery,* 68:158–164.
5. Bluming, A. Z., Vogel, C. L., Ziegler, J. L., Mody, N., and Kamya, G. (1972): Immunologic effects of BCG in malignant melanoma: Two modes of administration compared. *Ann. Intern. Med.,* 76:405–411.
6. Gutterman, J. U., Mavligit, G., McBride, C., Frei III, E., Freirich, E. J., and Hersh, E. M. (1973): Active immunotherapy with BCG for recurrent malignant melanoma. *Lancet,* 1:1208–1212.
7. Gehan, E. A. (1965): A generalized Wilcoxan test for comparing arbitrarily single censored samples. *Biometrika,* 52:203–233.
8. Kaplan, E. L. and Meier, P. (1969): Non-parametric estimation from incomplete observations. *J. Am. Stat. Assoc.,* 53:457–481.

Immunotherapy of Cancer: Present Status of Trials in Man, edited by W. D. Terry and D. Windhorst. Raven Press, New York © 1978.

A Randomized Prospective Trial Comparing Methyl-CCNU + Vincristine to Methyl-CCNU + Vincristine + BCG + Allogeneic Tumor Cells in Patients with Metastatic Malignant Melanoma

*Michael J. Mastrangelo, *Robert E. Bellet, **David Berd, and Edward Lustbader

*Institute for Cancer Research, Fox Chase Cancer Center; *Department of Medicine, Temple University School of Medicine; and **University of Pennsylvania School of Medicine, Philadelphia, Pennsylvania 19104*

Several chemotherapeutic regimens are of clinical benefit in the treatment of metastatic malignant melanoma (1). However, objective remissions are infrequent, most often partial, and usually of short duration. Active specific immunotherapy with tumor cells in combination with mycobacterial adjuvants has been of little value in patients with advanced malignant melanoma (3,5). The objective of the present study was to assess the influence of the addition of active specific immunotherapy to chemotherapy on objective response rate, remission duration, survival, and hematologic toxicity in patients with metastatic malignant melanoma.

MATERIALS AND METHODS

The criteria for entrance to this study were: (a) histologically documented, surgically incurable, measurable, metastatic malignant melanoma, (b) a life expectancy in excess of 2 months, (c) white blood cell count in excess of 4,000/mm³, (d) platelet count in excess of 100,000/mm³, (e) total serum bilirubin less than 2 mg%, and (f) serum glutamic oxaloacetic transaminase (SGOT) less than 50 units. Patients were excluded who (a) had brain metastases, (b) were receiving steroid therapy, (c) had prior pelvic irradiation therapy, or (d) had been previously treated with a nitrosourea.

Prior to the initiation of therapy, patients were evaluated to determine the extent and distribution of their metastatic disease. This evaluation included a history and physical examination, complete blood and platelet counts, blood urea nitrogen (BUN), liver function profile (total serum bilirubin, SGOT, LDH, alkaline phosphatase), chest X-ray, and liver, brain, and bone scans. Complete blood and platelet counts were repeated at 4, 6, and 8 weeks of each course of therapy. The chest X-ray, BUN, and liver function profile were repeated at 8-week intervals. Liver, brain, and bone scans were repeated when clinically indicated.

Before treatment, the immunologic status of each patient was evaluated by quantitation of immunoglobulins, serum hemolytic complement determination, sensitization (2 mg) and challenge (0.1 mg) with dinitrochlorobenzene (DNCB), and assessment of the cutaneous delayed hypersensitivity response to the following microbial antigens: purified protein derivative (PPD, intermediate strength, Connaught), *Candida* (Hollister-Steir Labs), *Tricophyton* (Hollister-Steir Labs), and streptokinase (Lederle). PPD-negative patients treated with Bacillus Calmette-Guérin (BCG) were retested at 8 weeks.

Methyl 1-(2-chloroethyl)-3-(4-methylcyclohexyl)-1-nitrosourea (methyl-CCNU; NSC 95441) was supplied by the Cancer Therapy Evaluation Branch, DCT, National Cancer Institute. Vincristine (Oncovin®) was purchased from Eli Lilly and Co. BCG, Glaxo strain, is an attenuated viable bovine tubercle bacillus purchased from Eli Lilly and Co. in the lyophilized state. Each vial (4 to 9 × 10⁶ organisms) is reconstituted to 1 ml with sterile water. One immunizing dose is 0.1 ml injected intradermally.

Tumor cells were prepared from tissue obtained from two donors with histologically documented metastatic malignant melanoma; the material was not pooled. Under sterile conditions, the tumor was trimmed of fat and connective tissue, minced, and forced through a 40-mesh wire screen. The viable cells were counted by use of trypan blue exclusion. The cell suspensions were then sedimented by centrifugation, resuspended in Prehn's modification of Eagle's medium (PEM) (Associated Biomedic Systems, Inc.) + 30% fetal calf serum + 12% DMSO to a concentration of 1 to 2 × 10⁸ viable cells/ml, and added in 1-ml amounts to plastic serum test tubes (A/S Nunc). The tubes were left at room temperature for 30 min, placed at −76°C for at least 2 hr and then stored in liquid nitrogen. On the day the cells were to be used, they were thawed quickly in 37°C water, transferred to Falcon 3002 Petri dishes with 5 ml Hank's balanced salt solution (HBSS), and exposed to 15,000 rads with a GE Maximar machine at 220 keV and 15 mAmps that delivered 450 rads/min. The irradiated cell suspensions were transferred to tubes with 5 ml HBSS, sedimented by centrifugation, washed once with 5 ml HBSS, and resuspended in HBSS for injection. Just prior to treatment, individual doses were prepared by adding 1 ml (1 to 2 × 10⁸) melanoma cells to 0.5 ml BCG (2 to 4.5 × 10⁶ organisms). The cell preparation was administered intradermally in the scapular areas in five divided doses.

Patients were stratified by age, sex, and site of tumor involvement (nonvisceral, lung with or without nonvisceral metastases, or nonpulmonary visceral metastases) and randomly allocated to one of two treatment regimens:

1. Chemotherapy (CT) alone
     Methyl-CCNU, 200 mg/m², p.o., on day 1
          plus
     Vincristine, 2 mg, i.v., on days 1 and 29
          or

2. Chemoimmunotherapy (CIT)
   Methyl-CCNU, 200 mg/m², p.o., on day 1
   plus
   Vincristine, 2 mg, i.v., on days 1 and 29
   plus
   1 to 2 × 10⁸ irradiated allogeneic tumor cells admixed with 0.5 ml
   BCG, i.d. (five divided doses), on days 1, 15, 29, 43, and 57.

An adequate trial consisted of completing 57 days of therapy. Treatment was continued, with cycles repeated every 8 weeks, until clinically evident progression of disease. A complete response was defined as the disappearance of all detectable tumor for at least 2 months. A partial remission was ≧ 50% decrease in the sum of the products of the longest perpendicular diameters of all measurable lesions of 2 months duration without the development of new lesions or deterioration in performance status. All other patients were categorized as nonresponders.

RESULTS

Fifty-five patients were entered into the study. Five were excluded because of the development of brain metastases that necessitated the administration of prednisone during the 57-day treatment period. Of the remaining 50 evaluable patients, 26 were treated with CT alone whereas 24 received CIT. The clinical profile of the evaluable patients is presented in Table 1. In single factor analyses, the groups did not differ significantly in the following clinical parameters of possible prognostic importance: sex, age at the initiation of current treatment, time from the initial diagnosis to entry into this study, prior CT or immunotherapy, location of the primary lesion, or distribution of sites of metastases. Ten multifactorial comparisons of potentially pertinent interactions (e.g., age by sex) were also performed. No significant differences were noted (Chi square tests of association). Thus the groups were judged sufficiently randomized and hence comparable. The immunologic profile of both groups of patients is presented in Table 2, and the groups are considered comparable.

Six objective remissions (two complete, four partial) were noted in 26 patients (23%) treated with CT alone as compared with four objective remissions (one complete, three partial) achieved in 24 patients (16.7%) treated with CIT (Table 3). For patients receiving CT, remissions were noted in 2 of 10 with only nonvisceral metastases and 4 of 14 with lung metastases (with or without nonvisceral metastases). For patients receiving CIT, remissions were noted in 2 of 9 with only nonvisceral metastases and 2 of 10 with lung metastases (with or without nonvisceral metastases). These response rates do not differ significantly. The durations of remission are presently similar in the two groups, but this could change since the median in the

TABLE 1. *Clinical profile of patient populations*

		CT (%)		CIT (%)		P
Total		26		24		
Male/female		19/7		15/9		NS
Age (yrs):	Mean	50.8		52.7		NS[c]
	Median	57		55		NS[c]
	Range	22–84		25–84		
Time (mos) diagnosis to						
treatment:	Mean	30.6		24		NS[c]
	Median	23		18		NS[c]
	Range	0–98		0–66		
Prior CT[a]		9/26	(34)	7/24	(29)	NS
Prior Immunotherapy[b]		5/26	(19)	4/24	(16)	NS
Location prime:	H & N	3/26	(11.5)	4/24	(16)	NS
	Back (U)	8/26	(31)	5/24	(21)	NS
	Back (L)	3/26	(11.5)	2/24	(8)	NS
	Chest	5/26	(19)	3/24	(12)	NS
	Abdomen	1/26	(4)	1/24	(4)	NS
	Arm	1/26	(4)	0/24	(0)	NS
	Leg	2/26	(8)	6/24	(25)	NS
	Other	3/26	(11.5)	3/24	(12)	NS
Metastasis:	Subcutaneous	12/26	(46)	9/24	(38)	NS
	Lymph node	15/26	(58)	11/24	(46)	NS
	Lung	11/26	(42)	11/24	(46)	NS
	Liver	1/26	(4)	2/24	(8)	NS
	Bone	1/26	(4)	2/24	(8)	NS
	Dermal	7/26	(27)	4/24	(16)	NS
	Other	2/26	(8)	2/24	(8)	NS

[a] DTIC.
[b] Intralesional or postsurgical adjuvant BCG.
[c] Mann-Whitney analysis.
H & N, head and neck; U, upper; L, lower; NS, $p > 0.05$ using Fisher's Exact Test.

TABLE 2. *Immune profile of patient populations*

	CT		CIT		P
Total	26		24		
DNCB sensitization	17/21	(81%)	20/24	(83%)	NS
$\geq$ 1 Skin tests positive	21/23	(91%)	21/24	(87%)	NS
IgG	15(N), 4($\uparrow$), 2($\downarrow$)		20(N), 1($\uparrow$), 2($\downarrow$)		NS
IgM	20(N), 1($\uparrow$), 0($\downarrow$)		21(N), 1($\uparrow$), 1($\downarrow$)		NS
IgA	19(N), 2($\uparrow$), 0($\downarrow$)		18(N), 4($\uparrow$), 1[a]($\downarrow$)		NS
CH$_{50}$	12(N), 0($\uparrow$), 1($\downarrow$)		17(N), 0($\uparrow$), 2($\downarrow$)		NS
PPD positive[b]	12/21	(57%)	11/24	(46%)	NS
PPD conversion[b]	—		9/11	(82%)	

[a] IgA absent on all determinations.
[b] PPD intermediate strength.
CH$_{50}$, serum hemolytic complement; N, normal; $\uparrow$, increased; $\downarrow$, decreased; NS, $p > 0.05$ using Fisher's Exact Test.

TABLE 3. *Response profile*

	CT	CIT	p
Total	26	24	
CR	2/26 (8%)	1/24 (4%)	NS
PR	4/26 (15%)	3/24 (13%)	NS
ORR	6/26 (23%)	4/24 (16.6%)	NS
95% CI	10.6–42.1%	5.9–34.7%	
Remission duration (mos)			
Median	4	5+	NS[b]
Range	3+–9	4–12+	
Survival[a] (mos)			
Median	6.0	8.0	NS[b]
Range	2–20	2–16	
Alive	5/26 (19%)	10/24 (42%)	

[a] Survival of those who have died.

[b] Mann-Whitney analysis.

CI, confidence interval; CR, complete remission; PR, partial remission; NS, $p > 0.05$ using Fisher's Exact Test; ORR, overall response rate.

CIT group has not yet been reached. The medians for survival for those patients who have died are similar. At this report, 10 of 24 patients treated with CIT are still alive as are 5 of 26 treated with CT alone. Nine of 11 PPD-negative patients treated with CIT converted to positive posttreatment (Table 2).

The intradermal immunotherapy produced the previously described (5) local abscess formation. However, systemic toxicity (flu-like symptoms) was minimal and only occurred in patients receiving multiple cycles of therapy. Only 4 of 50 patients experienced neurotoxicity from the vincristine during

TABLE 4. *Mean percent difference in white blood cell and platelet counts compared with pretreatment values*

	Day 29	Day 43	Day 57
White blood cell counts[c]			
CT	−16.3%	−29.4%	−21.5%
CIT	+ 3.7%	−38.0%	+13.7%
	(p = NS)	(p = NS)	(p = 0.01[a])
			(p = 0.002[b])
Platelet counts[c]			
CT	−39.2	+ 9.3	− 7.5
CIT	−43.5	+24.9	+29.7
	(p = NS)	(p = NS)	(p = 0.01[a])
			(p = 0.006[b])

[a] T test.

[b] Mann-Whitney test.

[c] Data from first cycle of therapy.

NS, $p > 0.05$.

the first cycle of therapy. With protracted vincristine therapy, dose modification was required. Methyl-CCNU produced the anticipated gastrointestinal toxicity, which did not require dose modification. The spectrum of hematologic toxicity induced by methyl-CCNU is summarized in Table 4. Both regimens produced significant depressions in white blood cell and platelet counts. However, recovery was more rapid on the CIT regimen. There were no drug related deaths.

DISCUSSION

Gutterman et al. (4) treated 89 patients with disseminated malignant melanoma with a combination of intravenous dimethyl triazeno imidazole carboxamide (DTIC) plus BCG administered by scarification (Pasteur Institute, 6×10^8 viable units on days 7, 12, and 17). The CIT-treated patients with lymph node (with or without subcutaneous) metastases had a remission rate of 55% (11/20) compared to 18% (3/17) for the historic controls treated with DTIC alone ($p = 0.025$). Patients with visceral metastases did not have an improved response rate to CIT. However, the durations of remission and survivals were significantly longer for all categories of patients treated with CIT than the historic controls treated with CT alone.

In the present study, the response rates for patients with nonvisceral metastases did not differ significantly (2/9 CIT, 2/10 CT). The median duration of remission for the CIT group and the medians for survival for both groups have not as yet been reached. With further follow-up, survival may be improved for patients receiving CIT. Our failure to confirm the observation of Gutterman et al. (4) of an improved objective response rate with CIT in patients with nonvisceral metastases may be the result of several factors. Methyl-CCNU is more immunosuppressive than DTIC and could have interfered with the immunotherapy (2,6). However, methyl-CCNU did not prevent 9 of 11 PPD-negative patients from converting to PPD positive following CIT. Secondly, no special effort was made to place the BCG + tumor cells in skin sites that would drain to involved lymph nodes. Finally, the dose, strain, and route of BCG administration differed.

The present study has failed to demonstrate an improved overall objective response rate for CIT as compared to CT alone. This may have resulted from a chance maldistribution of responses in our small sample (50 total patients). However, even if an additional 30 patients were entered and responses were achieved at a rate of 34.7% (upper limit of the 95% confidence interval) for CIT and 10.6% (lower limit of 95% confidence interval) for CT, no significant differences would be demonstrated. Further, based on the present data, there is only a 16.8% probability that the response rate for CIT is 5% greater (e.g., 20 versus 25%) than the response rate for CT.

In summary, methyl-CCNU + vincristine + BCG + tumor cells is not superior to methyl-CCNU + vincristine in inducing objective remissions in patients with metastatic malignant melanoma. There are as yet insufficient data to compare median durations of remission and survivals, but the latter may be improved for the CIT-treated group. Both regimens were well tolerated, and no unexpected toxicity was noted. Patients receiving CIT rebounded more quickly from their hematologic suppression than CT patients. This study is being continued to determine if remission duration and survival are prolonged by the addition of immunotherapy.

SUMMARY

Fifty patients with metastatic malignant melanoma were randomized to treatment with either (a) methyl-CCNU (200 mg/m², p.o., q 8 weeks) plus vincristine (2 mg, i.v., q 4 weeks), or (b) the same CT plus intradermal injections of irradiated (15,000 rads) allogeneic (fresh frozen) melanoma cells (1 to 2 × 10⁸) admixed with BCG (Glaxo, 2 to 4.5 × 10⁶ organisms) every 2 weeks. Treatment cycles were repeated every 8 weeks until tumor progression. Six (two complete, four partial) objective remissions were noted among 26 patients (23%) treated with CT alone, whereas 4 (one complete, three partial) objective remissions were noted among 24 patients (16.7%) treated with CIT (p = not significant). The median duration of remission has not yet been reached for both groups (4 and 5+ months, respectively). Further, the median survivals have also not been reached. The patients manifested no unexpected toxicity. Hematologic toxicity was experienced by patients on both regimens; however, those receiving CIT rebounded more quickly.

ACKNOWLEDGMENTS

This work was supported by U.S. Public Health Service grants no. CA-13456, CA-06927, and RR-05539 from the National Institutes of Health and by an appropriation from the Commonwealth of Pennsylvania.

REFERENCES

1. Bellet, R. E., Mastrangelo, M. J., and Berd, D. (1977): The chemotherapy of malignant melanoma. A review. In: *Malignant Melanoma,* Grune & Stratton, New York. (*In press.*)
2. Bruckner, H. W., Mokyr, M. B., and Mitchell, M. S. (1974): Effect of imidazole-4-carboxamide, 5-(3,3-dimethyl-1-triazeno) on immunity in patients with malignant melanoma. *Cancer Res.,* 34:181–183.
3. Gerner, R. E., and Moore, G. E. (1976): Feasibility of active immunotherapy in patients with solid tumors. *Cancer,* 38:131–143.
4. Gutterman, J. U., Mavligit, G., Gottlieb, J. A., Burgess, M. A., McBride, C. E., Einhorn, L., Freireich, E. J., and Hersh, E. M. (1974): Chemoimmunotherapy of disseminated malignant melanoma with dimethyl triazeno imidazole carboxamide and bacillus Calmette-Guerin. *N. Engl. J. Med.,* 291:592–597.
5. Mastrangelo, M. J., Bellet, R. E., Laucius, J. F., and Berkelhammer, J. (1976):

Immunotherapy of malignant melanoma. In: *Oncologic Medicine,* edited by A. I. Sutnick and P. F. Engstrom, pp. 71–93. Univ. Park Press, Baltimore, Md.

6. Mitchell, M. S., Mokyr, M. B., and Davis, J. M. (1974): Effect of chemotherapy and immunotherapy upon tumor-specific immunity in melanoma. *Proc. Am. Assoc. Cancer Res.,* 15:3 (Abstr. #11).

Question and Answer Session

Dr. Hersh: Were the immunizations given only during the first 57-day period, or with each 57-day cycle indefinitely?

Dr. Mastrangelo: The immunizations were continued throughout repeated cycles up to about the fourth cycle, at which time it was so toxic that it was cut down to one-half the dose. The patients were sick four or five days and they would not tolerate it.

Dr. Rosenberg: When did the studies start and what was the median duration of follow-up for the study?

Dr. Mastrangelo: The study started two years ago. I cannot tell you what the median duration of follow-up is; I do not know. I suspect it is about a year. The longest patients have been at risk for over two years.

Dr. Holland: What did the local immunizing lesion look like?

Dr. Mastrangelo: It is a tremendous abscess. Because of the volume of the tumor cells and the BCG, they have to be given in five separate locations so these people wind up getting five abscesses linearly down their back every two weeks.

Question: Did you observe brain metastases in the patients?

Dr. Mastrangelo: My impression is that 75 percent of the patients are dying of brain metastases. I have not formally analyzed it, but it is a very high percentage.

Immunotherapy of Cancer: Present Status of
Trials in Man, **edited by W. D. Terry and D. Windhorst.**
Raven Press, New York © 1978.

Chemoimmunotherapy of Disseminated Malignant Melanoma with BCG: Follow-Up Report

Jordan U. Gutterman, Evan M. Hersh, Giora M. Mavligit,
Michael A. Burgess, Stephen P. Richman, Max Schwarz,
Victorio Rodriquez, and Manuel Valdivieso

Department of Developmental Therapeutics, The University of Texas System Cancer Center, M. D. Anderson Hospital and Tumor Institute, Houston, Texas 77030

Chemotherapy of disseminated malignant melanoma continues to produce low response rates and very few long-term survivors. In April, 1972, we initiated our first trial of Bacillus Calmette-Guérin (BCG) immunotherapy plus dimethyl triazeno imidazole carboxamide (DTIC) chemotherapy for patients with disseminated melanoma. The initial results of this study were previously reported (6). The major conclusions of that study can be summarized as follows: (a) overall remission rates with DTIC plus BCG were not increased compared to DTIC alone; (b) there was an increased remission rate in areas regional to BCG scarification (tumor confined to lymph node regions in the DTIC-BCG trial) compared to DTIC chemotherapy alone; (c) there was a significant prolongation of remission duration with chemoimmunotherapy compared to chemotherapy alone; and (d) most notable was the significant prolongation of survival particularly among responding patients treated with DTIC-BCG compared to DTIC alone.

We report a 4½ year follow-up of our trial with DTIC plus BCG.

PATIENTS AND METHODS

A total of 101 consecutive patients with unresectable disseminated metastatic melanoma (stage IV) were entered on the study between April 15, 1972, and March 15, 1973. Before chemoimmunotherapy, patients were evaluated for metastatic disease with the following tests—physical examination, complete blood count, urinalysis, tests of liver and renal function, chest X-ray, liver scan, electroencephalogram, brain scan, and bone marrow biopsy. When specific symptoms indicated, a metastatic bone survey or X-ray examination of the gastrointestinal tract, or both, were done.

The experimental design of the chemoimmunotherapy was as follows—chemotherapy consisted of DTIC, 250 mg/m^2, intravenously on days 1 through 5. Fresh liquid Pasteur strain BCG, 6×10^8 viable units, was administered by scarification on days, 7, 12, and 17 of each course. Courses were repeated every 21 days if the blood counts permitted.

The BCG was shipped weekly from the Pasteur Institute (Paris, France) to our institution by air, stored at 4° C, and used within 10 days. The BCG was administered by scarification with an 18 gauge needle. The scarifications were applied in a rotating fashion on the upper arms and upper thighs as previously described (6). The total number of viable units administered was calculated from the number of viable units per vial as estimated by the manufacturers at the time of shipment.

The DTIC was adjusted as follows—if myelosuppression did not occur during the initial course, the dose of chemotherapy was increased by 50% during the subsequent course. If the white cell count was reduced to below 1,000/mm^3, the granulocyte count to 500 mm^3 or below, or the platelet count to 50,000/mm^3 or less, DTIC dosage was reduced by 25 to 50% during the next course.

The following definitions were used: (a) complete remission, complete disappearance of all objective and subjective disease manifestations; (b) partial remission, 50% or greater reduction in the area of all measurable tumor; (c) stabilization, less than 50% reduction or less than 25% increase in tumor size for at least 2 months; (d) progression, 25% or greater increase in tumor masses or appearance of any new masses; and (e) relapse, reappearance of a tumor mass.

Survival was measured from onset of the treatment to death or date of last follow-up examination. DTIC-BCG was continued for a minimum of two courses unless the patient died. The therapy was stopped only on evidence of progression.

The responses to therapy with DTIC-BCG were compared to the responses of a consecutive series of 111 patients treated in an identical fashion in combination with DTIC alone from March, 1967 to August, 1969. In the intervening period, August, 1969 to March, 1972, DTIC was used in combination with other drugs in two separate studies and therefore might not be suitable as historical controls. However, the clinical results of these groups were nearly identical to those receiving DTIC alone, and therefore, survival curves of these two studies also were used as supplemental historical controls. The first combination study was 1-3-bis-(2-chloroethyl)-1-nitrosourea (BCNU), vincristine, and DTIC (August, 1969 to August, 1971), and the second combination study was DTIC and procarbazine (August, 1971 to March, 1972).

Criteria for admission to all these studies were identical. All patients with clinical evidence of disseminated melanoma unresectable by surgery were admitted for therapy. Concurrent therapy with other modalities in the DTIC-BCG study was used only in six cases and included local radiotherapy for brain metastasis or other sites of metastases associated with severe pain.

Table 1 shows that the DTIC-BCG and DTIC groups were comparable in the major features known to be associated with prognosis. The distribution of visceral and nonvisceral metastases was similar. The frequency of pulmonary

TABLE 1. *Clinical features of 89 patients treated with DTIC-BCG and 111 treated with DTIC*

Clinical feature	DTIC-BCG		DTIC	
Median age (yr)	51 (25–88)[a]		50 (24–75)[a]	
Male (%)	57		53	
Female (%)	43		47	
Metastasis (%)				
Nonvisceral	27		21.6	
Visceral	73		78.4	
Pulmonary		31		31.4
Nonpulmonary		42		47
Site of primary tumor (%)				
Trunk	29		33	
Head and neck	20		11	
Extremities	25		30	
Unknown	26		26	
Duration of primary tumor to metastases (%)				
< 2 yr	33		30.5	
2–5 yr	36		40.5	
≥ 5 yr	18		12.0	
Unknown	13		17.0	
Prior immunotherapy (%)	9		< 1	
Prior chemotherapy (%)	< 1		< 1	

[a] Range.

and nonpulmonary metastases (liver, bone, and brain) was nearly identical in both groups. Also comparable were the sites of the primary melanoma as well as the interval from the primary tumor to onset of disseminated metastasis (stage IV). The only major difference between the two groups was the group of nine patients who had prior immunotherapy in the DTIC-BCG group as compared to patients who received DTIC alone. The difference, however, did not influence the results.

Statistical methods included the Chi square for testing differences in remission rate, a generalized Wilcoxon test, with a one-tailed analysis for testing differences between remission or survival curves (3), and the method of Kaplan and Meier for calculating and plotting remission and survival curves (9).

RESULTS

An overall remission rate of 27% among 89 evaluable patients was reported previously. This has not changed since the initial report. Table 2 shows an additional analysis of responses by age. The remission rate for patients under the age of 60 treated with DTIC alone was 19%. Forty-nine percent of these patients had progression of the disease. There was a modest

TABLE 2. *Chemoimmunotherapy of disseminated malignant melanoma—
response to treatment by age*

	< 60 Years		> 60 Years	
	DTIC	DTIC-BCG	DTIC	DTIC-BCG
CR + PR	15[a] (18)	16 (27)	1 (3)	8 (27)
Stable	26 (32)	21 (36)	8 (27)	6 (20)
Progression	40 (49)	22 (37)	21 (70)	16 (53)

[a] Number of patients; no. in parentheses = %.
CR, complete remission; PR, partial remission.

but statistically insignificant increase in remission rate among patients less
than 60 years of age treated with DTIC plus BCG. Thus, 16 of 59 (27%)
of these patients achieved remission.

However, there was a significant increase in the remission rates among
patients over the age of 60. Thus, only one of 30 (3%) treated with DTIC
alone achieved remission. In contrast, seven of 30 (27%) of the patients
treated with DTIC plus BCG achieved remission ($p = 0.05$).

The long-term follow-up of duration of remission for these two groups of
patients is shown in Fig. 1. As reported previously, all 16 remission patients
treated with DTIC alone relapsed within 12 months. Three of the 24 DTIC-

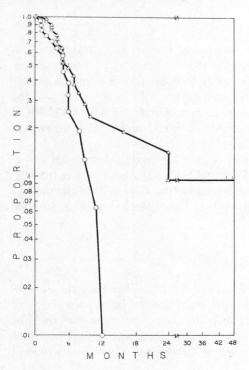

FIG. 1. Chemoimmunotherapy of disseminated
melanoma. Long-term follow-up of duration of
remission for patients on DTIC alone (O) and on
DTIC-BCG (△). Relapses were 16/16 and 21/24,
respectively. ($p = 0.1$.)

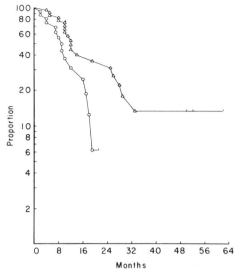

FIG. 2. Chemoimmunotherapy of disseminated melanoma. Survival of patients responding to treatment of DTIC alone (O) and DTIC-BCG (△). Deaths were 15/16 and 20/24, respectively. ($p = 0.01$.)

BCG responders are still in remission. One of these patients was lost to follow-up at 8 months. However, two of the patients are in remission at 46 and 52 months, respectively. These differences are at the borderline of statistical significance ($p = 0.1$).

The survival among responding patients is shown in Fig. 2. Thus, only one of 16 patients treated with DTIC was alive at the last follow-up. This patient has been lost to follow-up. Four of the 24 patients (16%) of the DTIC-BCG responders are still alive. One of these is the patient who, lost to follow-up, was alive at last contact. Three of 24 patients (12%) treated with DTIC-BCG are alive at 4 or more years. These differences are statistically significant ($p = 0.01$).

The survival of all patients treated with an adequate trial of DTIC and DTIC-BCG is shown in Fig. 3. Only two of the 111 patients treated with DTIC alone are alive. Five of 89 patients treated with DTIC-BCG are alive. One is the patient lost to follow-up. Four patients are alive at 4 years or greater. These differences are statistically significant in favor of the DTIC-BCG group compared to the DTIC group ($p = 0.001$).

In order to further illustrate the modest but definite benefit of BCG immunotherapy combined with DTIC chemotherapy among patients with disseminated melanoma, the survival of patients treated in three trials with chemotherapy and BCG immunotherapy carried out in our department at M. D. Anderson from 1971 until 1975 is shown in Fig. 4. The overall survival for patients treated with DTIC plus BCG, with methyl 1-(2-chloroethyl)-3-cyclohexyl-1-nitrosourea (methyl CCNU) plus BCG (7), and with DTIC-BCG plus one dose of transfer factor on day 12 (12) is combined in one curve. Similarly, the survival for the 274 patients treated with chemotherapy

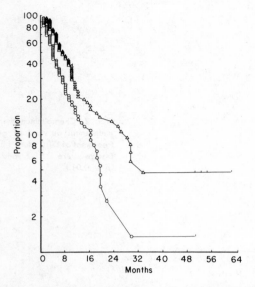

FIG. 3. Chemoimmunotherapy of disseminated melanoma. Survival of all patients treated with an adequate trial of DTIC alone (○) or DTIC-BCG (△). Deaths were 109/111 and 84/89, respectively. (p = 0.001.)

alone from 1967 to 1971 is combined in one curve (see ref. 6 for details of chemotherapy studies). Although there were only modest differences in the median survival, the curve broadens out so that by the 0.15 percentile there is a highly significant difference in the survival of the chemoimmunotherapy patients compared to chemotherapy (p = 0.001).

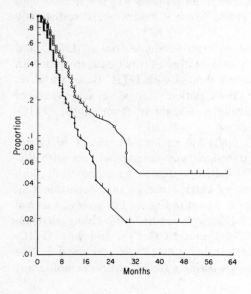

FIG. 4. Chemotherapy (●) during 1967–1971 and chemoimmunotherapy (○) during 1971–1975 of disseminated melanoma in patients at M. D. Anderson Hospital. Deaths were 260/274 and 174/204, respectively. See text for details.

DISCUSSION

Long-term follow-up evaluation of our initial study continues to show a significant advantage for patients treated with chemoimmunotherapy over those treated with DTIC chemotherapy alone. Several points need to be emphasized. Reexamination of response data suggests that the addition of BCG to DTIC chemotherapy was associated with higher rates among patients over the age of 60. However, the response rates in the overall program continue to be disappointingly low. The durations of remission continue to favor the group of patients treated with DTIC plus BCG. Although only a small fraction of patients continues in remission on chemoimmunotherapy, the fact that we have a detectable long-term remission duration is important.

Perhaps the most important effect of this study has been the improved survival among responding patients; 16% of responding patients on DTIC-BCG are still alive. This confirms experimental as well as recent clinical data that illustrate that immunotherapy has its most notable effect on survival of responding patients.

There are obviously major limitations with the present regimen for treating patients with disseminated malignant melanoma. The remission rates are low. Thus, additional new chemotherapeutic as well as new immunotherapeutic approaches are needed. There are leads in this direction. A recently reported trial suggested that active specific immunotherapy with tumor cells plus low doses of Glaxo BCG plus DTIC chemotherapy may have increased remission rates (2). Based on experimental work that intravenous immunotherapy is superior to intradermal immunotherapy for pulmonary metastases (1,8,10), we have been using intensive *Corynebacterium parvum* prior to and intermittent with chemotherapy. We have suggestive data that a combination of DTIC, actinomycin D, and intensive intravenous *C. parvum* may be producing higher remission rates and prolonged survival in advanced melanoma patients (4).

Improved results for chemoimmunotherapy of advanced melanoma are needed. In addition, the application of chemoimmunotherapy regimens as described in this chapter should be applied earlier in the course of melanoma when the tumor load is smaller and a greater chance for long-term survival exists (5,11).

ACKNOWLEDGMENTS

This work has been supported by contract NO1-CB-33888 and grants 05831 and 11520 from the National Cancer Institute, Bethesda, Maryland 20014. Drs. Gutterman and Mavligit are the recipients of career development awards (CA 71007–02 and CA 00130–01, respectively) also from the National Cancer Institute.

The authors gratefully acknowledge the excellent technical assistance of

Tonya Smith, Kathy Dandridge, Shirley Livingston, and Marty Marshall as well as the secretarial assistance of Darlene Hall in the preparation of this manuscript.

REFERENCES

1. Baldwin, R. W., and Pimm, M. V. (1973): BCG immunotherapy of pulmonary growths from intravenously transferred rat tumor cells. *Br. J. Cancer,* 27:48–54.
2. Currie, G. A., and Bagshawe, K. B. (1970): Active immunotherapy with C. parvum and chemotherapy in murine fibrosarcomas. *Br. Med. J.,* 1:541–544.
3. Gehan, E. A. (1965): A generalized Wilcoxon test for comparing arbitrarily singly-censored samples. *Biometrika,* 52:203–223.
4. Gutterman, J. U. (1977): *Proc. Am. Soc. Clin. Oncol. (Submitted for publication.)*
5. Gutterman, J. U., Mavligit, G. M., Burgess, M. A., Cardenas, J. O., Blumenschein, G. R., Gottlieb, J. A., McBride, C. M., McCredie, K. B., Bodey, G. P., Rodriquez, V., Freireich, E. J., and Hersh, E. M. (1976): Immunotherapy of breast cancer, malignant melanoma, and acute leukemia with BCG: Prolongation of disease free interval and survival. *Cancer Immunol. Immunother.,* 1:99–107.
6. Gutterman, J. U., Mavligit, G. M., Gottlieb, J. A., Burgess, M. A., McBride, C. M., Einhorn, L., Freireich, E. J., and Hersh, E. M. (1974): Chemoimmunotherapy of disseminated malignant melanoma with dimethyl triazeno imidazole carboxamide and Bacillus Calmette-Guerin. *N. Engl. J. Med.,* 291:592–597.
7. Gutterman, J. U., Mavligit, G. M., Reed, R., Burgess, M. A., Gottlieb, J., and Hersh, E. M. (1976): Bacillus Calmette-Guerin immunotherapy in combination with DTIC (NSC-45388) for the treatment of malignant melanoma. *Cancer Treat. Rep.,* 60:177–182.
8. Israel, L., Edelstein, R., Depierre, A., and Dimitrov, N. (1975): Daily intravenous infusions of Corynebacterium parvum in twenty patients with disseminated cancer: A preliminary report of clinical and biological findings. *J. Natl. Cancer Inst.,* 55:29–33.
9. Kaplan, E. L., and Meier, P. (1958): Nonparametric estimation from incomplete observations. *J. Am. Stat. Assoc.,* 53:457–481.
10. Milas, L., Gutterman, J. U., Basic, I., Hunter, N., Mavligit, G. M., Hersh, E. M., and Withers, H. R. (1974): Immunoprophylaxis and immunotherapy for a murine fibrosarcoma with C. granulosum and C. parvum. *Int. J. Cancer,* 14:493–503.
11. Morton, D. L., Eilber, F. R., Holmes, E. C., Sparks, F. C., and Ramming, K. P. (1976): Present status of BCG immunotherapy of malignant melanoma. *Cancer Immunol. Immunother.,* 1:93–98.
12. Schwarz, M., Gutterman, J. U., Hersh, E. M., Mavligit, G., and Bodey, G. (1977): Chemoimmunotherapy of disseminated malignant melanoma (DMM) with DTIC, BCG, transfer factor (TF) ± melphan (L-PAM). *Proc. Am. Assoc. Cancer Res. (Submitted for publication.)*

Question and Answer Session

Dr. LoBuglio: In your current study with *C. parvum* what proportion of those patients have visceral metastases?

Dr. Hersh: I can't give you the exact number. It is approximately the same as in our previous studies.

A Participant: In your *C. parvum* study, what is the incidence of myelosuppression compared to your previous studies?

Dr. Hersh: There is more myelosuppression.

A Participant: What kind of schedule do you use for *C. Parvum?*

Dr. Hersh: The ultimate dose is 2 mg/m², but we scale up to that over the first four days. We found when we started off with 2 mg/m² from day 1, we had very severe toxicity in terms of fever and chills. By starting with a lower dose and scaling up over the first four days, we avoid that very severe toxicity.

Dr. Rosenberg: In the comparison of the DTIC plus BCG group with your own historical controls you mentioned that patients had to complete at least one cycle of the DTIC-BCG to be eligible for this protocol.

Did you similarly go back and eliminate from your historical control group those patients that would not have completed a single cycle of this regimen?

Dr. Hersh: That's correct.

Immunotherapy of Cancer: Present Status of Trials in Man, edited by W. D. Terry and D. Windhorst. Raven Press, New York © 1978.

Effect of *Corynebacterium Parvum* on Combination Chemotherapy of Disseminated Malignant Melanoma

Cary A. Presant, *Alfred A. Bartolucci, **Richard V. Smalley, †W. Ralph Vogler

*Division of Hematology-Oncology, Washington University School of Medicine, The Jewish Hospital of St. Louis, St. Louis, Missouri 63110; *Department of Biometry and †Department of Medicine, Emory University, Atlanta, Georgia 30322; and **Department of Medicine, Temple University Health Science Center, Philadelphia, Pennsylvania 19104*

The management of metastatic malignant melanoma remains difficult. Standard therapy employing 5-(3,3-dimethyl-l-triazeno)-imidazole-4-carboxamide (DTIC) results in 24% complete or partial remissions and an overall median survival of only 4.6 months (3). In an attempt to improve the response rates, response durations, and total survival of patients with metastatic malignant melanoma, the Southeastern Cancer Study Group initiated a protocol employing cyclophosphamide plus DTIC with or without the addition of the *Corynebacterium parvum* vaccine. This chapter details the results of that study as of June, 1976.

The rationale for the use of *C. parvum* was based mostly on the work of Israel. *C. parvum* plus chemotherapy was found to produce longer remissions and survivals in patients with assorted tumors than patients receiving chemotherapy alone (9,12). A preliminary report by Reed (13) suggested that the addition of *C. parvum* plus innoculation of irradiated cultured tumor cells improved the response of liver and lung metastases to a treatment with DTIC, 1-[2-chloroethyl]-3-[4 methylcyclohexyl]-1-nitrosourea (methyl-CCNU), plus BCG. There is additional anecdotal evidence that *C. parvum* may have an antitumor effect itself without the use of additional chemotherapy (1,10,11). Several investigators have reported that the use of *C. parvum* with myelosuppressive chemotherapy may result in less hematological toxicity than the use of chemotherapy alone (6,9), although a preliminary report of a contradictory study has appeared (8).

The rationale for the choice of chemotherapy regimen was based on the independent activities of the two agents. DTIC is the standard chemotherapeutic agent in malignant melanoma (3). Cyclophosphamide has not been extensively tested in malignant melanoma, although reported objective response rates vary from 5 to 22% depending upon the criteria used to estab-

---

For The Southeastern Cancer Study Group.

lish objective response (2). A small study using cyclophosphamide with a single injection of DTIC plus vincristine demonstrated at least as high a response rate as DTIC alone (7). Therefore, cyclophosphamide plus 5 days of treatment with DTIC was employed as the chemotherapy regimen common to both of the treatment modalities in this study.

METHODS

Protocol 361 of the Southeastern Cancer Study Group was initiated in June, 1974. This report includes patients evaluated through June, 1976.

Patients were eligible for this study if they had not previously received any chemotherapy or immunomodulatory agents and had biopsy-proved malignant melanoma incurable by standard surgical techniques, regardless of their Karnofsky performance status. Each patient had at least one tumor measurable by physical examination or radiographic technique.

All patients who received at least one injection of chemotherapy were evaluable. Patients were inevaluable if cyclophosphamide, *C. parvum,* or DTIC was given in an incorrect schedule, if the patients refused further therapy, or if patients did not return for evaluation of antitumor or toxic effects. However, patients who died at home were considered evaluable.

Patients were randomized into either of two treatment regimens. Treatment regimen A consisted of cyclophosphamide 600 mg/m², i.v., on day 1 plus DTIC 200 mg/m², i.v., on days 1 through 5. Treatment regimen B consisted of the same chemotherapy as regimen A, with the addition of *C. parvum* 5 mg/m², i.v., on day 8 and 15. *Corynebacterium parvum* was supplied as Coparvax® by Burroughs Wellcome Co., Research Triangle Park, North Carolina 27709. Both treatment regimens were repeated every 21 days.

During either therapeutic regimen if the nadir granulocyte count was below 750 cells/mm³ or if the nadir platelet count was less than 50,000 cells/mm³, doses of cyclophosphamide and DTIC were reduced by 50% for the next course of chemotherapy. If the patient had exceptional chills or fever following *C. parvum,* acetaminophen and diphenhydramine were administered. Severe reactions persisting despite this therapy were treated with intravenous corticosteroids.

Antitumor response was evaluated 3 weeks following the third course of chemotherapy. Complete response consisted of complete disappearance of all objective evidence of disease and attainment of a 100% performance status. Partial response consisted of a 50 to 100% reduction in the sum of the products of the perpendicular diameters of all measurable lesions. Stable disease was defined as less than a partial response but no enlargement of measured tumors by more than 25% in the sum of the products of diameters, and no appearance of new lesions during therapy. All other patients were defined as having progression of tumor.

Toxic reactions were defined as mild, or moderate to severe. Mild anemia consisted of a 3- to 4.9-g fall in hemoglobin concentration. Moderate to severe toxicity consisted of greater than a 5-g fall in hemoglobin concentration. Mild thrombocytopenia was defined as a nadir platelet count of 50,000 to 100,000 cells/mm³. Moderate to severe thrombocytopenia consisted of a nadir platelet count of less than 50,000 cells/mm³. Mild granulocytopenia consisted of a nadir granulocyte count of 750 to 1,500 cells/mm³. Moderate to severe toxicity consisted of a nadir granulocyte count of less than 750 cells/mm³. A change in blood pressure was classified as mild if hypertension greater than 150/100 was observed in a previously normotensive patient. Moderate to severe blood pressure change was defined as hypotension less than 90/60 in a previously normotensive patient. Vomiting was defined as mild if antiemetics easily controlled the reaction or were not required. Vomiting was defined as moderate to severe if antiemetics did not control the reaction. Azotomia was defined as mild if the creatinine concentration rose to between 1.2 to 2.0 mg/dl. Moderate to severe reactions were defined as a rise in creatinine concentration greater than 2.0 mg/dl. Fever and chills were considered mild if the temperature rose to less than 101° and chills were described by the patient and physician observer as mild. A temperature elevation to above 101° or a more marked chill was defined as moderate to severe toxicity.

RESULTS

As of June, 1976, 101 patients had been entered into the treatment program, but only 69 patients had completed their trials. Of those 56 were evaluable by the criteria listed in the section on methods (81% evaluability). The number of patients entered, trials completed, and trials evaluable was similar in regimens A and B (Table 1). There was no significant difference between patients on regimen A or B with respect to mean age, sex distribution, frequency of visceral involvement, pretreatment performance status, or pretreatment presence of anergy [defined as absence of induration of greater than 5 mm in diameter within 72 hr following testing of delayed hypersensitivity with purified protein derivative (PPD), histoplasm, or mumps

TABLE 1. *Characteristics of patient populations*

	Regimen A	Regimen B
Number of patients entered	50	51
Number of trials completed	33	36
Number of trials evaluable	29	27
Mean age (years)	46	51
Males	72%	56%
Visceral involvement	75%	70%
Karnofsky performance status		
70% or above	72%	74%
Anergic	17%	21%

antigens]. Thus, the two treatment regimens consisted of patient populations that were apparently similar.

Complete or partial antitumor responses (Table 2) were obtained in eight of 29 patients on regimen A (28%), and nine of 27 patients on regimen B (33%). There was no significant difference in the response rates, distribution of complete or partial responses, median durations of remission (3.0 months in A, 2.6 in B), or median survival (5.6 months in A, 5.5 in B). In addition, analysis of the remission duration and survival curves for regimens A and B by a modified Wilcoxon analysis demonstrated no significant difference.

With regard to pretreatment variables, 21% of 19 patients who were not anergic had complete or partial remissions on regimen A, versus 40% of 15 patients on regimen B (not significantly different; the remaining patients were not evaluable for delayed hypersensitivity testing). Of the four anergic patients on regimen A, one had a partial response, and of the four anergic patients on regimen B, similarly one patient had a partial response.

Of patients who had cutaneous or lymph node involvement only (absence of visceral disease) three of seven patients on regimen A (43%) and four of eight patients on regimen B (50%) had complete or partial responses. The median survival in patients without visceral disease was 5.2 months on regimen A and greater than 7.0 months on regimen B, although these differences are not significant because of the limited number of patients studied.

In patients with visceral metastases, five of 21 patients on regimen A (24%) and five of 19 patients on regimen B (26%) had complete or partial responses. The median duration of these responses was 3.2 months and the median survival overall was 5.5 months, 4.0 months on regimen A, and 6.2 months on regimen B.

In patients with a performance status less than 70%, none of eight on regimen A and only one of seven on regimen B had a partial response. The median survivals were 1.0 month on regimen A and 3.4 months on regimen B.

Of 21 patients on regimen A with a performance status of 70% or better, eight achieved a complete or partial response (38%). Eight of 20 such patients on regimen B had a response (40%). The median survival for regimen A was 7.0 months, and for regimen B was 6.0 months. Despite the fact that there was not a large numerical difference, these curves were statistically

TABLE 2. *Antitumor response*

	Regimen A	Regimen B
Number of patients evaluable	29	27
Complete response	1 (3%)	3 (11%)
Partial response	7 (25%)	6 (22%)
Stable	3	2
Progression	18	16
Median duration of remission (months)	3.0	2.6
Median survival (months)	5.6	5.5

TABLE 3. *Percent of patients with toxic reactions*

Toxic reaction	Regimen A		Regimen B	
	Mild	Moderate or severe	Mild	Moderate or severe
Anemia	14	3	11	11
Granulocytopenia	17	0	11	4
Thrombocytopenia	7	0	7	0
Blood pressure change	0	0	7	7
Vomiting	41	28	48	37
Azotemia	3	3	0	4
Fever, chill	10	0	56	19

different by Wilcoxon analysis ($p < 0.05$), with regimen A slightly superior to regimen B.

Toxicity differed in each of the regimens (Table 3). Anemia, granulocytopenia, and thrombocytopenia were equal on either regimen. There was no tendency for patients on regimen B to have a decreased frequency of any of these reactions or to have more mild reactions. Vomiting, which was not associated with C. parvum administration, was equal in both regimens. However, hypertension and hypotension were only noted on regimen B. Although fever of mild severity was occasionally noted during cyclophosphamide plus DTIC therapy in patients on regimen A, 75% of patients receiving C. parvum had fever or chills. Two patients declined further therapy because of recurrent chills following C. parvum.

Although azotemia was no more frequent in regimen B, one patient after receiving the fifth dose of C. parvum had fever, chills, hypotension, and cyanosis. He then developed proteinuria with a rise in serum urine nitrogen from 9 to 73 mg/dl. At that time, creatinine clearance was 42 ml/min. He had red blood cell and white cell casts in his urine and decreased levels of C'3. All of these reactions were transient, and the patient's renal function and cardiovascular status returned completely to normal. The only other severe reaction to C. parvum consisted of severe hypotension (blood pressure 50/0), which responded to administration of intravenous cortisteroids and did not recur with subsequent treatments. However, that patient did develop proteinuria with a creatinine clearance of 43 ml/min that improved following discontinuation of therapy.

DISCUSSION

We conclude from the results presented that C. parvum failed to modify the therapeutic effect or hematological toxicity of cyclophosphamide plus DTIC in the management of patients with metastatic malignant melanoma. However, toxicity consisting of fever, chills, hypertension, hypotension, and occasionally azotemia were increased in patients receiving chemotherapy with

C. parvum. Therefore, the addition of *C. parvum* to cyclophosphamide plus DTIC therapy in patients with metastatic malignant melanoma is not recommended.

The failure of an immunomodulator (*C. parvum* in our study) to improve the results of response rate to chemotherapy has been previously observed by Costanzi (4) who found equivalent response rates to 1,3-bis-(2-chloroethyl)-1-nitrosourea (BCNU), hydroxyurea, plus DTIC with or without BCG. In contrast, Reed (13) demonstrated an improvement in the frequency of response of liver and lung metastases in metastatic melanoma if *C. parvum* and an injection of irradiated cultured tumor cells were added to a combination of DTIC, methyl CCNU, plus BCG. Our study failed to demonstrate an increased response rate either in patients with cutaneous and lymph node metastases or in patients with visceral metastases.

It is important to note that there may be other doses, schedules, or routes of administration of *C. parvum* that might produce an increase or decrease in therapeutic results of this or other chemotherapy combinations. However, a dosage of 5 mg/m² given at 1-week intervals between courses of chemotherapy was unsuccessful in this study. It may also be possible that with less tumor burden, (i.e., in an adjuvant setting) our route, dose, and schedule of *C. parvum* injections might enhance the therapeutic effects of cyclophosphamide plus DTIC. The effect of *C. parvum* as an adjuvant to surgery is currently under study in the Southeastern Cancer Study Group.

The results of cyclophosphamide plus DTIC, with or without *C. parvum,* demonstrated an objective response rate that compares favorably with the best reported experience from large, multiinstitutional studies (4,5). It should be noted that despite an overall objective response rate of 30% in our study, our patients were all evaluated at only one time point during their course (3 weeks after the third course of chemotherapy). Additional patients manifested partial antitumor responses but relapsed by the time of evaluation for this study. In addition, on regimen A, one patient with a partial response when evaluated continued chemotherapy and after three additional courses developed a complete remission. Two patients with stable disease on regimen A when evaluated subsequently had partial responses. The subsequent responses are not reflected in the results previously discussed. No patient on regimen B with continuation of chemotherapy plus *C. parvum* had an improvement in the quality of his antitumor response.

The duration of antitumor responses to cyclophosphamide plus DTIC was short. Despite an encouraging duration of survival in patients treated with a combination of BCNU, hydroxyurea, plus DTIC (5), a subsequent preliminary report (4) using the same therapy in the same institutional group produced durations of survival similar to those we observed using cyclophosphamide plus DTIC. Therefore, we conclude in addition that cyclophosphamide plus DTIC produces an objective response rate in metastatic malignant melanoma comparable to the best regimens yet reported from multiinstitutional studies and numerically higher than the reported response rates to DTIC alone (3). Despite this, response rates remain low and durations, remission, and survival remain short.

SUMMARY

In order to determine whether *C. parvum* modified the therapeutic or toxic effects of a chemotherapy regimen in patients with metastatic malignant melanoma, 29 evaluable patients were treated with regimen A, cyclophosphamide 600 mg/m² on day 1 plus DTIC 200 mg/² on days 1 through 5, and 27 patients were treated with regimen B, the same chemotherapy with *C. parvum* 5 mg/m², i.v., on days 8 and 15. Courses were repeated every 3 weeks, and patients were evaluated 3 weeks after the third course. Complete or partial responses were observed in 28% of patients on regimen A and 33% of patients on regimen B. Durations of remission and survival were equal. There was no therapeutic advantage in frequency of response, duration of survival, or length of remission for regimen B when patients were analyzed according to the presence or absence of visceral metastases, pretreatment performance status, or pretreatment evaluation of delayed hypersensitivity. Although myelosuppression was equal in both regimens, blood pressure changes, fever, chills, and azotemia were more frequent and/or more severe in patients on regimen B. Thus cyclophosphamide plus DTIC produces a low to moderate frequency of antitumor response in patients with metastatic malignant melanoma. However, the addition of *C. parvum* does not increase the therapeutic response, but does increase toxicity and is not recommended.

ACKNOWLEDGMENTS

This research was supported by U.S. Public Health Service research grants no. CA-03013, 15584, 03177, 05634, 03227, 16389, 05641, 13249, 15578, 12223, 12640, 17214, 07961, 13232, 17027, 03376, 15241, 19657, 11263, 12283, and FR36.

Ms. Mildred Rosenberg assisted in the preparation of this manuscript.

REFERENCES

1. Band, P. R., Jao-King, C., Urtason, R., and Haraphongse, M. (1975): A Phase I study of intravenous *Corynebacterium parvum* in solid tumors. *Proc. Am. Assoc. Cancer Res.*, 16:9.
2. Carter, S. K., and Livingston, R. B. (1975): Cyclophosphamide in solid tumors. *Cancer Treatment Rev.*, 2:295–322.
3. Comis, R. L., and Carter, S. (1974): Integration of chemotherapy into combined modality therapy of solid tumors. IV. Malignant melanoma. *Cancer Treatment Rev.*, 1:285–304.
4. Costanzi, J. J. (1976): Combination chemoimmunotherapy for disseminated malignant melanoma. *Proc. Am. Soc. Clin. Oncol.*, 17:241.
5. Costanzi, J. J., Vaitkevicius, V. K., Quagliana, J. M., Hoogstraten, B., Coltman,

    C. A., Jr., and Delaney, F. C. (1975): Combination chemotherapy for disseminated malignant melanoma. *Cancer*, 35:342–346.

6. Dimitrov, N. V., Singh, T., Conroy, J., and Suhrland, G. L. (1976): Combination therapy with *C. parvum* and adriamycin in patients with lung carcinoma. *Proc. Am. Soc. Clin. Oncol.*, 17:292.
7. Gardere, S., Hussain, S., and Cowan, D. H. (1972): Treatment of metastatic malignant melanoma with a combination of DTIC, cyclophosphamide and vincristine. *Cancer Chemother. Rep.*, 56:357–361.
8. Haskell, C. M., Ossurio, R. C., Sarna, G. P., and Fahey, J. L. (1976): Chemo-immunotherapy of metastatic breast cancer with *C. parvum:* A double blind randomized trial. *Proc. Am. Soc. Clin. Oncol.*, 17:265.
9. Israel, L., (1974): Nonspecific immunostimulation in bronchogenic cancer. *Scand. J. Respir. Dis. [Suppl.]*, 89:95–105.
10. Israel, L., and Edelstein, R. (1975): Immunological control of cancer. *Lancet*, 1:979–980.
11. Israel, L., Edelstein, R., DePierre, A., and Dimitrov, N. (1975): Daily intravenous infusions of *C. parvum* in 20 patients with disseminated cancer. *J. Natl. Cancer Inst.*, 55:29–33.
12. Israel, L., and Halpern, B. (1972): Le *Corynebacterium parvum* dans les cancers avances. *Nouv. Presse Med.*, 1:19–23.
13. Reed, R. C. (1976): Increased regression of liver and lung metastases by the addition of *C. parvum* to the DTIC, nitrosourea and BCG regimen. *Proc. Am. Assoc. Cancer Res.*, 17:214.

Question and Answer Session

Dr. Rosenberg: Why were one-third of the patients in each of the groups not evaluable?

Dr. Presant: The reason was that while we had 100 patients admitted to the study, only a limited number have been in long enough to be evaluable. We have not lost these patients; it's just too early.

Dr. LoBuglio: How many patients were able to tolerate that *C. parvum* dose? What do your statisticians tell you you can conclude? Can you discern a 50 percent improvement? Twenty percent?

Dr. Presant: The question is, what is the likelihood of missing a difference of 10 percent, or 20 percent, or 30 percent? Since this study, in contrast to some of the other studies that we've heard this morning, is still in progress, we've not taken the time to analyze that question. I think our final communication regarding this treatment program will address itself to that fact. You must realize that these are 28 patients out of a projected roughly 80 patients per treatment that will be evaluated. However, at the current time there is no trend toward a difference.

A Participant: You're using very high doses of *C. parvum* and you reported only 19 percent with chills and fever? Is that correct?

Dr. Presant: Three-quarters of the patients had chills and fever, but in 19 percent they were considered moderate or severe. All patients were premedicated with Tylenol and Benadryl, and these patients did, despite that, have fairly substantial chills and fever at the 5 mg/m² dose.

Three patients refused to take further therapy but most of the patients did tolerate continued therapy fairly well, and as has been observed by other investigators with continued *C. parvum* therapy, there is a gradual amelioration of the degree of side-effects, even though they may still have chills and fever.

A Participant: I'd like to emphasize the danger of evaluating multi-institution clinical trials early. I think that it is dangerous, and there can be fluctuating results.

How do you explain the toxicity of azotemia from either chemotherapy or the combined treatment?

Dr. Presant: The appearance of azotemia with *C. parvum* is something that has been recognized in several clinical trials, and it seems to be an immune nephritis. Complement levels decrease.

A Participant: But you had eight in your chemotherapy?

Dr. Presant: Those were patients who were observed to have an increase in their serum creatinine concentration, decreased creatinine clearance, and increases in BUN. The exact mechanism for this I don't know. Perhaps occasional patients with this particular combination do have some mild reversible decrease in renal function. These were reversible in these patients. I'm not certain what the origin is.

Dr. Powles: In view of your last statement, that the use of *C. parvum* in disseminated melanoma in this study is now not recommended, how can you justify the continuation of this trial?

Dr. Presant: The trial has been concluded, even though the results of the patients who have been entered on the study are not yet in.

Immunotherapy of Cancer: Present Status of
Trials in Man, edited **by W. D. Terry and D. Windhorst.**
Raven Press, New York © 1978.

Active Specific Immunotherapy for Advanced Melanoma Utilizing Neuraminidase-Treated Autochthonous Tumor Cells

Richard L. Simmons, Gerald V. Aranha, [1]Audolfur Gunnarsson, Theodor B. Grage, and Charles F. McKhann

Department of Surgery, University of Minnesota, Minneapolis, Minnesota 55455

We have previously demonstrated that transplantable and spontaneous syngenic solid murine tumors can be made to regress if the mice are challenged with tumor cells treated *in vitro* with *Vibrio cholerae* neuraminidase (VCN) (23). The regression is immunospecific, and the effect is not abrogated by pretreatment of the challenging cells with mitomycin C or irradiation to prevent the growth of the challenging inoculum. The vaccine does not lose potency by storage at $-70°C$ (13). Furthermore, the immunoregressive effect can be augmented by simultaneous inoculations of nonspecific immunostimulants, e.g., *Mycobacterium bovis* strain Bacillus Calmette-Guérin (BCG) (18,19), or by reduction of tumor mass by surgical excision (12) or local irradiation (27). Independent and generally confirmatory results have been achieved by other investigators (2,5). The present studies were designed to determine whether such therapy would be useful adjunctive therapy to the standard treatments of advanced melanoma.

MATERIALS AND METHODS

Patients with histologically proved advanced melanoma presenting at the University of Minnesota hospitals were treated by standard therapy with or without adjuvant immunotherapy. All patients have been followed for a minimum of 6 months and some for as long as 5 years.

There were two groups of patients in this series; patients with stage II melanoma were defined as those patients with regional lymph nodes, clinically, grossly, and histologically involved with metastatic melanoma but without evidence of more widespread disease. Such patients have been classified informally as clinical stage II disease, and their prognosis is generally regarded as far inferior to those patients without palpable involved lymph nodes but with microscopic metastases. Patients with microscopic involvement of regional lymph nodes but without gross evidence of palpable enlarged lymph

---

[1] Present address: Geitland 6, Fossvogur, Reykjavik, Iceland.

TABLE 1. *Schema for randomizing patients with clinical stage II rendered disease free by surgery*

1. Palpable clinically involved regional nodes
2. No dissemination
3. Stratify for sex, age, location, number of nodes
↓
"Surgical cure" by wide local excision
and regional node dissection

No adjuvant therapy   Immunotherapy
(BCG + VCN-treated
autochthonous cells)

nodes were not included in this study. Surgical treatment consisted of wide excision of the primary tumor and standard regional node dissection. All patients were clinically disease free at the termination of the operation. Patients were then randomized according to the scheme in Table 1. Other patients with clinical stage II melanoma were treated surgically but not randomized because of the unavailability of tumor cells that could be used for immunotherapy. Such patients were divided arbitrarily but *not randomly* into two groups consisting of surgery plus BCG or surgery plus chemotherapy as described below.

Patients with stage III melanoma were those with recurrent melanoma in which the recurrence was not limited to the regional lymph nodes or to local skin, i.e., those with brain, lung, liver, diffuse skin, or widespread nodal involvement. All such patients were treated with chemotherapy as described below. Those patients with available tumor tissue for preparation of tumor vaccine were strictly randomized by the scheme in Table 2. Patients who did not have available tumor cells, i.e., those with visceral metastases that would have required major surgery were arbitrarily but *not randomly* assigned to chemotherapy-alone or chemotherapy-plus-BCG treatment groups. In the section on results, such groups and subgroups are strictly distinguished.

TABLE 2. *Schema for randomizing patients with disseminated and recurrent melanoma not limited to one region*

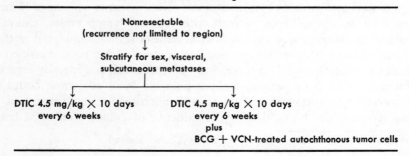

Nonresectable
(recurrence *not* limited to region)
↓
Stratify for sex, visceral,
subcutaneous metastases

DTIC 4.5 mg/kg × 10 days   DTIC 4.5 mg/kg × 10 days
every 6 weeks   every 6 weeks
plus
BCG + VCN-treated autochthonous tumor cells

Chemotherapy was administered to all stage III patients (and a few stage II patients as noted) in the form of imidazole carboxamide (DTIC) 4.5 mg/kg daily i.v. for 10 days at 6-week intervals. This was continued until recurrence of disease or drug toxicity.

Immunotherapy in the randomized studies consisted of *M. bovis* strain BCG with VCN-treated autochthonous tumor cells (Table 3). Some non-randomized patients received BCG without autochthonous vaccine. When BCG was administered it was always administered in the same way to all groups of patients. BCG consisted of the Tice strain (University of Illinois, Chicago, Illinois). Material was said to contain $5 \pm 3 \times 10^8$ colony-forming units (cfu) per vial. The entire contents of the vial were suspended in the smallest possible volume (approximately 0.3 ml) and placed as a drop on the skin. A heaf gun (Pan Ray Corp., Division of Ormont Drug & Chemical Co., Englewood, New Jersey) was utilized for intracutaneous administration of the vaccine. Six shots of the heaf gun were administered through the drop-let containing the entire vial of BCG material. The area was covered with a small piece of gauze that was left in place for 24 hr. BCG therapy was initiated as soon after surgical treatment as possible and always within 2 weeks. The BCG was administered weekly for 6 weeks, biweekly for 12 weeks, and monthly for life. When the heaf gun was not available, the tine technique utilizing the multiple puncture disc with magnet holder (Research Foundation, Chicago, Illinois) was used for inoculation.

Active specific immunotherapy utilized VCN-treated autochthonous cells in all cases. No cultured or allogeneic cells were utilized. The freshly excised tumors were minced and pressed through #45 mesh stainless steel screens in Medium 199 (M199) (Grand Island Biologicals, Grand Island, New York) without addition of trypsin. Cell clumps were then allowed to settle, and the supernatant single-cell suspensions were washed three times in M199 and counted in hemocytometers. Viability was not determined. VCN obtained from Behring Diagnostics (Somerville, New Jersey) is stated to contain 500 units enzyme/ml. (One unit of activity is equivalent to the release of 1 μg of N-acetyl neuraminic acid from a glycoprotein substrate at 37°C for 15 min at pH 5.5.) Numerous authors have previously shown that sialic acid is released

TABLE 3. *Outline of immunotherapy schedule using BCG- and VCN-treated autochthonous cells*

BCG $5 \pm 3 \times 10^8$ cfu—Tice
  Heaf gun
  Weekly $\times$ 6, biweekly $\times$ 6, monthly
VCN-treated autochthonous cells
  10,000 R, acetone-dry ice frozen, stored -70°C
  VCN 25 u/10^7 cells, 37°C, 1 hr
  ID—2×10^8 cells after conversion to PPD
  3 weeks after last chemotherapy

cfu, Colony-forming units; ID, intradermal

from cell surface of normal and malignant cells by VCN at neutral pH without affecting viability of the cell (14,16). Tumor cells in M199 (pH 7.2) were incubated for 1 hr at 37°C with 25 units VCN/ml/10^7 cells. The cells were then irradiated with 10,000 R (rads), snap frozen in acetone dry ice, and stored at −70°C. Cells were stored until skin tests with second strength purified protein derivative (PPD) demonstrated an area of induration 1 cm in diameter. At that time, 2×10^8 stored autochthonous cells were inoculated in multiple intradermal sites over a single area of about 36 cm², and a vial of BCG organisms was spread over the intradermal inoculation and inoculated into the areas directly over the cellular infiltrate with multiple punctures of the heaf gun. When immunotherapy was combined with chemotherapy, the immunotherapy was carried out 3 weeks after the last dose of DTIC. Immunotherapy with autochthonous cells was not carried out unless conversion to PPD had taken place, which usually occurred within 6 weeks of beginning the BCG therapy.

Actuarial survival curves were constructed by the methods of Merrell and Shulman (11).

RESULTS

Stage II Melanoma

Table 4 demonstrates that the randomized and nonrandomized patients with clinically palpable regional lymph nodes were comparable with respect to primary site except for an absence of patients with primaries of the head and neck among those randomized to treatment by surgery alone.

Figure 1 illustrates the actuarial rate of recurrence after "surgical cure" of patients with stage II melanoma. The patients randomized to surgical treatment alone had equivalent periods of disease-free status as those randomized to surgery plus BCG-VCN-treated autochthonous tumor cells. Patients not randomized because insufficient autochthonous tumor cells were available and, therefore, treated with surgery plus BCG or surgery plus DTIC chemotherapy had slightly but not significantly longer disease-free intervals.

The survival of these patients is shown in Fig. 2. Once again,

TABLE 4. *Number of patients with clinical stage II melanoma*

		Extremity (%)	Trunk (%)	Head & neck (%)	Total
Not randomized	Surgery + BCG	3 (21)	8 (57)	3 (21)	14
	Surgery + chemotherapy	4 (36)	5 (45)	2 (18)	11
Randomized	Surgery + BCG + VCN cells	2 (18)	5 (45)	4 (36)	11
	Surgery alone	5 (45)	6 (54)	0 (0)	11

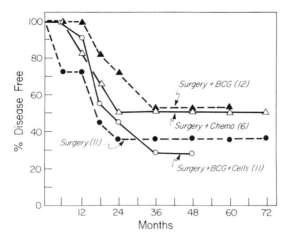

FIG. 1. Duration of disease-free status in patients with clinical stage II melanoma treated by four different arms. Patients treated with surgery alone or with surgery + BCG + cells were strictly stratified and randomized to the two treatment arms. Patients treated with surgery + BCG or with surgery + chemotherapy were not randomized because insufficient tumor cells were available to develop autochthonous tumor vaccine.

randomized to surgery alone or to surgery plus BCG-VCN-treated autochthonous tumor cells did not have significantly different survival rates. Those patients treated with surgery plus chemotherapy or surgery plus BCG (but not randomized) had slightly better but not statistically significant survival rates.

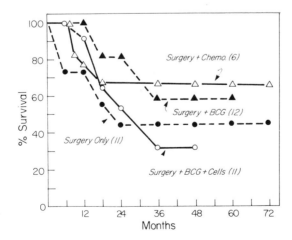

FIG. 2. Actuarial survival of patients with clinical stage II melanoma treated by four different arms. Patients treated with surgery alone or with surgery + BCG + cells were strictly stratified and randomized to the two treatment arms. Patients treated with surgery + BCG or with surgery + chemotherapy were not randomized because insufficient tumor cells were available to develop autochthonous tumor vaccine.

Stage III Melanoma

Figure 3 demonstrates the actuarial patient surival curves for stage III (disseminated) melanoma treated with chemotherapy and/or immunotherapy. This figure includes all the patients seen with stage III melanoma at the University of Minnesota during this period of time including randomized and nonrandomized patients. It is apparent that chemotherapy had some effect on patient survival when compared to five patients who refused all treatment. Neither immunotherapy with BCG nor immunotherapy with BCG plus VCN-treated tumor cells further improved results.

Figure 4 demonstrates the actuarial survival of patients *strictly randomized* to chemotherapy or to chemotherapy plus immunotherapy with BCG-VCN-treated tumor cells. In this analysis all nonrandomized patients were excluded. It is apparent that immunotherapy offered no improvement when compared with chemotherapy with DTIC alone.

Table 5 shows the response rate to chemotherapeutic treatment for patients with stage III disease depending on whether they received chemotherapy, chemotherapy plus BCG, or chemotherapy plus BCG-VCN-treated tumor cells. It is apparent that the response rate did not change with the therapy utilized. Table 6 divides the patients into those with node and subcutaneous

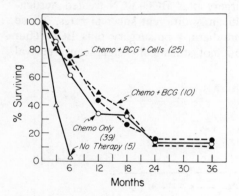

FIG. 3. Actuarial survival of all patients with disseminated melanoma as a function of method of treatment. All patients seen for the past 5 years (minimum follow-up = 6 months) are included.

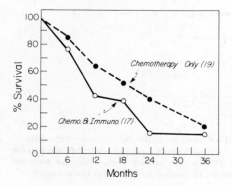

FIG. 4. Actuarial survival of randomized patients with disseminated melanoma treated by chemotherapy alone or by chemotherapy + immunotherapy with BCG + VCN-treated autochthonous tumor cells. Only patients strictly stratified and randomized are included.

TABLE 5. *Response to chemoimmunotherapy in patients with stage III disease according to type of treatment*

	Partial or complete (%)	No change (%)	Progression (%)	Total no. (% response)
Chemotherapy	12 (28)	0 (0)	31 (72)	43 (28)
Chemotherapy + BCG	5 (33)	2 (13)	8 (53)	15 (33)
Chemotherapy + BCG + cells	6 (26)	4 (17)	13 (56)	23 (26)

TABLE 6. *Percent response to chemoimmunotherapy in patients with stage III disease according to site of metastases*

	Node and subcutaneous	Lung	Liver	Brain
Chemotherapy	27 (4/15)	33 (3/9)	0 (0/4)	20 (1/5)
Chemotherapy + BCG	37 (3/8)	0 (0/2)	100 (1/1)	0 (0/4)
Chemotherapy + BCG + cells	25 (5/20)	25 (1/4)	0 (0/0)	0 (0/3)

metastases and those with lung, liver, or brain metastases. Here it is apparent that even when the patients are stratified for site of metastasis the response rate to chemotherapy did not differ depending on whether patients received chemotherapy alone, chemotherapy with BCG, or chemotherapy plus BCG-VCN-treated tumor cells. However, those patients with multiple nodal or subcutaneous metastases showed a higher response rate than those with brain and/or liver metastases.

DISCUSSION

The approach taken in this study is based on experimental observations demonstrating that VCN increases the immunogenicity of cells exposed to it *in vitro:* (a) fetal tissue incubated in VCN and injected into allogeneic recipients results in a greater degree of sensitization of those recipients than of animals injected with fetal tissue exposed to heat-inactivated VCN (17); (b) when nonimmunizing numbers of lymphoid cells were treated with VCN and injected into allogeneic recipients, donor skin grafts were rejected significantly more rapidly (24); (c) cyclophosphamide-prepared mice do not become tolerant of VCN-treated bone marrow cells (6); (d) human lymphocytes treated with VCN and mitomycin are severalfold more stimulating to allogeneic lymphocytes in one-way mixed lymphocyte culture than are lymphocytes treated with mitomycin alone (9,10); and (e) TA-3 tumor (15), Landschutz ascites tumor (3), L1210 leukemia (1), methylcholanthrene-induced fibrosarcoma (4,23,25), and Ehrlich ascites tumors (8) grow less well in normally susceptible recipients if the tumor cells have been incubated in VCN. Recipients that survive the primary tumor inoculum are rendered immune to subsequent inocula of untreated cells (4,8,25). We have shown that total immunospecific regression of firmly established methylcholanthrene fibrosarcomas and mammary tumors (26) can be induced by challenging the tumor-bearing animals with syngeneic tumor cells treated *in vitro* with VCN. The effect was shown to be due to the enzymatic action of VCN on the sialic acid residues of the tumor cell surfaces since heat-inactivation of the VCN or incubation of VCN and tumor cells with an excess of sialic acid or neuraminilactose (22) destroyed the ability of such cells to induce tumor regression (23). Similar results in murine leukemia systems have been obtained by Bekesi et al. (2) and Kollmorgan et al. (7).

Our approach here is based on two additional findings. First, the curative effect of VCN-treated tumor cells can be augmented by total or near-total excision of advanced transplantable mammary tumors or methylcholanthrene-induced fibrosarcomas (12). Excision of spontaneous mammary carcinomas in C3H/HeJ mice plus vaccination with VCN-treated autochthonous tumor cells markedly prolonged the survival of such mice treated by surgery alone (26). Local tumor irradiation plus VCN-treated tumor cells leads to better survival of mice than those treated with irradiation alone (27). Thus, the reduction of the mass of tumor to a minimal level permits this kind of active specific immunotherapy to work. The converse is also true. VCN-treated tumor cells are not effective once the tumors have reached any appreciable size. The critical size in mice appears to be a tumor of approximately 1 cm in diameter. Even subtotal excision leaving a rim of tumor will not be cured by VCN-treated tumor cells after excision of sizable tumors. These findings suggest one reason for the failure of the current experiments to demonstrate any prolongation of disease-free interval in patients with advanced melanoma. Patients with clinically, grossly, and histologically involved lymph nodes such as those treated as stage II tumors in this study have relatively short intervals of freedom from clinical disease. Such patients presumably already have extensive microscopic metastases and might be expected not to be good candidates for immunotherapy.

For the same reason, patients with stage III melanoma may not be good candidates for immunotherapy. The tumors are already widespread and diffuse; responses to DTIC chemotherapy have traditionally been poor, and total regression is rare. We and others have demonstrated that it is difficult to combine chemotherapy and immunotherapy effectively in immunotherapeutic animal model systems (20). In fact, we have been unable to demonstrate augmentation of the chemotherapeutic effect of any tumor with VCN-treated tumor cells even in animals that have good chemotherapeutic responses (*unpublished observations*). The correct choice of drug, dose of drug, and sequence of chemotherapy-immunotherapy that both reduces tumor mass and permits an appropriate immune response has not been found. Our choice to wait until immunologic competence was demonstrated by reactivity to PPD may not have been the best one by which to facilitate responses to the VCN-treated tumor cells. A similar argument could be brought to bear on the method of administration, the number of tumor cells given, their route of administration, their use of BCG, etc., and other critical variables in the experimental group that can not be systematically varied in a study involving fewer than several hundred patients.

Although challenge with VCN-treated tumor cells causes the regression of small transplantable and spontaneous tumors or larger tumors that have been reduced in size by surgery and radiation therapy, all tumors do not respond to this kind of treatment (22,25). It may be that the melanoma in man is a poor choice for treatment. It was chosen because of its availability and its rather prolonged course in its early stages, but its capacity to disseminate may make it difficult to cure once metastases become clinically apparent.

The use of autochthonous cells for active specific immunotherapy was governed by our finding that the response to VCN-treated tumor cells in tumor-bearing animals is highly specific. For example, VCN-treated mammary tumors that share mammary tumor virus-associated antigens will not cure each other, whereas VCN-treated cells will cause the regression of autochthonous tumors in the same mice (21). In contrast, Holland and Bekesi (5) have used allogeneic cells in experimental leukemias with success and utilize VCN-treated allogeneic leukemia cells in their human studies. Our use of autochthonous tumor vaccines imposes a severe burden on these patients and makes study of such an immunotherapeutic modality difficult. Patients with disseminated disease frequently do not have available tumor that can be excised with ease. If fresh tumor were required, repeated operations would be necessary. We have demonstrated in mice, at least, that freezing and storing VCN-treated autochthonous tumor cells does not reduce their immunogenicity (13), but this may not be true of human tumors. The technique using autochthonous cells is therefore cumbersome, and it would be preferable to use lines of cultured tumor cells if such cells could be shown to express critical cross-reactive antigens.

Active specific immunotherapy utilizing autochthonous cells has an additional disadvantage. In order to obtain sufficient cells for *in vitro* treatment and reinjection, only patients with grossly involved lymph nodes can be utilized. Such patients already have such a poor prognosis, presumably due to further dissemination beyond the nodal group, that they are less than ideal candidates for this kind of treatment. It would be much better to utilize patients with microscopic metastases, but the proof of microscopic metastases is not available until the tumor itself is destroyed by histologic study. For this reason, again, fresh or cultured allogeneic tumor cells would be far superior for the treatment of patients with minimal residual disease.

For these reasons, the future of active specific immunotherapy utilizing autochthonous tumors must remain in doubt, and although further study of this modality might possibly demonstrate efficacy, the clinical approach probably should be abandoned. If other studies demonstrate that fresh or cultured allogeneic cells share those tumor antigens essential to induce tumor regression or if autochthonous tumors can be reproducibly and reliably cultured without loss of immunogenicity, the technique should be revived.

ACKNOWLEDGMENT

This work was supported by contract NO1-CB-23885 from the National Cancer Institute, National Institutes of Health.

REFERENCES

1. Bagshawe, K. D., and Currie, G. A. (1968): Immunogenicity of L1210 murine leukemia cells after treatment with neuraminidase. *Nature,* 218:1254–1255.
2. Bekesi, J. G., St-Arneault, G., and Holland, J. F. (1971): Increase of leukemia L1210 immunogenicity by *Vibrio cholerae* neuraminidase treatment. *Cancer Res.,* 31:2130–2132.
3. Currie, G. A., and Bagshawe, K. D. (1968): The role of sialic acid in antigenic expression: Further studies of the Landschutz ascites tumour. *Br. J. Cancer,* 22:843–853.
4. Currie, G. A., and Bagshawe, K. D. (1969): Tumor-specific immunogenicity of methylcholanthrene-induced sarcoma cells after incubation in neuraminidase. *Br. J. Cancer,* 23:141–149.
5. Holland, J. F., and Bekesi, J. G. (1976): Immunotherapy of human leukemia with neuraminidase modified cells. *Med. Clin. North Am.,* 60:539–549.
6. Im, H. M., and Simmons, R. L. (1971): Modification of graft-versus-host disease by neuraminidase treatment of donor cells: Decreased tolerogenicity of neuraminidase-treated cells. *Transplantation,* 12:472–478.
7. Kollmorgen, G. M., Erwin, D. N., Killion, J. J., Hoge, A. F., and Sansing, W. A. (1973): Combination chemotherapy and immunotherapy of transplantable murine leukemia. *Proc. Am. Assoc. Cancer Res.,* 14:69.
8. Lindemann, J., and Klein, P. A. (1967): Immunological aspects of viral oncolysis. *Recent Results Cancer Res.,* 9:66–67.
9. Lundgren, G., Jeitz, L., Lundin, L., and Simmons, R. L. (1971): Increased stimulation by neuraminidase treated cells in mixed lymphocyte cultures. *Fed. Proc.,* 30:395.
10. Lundgren, G., and Simmons, R. L. (1971): Effect of neuraminidase on the stimulatory capacity of cells in human mixed lymphocyte cultures. *Clin. Exp. Immunol.,* 9:915–926.
11. Merrell, M., and Shulman, L. E. (1955): Determination of prognosis in chronic disease, illustrated by systemic lupus erythematosus. *J. Chronic Dis.,* 1:12–32.
12. Rios, A., and Simmons, R. L. (1974): Active-specific immunotherapy of minimal residual tumors: Excision plus neuraminidase treated tumor cells. *Int. J. Cancer,* 13:71–81.
13. Rios, A., and Simmons, R. L. (1974): Experimental cancer immunotherapy using a neuraminidase treated non-viable frozen tumor vaccine. *Surgery,* 75:503–507.
14. Rosenberg, S. A., and Einstein, A. B. (1972): Sialic acids on the plasma membrane of cultured human lymphoid cells: Chemical aspects of biosynthesis. *J. Cell. Biol.,* 53:466–473.
15. Sanford, B. H. (1967): An alteration in tumor histocompatibility induced by neuraminidase. *Transplantation,* 4:1273–1279.
16. Sanford, B. H., and Codington, J. F. (1971): Further studies on the effect of neuraminidase on tumor cell transplantability. *Tissue Antigens,* 1:153–161.
17. Simmons, R. L., Lipschultz, M. L., Rios, A., and Ray, P. K. (1971): Failure of neuraminidase to unmask histocompatibility antigens on trophoblast. *Nature,* 231:111–112.
18. Simmons, R. L., and Rios, A. (1971): Immunotherapy of cancer: Immunospecific

rejection of tumors in recipients of neuraminidase-treated tumor cells plus BCG. *Science,* 174:591–593.

19. Simmons, R. L., and Rios, A. (1972): Immunospecific regression of methylcholanthrene fibrosarcoma using neuraminidase. II. Intratumor injections of neuraminidase. *Surgery,* 71:556–564.

20. Simmons, R. L., and Rios, A. (1973): Immunospecific regression of methylcholanthrene fibrosarcoma using neuraminidase. IV. Chemotherapeutic agents reverse the effects of tumor immunotherapy. *Bull. Bell Museum Pathol.,* 3:28–30.

21. Simmons, R. L., and Rios, A. (1973): Differential effect of neuraminidase on the immunogenicity of viral associated and private antigens of mammary carcinomas. *J. Immunol.,* 111:1820–1825.

22. Simmons, R. L., and Rios, A. (1974): Immunospecific regression of methylcholanthrene fibrosarcoma with the use of neuraminidase. V. Quantitative aspects of the experimental immunotherapeutic model. *Isr. J. Med. Sci.,* 10:925–938.

23. Simmons, R. L., Rios, A., Lundgren, G., Ray, P. K., McKhann, C. F., and Haywood, G. R. (1971): Immunospecific regression of methylcholanthrene fibrosarcoma with the use of neuraminidase. *Surgery,* 70:38–46.

24. Simmons, R. L., Rios, A., and Ray, P. K. (1971): Immunogenicity and antigenicity of lymphoid cells treated with neuraminidase. *Nature,* 231:179–181.

25. Simmons, R. L., Rios, A., Ray, P. K. and Lundgren, G. (1971): Effect of neuraminidase on the growth of methylcholanthrene fibrosarcoma in normal and immunosuppressed syngeneic mice. *J. Natl. Cancer Inst.,* 47:1087–1094.

26. Simmons, R. L., Rios, A., and Trites, P. (1976): Modified tumor cells in the immunotherapy of solid mammary tumors. *Med. Clin. North Am.,* 60:551–565.

27. So, S. K. S., Song, C. W., Rios, A., and Simmons, R. L. (1977): The combined effect of radiotherapy and neuraminidase-treated tumor cells on 3-methylcholanthrene-induced fibrosarcoma. *J. Surg. Oncol.,* (November).

Question and Answer Session

Dr. Rosenberg: Were stage III patients treated with autologous treated cells as well?

Dr. Simmons: Yes, the reason we went to autologous cells was because the data in mice indicated that autologous cells were useful.

*Immunotherapy of Cancer: Present Status of
Trials in Man,* edited by W. D. Terry and D. Windhorst.
Raven Press, New York © 1978.

Serotherapy of Malignant Melanoma

Peter W. Wright, Karl Erik Hellström, Ingegerd Hellström,
*Glenn Warner, Ross Prentice, and **Robert F. Jones

*Division of Tumor Immunology and Program in Epidemiology and Biostatistics, Fred
Hutchinson Cancer Research Center, Seattle, Washington 98104; *Tumor Institute,
Swedish Hospital Medical Center, Seattle, Washington 98104; and **Department of
Medicine, Division of Oncology, and Department of Surgery, University of
Washington School of Medicine, Seattle Washington 98104*

Interest in the serotherapy of malignant melanoma has existed from the early report of Sumner and Foraker demonstrating complete regression of metastatic malignant melanoma in a patient receiving 250 ml of whole blood from a donor who had previously undergone a spontaneous regression of melanoma (13). A similar experience was later reported by Teimoorian and McCune (14). These sporadic case reports and more recent evidence for reactivity to melanoma-associated antigens *in vitro* have prompted a more systematic evaluation of serotherapy in patients with malignant melanoma. The rationale for our studies has been based on the observation that lymphocytes from melanoma patients usually show significant cytotoxicity against melanoma target cells *in vitro*. Cytotoxicity has been demonstrated in patients with varying stages of disease, although the cytotoxicity of lymphocytes in patients with advanced disease may be quantitatively depressed compared to patients with more localized tumor or those with no evident disease (5). Measurement of serum-blocking activity *in vitro* has been shown to parallel disease activity (5,8). Significant serum-blocking activity has been detected in a majority of patients with clinically evident disease. By contrast, serum-blocking activity has been infrequently present in patients considered to be clinically in remission. This correlation between a patient's clinical course and the measurement of serum-blocking activity has suggested that serum-blocking factors that specifically inhibit cellular immune responses *in vitro* may exert a similar effect *in vivo,* serving to prevent immunologic destruction of tumor cells.

This postulate has been strengthened by the demonstration of "unblocking" activity in the serum of a patient who had undergone a spontaneous regression of melanoma. Sera from this patient could be shown to specifically counteract the blocking effect of serum taken from other patients with evident melanoma (6). Thus, the possibility was raised that transfer of such sera to a patient with evident tumor might have some potential therapeutic benefit.

The chance observation that plasma from normal black (North American Negro) donors usually had unblocking activity to melanoma-associated antigens with a specificity identical to that observed in melanoma patients who had undergone spontaneous regression of their tumor (7) has allowed procurement of plasma with unblocking activity in sufficient amounts to undertake a clinical trial to evaluate the potential efficacy of such plasma in patients with malignant melanoma.

PATIENTS AND TREATMENT

In an initial trial, patients with regional lymph node involvement (stage II) or disseminated (stage III) melanoma were randomly allocated to treatment with either (a) Bacillus Calmette-Guerin (BCG) scarification and unblocking (black) plasma, (b) BCG scarification and normal (Caucasian) plasma, or (c) "conventional" therapy. Conventional therapy included no treatment in patients with stage II disease or treatment with surgery, radiotherapy, or chemotherapy (but no form of immunotherapy) in patients with stage III disease. The plasma was coded and administered in a "blind" fashion, its source unknown to anyone associated with the clinical trial. This particular design was selected not only because it would presumably allow for an evaluation of the effect of treatment with unblocking (black) versus normal plasma, but also because it would provide a comparison between groups receiving BCG and no form of immunotherapy. Patients with stage II disease or stage III disease with no clinically evident tumor at the time of randomization received immunotherapy consisting of plasma, 250 ml intravenously, and BCG scarification (Tice strain, 10^8 colony forming units (CFU) per dose) on alternate weeks. Stage III patients with nonresectable disease at the time of randomization received the same immunotherapy and systemic chemotherapy with dimethyl triazeno imidazole carboxamide (DTIC) in standard doses. Patients were stratified for several important prognostic factors that included

TABLE 1. *Serotherapy of malignant melanoma*

	Stage	Stratification	Therapy
Pretherapy evaluation + surgery	II	± ≥ 3 Involved nodes	Protocol schedule A 1 BCG + UBP 2 BCG + NP
	III$_{NED}$	± Visceral disease − Evident disease	Protocol schedule A 1 BCG + UBP 2 BCG + NP
	III$_{ED}$	± Visceral disease + Evident disease	Protocol schedule B 1 DTIC + BCG + UBP 2 DTIC + BCG + NP

UBP, unblocking (black) plasma; NP, normal Caucasian plasma. NED, no evident disease; ED, evident disease.

age, sex, stage, site of primary tumor, and evident tumor at the time of randomization.

Between July 1, 1973 and December 31, 1974, 42 patients (15 patients receiving BCG + coded plasma 1, 12 patients receiving BCG + coded plasma 2, and 15 patients receiving conventional therapy) were entered on this protocol. A second protocol was activated in January, 1975. The design of this second study was identical to the first, except that the conventional nonimmunotherapy control arm was discontinued. The treatment scheme is shown in Table 1. An additional 66 patients (41 stage II, and 25 stage III; 34 BCG + coded plasma 1, and 32 BCG + coded plasma 2 patients) have been entered on the second protocol through June 10, 1976.

STATISTICAL ANALYSIS AND RESULTS

The current analysis was based on the 108 evaluable patients included in both protocols. The follow-up time varies from 36 to 1 month. Additional descriptors of the population studied are included in Table 2. The median times to objective progression and median survival times by treatment and stage for all patients are shown in Table 3. These data show most dramatically the effect of evident or residual disease on patients compared with patients who are tumor free at the time of randomization. For example, of 34 patients with evident disease at the time of randomization, 30 had objective tumor progression and 24 died during the period of observation. By contrast,

TABLE 2. *Description of patient population*

		Control	BCG + plasma (1)	BCG + plasma (2)
Treatment		15	49	44
Progressions		11	26	23
Deaths		8	15	15
Stage				
II	58			
III	50			
Evident disease at randomization				
No	74			
Yes	34			
Age				
≥ 45	38			
< 45	70			
Sex				
F	46			
M	62			
Site				
Trunk	64			
Extremity	28			
Unspecified	16			

TABLE 3. *Median progression and survival time estimates (months)*

	All 108 patients			66 Patients not progressing in first 3 months		
	Control	BCG + PI (1)	BCG + PI (2)	Control	BCG + PI (1)	BCG + PI (2)
Objective Progression						
Stage II	20.8	15.3	8.3	20.8	15.3	> 8.3
	(3/7)	(10/26)	(10/25)	(3/7)	(5/19)	(7/20)
Stage III	1.9	2.5	3.1	5.5	11.4	14.8
	(8/8)	(16/23)	(13/19)	(3/3)	(3/7)	(4/10)
Stage III ⎰No residual ⎱ disease	—	> 11.4	14.8	—	> 11.4	14.8
	(0/0)	(3/9)	(4/7)	(0/0)	(1/5)	(2/5)
Stage III ⎰Residual ⎱ disease	1.9	1.4	2.3	5.5	4.2	> 4.5
	(8/8)	(13/14)	(9/12)	(3/3)	(2/2)	(2/5)
Survival						
Stage II	29.9	> 8.9	> 14.9	29.9	> 8.9	> 14.9
	(1/7)	(4/26)	(5/25)	(1/7)	(2/19)	(2/20)
Stage III	6.3	11.7	9.1	13.4	> 13.3	11.0
	(7/8)	(11/23)	(10/29)	(2/3)	(1/7)	(2/10)
Stage III ⎰No residual ⎱ disease	—	> 13.3	> 6.6	—	> 13.3	> 6.6
	(0/0)	(2/9)	(2/7)	(0/0)	(0/5)	(0/5)
Stage III ⎰Residual ⎱ disease	6.3	4.9	6.6	13.4	> 6.7	11.0
	(7/8)	(9/14)	(8/12)	(2/3)	(1/2)	(2/5)

The number of progressions or deaths and the number of individuals at risk are indicated as a ratio in parentheses below each median estimate. The "greater than" sign indicates that the number of progressions or deaths was too small to obtain the "product-limit estimate" of the median.

PI, plasma.

of 16 patients with no evident disease at the time of randomization, seven had objective tumor progression and only two died during the same interval. The median survival time was only 5.7 months for patients with evident disease and > 14 months for patients with no evident disease at the time of randomization. No significant differences for either progression or survival are noted among the various treatment groups. A similar analysis undertaken for the 66 patients in all stages who were followed for a minimal period of 3 months before progression resulted in similar conclusions.

In Table 4, the data are presented in terms of the estimated mean time to progression or death. The quantities shown represent the total accumulated time to progression or death divided by the number of progressions or deaths that have actually occurred during the study interval. The conclusions drawn from this analysis are similar to those mentioned in discussion of Table 3.

A more formal comparison of the treatments was undertaken using the regression model of Cox (4). This approach supposes that progression or death rates can be written as a multiplicative function of prognostic factors (stage, age, evident disease, sex, and treatment were used in the present analysis) and uses the data to estimate the multiplicative effect of each factor

TABLE 4. *Estimated mean times to progression and death (months)*

	All 108 patients			66 Patients not progressing in first 3 months		
	Control	BCG + PI (1)	BCG + PI (2)	Control	BCG + PI (1)	BCG + PI (2)
Objective progression						
Stage II	36.5	20.0	19.8	36.5	37.1	26.3
	(3/7)	(10/26)	(10/25)	(3/7)	(5/19)	(7/20)
Stage III	2.7	8.4	10.5	5.1	36.3	30.9
	(8/8)	(16/23)	(13/19)	(3/3)	(3/7)	(4/10)
Stage III { No residual disease	— (0/0)	36.6 (3/9)	22.7 (4/7)	— (0/0)	100.3 (1/5)	43.8 (2/5)
Stage III { Residual disease	2.7 (8/8)	1.9 (13/14)	5.1 (9/12)	5.1 (3/3)	4.3 (2/2)	18.0 (2/5)
Survival						
Stage II	142.4	68.3	51.1	142.4	104.7	107.8
	(1/7)	(4/26)	(5/25)	(1/7)	(2/19)	(2/20)
Stage III	10.2	18.4	18.6	23.3	124.9	75.1
	(7/8)	(11/23)	(10/29)	(2/3)	(1/7)	(2/10)
Stage III { No residual disease	— (0/10)	65.7 (2/9)	58.2 (2/7)	— (0/0)	103.9 (0/5)	105.8 (0/5)
Stage III { Residual disease	10.2 (7/8)	7.9 (9/14)	8.7 (8/12)	23.3 (2/3)	21.0 (1/2)	22.2 (2/5)

PI, plasma.

in reference to the others. For example, using this approach it is possible to estimate the effect of treatment on the progression or death rate while other factors such as stage, evident disease, etc., are taken into account. Such an analysis was carried out for (a) all 108 evaluable patients, (b) the 66 patients receiving therapy for 3 months or more before progression, (c) the 58 stage II patients alone, and (d) the 46 stage II patients receiving therapy for 3 months or more before progression. The results of this analysis are included in Table 5. The significance of the value of each coefficient listed can be determined by comparing the absolute value of the coefficient with its standard error. For example, with objective progression and all 108 patients, the coefficient 1.02 opposite age can be interpreted by the ratio 1.02/0.33 = 3.09. Ratios of the coefficient to standard error that exceed 2.57, 1.96, and 1.65 in absolute value are significant at the 1, 5, and 10% levels, respectively. Since 3.09 exceeds 2.57, age is shown to be a significant factor in progression at the 1% level of significance. Using this approach, it can be seen that analysis of objective progression for all 108 patients also demonstrates that male patients also have a significantly higher progression rate than females. Residual disease at the time of randomization has a dramatic effect in all analyses.

Using this approach, no significant differences in progression rate were observed among treatment groups, although the progression rates of both

TABLE 5. *Regression analysis of times to progression and death (all 108 patients)*

	All 108 patients		66 Patients without early progression		58 Stage II patients		46 Stage II patients without early progression	
	Coefficient	SD	Coefficient	SD	Coefficient	SD	Coefficient	SD
Objective progression								
Age ($<$ 45 vs. $\geq$ 45)	1.02	0.33	1.07	0.53	0.95	0.56	0.33	0.61
Sex (F vs. M)	0.68	0.29	0.78	0.46	0.28	0.46	0.58	0.58
Stage (II vs. III)	0.36	0.46	−0.08	0.69	—		—	
Residual disease								
(No vs. Yes)	1.95	0.47	2.13	0.80	—		—	
Control vs. BCG + PI(1)	0.61	0.39	0.28	0.62	0.74	0.66	0.14	0.76
Control vs. BCG + PI(2)	0.29	0.39	0.22	0.54	0.64	0.67	0.42	0.71
BCG + PI(1) vs. BCG + PI(2)	−0.33	0.29	−0.06	0.49	−0.10	0.45	0.28	0.59
Survival								
Age ($<$ 45 vs. $\geq$ 45)	0.19	0.37	−0.41	0.80	−0.04	0.70		
Sex (F vs. M)	1.22	0.37	1.60	0.77	1.03	0.61		
Stage (II vs. III)	0.20	0.63	—		—		(Too few deaths	
Residual disease							for this	
(No vs. Yes)	2.39	0.62	2.54	0.77	—		analysis)	
Control vs. BCG + PI(1)	0.47	0.48	−0.29	1.14	0.54	1.16		
Control vs. BCG + PI(2)	0.55	0.48	0.30	0.95	1.03	1.14		
BCG + PI(1) vs. BCG + PI(2)	0.08	0.37	0.59	0.82	0.49	0.71		

PI, plasma; SD, standard deviation.

immunotherapies are in the direction of being larger than those of controls and an overall test for equality of progression rates in all three treatments is just significant at the 10% level (Chi square = 4.2). A comparison of the two immunotherapy (BCG + coded plasma 1 versus BCG + coded plasma 2) groups shows no significant differences in any of the analyses conducted. Thus, there is no evidence to favor one immunotherapy regimen over the other. The regression analyses based on time to death yield similar results with regard to treatment comparison.

Even though these present data are not suggestive of a difference in effect between the two immunotherapies, it should be noted that the numbers of patients entered in the trial to date are too small to exclude potential treatment differences of substantial magnitude. For example, objective progression has been observed in only 23 of 50 or 40% of stage II patients. Analysis based on this small patient sample is consistent with treatment differences that range between a 40% reduction or 40% increase in progression rates for BCG + plasma 1 versus BCG + plasma 2. An additional 29 stage II patients (86 total patients) would have to be randomized with complete follow-up to determine that a difference greater than 25% did not exist between the progression rates for the two treatment groups (at the 90% level of confidence).

TOXICITY

No unexpected toxicity was encountered in patients receiving BCG scarification (11). Significant systemic febrile responses (temperature $\geq 101°F$) were observed infrequently. BCG was discontinued in two patients because of persistent marked local and systemic reactions to scarification. Disseminated BCG infection was not observed. Mild immediate hypersensitivity reactions (hives) associated with plasma infusion were encountered frequently and were usually responsive to treatment with antihistamines. Two patients, however, developed significant hypotension associated with plasma infusions, and one required hospitalization. No anaphylactic deaths were observed. Clinical hepatitis was encountered in five patients. Transient liver function abnormalities were noted in an additional six patients. No patient has developed persistent liver function abnormalities. The development of clinical hepatitis, however, represents the most significant risk of the treatment regimen.

DISCUSSION

The present study reveals no significant differences to date in progression rates or survival in patients with malignant melanoma receiving unblocking (black) plasma as compared to control Caucasian plasma. Despite this negative conclusion, the results of our experience have several practical implications for future serotherapy trials.

1. Future serotherapy trials in man should be based on the best available animal model tumor systems. For example, Hersey has recently described methods for producing xenogeneic antisera that were rendered specific after appropriate adsorption for antigens expressed on leukemic, but not normal, rat cells. Administration of this antiserum had a clear antileukemic effect *in vivo* (9). Procedures described by Hersey could well be adapted for the production of antisera to human leukemic cell lines and would seem to provide intelligent guidelines were such an approach adopted in the treatment of human leukemia.

2. Future serotherapy trials should include *in vitro* monitoring. The specific immunologic activity of the serum should be determined prior to, and at various times after, its administration. For example, Sjögren and co-workers have shown inhibition of growth of primary polyoma virus-induced tumors in W/Fu rats treated with an unblocking antipolyoma serum. Sufficient amounts of the serum were administered to result in the disappearance of blocking activity and the appearance of unblocking activity in serum recipients demonstrable by *in vitro* assays (1,2).

3. Attempts should be made in the future to better characterize and hopefully concentrate antibodies responsible for antitumor effects *in vivo*. Antiserum obtained from tumor-immune rats and mice have been shown to contain factors capable of either retarding or accelerating tumor growth *in vivo*.

Fractionation of these sera has been required to isolate those antibodies responsible for tumor growth inhibition (3,10). Fractionation of tumor sera, isolation and concentration of those antibodies responsible for inhibition of tumor growth *in vivo,* and removal of serum factors that could potentially result in enhancement of tumor growth may substantially increase the efficacy of such serum preparations. For example, fractionation of sera from rats bearing polyoma virus-induced sarcomas or carcinogen-induced carcinomas of the colon has shown that serum-blocking activity is associated with IgG. Removal of IgG from serum by immunoadsorbents has shown that the adsorbed serum has no blocking activity but retains specific unblocking activity (12). Utilization of selected immunoadsorbents on a larger scale may provide a simple means of preparation of antisera for future serotherapy trials.

4. Serotherapy in man must be considered experimental. If serum therapy is to be given at all, such treatment must be given under defined, well-controlled circumstances. The potential efficacy of serotherapy is unknown and will remain so until competent, controlled trials are conducted.

SUMMARY

The effect of administration of "unblocking" plasma from normal black donors was compared to that of control Caucasian plasma in a prospective, randomized, double-blind trial in patients with stage II (regional lymph node involvement) and stage III (disseminated) melanoma. Stage II patients and stage III patients with no clinically evident disease at randomization received plasma and BCG scarification on alternate weeks. Stage III patients with non-resectable disease received the same immunotherapy, combined with systemic chemotherapy (DTIC). A conventional nonimmunotherapy control group was included in the first year of study. One hundred and eight evaluable patients (58 stage II and 50 stage III patients) were studied. No difference in progression rate or survival was observed in patients receiving unblocking plasma compared to control plasma. Similarly, no differences have been observed when patients receiving immunotherapy were compared with patients in a nonimmunotherapy control group. The numbers of patients included in the study to date have been too small, however, to exclude potential treatment differences of substantial magnitude.

ACKNOWLEDGMENTS

This investigation was supported by contract number NO1-CB-64018, awarded by the National Cancer Institute, Department of Health, Education, and Welfare. A portion of this work was conducted through the Clinical Research Center of the University of Washington, supported by National Institutes of Health grant number RR-37.

The authors gratefully acknowledge the support and varied contributions made to our immunotherapy program by Drs. William B. Hutchinson, Fred Hutchinson Cancer Research Center; Roger Moe, University of Washington; Dennis Donohue, Puget Sound Blood Center; H. Clark Hoffman, Swedish Hospital; and Edmund R. Clarke, Jr., Group Health Cooperative of Puget Sound, Seattle, Washington.

The plasma used in this program was provided by volunteer donors through the cooperation of the Puget Sound Blood Center, a National Demonstration Center of the National Heart, Lung, and Blood Institute.

REFERENCES

1. Bansal, S. C., and Sjögren, H. O. (1971): "Unblocking" serum activity in vitro in the polyoma system may correlate with antitumor effects of antiserum in vivo. *Nature [New Biol.]*, 233:76–78.
2. Bansal, S. C., and Sjögren, H. O. (1972): Counteraction of the blocking of cell-mediated tumor immunity by inoculation of unblocking sera and splenectomy: Immunotherapeutic effects on primary polyoma tumors in rats. *Int. J. Cancer*, 9:490–509.
3. Bubenik, J., and Koldovsky, P. (1965): Factors influencing the induction of enhancement and resistance to methylcholanthrene-induced tumours in a syngeneic system. *Folia Biol. (Praha)*, 1: 258–265.
4. Cox, D. R. (1972): Regression models and life-tables (B). *J. R. Stat. Soc.*, 34:187–202.
5. Hellström, I., and Hellström, K. E. (1973): Some recent studies on cellular immunity to human melanomas. *Fed. Proc.*, 32:156–159.
6. Hellström, I., Hellström, K. E., Sjögren, H. O., and Warner, G. A. (1971): Serum factors in tumor-free patients cancelling the blocking of cell-mediated tumor immunity. *Int. J. Cancer*, 8:185–191.
7. Hellström, I., Hellström, K. E., Sjögren, H. O., and Warner, G. A. (1973): Destruction of cultivated melanoma cells by lymphocytes from healthy Black (North American Negro) donors. *Int. J. Cancer*, 11:116–122.
8. Hellström, I., Warner, G. A., Hellström, K. E., and Sjögren, H. O. (1973): Sequential studies on cell-mediated tumor immunity and blocking serum activity in ten patients with malignant melanoma. *Int. J. Cancer*, 11:280–292.
9. Hersey, P. (1973): New look at antiserum therapy of leukemia. *Nature [New Biol.]*, 344:23–24.
10. Möller, G. (1974): Effect on tumor growth in syngeneic recipients of antibodies against tumor-specific antigens in methylcholanthrene-induced mouse sarcomas. *Nature*, 204:846–847.
11. Sparks, F. C. (1976): Hazards and complications of BCG immunotherapy. *Med. Clin. N. Am.*, 60:499–509.
12. Steele, G., Jr., Ankerst, J., and Sjögren, H. O. (1974): Alterations of in vitro antitumor activity of tumor-bearing sera by absorption with Staphylococcus aurea, Cowan 1. *Int. J. Cancer*, 14:83–92.
13. Sumner, W. C., and Foraker, A. G. (1960): Spontaneous regression of human melanomas: Clinical and experimental studies. *Cancer*, 13:79–81.
14. Teimoorian, B., and McCune, W. S. (1963): Surgical management of malignant melanoma. *Am. Surg.*, 29:515–519.

DISCUSSION: DISSEMINATED MELANOMA

Dr. Rosenberg: In the second set of reports on melanoma, all of the authors, with the exception of one, have reported negative trials in the use of immunotherapy in patients with disseminated disease (Table 1). I'd like to try to pinpoint those factors that may be involved in obtaining a positive result in the hands of one investigator and negative results in others.

In your study, Dr. Constanzi, with almost 100 patients in each group, there appears to be no difference between patients receiving any of the regimens. BCG seems to add nothing to your three-drug regimen. A similar result was obtained when *C. parvum* was added to the combination of DTIC + cytoxan. No significant differences were found. In Dr. Hersh's study, however, BCG + DTIC appeared better than DTIC alone.

Now I'd like to ask the members of the panel to address the fact that in the one nonrandomized study, we are seeing positive effects of immunotherapy but we are not seeing them in very large randomized prospective trials.

Dr. Hersh: Our patient groups were comparable to those of Dr. Costanzi's as far as we could determine. We compared our patients to his patients and found them to be essentially identical.

I think that Dr. Costanzi's study is large enough to overcome any of the usual problems with randomized trials. From the point of view of being convinced that BCG immunotherapy is beneficial in metastatic melanoma, one looks at the BHD-BCG study and asks the question: what are the factors in that study which interfered with the activity of BCG? We are becoming more and more aware that there are interactions between the immunotherapeutic agents and the chemotherapeutic agents, one area being an effect on the hepatic microsomal enzyme function. But beyond that, I really can't say—I can't see any other basic ingredients which have resulted in one study being positive and one being negative.

TABLE 1. *General discussion of disseminated melanoma*

Treatment	Response Rate	Remission Duration	Survival	Author
BHD ± BCG or DTIC + BCG	No change	No change	No change	Costanzi
Methyl CCNU + VCR ± Tumor cells + BCG	No change	Undetermined	Undetermined	Mastrangelo
DTIC ± BCG	2x increase (14% vs 27%)	2x increase (4 to 8 months)	2x increase (6 to 11 months)	Hersh
CTX and DTIC ± C. parvum	No change	No change	No change	Presant
VCN treated tumor cells ± BCG	No change	No change	No change	Simmons
Unblocking plasma vs control plasma	No change	No change	No change	Wright

BHD, BCNU + hydroxyurea + DTIC; UCR, vineristine; CTX, cytoxan; VCN, vigrio cholera neuraminidase; TC, tumor cells.

My own inclination would be not to attribute it to the randomized vs the historical nature of the trials, because the number of patients in both studies is large enough to overcome the disadvantages of both types of trials.

Dr. Rosenberg: Is the administration of BCG comparable in the two studies?

Dr. Hersh: I think it's fairly comparable in the sense that the Southwest Group used scarification and we used scarification. Clearly there are going to be differences in the aggressiveness with which BCG is administered at any given treatment, but I can't say that it was administered more or less aggressively by us or by the Southwest Group. The only difference that I can think of is that after remission was achieved, the frequency of BCG administration was reduced in the Southwest Group study and was not reduced in our study. They used Connaught BCG which, by various studies carried out by George Mackaness, is an excellent BCG preparation with the biological characteristics that one normally associates with good efficacy. We used, if anything, an inferior product. The study, having been done a number of years ago, used liquid Pasteur BCG. This material had to be sent by air from the Pasteur Institute and it has a shelf life of only a couple of weeks.

Dr. Rosenberg: Dr. Costanzi, in your study the DTIC-BCG combination had lower response rates and durations of survival than in the other arms. How do you explain this difference in results?

Dr. Costanzi: I can't come up with a concrete answer, but I think there are some important differences. First of all, I want to reiterate that when Dr. Hersh and I looked at our data a few years ago, as far as patients were concerned, I can reassure you they were comparable populations. But I think there are three major differences here which, when put together, may account for this difference.

First of all, in a cooperative group you are dealing with many institutions. There are 39 institutions in the Southwest Group, and of course we analyze the data from all of these. Although we do have a good quality control system, I think that there could be some advantage in a study done with a large number of patients at one institution as compared to a multi-institutional study. This may be a variable between the two studies. The second thing alluded to is the difference in the BCG strength. We used lyophilized Connaught, and Dr. Hersh used the Pasteur preparation.

One other item that may be important is that Dr. Hersh's patients got more drug. His schedule of DTIC was 250 milligrams per meter square daily for five days every 21 days, and his BCG was given on days 7, 12, and 17. Our regimen for DTIC was the same, but it was administered every four weeks. Over a period of time there would be an extra week or two of therapy administered. I can't see any other difference in the two studies.

Dr. Hersh: Another factor to which I alluded before, which we really need to investigate very intensively in animal models, is the question of the relationship between immunosuppressive drugs and immunopotentiating agents.

We find that DTIC is not very immunosuppressive. Other drugs might modify the effects of BCG by suppressing or preventing the activation of whatever host defense mechanisms are important. Perhaps also the immuno-stimulation followed by an immunosuppressant drug would be more immuno-suppressive than the administration of the chemotherapeutic agent alone. I know that Georges Mathé has been concerned about this and written about it a number of times.

Dr. Holland: I think Dr. Costanzi's DTIC + BCG arm and Dr. Hersh's arm should be compared.

Dr. Rosenberg: Okay, let's take a look at that in terms of the response rate to DTIC and BCG.

Dr. Costanzi: The response rate to that regimen was 17 out of 96 for 18 percent.

Dr. Rosenberg: And Dr. Hersh?

Dr. Hersh: Ours was 26.9 percent.

Dr. Rosenberg: So there was a difference in response rates between 18 and 27 percent. How about median durations of remission and survival?

Dr. Costanzi: They were similar in the two studies. As a matter of fact, we looked at this the other day, and Dr. Hersh's curve and our curve were almost superimposable.

Dr. Presant: Could I ask Dr. Hersh and Dr. Costanzi to break that down with respect to visceral disease vs skin and lymph node, because clearly, Dr. Hersh's data are also distinctly different for those two subgroups. I would like to know if Dr. Costanzi's is also broken down into skin and lymph node disease vs non-skin and lymph node disease.

Dr. Hersh: Let me clarify that point because that has been misinterpreted before. A patient may have pulmonary metastases and lymph node and skin metastases. The response of metastases to the lymph nodes and skin increased from 18 to 55 percent. The response of metastases to the viscera didn't change. It was 13 percent in one group and 17 percent in the other. But that is looking only at sites of response, not total response. There were 26 percent of patients who showed complete or partial remission of all disease.

Dr. Costanzi: Here is a major difference because in our nonvisceral, which would be just lymph node and/or skin, the response rate with DTIC-BCD was 25 percent, 7 out of 28, whereas it was 18 percent overall (including patients with visceral and nonvisceral metastases). So that is not a significant increase.

Dr. Rosenberg: I'd like to emphasize as we carry out this discussion that we do not have available anywhere a prospective randomized comparison between DTIC alone and DTIC + BCG.

Dr. Holmes (Westminster): There was one just published using exactly the schedules proposed by M.D. Anderson Hospital. In that study there is no significant difference between the two and the response rate is 27 in one and 28 in the other.

Dr. Rosenberg: Could you tell us a little bit more about the study: the kinds of patients, the number of patients, the duration?

Dr. Holmes: Fifty-nine patients were compared. I think the big difference now is Dr. Hersh's historical control group. He only had a 14 percent response to DTIC. From my colleagues in Europe and others in Britain, I would think this was abnormally low.

Dr. Hersh: We observed a similar response rate with other regimens with relatively large numbers of patients, so that is the kind of response rate we have observed at the M.D. Anderson to DTIC alone, or to DTIC + other drugs. I am well aware of the fact that most groups have obtained approximately a 20 percent response rate with DTIC, regardless of the schedule.

Dr. Rosenberg: The most powerful statement that comes from the Southwest Oncology Group trials with regard to immunotherapy is that adding BCG to the three-drug regimen does not improve it.

Dr. Holland: Dr. Costanzi, did you ever study DTIC alone in the Southwest Group in the past, and can you go back and make the same manipulation that Dr. Hersh does to look at a historical control and see if you can demonstrate the DTIC activity?

Dr. Costanzi: We never used DTIC alone in our group.

Dr. Peto: I just want to point out at the beginning of 1975, there were 68 different trials of immunotherapy of melanoma in progress. Since then, many more have started. One would expect from such an array of trials in progress around the world a dozen significant results by chance alone even if immunotherapy has no value whatsoever. This is about the proportion that we observe. There are two studies which are significant at about the 5 percent level, and, you know, this is just what one expects if this modality is not useful at all.

Dr. Rosenberg: I don't think that that is an entirely fair comment. The point in performing the well-designed trials is an attempt to see differences. When a difference is seen, for example, if Dr. Morton's difference is real—well, then, that's something that points the way for repetition by other groups. The point of presenting these studies in a forum such as this is to see what the current leads are. Any individual result can clearly be wrong, but it points the way to things that can be repeated and confirmed.

Dr. Morton: I'd like to point out that as has been mentioned repeatedly, there are no uniform criteria in all these hundred trials. Each one has a different way of stratifying the patients or of administering the immunotherapy. I think the real question is if we have uniformity in stratification factors and in approach to the disease, can we show an effect? If we think about the natural history of melanoma, stage II disease or even stage III disease, it is clear that there is a significant proportion of patients—let's talk about stage II disease—that are going to remain free of disease regardless of whether they get immunotherapy or not. That will be about 30 percent of the population. There is another population of patients that are going to recur promptly, and immunotherapy is not going to affect their rate of recurrence or death at all. Now, there is a third population (on the order of perhaps 30 percent or 40 percent) where immunotherapy in fact influences the natural history of the disease. Well, when you're taking a group of patients that are the whole, and you only can influence a small proportion of the whole—which you cannot select out by any known criteria today—the analysis becomes very difficult.

I wanted to ask Dr. Wright a question regarding the unblocking plasma. In our data, we consistently find that a certain proportion of the population (they don't have to be black) have antibodies that appear to be directed against antigens associated with melanoma. I was wondering, therefore, if you preselected your non-black plasma on the basis that they had no serologic reactivity to melanoma cells, or did you just take the plasma as it came, without preselecting it?

Dr. Wright: These tests were done in Dr. Hellstrom's lab, and I am not familiar with all the details. It was my understanding that the initial studies involving approximately 100 blacks, as well as 100 whites, were systematically analyzed for the presence or absence of unblocking activity. These data indicated that approximately 90 percent of normal blacks manifested the activity. As far as I know, this was not shown in any of the Caucasian serum.

Dr. Gehan: I'd like to make a couple of comments on randomized vs nonrandomized studies. In randomized studies, we have to ask the question, were the patient numbers adequate enough to detect reasonable amounts of difference? If one is looking for an advantage for one group over another— and I think that's what people are looking for in a BCG vs a no-BCG trial— to find a 20 percent difference, you need something on the order of 75 patients in each group. To find a 30 percent difference, you need 37 patients in each group, and to find a 40 percent difference, about 23 patients are needed in each group.

The point that Dr. Morton made was especially pertinent. If only an undefined subgroup of patients are going to benefit from immunotherapy, the randomized studies presented would have very little chance of detecting that benefit.

Other types of questions must be asked about nonrandomized studies. For instance, what attempts have been made to adjust for prognostic factors, and how comparable are the control and treatment groups?

Immunotherapy of Cancer: Present Status of
Trials in Man, edited by W. D. Terry and D. Windhorst.
Raven Press, New York © 1978.

Lung Cancer: Prognostic Factors and Adjuvant Therapy Results

Martin H. Cohen

National Cancer Institute-Veterans Administration Medical Oncology Branch,
Veterans Administration Hospital, Washington, D.C. 20422

Presently about 5 to 10% of an estimated 91,000 American patients developing lung cancer this year can expect to survive 5 years (1–3). For patients having surgical resection the 5-year survival increases to 25 to 30% (4,5). For the most favorable surgical patients, with small tumors confined to the lung, the 5-year survival is approximately 50% (6). For patients who are nonresectable at presentation, some benefit may be achieved by radiation therapy and chemotherapy but expected median survival is less than 1 year (7).

There are obvious possibilities for improving these statistics. Early diagnosis, at a time when the tumor is confined to the lung, would improve surgical curability. For more advanced tumors surgical adjuvant therapy to destroy residual regional or systemic tumor cells might be beneficial. The choice of therapeutic modalities for adjuvant studies is determined, in part, by the frequency of regional versus systemic tumor recurrence. Thus for epidermoid lung cancer, which has the lowest metastatic potential of the four major histologic subtypes of lung cancer (8,9), radiation therapy might be appropriate. For adenocarcinoma and large cell anaplastic carcinoma, where surgical failure is more often due to unsuspected systemic metastases (8,9), chemotherapy is an appropriate adjuvant. Small cell anaplastic lung cancer is generally not a surgical disease, and treatment consists of chemotherapy with or without radiation therapy (10,11). Immunotherapy alone or with radiation therapy or chemotherapy might be beneficial in all stages and histologies of lung cancer because of the immunosuppressive potential of the latter two therapies (12) and because of the depressed immune reactivity of the lung cancer patient (13). Although previous trials have investigated some of the above questions, interpretation of reported results is often difficult. Frequently study populations have not been adequately defined with regard to important prognostic variables. Detailed statistical analysis of trials with emphasis on subgroups of patients that might have benefited from treatment is also not usually available. The following discussion considers important prognostic variables and reviews published results of randomized trials utilizing chemotherapy or radiation therapy as surgical adjuvants. Hopefully this information will be useful in the design and evaluation of future lung cancer trials.

PROGNOSTIC FACTORS

Stage of Disease

The purpose of staging is to group patients who have similar prognoses. Thus patients in a numerically or alphabetically lower staging category have a better prognosis than those in a higher category (14). Staging may be based on clinical evaluation, on surgical evaluation, or on pathologic evaluation of resected tissue after surgery. Precision of staging, if adequate material is submitted to the pathologist, is greatest for pathologic staging. Since clinical staging methods tend to understage disease (15) patients staged pathologically have better prognoses than patients staged clinically.

Stage of disease is frequently recorded in the tumor-node-metastases (TNM) system (Table 1). This staging system is valid for epidermoid carcinoma, adenocarcinoma, and large cell anaplastic bronchogenic carcinoma. For small cell carcinoma, except possibly when it presents as a peripheral

TABLE 1. *TNM classification and staging*

| | | | Primary tumor | Extra pulmonary involvement | |
| | | | Bronchoscopy | | |
Category	Tumor diameter	Atelectasis and/or obstructive pneumonitis	finding: most proximal tumor extension	Pleural effusion	Local extension-Chest wall, mediastinum, etc.
T1	≤3 cm	None	Lobar bronchus	None	None
T2	>3 cm	<Entire lung	≥2 cm from carina	None	None
T3	Any size	Entire lung	<2 cm from carina	Present or absent	Present or absent

Category	Regional nodes — Ipsilateral hilar	Mediastinal
N0	None	None
N1	Present	None
N2	Present or absent	Present

Category	Metastases
M0	No metastases
M1	Extrathoracic or contralateral thoracic metastases

STAGE

I	II	III
T1 N0 M0	T2 N1 M0	T3 any N or M
T1 N1 M0		N2 any T or M
T2 N0 M0		M1 any T or N

M, metastases; N, regional nodes; T, primary tumor.

lung nodule (16), clinical staging underestimates the extent of tumor dissemination (14).

For the primary tumor (T) prognostic factors include the diameter of the lesion, the most proximal extent of the tumor on bronchoscopy, the presence or absence of tumor extension into adjacent structures including the chest wall or mediastinum, and the presence or absence of bronchial obstruction with associated atelectasis or pneumonitis, or both. Further subdivision of the T category may be necessary as more asymptomatic individuals with normal chest roentgenograms are identified in early diagnosis studies. These studies utilize serial chest X-ray and sputum cytology examinations at 4- to 6-month intervals (17–19). When a malignant cytology is obtained intrabronchial tumor is identified either by fiberoptic bronchoscopy (20) or tantalum bronchography (21). Patients identified in early detection studies are likely to have a better prognosis than individuals identified because of the development of symptoms or because of the finding of an abnormal chest roentgenogram. Presumably the earlier a tumor is detected the more likely it is to be localized and amenable to complete surgical resection. Even if the natural history of disease is unaffected by early diagnosis, however, the time frame for therapeutic evaluation of the patient is shifted to an earlier period.

Regional disease staging is principally concerned with the status of hilar and mediastinal lymph nodes. Besides the importance of assessing these nodes for their influence on complete tumor resection, it would also be important to have accurate information on nodal status if a preoperative tumoricidal therapy was planned. Mediastinoscopy is the best technique for determining paratracheal node metastasis from tumors arising in all lung regions except for the left upper lobe and left hilum (22,23). Tumors arising in these two regions drain to anterior mediastinal lymph nodes that are best evaluated by anterior mediastinotomy (24). Angiographic staging procedures are associated with a greater percentage of false negative results than are surgical procedures (25,26), and thus they probably should not be used alone for regional disease staging. The combination of mediastinoscopy and pulmonary angiography is probably the most accurate preoperative means of mediastinal evaluation (27), as pulmonary angiography demonstrates the main pulmonary vessels, pericardium, and right atrium—areas not well seen on mediastinoscopy.

The principal problem regarding staging relates to the detection of extrathoracic metastasis (M). Systemic metastasis in the absence of regional lymph node involvement is frequent. Autopsies performed in a group of 202 patients who died within 30 days of an apparently curative surgical resection revealed previously undetected distant metastases in 25% (9). Yashar (28) and Bell (29), by performing abdominal explorations at the time of, or prior to, thoracotomy in clinically resectable patients, were able to document hepatic metastases in 14.9 and 13.6% of patients, respectively. In addition Bell also found metastases in abdominal lymph nodes in four patients and adrenal and rib metastases in one patient each. Hansen and Muggia demonstrated bone marrow involvement in four of 63 patients with non-small cell lung cancer in whom disease was clinically confined to the thorax (30), whereas Newman and Hansen, in a similar patient population, detected asymptomatic or symptomatic brain metastases at presentation in 18 of 201 patients (31). It is clear from the above data that the more one looks for extrathoracic disease in potentially operable patients the more likely one is to find it. Thus in comparing patient groups in different trials it is important to know the thoroughness with which clinical staging was performed.

Completion of clinical staging allows one to separate patients into potentially resectable and nonresectable groups. The former includes stages I and II epidermoid, adeno, and large cell anaplastic carcinoma and possibly stage III epidermoid carcinoma (based on ipsilateral mediastinal lymph nodes) (Table 1) (6). Nonresectable patients are those with small cell carcinoma, except possibly when disease presents as an asymptomatic pulmonary nodule (16), most patients with advanced primary tumors (T3), patients with ipsilateral mediastinal nodes in which tumor has spread to perinodal tissues or where nodes are located high in the mediastinum, and patients in whom the tumor has spread beyond the ipsilateral hemithorax.

In potentially resectable patients who are physiologically able to withstand the anticipated surgery more detailed staging can be performed. The precision of surgical staging depends in part on the type of pulmonary resection performed. Wedge or segmental resection represents a conservative and generally unsatisfactory lung cancer operation. This procedure is usually reserved for patients with peripheral lesions who have borderline pulmonary function. Little additional information on the status of hilar and mediastinal nodes is obtained from the operation. Lobectomy and pneumonectomy, performed in standard fashion or as radical procedures, are more acceptable lung cancer operations. Radical surgery involves either mediastinal node dissection or extension of the resection into the pericardium, to the chest wall, or to the diaphragm (32). It is evident that patients surviving radical surgery would be most accurately staged and would therefore be expected to have a better prognosis than individuals staged clinically or by lesser surgical procedures.

The pathologist is the final individual involved in the determination of stage and prognosis. There are four principal questions for the pathologist: (a) Is tumor present at the resection margin? (b) Is there blood vessel or lymphatic invasion? (c) Does tumor extend through the lymph node capsule into perinodal tissues? and (d) What is the degree of metaplasia of bronchial mucosa distant to tumor? Positive answers to any or all of the first three questions indicate a worse prognosis for the patient (33). Concerning the last question early diagnosis studies indicate that patients may present with multiple primary tumors or that they may have carcinoma *in situ* or severe squamous metaplasia in areas distant from the primary tumor. Second primary

TABLE 2. *Stratification for clinical trials*

Patients having curative resection	Nonresectable patients
Type of surgery	Histology
Stage of disease	Stage of disease
Pathologic evaluation	Performance status
Age $\leq$ 60 vs. > 60	Immune status
Sex	

tumors were noted in seven of 27 patients in the Mayo Clinic series (18) and in seven of 26 patients from Memorial Hospital (19). The high frequency of multiple primaries indicates the need to conserve as much functioning pulmonary tissue as possible at the original surgery (18,19).

Age and sex are also important prognostic factors for curative lung resection. The Veterans Administration Surgical Adjuvant Group demonstrated that patients less than 60 years old did better than individuals above this age (34). Similar results were obtained by Bergh (35). Females had a better prognosis than males probably because of the higher frequency of peripheral adenocarcinoma and especially bronchioloalveolar carcinoma in the female population (36,37).

Table 2 summarizes the prognostic variables that are useful for stratification in adjuvant trials after curative resection and in trials studying therapy of nonresectable patients. In the former group of trials, excluding small cell carcinoma, histology is not included as there is little difference in 5-year survival by cell type (Table 3) (16,32,36,38–40). For trials involving nonresectable patients histology is important because of differences in sensitivity to radiation therapy and chemotherapy by cell type (41,42). Performance status is of major prognostic significance. Asymptomatic individuals can expect survivals about three times longer than patients who are bedridden because of tumor symptoms (43). Reactivity to recall-delayed type hypersensitivity skin tests is also associated with better prognosis when compared with survival of anergic individuals (44).

Turning from prognostic factors to therapeutic results, data are available on the use of chemotherapy and radiation therapy as adjuvants to pulmonary resection. In designing a chemotherapy adjuvant program, current concepts indicate that the drugs used should be given intermittently to avoid a prolonged immunosuppressive effect and that they should be given for 18 to 24 months to ensure tumor eradication (45). Table 4 lists trials where patients

TABLE 3. *Lung cancer survival after curative resection—effect of histology*

Cell type	Number of patients	5-Year survival (%)
Epidermoid	1,767	30
Adenocarcinoma	557	32
Anaplastic	593	25

TABLE 4. Surgical adjuvant chemotherapy trials

Drug	Dose	Schedule	Treatment duration	Stratification	Results	Ref.
Cyclophosphamide (Cytoxan)	6 mg/kg	Daily × 5	Postoperative + week 5	None	Benefit in small cell carcinoma	51
Cyclophosphamide	1 g	Every 5 days	6–8 weeks	None	Benefit except in adenocarcinoma	49
Cyclophosphamide	8 mg/kg	Daily × 5 every 5 weeks	18 months	None	No benefit	54
Cyclophosphamide	12 mg/kg	Weekly for 8–9 doses every 4 months	2 years	None	Cyclophosphamide worse	50
Cyclophosphamide	75–200 mg	Daily	2 years	Histology	No benefit	46
Cyclophosphamide	50–200 mg	Daily	21 months	Histology	Benefit for epidermoid	47
Vinblastine	0.1 mg/kg	Weekly	3 months	Histology	Benefit for small cell and other pts. with positive nodes	52
Busulfan	1.0–4.0 mg	Daily	2 years	Histology	No benefit	46
Nitrogen mustard	0.3–0.4 mg/kg	Daily	3–4 days	Stage	No benefit	53,54
Cyclophosphamide alt. with methotrexate	8 mg/kg 10 mg/d	Daily × 5 Daily × 5	18 months	None	No benefit	55
Cyclophosphamide 5-fluorouracil, methotrexate, vinblastine	—	—	3 years	Histology; stage	Possible benefit stage I	56

were randomized either to chemotherapy or to a placebo. As indicated the only drug used in more than one trial was cyclophosphamide. Even with this drug, using the aforementioned concepts for adjuvant drug administration, only one of the six cyclophosphamide trials was done optimally. Two studies used daily oral drug administration (46,47), two treated only for a short period of time (48,49), and in one study drug was administered weekly for 8 or 9 weeks every 4 months (50). An additional difficulty in interpreting the results of these studies was the lack of stratification of patients by appropriate prognostic variables, especially histology and stage of disease. Thus it is difficult to assess the role of cyclophosphamide in surgical adjuvant therapy. The drug appears to be useful in resected small cell carcinoma, but few of these patients ever come to surgery (51). For the other studies suggesting therapeutic benefit, patient follow-up was either brief or incompletely documented. Neither vinblastine, nitrogen mustard, or busulfan seem beneficial as adjuvant treatments although, again, drug administration was not optimal (46,52–54).

There has been one adjuvant study using sequential administration of cyclophosphamide and methotrexate where no benefit of therapy was noted (55). A single study of combination chemotherapy utilized cyclophosphamide, 5-fluorouracil, methotrexate, and vinblastine. Although results were promising in this study, only small numbers of patients were studied (56).

The development of future surgical adjuvant chemotherapy trials is dependent upon the identification of new active single drugs and drug combinations. Until greater chemotherapeutic efficacy is demonstrated, it appears unreasonable to conduct such trials in stage I and probably stage II patients.

Radiation therapy has been given preoperatively or postoperatively. These trials are listed in Table 5 (49,57–61). Only one of these six trials demonstrated therapeutic benefit for radiation therapy (49). As in the chemotherapy trials, however, evaluation of results is difficult because of lack of adequate staging data in four of the six studies. Preoperative or postoperative radiation therapy should be most useful in patients with epidermoid carcinoma who have positive mediastinal lymph nodes (8,9,62). Only two of the above studies gives enough information to allow evaluation of this subgroup of pa-

TABLE 5. Preoperative and postoperative radiation therapy

RT Given	Dose/treatment duration	Stratification	Conclusion	Ref.
Preoperative	4,000–5,200r/4–6 weeks	Histology	No benefit	57
Preoperative	4,000–5,000r/4–6 weeks	Histology	No benefit	58
Preoperative	5,500r/4–5 weeks Some large fractions	Histology	No benefit	59
Postoperative	4,500r/5 weeks	Histology	No benefit	60
Postoperative	4,500r/4 weeks	Histology	No benefit	61

RT, radiation therapy.

tients. One study demonstrated survival gain from radiation therapy (49), whereas the other did not (60). Further studies in the patient group are clearly indicated.

Another problem in evaluating adjuvant studies is the lack of adequate patient numbers, especially for stage I disease. In this stage one would expect an approximate 50% 5-year survival from surgery. Further of the 50% of patients who die, approximately 14% die of causes unrelated to cancer (34). Consequently adjuvant therapy might be expected to benefit only one-third of all study patients. For stage II with a 5-year survival of 25% and with 14% of deaths unrelated to cancer, about 60% of patients might benefit from adjuvant therapy. For stage III disease with a 5-year survival under 10%, one might expect benefit in over 75% of patients.

Development of new lung cancer studies would also be facilitated if we had detailed information for previous trials on failure patterns for each histology and presenting stage of disease. This would allow for more proper use of local and systemic cytotoxic and immunologic therapies. Since detection of failure requires prompt recognition of disease recurrence, strategies and techniques have to be developed to recognize recurrence early. Perhaps biologic markers such as carcinoembryonic antigen (CEA) or big adrenocorticotrophic hormone might be useful (63–65). Other promising techniques include computerized axial tomography (66) and diagnostic ultrasound (67). Because of the risk of development of second primary lung cancers in the patient population, careful follow-up of sputum cytology will also be necessary.

REFERENCES

1. American Cancer Society (1975): *Cancer Facts and Figures.*
2. Maloney, J. V., Bennett, L. R., Longmire, W. P., Madden, S. C., Rigler, L. G., Simmons, D. H., Steele, J. D., Stein, J. J., Troup, G. M., and Weber, A. P. (1966): Carcinoma of the lung. *Ann. Intern. Med.,* 64:165–188.
3. Senior, R. M., and Adamson, J. S. (1970): Survival in patients with lung cancer. *Arch Intern. Med.,* 125:975–980.
4. Selawry, O. S., and Hansen, H. H. (1973): Lung cancer. In: *Cancer Medicine,* edited by J. F. Holland and E. Frei, III, pp. 1473–1518. Lea & Febiger, Philadelphia.
5. Benfield, J. R., Julliard, G. J. F., Pilch, Y. H., Rigler, L. G., and Selecky, P. (1975): Current and future concepts of lung cancer. *Ann. Intern. Med.,* 83:93–106.
6. Mountain, C. F. (1974): Surgical therapy of lung cancer: Biologic, physiologic and technical determinants. *Semin. Oncol.,* 1:253–258.
7. Carbone, P. P., Frost, J. K., Feinstein, A. R., Higgins, G. A., Jr., and Selawry, O. S. (1970): Lung cancer: Perspectives and prospects. *Ann. Intern. Med.,* 73:1003–1024.
8. Line, D. H., and Deeley, T. J. (1971): The necropsy findings in carcinoma of the bronchus. *Br. J. Dis. Chest.,* 65:238–242.
9. Matthews, M. J., Kanhouwa, S., Pickren, J., and Robinette, D. (1973): Frequency of residual and metastatic tumor in patients undergoing curative surgical resection for lung cancer. *Cancer Chemother. Rep.,* 4:63–67.
10. Mountain, C. F. (1973): Keynote address on surgery in the therapy for lung cancer: Surgical prospects and priorities for clinical research. *Cancer Chemother. Rep.,* 4:19–24.

11. Cohen, M. H. (1975): Lung cancer: A status report. *J. Natl. Cancer Inst.,* 55: 505–511.
12. Hersh, E. M., Mavligit, C. M., and Gutterman, J. U. (1974): Immunotherapy as related to lung cancer: A review. *Semin. Oncol.,* 1:273–278.
13. Dellon, A. L., Potvin, C., and Chretien, P. B. (1975): Thymus dependent lymphocyte levels in bronchogenic carcinoma: Correlations with histology. Clinical stage and clinical course after surgical treatment. *Cancer,* 35:687–694.
14. Mountain, C. F., Carr, D. T., and Anderson, W. A. D. (1974): A system for the clinical staging of lung cancer. *Am. J. Roentgenol. Radium Ther. Nucl. Med.,* 120:130–138.
15. Cliffton, E. E., Martini, N., and Beattie, E. J., Jr. (1973): A classification of lung cancer: Value for prognosis and comparison of series and methods of treatment. *Proc. Seventh Natl. Cancer Conf.,* 7:729–737.
16. Higgins, G. A., Shields, T. W., and Keehn, R. J. (1975): The solitary pulmonary nodule. Ten years follow-up of Veterans Administration-Armed Forces Cooperative study. *Arch. Surg.,* 110:570–575.
17. Baker, R. R., Stitik, F. P., and Marsh, B. R. (1975): The clinical assessment of selected patients with bronchogenic carcinoma. *Ann. Thorac. Surg.,* 20:520–528.
18. Fontana, F. S., Sanderson, D. R., Woolner, L. B., Miller, W. E., Bernatz, P. E., Payne, W. S., and Taylor, W. F. (1975): The Mayo lung project for early detection and localization of bronchogenic carcinoma: A status report. *Chest,* 67:511–522.
19. Martini, N., Beattie, E. J., Jr., Cliffton, E. E., and Melamed, M. R. (1974): Radiologically occult lung cancer: Report of 26 cases. *Surg. Clin. North Am.,* 54:811–823.
20. Marsh, B. R., Frost, J. K., Erozan, Y. S., and Carter, D. (1974): Role of fiberoptic bronchoscopy in lung cancer. *Semin. Oncol.,* 1:199–203.
21. Stitik, F. P., and Proctor, D. F. (1975): Delayed clearance of tantalum by radiologically occult cancer. *Ann. Otol.,* 84:589–595.
22. Pearson, F. G., Nelems, J. M., Henderson, R. D., and Delarue, N. C. (1972): The role of mediastinoscopy in the selection of treatment for bronchial carcinoma with involvement of superior mediastinal lymph nodes. *J. Thorac. Cardiovasc. Surg.,* 64:382–387.
23. Fishman, N. H., and Bronstein, M. H. (1975): Is mediastinoscopy necessary in the evaluation of lung cancer? *Ann. Thorac. Surg.,* 20:678–685.
24. Jolly, P. C., Hill, L. D., III, Lawless, P. A., and West, T. L. (1973): Parasternal mediastinotomy and mediastinoscopy. Adjuncts in the diagnosis of chest disease. *J. Thorac. Cardiovasc. Surg.,* 66:549–555.
25. Benfield, J. R., Bonney, H., Crummy, A. B., and Cleveland, R. J. (1969): Azygograms and pulmonary arteriograms in bronchogenic carcinoma. *Arch. Surg.,* 99:406–409.
26. Janower, M. L., Dreyfuss, J. E., and Skinner, D. W. (1966): Azygography in lung cancer. *New Engl. J. Med.,* 275:803–808.
27. Delarue, N. C., Sanders, D. E., and Silverberg, S. A. (1970): Complementary value of angiography and mediastinoscopy in individualizing treatment for patients with lung cancer. *Cancer,* 26:1370–1378.
28. Yashar, J. (1966): Transdiaphragmatic exploration of the upper abdomen during surgery for bronchogenic carcinoma. *J. Thorac. Cardiovasc. Surg.,* 52:599–603.
29. Bell, J. W. (1968): Abdominal exploration in one hundred lung carcinoma suspects prior to thoracotomy. *Ann. Surg.,* 167:199–203.
30. Hansen, H. H., and Muggia, F. M. (1972): Staging of inoperable patients with bronchogenic carcinoma with special reference to bone marrow examination and peritoneoscopy. *Cancer,* 30:1395–1401.
31. Newman, S. J., and Hansen, H. H. (1974): Frequency, diagnosis, and treatment of brain metastases in 247 consecutive patients with bronchogenic carcinoma. *Cancer,* 33:492–496.
32. Watson, W. L. (1968): Extended surgical procedures at Memorial Hospital. In: *Lung Cancer: A Study of 5000 Memorial Hospital Cases,* edited by W. L. Watson, pp. 299–307. Mosby, St. Louis, Mo.
33. Spjut, H. J., Roper, C. L., and Butcher, H. R. (1961): Pulmonary cancer and its

prognosis. A study of the relationship of certain factors to survival of patients treated by pulmonary resection. *Cancer,* 14:1251–1258.

34. Shields, T. W., Higgins, G. A., and Keehn, R. J. (1972): Factors influencing survival after resection for bronchial carcinoma. *J. Thorac. Cardiovasc. Surg.,* 64:391–399.

35. Bergh, N. P., and Schersten, T. (1965): Bronchogenic carcinoma. A follow-up study of a surgically treated series with special reference to the prognostic significance of lymph node metastases. *Acta Chir. Scand. [Suppl.],* 347:1–42.

36. Ashor, G. L., Kern, W. H., Meyer, B. W., Lindesmith, G. G., Stiles, Q. R., Tucker, B. L., and Jones, J. C. (1975): Long term survival in bronchogenic carcinoma. *J. Thorac. Cardiovasc. Surg.,* 70:581–589.

37. Connelly, R. R., Cutter, S. J., and Baylis, P. (1966): End results in cancer of the lung: Comparison of male and female patients. *J. Natl. Cancer Inst.,* 36:277–287.

38. Siddons, A. H. M. (1962): Cell type in the choice of cases of carcinoma of the bronchus for surgery. *Thorax,* 17:308–309.

39. Shields, T. W., Yee, J., Conn, J. H., and Robinette, C. D. (1975): Relationship of cell type and lymph node metastasis to survival after resection of bronchial carcinoma. *Ann. Thorac. Surg.,* 20:501–510.

40. Vincent, R. G., Takita, H., Lane, W. W., Gutierrez, A. C., and Pickren, J. W. (1976): Surgical therapy of lung cancer. *J. Thorac. Cardiovasc. Surg.,* 71:581–591.

41. Salazar, D. M., Rubin, P., Brown, J. C., Feldstein, M. L., and Keller, B. E. (1936): Predictors of radiation response in lung cancer. A clinico-pathobiological analysis. *Cancer,* 37:2636–2650.

42. Selawry, O. S. (1974): The role of chemotherapy in the treatment of lung cancer. *Semin. Oncol.,* 1:259–272.

43. Zelen, M. (1973): Keynote address on biostatistics and data retrieval. *Cancer Chemother. Rep.,* 4:31–42.

44. Israel, L., Mugica, J., and Chahinian, P. H. (1973): Prognosis of early bronchogenic carcinoma. Survival curves of 451 patients after resection of lung cancer in relation to the results of preoperative tuberculin skin test. *Biomedicine,* 19:68–72.

45. Carter, S. K. (1973): Some thoughts on surgical adjuvant studies in lung cancer. *Cancer Chemother. Rep.,* 4:109–117.

46. Medical Research Council Working Party (1971): Study of cytotoxic chemotherapy as an adjuvant to surgery in carcinoma of the bronchus. *Br. Med. J.,* 2:421–428.

47. Poulsen, O. (1962): Cyclophosphamide. An evaluation of its cytostatic effects on surgically treated carcinoma of the lung. *J. Int. Coll. Surg.,* 37:177–187.

48. Higgins, G. A., Humphrey, E. W., Hughes, F. A., and Keehn, R. J. (1969): Cytoxan as an adjuvant to surgery for lung cancer. *J. Surg. Oncol.,* 1:221–228.

49. Pavlov, A., Pirogov, A., Trachtenberg, A., et al. (1973): Results of combination treatment of lung cancer patients: Surgery plus radiotherapy and surgery plus chemotherapy. *Cancer Chemother. Rep.,* 4:133–135.

50. Brunner, K. W., Marthaler, T., and Muller, W. (1971): Unfavorable effects of long term adjuvant therapy with Endoxan in radically operated bronchogenic carcinoma. *Eur. J. Cancer,* 7:285–294.

51. Higgins, G. A. (1972): Use of chemotherapy as an adjuvant to surgery for bronchogenic carcinoma. *Cancer,* 30:1383–1387.

52. Crosbie, W. A., Kamdar, H. H., and Belcher, J. R. (1966): A controlled trial of vinblastine sulphate in the treatment of cancer of the lung. *Br. J. Dis. Chest,* 60:28–35.

53. Slack, N. H. (1970): Bronchogenic carcinoma: Nitrogen mustard as a surgical adjuvant and factors influencing survival. University Surgical Adjuvant Lung Project. *Cancer,* 25:987–1002.

54. Shields, T. W. (1973): Status report of adjuvant chemotherapy trials in the treatment of bronchial carcinoma. *Cancer Chemother. Rep.,* 4:119–124.

55. Shields, T. W., Robinette, D., and Keehn, R. J. (1974): Bronchial carcinoma treated with adjuvant cancer chemotherapy. *Arch. Surg.,* 109:329–333.

56. Karrer, K., Pridun, N., and Zwintz, E. (1973): Chemotherapeutic studies in bronchogenic carcinoma by the Austrian Study Group. *Cancer Chemother. Rep.,* 4:207–213.

57. Warram, J. (1975): Preoperative irradiation of cancer of the lung: Final report of a therapeutic trial. A collaborative study. *Cancer*, 36:914–925.
58. Shields, T. W. (1972): Preoperative radiation therapy in the treatment of bronchial carcinoma. *Cancer*, 30:1388–1393.
59. Eichorn, H. J., Eule, H., Lessel, A., and Matschke, S. (1975): Results of a controlled clinical trial for evaluation of intensive preoperative irradiation in operable bronchial carcinoma. *Arch. Geschwulstforsch.*, 45:376–384.
60. Bangma, P. J.: (1971): Post operative radiotherapy. In: *Modern Radiotherapy. Carcinoma of the Bronchus*, edited by T. J. Deeley, pp. 163–170. Appleton-Century-Crofts, New York.
61. Paterson, R., and Russell, M. H. (1962): Clinical trials in malignant disease. IV. Lung cancer. Value of post-operative radiotherapy. *Clin. Radiol.*, 13:141–144.
62. Kirsh, M. M., Kahn, D. R., Gago, O., Lampe, I., Fayos, J. V., Prior, M., Moores, W. Y., Haight, C., and Sloan, H. (1971): Treatment of bronchogenic carcinoma with mediastinal metastases. *Ann. Thorac. Surg.*, 12:11–18.
63. Vincent, R. G., and Chu, T. M. (1973): Carcinoembryonic antigen in patients with carcinoma of the lung. *J. Thorac. Cardiovasc. Surg.*, 66:320–328.
64. Pauwels, R., and van der Streten, M. (1975): Plasma levels of carcinoembryonic antigen in bronchial carcinoma and chronic bronchitis. *Thorax*, 30:560–562.
65. Ayvazian, L. F., Schneider, B., Gewirz, G., and Yalow, R. S. (1975): Ectopic production of big ACTH in carcinoma of the lung. *Am. Rev. Respir. Dis.*, 111:279–287.
66. Twigg, H. L., Axelbaum, S. P., and Schellinger, D. (1975): Computerized body tomography with the ACTA scanner. *JAMA*, 234:314–317.
67. Carson, P. L., Wenzel, W. W., Avery, P., and Hendee, W. R. (1975): Ultrasound imaging as an aid to cancer therapy. I. *Int. J. Radiat. Oncol.*, 1:119–132.

Immunotherapy of Cancer: Present Status of
Trials in Man, edited by W. D. Terry and D. Windhorst.
Raven Press, New York © 1978.

Regional Immunotherapy of Lung Cancer Using Postoperative Intrapleural BCG

Martin F. McKneally, Carole M. Maver, and Harvey W. Kausel

Albany Medical College, Albany, New York 12208

We based our approach to immunotherapy on the clinical observation that patients who develop postoperative empyema have a higher survival rate than those who do not develop this complication (1), and on experimental observations from the laboratories of Herbert Rapp (2,3) and George Mackaness (4). These experimental studies suggest that simultaneous presentation of an immunostimulant with tumor antigen may be the most efficient way to stimulate an immune response against the tumor. Studies in our own laboratories confirmed the safety of intrapleural Bacillus Calmette-Guérin (BCG) when given immediately following pulmonary resection (5,6) and established that there is an optimal dose range (6,7). We also found that complementary use of isoniazid (INH) after a suitable interval reduced the toxicity of BCG (7) and improved the efficiency of intrapleural BCG as an antitumor agent (8).

PATIENTS

Preliminary toxicity studies were carried out in 1972 in patients with pleural effusions secondary to proven malignancy in the pleural space. Of five such patients treated solely with intrapleural BCG, four experienced complete control of their effusions by this agent without significant toxicity. The fifth patient, who had a malignant mesothelioma, was not improved. In April, 1973 a randomized prospective study was begun at the affiliated hospitals of the Albany Medical College. All patients admitted to the cardiothoracic service for surgical resection of lung cancer were eligible for study. Preliminary evaluation included measurement of pulmonary function, routine blood chemical testing, and skin tests with recall antigens. Included were mumps, histoplasmin, old tuberculin, purified protein derivative, *Candida,* trychophyton, varidase, and phytohemagglutinin (PHA). All resections were performed by the same surgical group using uniform surgical criteria and techniques. Following resection the patients were separated by cell type into three groups: anaplastic carcinoma, adenocarcinoma, and squamous carcinoma. "Oat cell" or small cell anaplastic cancers were excluded from the study. Postsurgical staging and histologic typing of the resected tumors were done by one observer (H.W.K.) without knowledge of treatment category of the patient. The staging followed the American Joint Committee on Cancer

TABLE 1. *Postsurgical staging of lung cancer (Albany Medical Center Hospital)*

Stage I	Tumor 3.0 cm in diameter or less. Hilar lymph nodes may contain metastatic tumor or they may not. **OR** Tumor greater than 3.0 cm in diameter without involvement of adjacent structures or hilar lymph nodes.
Stage II	Tumor greater than 3.0 cm in diameter. Hilar lymph nodes contain metastatic tumor.
Stage III	Tumor invading mediastinal structures or chest wall, or mediastinal lymph nodes contain metastatic tumor.

This staging system is simplified from the system described by Mountain (ref. 9).

Staging criteria as modified for surgical patients by Mountain (9). Because this is a prospective study that requires staging of the patient at the time of removal of the chest catheter, it was often necessary to stage the patients within 2 to 3 days of surgical resection. A complete pathology report and detailed operative note were not always available at the time of staging. For this reason a simplified form of the staging system was derived (Table 1). As soon as the histologic diagnosis was confirmed and the tumor size and status of the lymph nodes reported, but before the patient's chest drainage tubes were removed, informed consent for entry into the study was obtained. The patients were assigned by a sealed-envelope technique into control or BCG-treated groups. An analysis of the significant prognostic factors in the BCG-

TABLE 2. *Distribution of significant prognostic factors in lung cancer patients*

Prognostic factors	BCG + INH (N = 47)	INH Control (N = 48)
Cell type		
Squamous	24	27
Adenocarcinoma	15	15
Anaplastic	8	6
Operation		
Pneumonectomy	18	13
Bilobectomy	6	3
Lobectomy	21	29
Segmental resection	2	3
Other		
Age > 60 years	37	23
Weight loss > 10 lbs.	2	6
Operation of left	20	22
Metastatic tumor in		
hilar lymph nodes	18	18

Modified from Shields et al. (ref. 18).

treated and control groups is presented in Table 2. There were no significant differences that favored the BCG and INH group.

TREATMENT

BCG-treated patients were given a single intrapleural injection of 10^7 colony-forming units BCG vaccine (Tice strain, University of Illinois). The injection was given through the chest tube just prior to its removal in patients undergoing lobectomy and by thoracentesis in patients undergoing pneumonectomy (usually on postoperative day 4 to 6). The patients were treated with aspirin and benadryl for 48 hr to reduce the discomfort of the "influenzal" syndrome of fever and malaise that regularly occurred following BCG injection. They were discharged on approximately the fifth postinjection day. Fourteen days following injection of BCG, INH 300 mg/day was begun and continued for 12 weeks to prevent overgrowth of BCG organisms. Control patients began INH 300 mg/day on the 14th day following discharge from the hospital and continued this medication for 12 weeks. They did not receive a placebo injection intrapleurally. At 2, 4, 12, 26, and 52 weeks, and at 6-month intervals thereafter, all patients returned to the thoracic surgical outpatient office for follow-up by physical examination, chest X-rays, skin tests, blood chemical testing, and measurement of lymphocytotoxicity against lung tumor cells *in vitro*. Patients who developed metastases or local recurrence were treated by X-irradiation, if appropriate, in the division of radiotherapy but continued to be followed in the division of thoracic surgery. Any patient who was treated with adrenal cortical steroids for a subsequent brain metastasis was simultaneously treated with INH if he received BCG in the postoperative interval.

STATISTICAL ANALYSIS

Survival curves were prepared by the method of Kaplan and Meier (10) and the significance of differences observed computed by the technique of Gehan (11). The follow-up period was defined from the time of surgery. The time of recurrence was defined as the first entry in the chart of a symptom, sign, or radiographic finding that subsequently proved to be related to recurrent cancer.

RESULTS

The data base includes 95 patients, of whom 47 were treated with BCG and 48 are in the control group. Of the total of 95 patients 62 have been followed for more than 1 year and 39 have been followed for more than 2 years. No patients have been lost to follow-up.

There was a reduction in the incidence of tumor recurrence in stage I patients undergoing resection followed by intrapleural administration of BCG. Of 26 such patients, one has died from recurrent cancer. A second one has recently developed a new lesion in another lobe, which may be a new primary or a recurrence developing 18 months after its original resection and BCG treatment. Of 32 stage I control patients, nine have developed recurrent cancer in the same interval. The difference observed between the groups is statistically significant ($p = <0.01$), and is illustrated graphically in Figs. 1 and 2. We have studied a smaller number of patients with more advanced disease in stages II and III. The results of treatment in these patients are recorded in Fig. 3. Although no firm inferences can be made from the pre-

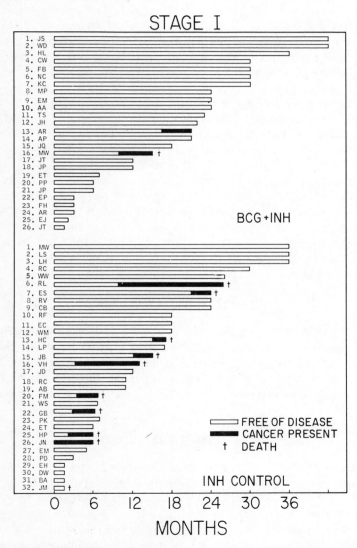

FIG. 1. Recurrences were less frequent and appeared to occur later in patients treated with BCG and INH when compared to those treated with INH alone ($p = <0.01$).

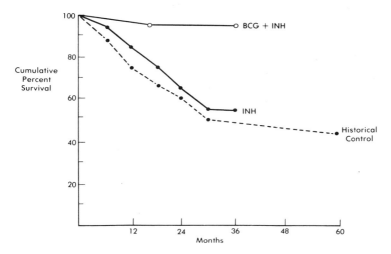

FIG. 2. Survival curves, stage I. The survival fraction in patients treated with BCG and INH was significantly improved when compared with patients treated with INH alone or with historical control patients (*p* = <0.01).

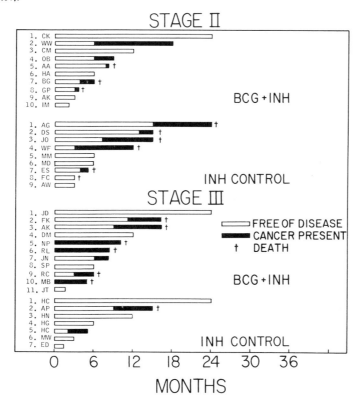

FIG. 3. Patients with more advanced but resected lung cancers in stage II and stage III did not appear to be improved by treatment with BCG and INH.

liminary data in these groups, it appears that BCG as administered in this program does not improve the prognosis in patients with more advanced disease.

The tuberculin test converted to positive (induration greater than 10 mm) in 30 of 32 BCG treated patients. The PHA skin test proved a vague predictor of prognosis, in that 14 of 23 patients with a negative PHA skin test (induration less than 10 mm) developed recurrent cancer, whereas cancer recurred in only 11 of 52 patients with a positive skin test. Skin test reactivity to recall antigens and lymphocytotoxicity against cultured tumor cells did not reflect or predict the clinical course.

SIDE EFFECTS OF TREATMENT

Intrapleural BCG caused transient fever and malaise in most patients. The average temperature elevation was to 101.3°F and the highest temperature observed was 104°F. For this reason patients who were hemodynamically unstable in the immediate postoperative interval were excluded from randomization to prevent further compromise of their clinical condition that might be induced by a febrile response to BCG. Six such patients were excluded of whom two died of respiratory insufficiency and one of myocardial infarction in the immediate postoperative period. One excluded patient died from a second primary carcinoma that developed 18 months after his original resection. One patient who underwent simultaneous coronary bypass surgery was excluded since the effect of intrapleural BCG on vein grafts and vascular anastamoses has not been studied. The duration of hospitalization was prolonged by 5.3 ± 1.7 days in patients treated with BCG. In addition to fever and malaise, 11 postoperative complications occurred in the BCG group. These included: atrial dysrhythmia 2, minor nonmycobacterial wound infection 3, chylothorax prior to BCG 1, atelectasis 1, incarcerated inguinal hernia 1, and infected drain site 2. One patient developed postpneumonectomy empyema in the sixth postoperative month, from which *Escherichia coli* was cultured. Mycobacteria were not present. This patient was treated by open drainage for 10 weeks, after which the pleural space was irrigated repeatedly with neomycin and closed, using Clagett's technique (12). He is well 3 years after his surgical resection. All patients receiving BCG intrapleurally developed transient elevation of the alkaline phosphatase level, without evidence of jaundice or liver tenderness. This was felt to represent an asymptomatic, controlled form of BCG-induced granulomatous hepatitis, as described by Hunt (13) (Fig. 4). The presence of diabetes mellitus in two BCG-treated patients did not adversely affect the response to the vaccine. Eight postoperative complications occurred in the control group, including: atrial dysrhythmia 3, pulmonary embolus 1, wound disruption 1, contralateral spontaneous pneumothorax 1, INH-induced peripheral neuropathy 1, compression induced peripheral neuropathy 1. There was elevation of the serum

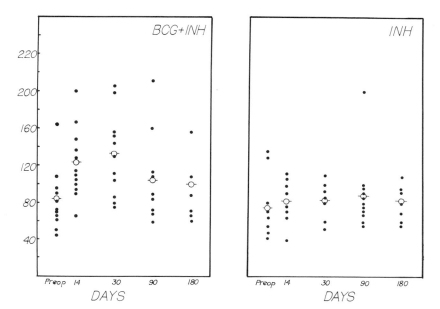

FIG. 4. There was transient elevation of the alkaline phosphatase in BCG treated patients, probably reflecting asymptomatic granulomatous hepatitis.

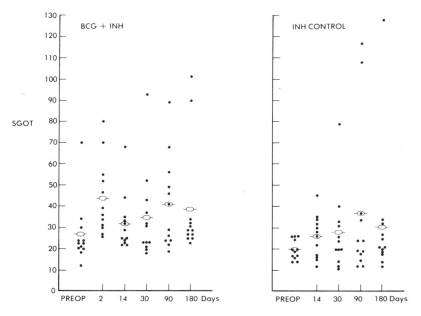

FIG. 5. There was transient elevation of the SGOT above 100 units in five patients treated with INH or INH and BCG. No patients developed jaundice or clinical evidence of hepatitis.

glutamic oxaloacetic transaminase (SGOT) level above 100 units in three patients treated with INH alone, and in two patients treated with BCG and INH (Fig. 5). No significant liver toxicity was evident clinically.

We have recently been informed of three patients at other institutions who have developed severe life-threatening systemic BCG infections following intrapleural administration of much higher doses of BCG than we have used in this study. It is most important that the dose of organisms administered should not exceed 10^7 colony-forming units (approximately 2 mg wet weight). An overdose of this agent, as with many effective remedies, may do great harm.

DISCUSSION

Analysis of our preliminary results at this time reveals an increase in the survival fraction following resection and intrapleural BCG treatment of patients with lung cancer limited to the lung and hilar lymph nodes. The patients with more advanced cancer, though resectable, died early in both BCG-treated and control groups. Adjunctive immunotherapy alone, as administered in this program, probably has a limited capacity to complete the elimination of residual tumor. Our observations suggest that additional cytoreductive agencies, such as chemotherapy, should be added to the therapeutic program to achieve local control of the malignant process in such patients. It seems likely that a responsive immune system is a necessary adjunct but is unable to eliminate a locally invasive process alone or in concert with surgery. Similar rules apply when surgery is employed in the treatment of infectious disease in the lung.

We prefer the intrapleural route of administration of BCG in lung cancer patients because it most clearly mimics the natural experiment of postoperative empyema following lung resection. On theoretical grounds, stimulation in the field of lymphatic drainage of the tumor seems especially appropriate because undetected residual tumor cells may be present in unexcised lung and local lymphoid tissue after surgical resection. Activation of macrophages and release of tumoricidal lymphokines in the region of the residual tumor may help to destroy such cells by nonspecific mechanisms. Furthermore, residual tumor-specific transplantation antigens already entrained in the regional lymph nodes may be driven through the immunologic apparatus under the potentiating influence of BCG. This may result in the generation of tumor-specific immunity locally and systemically as well. If lung cancer proves to be cross-reactive with BCG, and if its antigens are clearly expressed on the cell surface and readily recognized by the immune system, distant immunization may prove to be as effective as regional immunization. However, since tumor cells are minimally or cryptically antigenic, it seems logical to attempt to generate a response to them by intensive stimulation of the lymphatic system in which they reside, rather than by relying solely on re-mote activation of the lymphoid tissues at more distant sites. The hypothesis that regional immunopotentiation with intrapleural BCG is more efficient than its use by other routes was not tested in our clinical study. Baldwin has found the intrapleural route more effective than the cutaneous route in a rat lung tumor system (14). We have not been able to consistently demonstrate superiority of the intrapleural route in our animal tumor studies (6).

In the present protocol, BCG was given only once, during a period of relative immunodepression related to the postoperative state. It may be appropriate to restimulate these patients subsequently by cutaneous immunization. In sensitized patients, cutaneous injection would probably result in a recall flare of immunologic activity in the pleural space. The addition of levamisole to the therapeutic program might prove beneficial in reducing systemic spread of the tumor, in view of Amery's observations that this agent is helpful in patients with locally advanced tumors (15).

Isoniazid did not influence the rate of tumor recurrence in the control group when compared to the usual course of surgically resected patients. Co-administration of INH with BCG does not interfere with its antineoplastic action in mice (16), and recent work suggests that it may work synergistically with BCG in some animal tumor systems (8,17). Although the mechanism of synergy is unclear, INH may serve to prevent the proliferation of the organism while maintaining a steady state of chronic stimulation of the immune response in a favorable BCG dose range.

In summary, we have attempted to reproduce the beneficial effect of postoperative empyema in patients undergoing surgical resection for lung cancer by administering BCG intrapleurally in the immediate postoperative interval. A randomized, prospective study of this mode of therapy suggests that stimulation of the regional lymph nodes by this technique may be beneficial to patients with stage I lung cancer. Although our experience with intrapleural BCG is encouraging, we emphasize that this is a preliminary report of what appears to be a small advance in the treatment of the most favorable group of lung cancer patients. The bulk of patients with lung cancer have disease so far advanced at the time of presentation, that they do not qualify for surgical resection. We emphasize the need for caution in the interpretation of our findings, lest false hopes be raised that cannot be realized with current treatment programs.

SUMMARY

Ninety-five patients have been entered into a prospective randomized study of postoperative intrapleural BCG therapy after complete surgical resection of lung cancer. Using a single injection of 10^7 colony-forming units of Tice strain BCG, we found that there was a reduction in the incidence of recurrent cancer and a prolongation of disease-free survival in patients with stage I lung cancer. With a median duration of observation of 20 months, there have been two recurrences among 26 treated, stage I patients and nine recurrences among 32 control patients. There has been no evidence of improved survival in patients with more advanced disease treated by this method.

ACKNOWLEDGMENTS

The research for this study was supported in part by the New York State Kidney Disease Institute (Unit of New York State Department of Health), The Thoracic Surgical Research Fund, The Laurence M. Warner Fund, and by National Institutes of Health grants RO1-CA-17346, MO1-RR00749, and NO1-CB-5394.

REFERENCES

1. Ruckdeschel, J. C., Codish, S. D., Stranahan, A., and McKneally, M. F. (1972): Postoperative empyema improves survival in lung cancer: Documentation and analysis of a natural experiment. *N. Engl. J. Med.,* 287:1013.
2. Bast, R. C., Zbar, B., Borsos, T., and Rapp. H. (1974): BCG and cancer. *N. Engl. J. Med.,* 290:1413, 1458.
3. Smith, H. G., Bast, R. C., Zbar, B., and Rapp, H. (1975): Eradication of microscopic lymph node metastases after injecting living BCG adjacent to the primary tumor. *J. Natl. Cancer Inst.,* 55:1345.
4. Mackaness, G. B., Lagrange, D. H., and Ishibashi, I. (1974): The modifying effect of BCG on the immunological induction of T cells. *J. Exp. Med.,* 139:1540.
5. McKneally, M. F., Maver, C., Civerchia, L., Codish, S., Kausel, H. W., and Alley, R. D. (1975): Regional immunotherapy for lung cancer using intrapleural BCG. In: *Neoplasm Immunity: Theory and Application,* edited by R. G. Crispen, pp. 153–159. ITR, Chicago.
6. McKneally, M. F., Howard, R. K., Civerchia, L., Codish, S. D., Maver, C. M., and Filardi, M. (1977): *In preparation.*
7. Codish, S. D., and McKneally, M. F. (1972): Dynamics and control of intrapleural BCG infection. *Fed. Proc.,* 31:658.
8. McKneally, M. F., and Filardi, M. (1977): *In preparation.*
9. Mountain, C. F., Carr, D. T., and Anderson, W. A. D. (1974): A system for the clinical staging of lung cancer. *Am. J. Roentgenol. Radium Ther. Nucl. Med.,* 1:130.
10. Kaplan, E. L., and Meier, P. (1958): Nonparametric estimation from incomplete observations. *J. Am. Stat. Assoc.,* 53:457–481.
11. Gehan, E. A. (1965): A generalized Wilcoxon test for comparing arbitrarily singly-censored samples. *Biometrika,* 52:203–223.
12. Clagett, O. T., and Geraci, J. E. (1963): A procedure for the management of postpneumonectomy empyema. *J. Thorac. Cardiovasc. Surg.,* 45:141.
13. Hunt, J. S., Sparks, F. C., Pilch, Y. H., Silverstein, M. J., Haskell, C. M., and Morton, D. L. (1973): Granulomatous hepatitis: A complication of BCG immunotherapy. *Lancet,* 2:820.
14. Pimm, M. V., and Baldwin, R. W. (1975): BCG therapy of pleural and peritoneal growth of transplanted rat tumors. *Int. J. Cancer,* 15:260–269.
15. Amery, W. K. (1976): Levamisole in resectable human bronchogenic carcinoma. In: *Clinical Tumor Immunology,* edited by J. Wybran and M. Staquet. Pergamon Press, Oxford.

16. Mackaness, G. B., Auclair, D. J., and Lagrange, P. H. (1973): Immunopotentiation with BCG. I. Immune response to different strains and preparations. *J. Natl. Cancer Inst.,* 51:1655.
17. Sparks, F. C., and Albert, N. E. (1975): Does isoniazid decrease the effect of BCG on local tumor growth? *Surg. Forum,* 26:162.
18. Shields, T. W., Higgins, G. A., Keehn, R. J. (1972): Factors influencing survival after resection for bronchial carcinoma. *J. Thorac. Cardiovasc. Surg.,* 64:391.

Immunotherapy of Cancer: Present Status of
Trials in Man, edited by W. D. Terry and D. Windhorst.
Raven Press, New York © 1978.

Immunotherapy of Lung Cancer with Oil-Attached Cell Wall Skeleton of BCG

Yuichi Yamamura

The Third Department of Internal Medicine, Osaka University Medical School, Fukushima, Osaka 553, Japan

Live Bacillus Calmette-Guérin (BCG) has been generally used as the most effective immunopotentiator in the immunotherapies of human malignant tumor. Many investigators, however, have noticed various kinds of serious side effects due to such therapy (1–6).

In previous studies we have demonstrated a potent anticancer effect for oil-attached cell wall skeleton of BCG (BCG-CWS) on human malignant melanoma as well as on transplantable and autochthonous tumors in animals (7–10). The present study was conducted to explore possible clinical value of immunotherapy with BCG-CWS in patients with lung cancer.

MATERIALS AND METHODS

Patients

Two hundred and sixty-one patients with lung cancer admitted to the Kyushu Cancer Center from May, 1972 to June, 1976 were used in the present study. One hundred and fifty-seven patients treated with conventional therapy alone were referred to a control group. One hundred and four patients received conventional therapy as well as treatment with BCG-CWS therapy. There were no considerable differences in average age, ratio of males to females, operability, and mode of conventional therapies, such as irradiation therapy, chemotherapy, and surgery, between patients of the control and BCG-CWS-treated groups. The clinical stage and histological types of patients are summarized in Table 1. The clinical staging of the patients was

TABLE 1. *Clinical stages and histological types of patients with lung cancer*

Groups of patients	Clinical stage				Histological type			
(No. of patients)	I	II	III	IV	Adeno-carcinoma	Squa-mous	Ana-plastic	Misc.
Control (157)	16	26	72	43	68	58	29	2
BCG-CWS-treated (104)	10	8	56	30	53	30	19	2

TABLE 2. *Clinical staging of lung cancer*

| Stage | Metastasis to intrathracic lymph node | | Intrathracic invasion | Distant metastasis |
	Hilum	Mediastinum		
I	−	−	−	−
II	+	−	−	−
III	+ or −	+	+	−
IV	+ or −	+ or −	+ or −	+

Japanese Lung Cancer Society.

based on the classification proposed by the Japanese Lung Cancer Society (Table 2).

Oil-Attached BCG-CWS

Cell wall skeleton of BCG was prepared by the method indicated in Fig. 1 (7,11). The chemical structure of BCG cell wall skeleton obtained is illustrated in Fig. 2.

Oil-attached cell wall skeleton (BCG-CWS) was prepared as follows. Briefly, 0.02 ml of light mineral oil (Drakeol 6VR, Pennsylvania Rifing Co., Batler, Pa.) was added to 5 mg of BCG-CWS and 5 ml of saline containing 0.2% of Tween 80 and ground to a smooth paste in a tissue grinder tube.

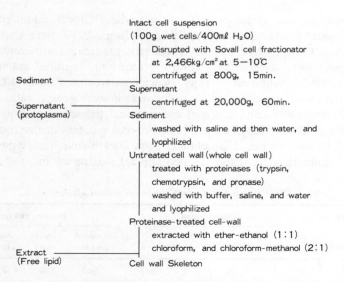

FIG. 1. Purification of cell wall skeleton from the cells of mycobacteria.

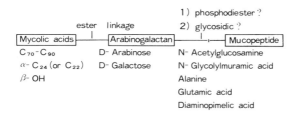

FIG. 2. Chemical structure of cell wall skeleton prepared from M. *bovis* strain BCG.

The resulting suspension of BCG-CWS was sterilized by incubation at 60°C for 30 min before use.

Procedure of Immunotherapy with BCG-CWS

The protocol of immunotherapy with BCG-CWS consisted of three groups as summarized in Table 3. In every group, 300 μg of BCG-CWS was injected once as induction therapy. In group 1, all of the patients received radical resection of the primary tumor beforehand. BCG-CWS was injected intradermally 7 to 10 days after the resection with 1×10^8 irradiated autologous tumor cells prepared from the resected tumor.

In group 2, BCG-CWS was injected intralesionally into the nonresectable primary tumor at exploratory thoracotomy, the superficial metastatic tumor, or the pleural cavity involved with malignant pleurisy.

In group 3, BCG-CWS was injected into the skin.

The induction therapy was followed by intradermal injection of 200 μg BCG-CWS every 2 weeks for 30 weeks and monthly thereafter as maintenance therapy. In some cases BCG-CWS was injected intralesionally during maintenance therapy.

TABLE 3. *Protocol for immunotherapy of lung cancer with BCG-CWS*

Group no.	Mode of immunotherapy
1	I , 300 μg BCG-CWS $+ 1 \times 10^8$ irradiated autologous tumor cells[a] M , 200 μg BCG-CWS, intradermally
2	I , 300 μg BCG-CWS, intralesionally (primary and metastatic tumor, pleural cavity involved with malignant pleurisy) M , 200 μg BCG-CWS, intradermally and/or intralesionally
3	I , 300 μg BCG-CWS, intradermally M , 200 μg BCG-CWS, intradermally

[a] Prepared from the tumor resected by curative surgical operation.
I , induction; M , maintenance; biweekly/30 weeks, thereafter monthly.

RESULTS

Survival Period of the Patients

The survival rates of the patients after admission to the Kyushu Cancer Center was determined monthly by a life table method. When the patients were treated at an early stage, i.e., stages I and II, the survival rates in both groups of patients were still so high that it was too early to evaluate the effect of the therapy.

When BCG-CWS was given to patients at a later stage, i.e., stage III and IV, distinct prolongation of the survival was observed as shown in Fig. 3. In control groups, median survival period was approximately 7 months in stage III and 4 months in stage IV, whereas it was 18 and 12 months, respectively, in BCG-CWS-treated groups. None of the patients treated with conventional therapy alone at stage IV survived 13 months. Median survival in each stage was analyzed according to histological types of the tumors, and similar results were obtained.

Survival periods of patients with malignant pleurisy were prolonged, espe-

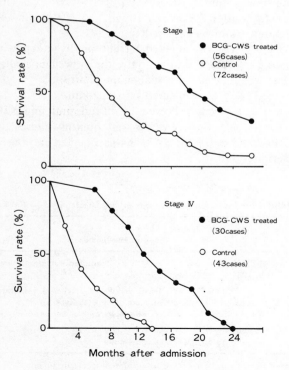

FIG. 3. Survival rate of patients with lung cancer.

TABLE 4. *Analysis of patients treated with intrapleural administration of BCG-CWS*

Group	Patient	Stage	Histological type	Survival period (months)	Status
Control	S.I.	III	large cell carcinoma	13	dead
	K.H.	III	adenocarcinoma	9	dead
	S.F.	III	adenocarcinoma	9	dead
	K.K.	III	adenocarcinoma	6	dead
	S.K.	III	adenocarcinoma	4	dead
	Y.M.	III	squamous cell carcinoma	4	dead
	Y.I.	III	squamous cell carcinoma	3	dead
	N.H.	IV	adenocarcinoma	8	dead
	Y.K.	IV	large cell carcinoma	7	dead
	S.K.	IV	adenocarcinoma	6	dead
	M.K.	IV	adenocarcinoma	5	dead
	H.N.	IV	adenocarcinoma	4	dead
	A.I.	IV	adenocarcinoma	4	dead
	T.N.	IV	adenocarcinoma	3	dead
	T.K.	IV	squamous cell carcinoma	3	dead
	T.M.	IV	adenocarcinoma	1	dead
BCG-CWS-treated	M.M.	III	adenocarcinoma	27	alive
	S.N.	III	adenocarcinoma	23	alive
	K.I.	III	adenocarcinoma	18	dead
	M.O.	III	adenocarcinoma	11	dead
	H.F.	III	adenocarcinoma	9	dead
	Y.N.	III	adenocarcinoma	7	dead
	M.K.	IV	adenocarcinoma	12	dead
	I.Y.	IV	adenocarcinoma	8	dead
	A.K.	IV	adenocarcinoma	8	dead
	I.K.	IV	adenocarcinoma	7	dead
	K.Y.	IV	adenocarcinoma	5	dead
	T.S.	IV	adenocarcinoma	5	dead
	T.S.	IV	squamous cell carcinoma	4	dead

cially in stage III, by BCG-CWS therapy as shown in Table 4. The mean survival period of the patients was 5.6 months in the control group, 11.0 months in the BCG-CWS-treated group. The difference between the groups was statistically significant ($p < 0.02$), even if the survival periods of two survivors under BCG-CWS therapy were assumed to be 23 and 27 months as indicated in the table. Tumor cells were found in the pleura of all patients before therapy and disappeared in approximately 70% of patients during therapy.

Side Effect of BCG-CWS Therapy

Small ulcerations were induced at the injected sites of the skin in almost all patients. After intrapleural or intralesional injection of BCG-CWS, fever up to 38°C for 3 to 4 days was often encountered. However, no serious harmful side effect was detected throughout the study.

DISCUSSION

Survival of patients with stage III and IV lung cancer was remarkably prolonged with BCG-CWS therapy. The effect was most pronounced in patients with malignant pleural effusion when BCG-CWS was administered intrapleurally and intradermally. The therapeutic effects during BCG-CWS therapy were observed to correlate with augmentation of various kinds of nonspecific immune reactivity of the patients, although the results are not described here (12). Thus, BCG-CWS secms to act by stimulating some immune reactions against tumor, as indicated in our previous experimental studies (7–10).

Intrapleural injection of BCG-CWS led to another important success in management of malignant pleural effusion. After the first application of BCG-CWS the effusion increased transiently and then diminished remarkably resulting in a decrease in frequency of therapeutic aspiration of the effusion. A similar effect commonly observed by another clinical group is reported in more detail (13).

The side effects of the treatment, such as fever and cutaneous ulceration, were not so serious as those induced by live BCG and were easily controlled in most cases.

In our laboratories further studies are being undertaken to develop the new synthetic immunopotentiators that will avoid the side effect and pharmaceutical disadvantages of live BCG.

SUMMARY

The therapeutic effect of oil-attached cell wall skeleton of BCG (BCG-CWS) was studied in terms of survival periods of lung cancer patients at various clinical stages.

Three hundred micrograms of BCG-CWS was injected intralesionally or intradermally into the patients who had been treated with conventional therapy. Maintenance therapy with intradermal injections of 200 μg of BCG-CWS followed biweekly for 30 weeks and monthly thereafter.

The mean survival rate of 104 patients treated with BCG-CWS was significantly prolonged compared with that of 157 patients who had been treated with conventional therapy alone as the control.

Usual side effects were fever up to 38°C after intralesional injection of BCG-CWS and small cutaneous ulcerations in the sites injected with BCG-CWS. Harmful side effects were not observed throughout the study.

REFERENCES

1. Morton, D. L. (1972): Immunotherapy of human melanomas and sarcomas. *Natl. Cancer Inst. Monogr.,* 35:375–378.
2. Gutterman, J. V., Mavligit, G., McBride, C., Frei, E., III, Freireich, E. J., and Hersh, E. M. (1973): Active immunotherapy with BCG for recurrent malignant melanoma. *Lancet,* 1:1208–1212.

3. Bast, R. C., Zbar, B., Borsos, T., and Rapp, H. J. (1974): Medical progress, BCG and cancer. *New Engl. J. Med.,* 290:1413–1420.
4. Lieberman, R., Wybran, J., and Epstein, W. (1975): The immunologic and histo-pathologic changes of BCG-mediated tumor regression in patients with malignant melanoma. *Cancer,* 35:756–777.
5. Sparks, F. C., Silverstein, M. J., Hunt, J. S., Haskell, C. M., Pilch, Y. H., and Morton, D. L. (1973): Complication of BCG immunotherapy in patients with cancer. *New Engl. J. Med.,* 289:827–830.
6. Rosenberg, E. B., Kanner, S. P., and Schwartzman, R. J. (1974): Systemic infection following BCG therapy. *Arch. Intern. Med.,* 134:769–773.
7. Azuma, I., Taniyama, T., Hirao, F., and Yamamura, Y. (1974): Antitumor activity of cell-wall skeletons and peptidoglycolipids on mycobacteria and related micro-organisms in mice and rabbits. *Gann,* 65:493–505.
8. Yamamura, Y., Yoshizaki, K., Azuma, I., Takayasu, Yagura, T., and Watanabe, T. (1975): Immunotherapy of human malignant melanoma with oil-attached BCG cell-wall skeleton. *Gann,* 66:355–363.
9. Tokuzen, R., Okabe, M., Nakahara, W., Azuma, I., and Yamamura, Y. (1975): Effect of Nocardia and Mycobacterium cell-wall skeleton on autochthonous tumor graft. *Gann,* 66:433–435.
10. Yoshimoto, T., Azuma, I., Sakatani, M., Nishikawa, H., Ogura, T., Hirao, F., and Yamamura, Y. (1975): Effect of oil-attached BCG cell-wall skeleton on the induction of pleural fibrosarcomas in mice. *Gann,* 67:441–445.
11. Azuma, I., Ribi, E. E., Meyer, T. M., and Zbar, B. (1974): Biologically active components from mycobacterial cell walls. I. Isolation and composition of cell wall skeleton and component P_3. *J. Natl. Cancer Inst.,* 52:95–101.
12. Yasumoto, K., Manabe, H., Ueno, M., Ohta, M., Ueda, H., Iida, A., Nomoto, K., Azuma, I., and Yamamura, Y. (1976): Immunotherapy of human lung cancer with BCG cell wall skeleton. *Gann,* 67:787–796.
13. Yamamura, Y., Ogura, T., Yoshimoto, T., Nishikawa, H., Sakatani, M., Itoh, M., Masuno, T., Namba, M., Yazaki, S., Hirao, F., and Azuma, I. (1976): Successful treatment of malignant pleural effusion with BCG cell-wall skeleton. *Gann,* 67:669–677.

Question and Answer Session

Dr. Peto: The big difference in survival curves was only for the first four months. Then the curves looked the same. How do you explain this? Can you tell us anything about the way patients were selected for these two series? I don't understand why you should get a very rapid difference in survival mainly in the first four months.

Dr. Yamamura: I haven't made a selection but I have used historical controls. All the patients who are admitted to our hospital are treated by BCG-CWS. We haven't made any selection.

Dr. Hersh: Professor Yamamura, did the patients with stage III or IV tumors receive therapy in addition to the cell wall skeleton? Did they also receive chemotherapy or radiotherapy?

Dr. Yamamura: That is a very important point. The same therapy, such as surgery, chemotherapy or radiation, was given to those patients who were treated with cell wall skeleton, as well as to the control patients.

Dr. Hersh: Did the same proportions of patients receive approximately the same radiotherapy or the same drugs in combination in the two periods of time?

Dr. Yamamura: Yes.

Immunotherapy of Cancer: Present Status of
Trials in Man, edited by W. D. Terry and D. Windhorst.
Raven Press, New York © 1978.

Combination Therapy with *Corynebacterium Parvum* and Doxorubicin Hydrochloride in Patients with Lung Cancer

Nikolay V. Dimitrov, *James Conroy, Leife G. Suhrland, Trevor Singh, and Howard Teitlebaum

*Department of Medicine, Michigan State University, East Lansing; Saginaw Cooperative Hospitals, Saginaw, Michigan 48824; and *Cancer Institute— Hahnemann Medical College, Philadelphia, Pennsylvania 15261*

Previous studies have indicated that doxorubicin hydrochloride (Adriamycin®) used as a single agent is of clinical value in advanced bronchogenic carcinoma in response rates ranging from 8 to 37% (1–3). In general, other agents have been less effective. Reports by Israel and his co-workers have indicated that *Corynebacterium parvum* (*C. parvum*) alone or in combination with chemotherapeutic agents may be beneficial in the treatment of cancer patients (4,5). These reports have suggested a need to evaluate more completely the role of *C. parvum* as an adjuvant to the chemotherapy of human cancer, and particularly bronchogenic carcinoma.

Therefore, a pilot study was designed to investigate the effects of *C. parvum* in combination with doxorubicin hydrochloride compared to the use of doxorubicin hydrochloride as a single agent in treatment of selected patients with bronchogenic carcinoma in a randomized trial.

MATERIALS AND METHODS

Sixty-six patients with histologically proven, inoperable bronchogenic carcinoma from four institutions were placed on protocol to study the effect of *C. parvum* as an adjuvant to treatment with doxorubicin hydrochloride. The patients were treated in Philadelphia (Hahnemann Hospital and Philadelphia General Hospital), Saginaw (Saginaw Cooperative Hospitals), and Lansing (Michigan State University Affiliated Hospitals). There were 59 men and seven women with a mean age of 59 years (range 42 to 70 years). Forty-one patients had squamous cell carcinoma, 18 had adenocarcinoma, and seven had large cell anaplastic carcinoma. Patients with small cell carcinoma were excluded. The median interval from diagnosis to entering the protocol was 38 days.

Previous treatment consisted of radiation therapy and chemotherapy.

Thirteen patients had radiation to the lung and contiguous lymph node areas with either no tumor response or appearance of new lesions in the contralateral side, bone, or pleura. Eight patients received local radiation therapy to painful bony metastasis. One patient was treated with nitrogen mustard as a single agent with excellent response but became resistant to the therapy after being in complete remission for 6 months. Two other patients were treated with cyclophosphamide (Cytoxan®) and methotrexate with no therapeutic response. Fourteen patients had previous thoracotomy. All patients were ambulatory.

Criteria for selection of patients were as follows: (a) progressive inoperable regional or distant metastatic disease, other than brain, liver, or bone marrow involvement, (b) expected survival time of at least 3 months, (c) measurable or evaluable disease present, (d) patient recovery from the effect of prior therapy, and (e) no evidence of active infection. Patients with history of heart disease or having an abnormal electrocardiogram were not eligible to enter the protocol, and patients with leukopenia below $4,500/mm^3$ were likewise excluded.

The extent of the disease was defined by clinical measurement, bone marrow examination, roentgenological study, and biochemical profile. The staging in all patients was done according to the directions of the American Joint Committee for Cancer Staging using TNM system. All patients were in stage III (Table 1).

The protocol was designed to evaluate the therapeutic response during 6 months of observation. Tumor measurements were recorded every 3 weeks during the first 3 months and every 6 weeks thereafter. The evaluation of response to therapy was based on objective changes. The criteria of response were: (a) complete remission (CR)—disappearance of all clinical evidence of disease, (b) partial remission (PR)—greater than 50% decrease in the lesion or lesions and the absence of appearance of new lesions or tumor progression elsewhere, (c) no change—neither response nor progression after completion of the treatment, and (d) progression—greater than 25% increase in tumor size from the original measurement or appearance of new lesions. If tumor progression was recorded, at least one or two more courses were administered before the patient was classified as a nonresponder.

The therapeutic schedule is shown in Table 2. The dose of doxorubicin hydrochloride used in this study was 60 mg/m^2 per treatment equally divided

TABLE 1. *The distribution of patients using TNM system (stage III)*

Classification	Number	Percent
$T_2 N_{1,2} M_1$	28	42.4
$T_3 N_{1,2} M_0$	21	31.8
$T_3 N_{1,2} M_1$	17	25.7

TABLE 2. *Therapeutic schedule for the treatment of bronchogenic carcinoma*

Cell type	R A N D O M I Z A T I O N		
Squamous cell carcinoma ———		———	Doxorubicin hydrochloride 60 mg/m² i.v. every 3 weeks
Adenocarcinoma ———			
Large cell carcinoma ———		———	Doxorubicin hydrochloride 60 mg/m² i.v. every 3 weeks + C. Parvum, 4.2 mg s.c. every week

into three consecutive daily intravenous injections. The administration was given as a push injection with simultaneously running dextrose 5% in water 250 cc. The total dose of doxorubicin hydrochloride received during the 6-month treatment was between 420 to 490 mg/m² per patient.

The amount of *C. parvum* vaccine administered was 4.2 mg/week given as multiple subcutaneous and intradermal inoculations. The Burroughs-Wellcome vaccine (4.2 mg = 0.6 cc) was mixed with 1.4 cc of 2% lidocaine (Xylocaine®). Six subcutaneous injections with 0.3 cc of the mixture were injected along the posterior axillary line. In addition, two intradermal injections of 0.1 cc of the same mixture were applied in the same area.

The initial protocol of this pilot study was designed to evaluate the effect of one (4.2 mg) and two weekly injections of *C. parvum* (8.4 mg) using the same dose of doxorubicin hydrochloride. Occurrence of severe pain at the injection site that was intolerable for the patients forced us to eliminate this arm from the study.

Doxorubicin hydrochloride was repeated every 3 weeks; however, if the leukocyte count and platelet count fell below 3,000/mm³ and 50,000/mm², respectively, before the next treatment, the succeeding dose of doxorubicin hydrochloride was reduced 75%. For leukocyte counts below 2,000/mm³, the drug was withheld until recovery to 5,000/mm³. After the therapeutic schedule was completed, patients from the combination therapy were placed on a monthly schedule with *C. parvum* and the patients treated with doxorubicin hydrochloride were placed on a monthly schedule with cyclophosphamide 500 mg/m² i.v. Five patients, however, from the doxorubicin hydrochloride group and 11 patients from the combination therapy group have received, after the 6-month mark, other chemotherapeutic agents including methotrexate, vincristine, and bleomycin.

Patients were monitored with a complete blood count and platelet count every 3 weeks before the next course of treatment. An SMA-12 was obtained at 6-week intervals. Skin tests were performed before initiation of therapy and thereafter every 3 months. The antigens used in the skin tests were varidase, candidine, and purified protein derivative (PPD). Since the subjects for this study were randomly assigned to one of the two experimental groups, the Fisher Exact Test was used for analysis of data (6).

RESULTS

Seventy-three patients were randomized in two arms to study the effect of *C. parvum* as an adjuvant. Only 66 patients were eligible for evaluation.

The therapeutic response is presented in Table 3, which compares the CR, PR, no change, and progression of the two treatment groups. Only one patient from the group treated with combination therapy achieved CR, whereas no CR was observed in the group treated with doxorubicin hydrochloride alone. There appeared to be no difference between the two groups for PR. In the category of no change, the group treated with combination therapy showed 51.4% compared to 37.9% in the doxorubicin hydrochloride alone group. In contrast, a smaller percentage (32.4%) of patients with progressive disease was found in the group of combination therapy than in the group treated with doxorubicin hydrochloride alone (44.8%).

The objective response in both groups lasted from 5 to 12 months. There was no significant difference in the duration of response between the two therapeutic schedules. Since the number of patients is small, it is impossible to evaluate the relationship between the histological type of tumor and the occurrence and duration of objective remission. It should be noted that the majority of patients (12) who received radiation therapy were in the group of no change and PR.

The overall median survival time of the patients cannot be evaluated because some of the patients from both groups are still alive. In addition, such evaluation would be inaccurate because the patients surviving the 1-year mark have been placed on various chemotherapeutic combinations and the effect of such inference cannot be ignored.

The 12-month survival curve as presented in Fig. 1 shows that 50% of

TABLE 3. *Therapeutic response*

Response	Doxorubicin hydrochloride + C. parvum	Doxorubicin hydrochloride
CR	1/37 (2.7%)	0/29 —
PR	5/37 (13.5%)	5/29 (17.5%)
No change	19/37 (51.4%)	11/29 (37.9%)
Progression	12/37 (32.4%)	13/29 (44.8%)

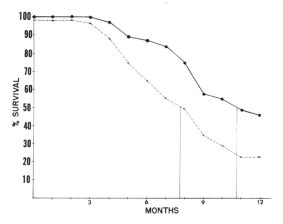

FIG. 1. Survival time in months in 37 patients treated with doxorubicin hydrochloride and C. *parvum* and 29 patients treated with doxorubicin hydrochloride alone (randomized groups). ●—●, Doxorubicin hydrochloride + C. *parvum*; ▶--- ▶, doxorubicin hydrochloride.

the patients treated with doxorubicin hydrochloride alone were alive at 7.8 months, whereas in the combination therapy group, the time was 10.7 months. At the end of 12 months, 25.2% of the patients treated with doxorubicin hydrochloride alone were living and 46% in the combination therapy group were alive. The statistical analysis of data revealed a probability level of $p <$ 0.07, which is not significant. In addition to the randomized patients, we have treated 16 more patients with C. *parvum* and doxorubicin hydrochloride and two more patients with doxorubicin hydrochloride alone, following the same criteria for patient selection. When these patients were added to the randomized group, the analysis of data showed a similar probability level of $p < 0.06$ —not significant (Fig. 2).

When the group showing no change and the group of responders are combined, the survival time of these two groups is significantly longer in patients receiving doxorubicin hydrochloride and C. *parvum* ($p < 0.05$). The results from the toxicity of doxorubicin hydrochloride are shown in Table 4. The side effects observed during this study do not differ from those described by other investigators (7). The most significant observation is the low incidence of leukopenia in patients treated with doxorubicin hydrochloride and C. *parvum*. Some differences noted in the other side effects are not significant.

Special attention was given to the side effects resulting from the administration of the vaccine; these are presented in Table 5. The total dose of C. *parvum* received during the 6-month period of observation is presented in Table 6. Eighty-nine percent of the patients experienced various degrees of local pain when multiple subcutaneous injections were applied. The duration of the pain was between 1 and 7 days. This includes the sites of intradermal application as well. No dermatitis or abscesses were observed. Fever in the range of 100 to 103°F developed in 56.7% of the treated patients with

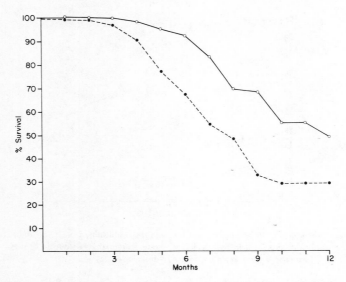

FIG. 2. Survival time in months in 53 patients treated with doxorubicin hydrochloride and C. *parvum* and 31 patients treated with doxorubicin hydrochloride alone (total amount of treated patients). O—O, doxorubicin hydrochloride + C. *parvum* (53); ●−−−●, doxorubicin hydrochloride (31).

duration between 12 and 48 hr. In some cases, a double peak temperature curve on alternate days was observed. A few patients developed chills. Malaise was a general complaint and appears to be the most bothersome for the patient.

Pretreatment and posttreatment skin tests, determination of the immunoglobulin levels, and biochemical profile of the serum (SMA-12) did not reveal any significant differences. Decreased and low normal phytohemagglutinin stimulation index was found in all 26 patients before the initiation

TABLE 4. *Side effects*

	Doxorubicin hydrochloride		Doxorubicin hydrochloride + C. *parvum*	
	Number of patients	Percentage	Number of patients	Percentage
Leukopenia				
4,000–2,500/mm³	16/29	55.1	5/37	13.5
Below 2,500/mm³	10/29	34.4	0/37	0
Anemia	9/29	31.0	15/37	40.5
Thrombocytopenia	3/29	10.3	5/37	13.5
EKG changes	9/29	31.0	5/37	13.5
Congestive heart failure (mild)	2/29	6.9	0/37	0
Alopecia	29/29	100.0	37/37	100.0
Nausea, vomiting, dysphagia	4/29	13.8	6/37	16.2

TABLE 5. *Frequency of side effects of C. parvum*

Side effect	Number	Percentage
Local pain	33/37	89
Fever	21/37	57
Chills	8/37	22
Malaise	34/37	92

TABLE 6. *Amount of C. parvum administered during the first 6 months*

Amount of vaccine	Medium	Number of patients
92–109 mg	96 mg	6
71–89 mg	79 mg	24
50–68 mg	61 mg	7

of the treatment, however, four patients in the *C. parvum* group showed a marked increase in the stimulation index at the end of the sixth month.

DISCUSSION

The results from this study, although far from conclusive, do indicate some differences between the two treatment schedules attributed to the use of *C. parvum* vaccine. Since this is a pilot study with a limited number of patients, it would be helpful to extract only the significant findings. Thus, the significantly longer survival over a 1-year observation period among patients in the two groups of responders plus no change treated with *C. parvum* and doxorubicin hydrochloride deserves further attention. Better analysis of the patients before treatment may provide additional information for explanation of such findings. Response to combination therapy of *C. parvum* and doxorubicin hydrochloride has been observed in experimental tumors with significant prolongation of the survival time of the animals compared to the control group treated with doxorubicin hydrochloride alone (8). The mechanisms involved in this drug potentiation are not clear.

Another interesting observation is the lower incidence of leukopenia in the group of patients treated with *C. parvum*. Although several experimental reports clearly indicate the stimulatory effect of *C. parvum* on the bone marrow colony-forming capacity, the preliminary experience with *C. parvum* in humans raises some questions regarding the myelostimulatory effect of the vaccine (9,10). In our protocol we have used a single chemotherapeutic agent, whereas studies by others include the use of combination chemotherapy (11). Additional studies are needed to elucidate the effect of *C. parvum* on the bone marrow function related to the time schedule and route of administration. Application of two weekly subcutaneous injections is impractical because of the great discomfort for the patient. Our limited experience indicates that the therapeutic value of such schedule is questionable as well.

This pilot study indicates that *C. parvum* may be a useful adjuvant in treatment of bronchogenic carcinoma.

SUMMARY

Sixty-six patients with stage III bronchogenic carcinoma were randomized in two arms: (a) doxorubicin hydrochloride 60 mg/m^2 i.v. every 3 weeks, and (b) doxorubicin hydrochloride 60 mg/m^2 i.v. every 3 weeks plus *C. parvum* 4.2 mg weekly as multiple subcutaneous injections. No difference in CR and PR was demonstrated. High percentages of the patients treated with combination therapy showed no change in status. Patients treated with doxorubicin hydrochloride and *C. parvum* had a significantly lower incidence of leukopenia compared to those treated with doxorubicin hydrochloride alone. The survival time at 1 year appeared to be longer for the group with combination therapy, but the difference is not statistically significant for the number of patients evaluated.

REFERENCES

1. O'Bryan, R., Luce, J., Talley, R., Gottlieb, J., Baker, L., and Bonadonna, G. (1973): Phase II evaluation of Adriamycin in human neoplasia. *Cancer,* 32:1–8.
2. Cortex, E. P., Hiroshi, T., and Holland, J. F. (1974): Adriamycin in advanced bronchogenic carcinoma. *Cancer,* 34:518–525.
3. Selawry, V. S. (1975): Response of bronchogenic carcinoma to Adriamycin (NSC-123127). *Cancer Chemother. Rep.,* 6:349–351.
4. Israel, L., and Halpern, B. N. (1973): Le Corynebacterium Parvum dans les cancers avances. *Nouv. Presse Med.,* 1:19–23.
5. Israel, L., Edelstein, R., Depierre, A., and Dimitrov, N. (1975): Daily intravenous infusions of Corynebacterium parvum in twenty patients with disseminated cancer: A preliminary report of clinical and biologic findings. *J. Natl. Cancer Inst.,* 55:29–33.
6. Bradley, J. V. (1968): *Distribution—Free Statistical Tests.* Prentice-Hall, Englewood Cliffs, N.J.
7. Benjamin, R. S. (1975): A practical approach to Adriamycin (NSC-123127) toxicology. *Cancer Chemother. Rep.,* 6:191–194.
8. Houchens, D. P., and Gaston, M. R. (1977): Therapy of experimental tumors with Corynebacterium parvum alone and in combination with Adriamycin. *Cancer Chemother. Rep.* (*In press.*)
9. Ossorio, C., Craddock, C., Brosman, J., and Plotkin, D. (1976): Bone marrow colony forming capacity and Adriamycin levels in patient receiving Corynebacterium parvum. *Proc. AACR,* 17:199.
10. Dimitrov, N. V., Singh, T., Conroy, J., and Suhrland, G. L. (1976): Combination therapy with C. parvum and Adriamycin in patients with lung carcinoma. *Proc. ASCO,* 17:292.

11. DeJager, R., Pinsky, C., Kaufman, R., Ochoa, M., Oettgen, H., and Krakoff, I. (1976): Chemotherapy of advanced breast cancer with a combination of cyclophosphamide, Adriamycin, methotrexate and 5-fluorouracil. *Proc. ASCO,* 17:296.

Question and Answer Session

Dr. Pinsky: What did you mix C. *parvum* with? Also, you said that in the overall groups there was no statistically significant difference in the survival, but you mentioned a subgroup where there was. Could you clarify that?

Dr. Dimitrov: 0.6 cc is equal to 4.2 mg of C. *parvum* and is mixed with 1.42 xylocaine.

When we combine the group of no change and the group with the responses, there was a statistically significant difference ($p = 0.05$) between survival in the C. *parvum* plus adriamycin® group versus adriamycin® alone.

Dr. Powles: Just following that point you have made, I think you must stress that, including the complete and partial remissions, you have five patients in one group and six in the other, so I think it makes a value of 0.05 somewhat artificial.

Dr. Dimitrov: The complete remission and partial remission from C. *parvum* and adriamycin® when compared to the same with adriamycin® alone are not significant, but if you take the complete remission, partial remission and no change in status and compare those two groups, there is significance.

Dr. Amery: It has been said that C. *parvum* influences the metabolism of other drugs. Could this possibly be the explanation for the lower degree of granulocyte drop in your study?

Dr. Dimitrov: Yes, we are very much involved now in adriamycin® metabolism to see if this is the case. I should say that C. *parvum* stimulates B cells and antibody production. Also, there is a publication by Hutchin which shows that if you combine C. *parvum* with adriamycin® you increase the effects, but adriamycin® or C. *parvum* alone has very little effect. Probably there is some synergism.

Dr. Woodruff: Could I ask why you gave C. *parvum* subcutaneously? There is a great deal of evidence that this is a poor way to give C. *parvum*. I can't think of any animal model where there is any convincing evidence that C. *parvum* is of value when given subcutaneously.

Dr. Dimitrov: That's because people have injected C. *parvum* as one injection. We have done studies with radioisotopes, doing multiple subcutaneous injections in the foot pad, and compared that to one subcutaneous injection. There is a great difference in the absorption of the radioactivity by the liver, by the spleen and other organs. This was the reason that we have chosen multiple subcutaneous injections in small doses to allow absorption, and that's why we probably have better results. I'm not sure about this.

Dr. Beretta: I would like to know if you had a lot of skin reaction after C. *parvum*. We frequently observe subcutaneous nodules after injection.

Dr. Dimitrov: If we inject the small doses that we are using, from time to time we can observe small subcutaneous nodules, but most of the patients don't have subcutaneous nodules. The intradermal injection of *C. parvum* does absolutely the same thing as BCG. The amount here is small, so that we don't have a difference in the appearance of that lesion.

Immunotherapy of Cancer: Present Status of Trials in Man, edited by W. D. Terry and D. Windhorst. Raven Press, New York © 1978.

A Placebo-Controlled Levamisole Study in Resectable Lung Cancer

Willem K. Amery[1]

Janssen Pharmaceutica, B-2340 Beerse, Belgium

Levamisole, an imidazo-thiazole derivative which has been used for years as an anthelmintic, was found some 5 years ago to possess immunotropic properties (6). Its effects on host defense mechanisms have repeatedly been reviewed in the meantime and may best be described as those of an anti-anergic chemotherapeutic agent (5,8). As host defense is probably implicated in the prognosis of cancer patients, it seemed logical to test levamisole as an adjunct to surgery in lung cancer patients, since prognosis in this type of patient is still far from satisfactory and since no effective adjuvant treatment is known for this disease.

PATIENTS

Only those 178 patients who had been operated on at least 1 year before this interim analysis have been included in the present evaluation. The patients' characteristics are summarized in Table 1. The two treatment groups are quite comparable except for the number of patients with squamous cell carcinoma, which was more frequently found ($p = 0.05$) among the levamisole-treated patients. The patients entered the study medially 2 years before this analysis.

Concerning the assessment of the tumor extent, three measures were adopted: (a) the largest tumor diameter was measured after its fixation by the local pathologist; (b) a category grouping system was adopted describing the regional extent of the tumor; within this system, category 1a is the only category where there is no evidence that the tumor could have left or has already left the primary site; and (c) a grading system was adopted combining the previous two assessments and giving a rough estimate of the preoperative tumor burden (grade I is assigned to patients with a smaller tumor burden).

---

[1] Chairman of the Study Group for Bronchogenic Carcinoma, whose composition is as follows: Cooperating investigators: Prof. J. Swierenga, Dr. H. C. Gooszen and Dr. R. G. Vanderschueren (Utrecht); Prof. J. Cosemans and Dr. A. Louwagie (Leuven); Dr. J. Stam, Prof. E. Lopes Cardozo and Dr. R. W. Veldhuizen (Amsterdam). Consultants: Dr. W. Tanghe, Dr. P. A. J. Janssen, Prof. A. Drochmans, J. Dony, Dr. L. Desplenter and G. De Ceuster. Coordination: E. Denissen.

TABLE 1. *Patients' characteristics*

Characteristics		Levamisole group (N = 82)[a]		Placebo group (N = 96)[a]	
Sex:	Male	79/82	(96)[b]	91/96	(95)
	Female	3/82	(4)	5/96	(5)
Age (years)	≤ 60	31/82	(38)	44/96	(46)
	> 60	51/82	(62)	52/96	(54)
Weight (kg)	≤ 70	35/81	(43)	41/92	(45)
	> 70	46/81	(57)	51/92	(55)
ESR	≤ 20 mm	40/81	(49)	42/94	(45)
	> 20 mm	41/81	(51)	52/94	(55)
Initial skin tests					
Diameter with PPD	< 10 mm	26/69	(38)	28/76	(37)
	≥ 10 mm	43/69	(62)	48/76	(63)
DNCB 50 μg	No induration	25/56	(45)	27/65	(42)
	Induration	31/56	(55)	38/65	(58)
DNCB 100 μg	No induration	11/51	(22)	6/54	(11)
	Induration	40/51	(78)	48/54	(89)
Daily use of cigarettes	≤ 10	24/76	(32)	24/88	(27)
	> 10	52/76	(68)	64/88	(73)
Tumor location	Right	48/82	(59)	45/95	(47)
	Left	34/82	(41)	50/95	(53)
	Peripheral	40/74	(54)	50/83	(60)
	Central	34/74	(46)	33/83	(40)
Type of surgery	Lobectomy	57/81	(70)	63/95	(66)
	Pneumonectomy	23/81	(29)	30/95	(32)
	Other	1/81	(1)	2/95	(2)
Histology	Squamous cell carcinoma	57/82	(69)	56/96	(58)
	Adenocarcinoma	12/82	(15)	26/96	(27)
	Others or mixed	13/82	(16)	14/96	(15)
Largest tumor diameter	≤ 3 cm	28/74	(38)	29/88	(33)
	≥ 4 cm	46/74	(62)	59/88	(67)
Grouping category	1 a	41/79	(52)	46/93	(49)
	Others	38/79	(48)	47/93	(51)
Total grading for extent	I	40/71	(56)	42/85	(49)
	II	31/71	(44)	43/85	(51)

[a] The totals are not always 82 and 96 as some data are unknown for some patients.
[b] Figures in parentheses are percentages.
DNCB, dinitrochlorobenzene; PPD, purified protein derivative; ESR, erythrocyte sedimentation rate.

More details about these assessments have been described in previous reports (1,2,7).

TREATMENT

The patients are randomly allocated to treatment with either levamisole or placebo, but randomization is stratified in the three cooperating centers to flatten out possible differences in the surgical and anesthesiological approach.

The medication is strictly double blind and individually coded in sufficient amounts for the entire duration of the trial.

One tablet of the double-blind supply, containing either 50 mg of levamisole or placebo, is given three times daily on the last 3 days before surgery (in an attempt to prevent immunosuppression caused by the operation), and a similar 3-day course is repeated every second week thereafter for 2 years after surgery, unless relapse is evident. In the latter case, appropriate cytoreductive therapy is given, but until recurrence is proved, the use of cytostatics, corticosteroids, and radiotherapy is prohibited.

STATISTICAL ANALYSIS

The end points of the study are the first sound suspicion of recurrence, the first proof of relapse, and carcinomatous death. All data are stored in an IBM 370/135 computer, and the statistical analysis is performed by means of the Fisher exact probability test, two-tailed, using a Wang 2200, except for the actuarial analysis where Student's t-test, two-tailed probability is used as programmed (4).

RESULTS

For the total population studied, a slight trend in favor of levamisole was found for the three end points, reaching statistical significance at the 5% level only 18 months postsurgery for suspected recurrence and for carcinomatous deaths and 21 months for disease mortality when analyzed by means of the actuarial method (Fig. 1). Also, a favorable trend was present in the data from each cooperating center.

However, since in the previous interim analyses (2,3) several patients were found to have been underdosed in this trial, the results were reanalyzed with respect to the weight of the patients. Exactly as on these previous occasions, no difference was found at all between levamisole and placebo in patients weighing above 70 kg; however, striking differences in favor of levamisole were found in those who had an initial body weight of 70 kg or below (Fig. 2).

In view of this decisive importance of the patient's weight, a search into other possibly predictive factors was limited to data obtained in patients weighing $\leq$ 70 kg.

1. *Initial skin tests* (Table 2). There is a tendency for good responders to do relatively better with levamisole than bad responders, but the beneficial trend present among the latter, too, and the small sample size preclude a sensible conclusion.

2. *Tumor histology* (Table 3). The efficacy of levamisole proves to be similarly distributed over the different types of cancer.

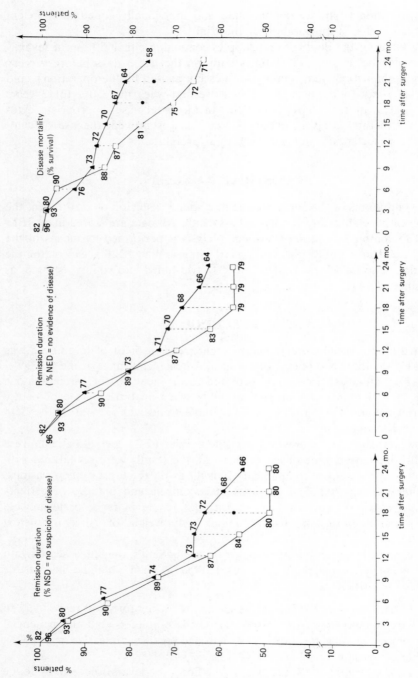

FIG. 1. Actuarial analysis of remission duration and survival. Eighty-two is the effective sample size. By the Student's t-test, two-tailed probability, * = $p \leq 0.05$, ** = $p \leq 0.01$, and *** = $p \leq 0.001$. ▲, Levamisole; □, placebo.

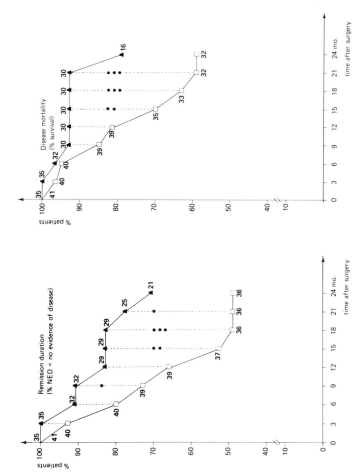

FIG. 2. Actuarial analysis of remission duration and survival in patients weighing ≤ 70 kg. Thirty-five is the effective sample size. By the Student's *t*-test, two-tailed probability, * = *p* ≤ 0.05, ** = *p* ≤ 0.01, and *** = *p* ≤ 0.001. ▲, Levamisole; □, placebo.

TABLE 2. *Results as related to initial skin test reactivity (patients $\leq$ 70 kg)*

Parameter	p Value[a]: levamisole vs. placebo	
	Proven relapses	Carcinomatous deaths
Initial PPD		
< 10 mm	NS	NS
	(4/13 vs. 8/13)	(2/13 vs. 6/13)
$\geq$ 10 mm	0.066	0.10
	(2/14 vs. 10/20)	(1/14 vs. 7/20)
Initial DNCB 50 μg		
No induration	NS	0.061
	(1/6 vs. 9/15)	(0/6 vs. 7/15)
Induration	0.036	NS
	(2/12 vs. 7/11)	(2/12 vs. 4/11)
Initial DNCB 100 μg		
No induration	NS	NS
	(1/2 vs. 1/3)	(0/2 vs. 1/3)
Induration	0.012	NS
	(2/15 vs. 10/17)	(2/15 vs. 7/17)

[a] Fisher exact probability test, two-tailed (the total number of patients is not always 35 for levamisole and 41 for placebo as some data were not available for some patients).

DNCB, dinitrochlorobenzene; NS, not significant; PPD, purified protein derivative.

3. *Initial tumor extent* (Table 4). Although a slight favorable trend is present with levamisole in those patients who had a smaller tumor burden preoperatively, the drug proves much more effective in preventing relapse and carcinomatous death in patients having more extended tumors at the time of operation.

Last but not least, the site of the first recurrence was analyzed in the patients with an initial weight of 70 kg or below, in order to evaluate the possible differential effect of levamisole on hematogenous metastases and on intrathoracic relapses (Table 5). Although the effect on the latter was limited, levamisole proved especially effective in controlling blood-borne sec-

TABLE 3. *Results as related to histological diagnosis (patients $\leq$ 70 kg)*

Parameter	p Value[a]: levamisole vs. placebo	
	Proven relapses	Carcinomatous deaths
Squamous cell carcinoma	NS	NS
	(6/26 vs. 10/23)	(4/26 vs. 7/23)
Adenocarcinoma	NS	NS
	(0/4 vs. 4/11)	(0/4 vs. 4/11)
Other + mixed	0.072	0.081
	(1/5 vs. 6/7)	(0/5 vs. 4/7)

[a] Fisher exact probability test, two-tailed.

TABLE 4. *Results relating to initial extent of tumor (patients ≤ 70 kg)*

Parameter	p Value[a]: levamisole vs. placebo	
	Proven relapses	Carcinomatous deaths
Largest tumor diameter		
≤ 3 cm	NS	NS
	(0/11 vs. 4/14)	(0/11 vs. 3/14)
≥ 4 cm	0.040	0.052
	(6/19 vs. 16/25)	(3/19 vs. 12/25)
Regional extent		
Grouping category 1 a	NS	NS
	(4/20 vs. 4/14)	(3/20 vs. 2/14)
Other categories	0.046	0.015
	(3/13 vs. 16/27)	(1/13 vs. 13/27)
Total grading		
Grade I	NS	NS
	(1/16 vs. 4/16)	(1/16 vs. 2/16)
Grade II	NS	0.034
	(5/12 vs. 16/23)	(2/12 vs. 13/23)

[a] Fisher exact probability test, two-tailed (the total number of patients is not always 35 for levamisole and 41 for placebo as some data were not available for some patients).

TABLE 5. *Site of first recurrence (patients ≤ 70 kg)*

	Levamisole group	Placebo group	Levamisole vs. placebo[a]
Intrathoracic relapses	4/35	7/41	NS
Distant metastases	3/35	13/41	0.022

[a] Fisher exact probability test, two-tailed.

ondaries. It may be of interest to note that one of the three patients who had a distant metastasis had temporarily interrupted his double-blind treatment 2 months before he developed clinical liver metastases. Also it is worth mentioning here that levamisole proved effective in controlling distant metastases, regardless of their sites (the metastases with placebo were distributed as follows: five in bone, three in liver, four in brain, and one in kidney; the respective figures with levamisole were: one, one, one, and zero).

ACCEPTABILITY OF THE TREATMENT

The noncancer mortality with levamisole proves quite comparable to that with placebo (Table 6). In particular, the risk of surgical mortality does not seem affected by preoperative levamisole treatment, nor does prolonged treatment seem to change general mortality (mainly cardiovascular).

Also, side effects do not seem to be a major obstacle to levamisole treatment (Table 7). Probably, the most frequently observed levamisole-related

TABLE 6. Overall mortality

	Levamisole group (N = 82)	Placebo group (N = 96)
Surgical mortality	3	4
Disease mortality	16	30
Other known cause of death	6	4
Unknown cause of death	1	2

TABLE 7. Survey of side effects

Type of side effect	% of patients on levamisole (N = 82)	% of patients on placebo (N = 96)
Gast. oenterological		
Sialorrhea	1.2	0.0
Nausea, vomiting, malaise	19.5[a]	8.3[a]
Foul taste	0.0	1.0[a]
Lack of appetite	4.9	1.0
Gastric complaints	3.7	4.2
Pyrosis	1.2	0.0
Abdominal pain	0.0	1.0
Diarrhea or intestinal complaints	3.7[a]	3.1
Anomalies in hepatic tests	0.0	1.0
Loss of weight	0.0	2.1
Weight gain	1.2	3.1
Total: gastroenterological	24.4	20.8
CNS phenomena		
Fatigue	7.3[a]	5.2
Apathy, inertia, adynamia	2.4	2.1
Nervousness, sleep disorders	4.9	2.1
Feeling of oppression	1.2	0.0
Fever, subfebrility, shivering	4.9	2.1
Paresthesia	0.0	2.1
Dizziness, vertigo	2.4[a]	1.0
Total: CNS	22.0	13.5
Miscellaneous		
Migraine	1.2[a]	0.0
Aching joints	0.0	2.1
Muscular cramps in the legs	0.0	1.0
Excessive perspiration	2.4	0.0
Skin rash	0.0	3.1[a]
Depigmentation	1.2	0.0
Total: miscellaneous	4.9	6.3
TOTAL: ALL SIDE EFFECTS	39.0	28.1

[a] Treatment discontinued because of these side effects: 7 patients with levamisole (but persistence of side effects in 4), 4 patients with placebo (no persistence of side effects).
CNS, central nervous system.

side effects are gastric intolerance, nervousness (sometimes causing sleep disturbances), and shiverings with or without fever.

DISCUSSION

The data reported here seem very encouraging and call for a broad clinical evaluation of levamisole used as an adjunct to classical anticancer treatment. However, in future trials the dose of levamisole ought to be adapted to the patients' weight (estimated daily dose, 2.5 mg/kg) or, probably still better, their body surface (approximately 100 mg/m² daily). In these investigations, careful attention should be paid to such features as the initial tumor load and the site of the first recurrence since these may provide further insight into the mechanism of action of the drug and its field of application in the clinic.

SUMMARY

The fourth interim analysis is reported of a prospective randomized placebo-controlled double-blind study with levamisole as an adjunct to surgery in resectable lung cancer. The data considered for this analysis are those obtained in the 82 levamisole-treated patients and the 96 placebo controls who were operated on at least 1 year before this evaluation.

Levamisole 50 mg t.i.d. or placebo is given for 3 consecutive days every fortnight, and the follow-up lasts for 2 years after surgery.

The dosage of levamisole fails to affect the prognosis in patients weighing more than 70 kg before surgery, but is strikingly effective compared with placebo in patients weighing 70 kg or less. In the latter group of patients, levamisole proved especially effective in controlling hematogenous metastases and in preventing relapse in patients having more extended tumors at the time of the operation.

Levamisole ought to be widely studied as an adjunct to classical anticancer treatment, but its dose should be adapted to the weight or the body surface of the patients.

REFERENCES

1. Amery, W. (1976): Levamisole in resectable human bronchogenic carcinoma. In: *Clinical Tumor Immunology,* edited by J. Wybran, and M. Staquet. Pergamon Press, Oxford.
2. Amery, W. (1976): Double-blind levamisole trial in resectable lung cancer. *Ann. NY Acad. Sci.,* 277:260–268.
3. Amery, W. (1976): Double-blind trial with levamisole in resectable lung cancer. In: *Proc. 9th Int. Congr. Chemotherapy.* Plenum, New York.
4. Dixon, W. J. (editor) (1973): *B. M. D., Biomedical Computer Programs.* Univ. California Press, Berkeley.
5. Janssen, P. A. J. (1976): The levamisole story. In: *Fortschritte in Arzneimittel-*

Forschung/Progress in Drug Research, Vol. 20, edited by E. Jucker, pp. 347–383. Birkhäuser Verlag, Basel.
6. Renoux, G., and Renoux, M. (1971): Effet immunostimulant d'un imidothiazole dans l'immunisation des souris contre l'infection par Brucella abortus. *CR Acad. Sci. Paris,* 272:349–350.
7. Study Group for Bronchogenic Carcinoma (1975): Immunopotentiation with levamisole in resectable bronchogenic carcinoma: A double-blind controlled trial. *Br. Med. J.,* 3:461–464.
8. Symoens, J. (1976): Levamisole: An anti-anergic chemotherapeutic agent. In: *Control of Neoplasia by Modulation of the Immune System,* edited by M. A. Chirigos. Raven Press, New York.

Question and Answer Session

Dr. Wright: One of the most important issues concerns the comparability of your treatment and control groups. Could you provide any additional information documenting the comparability of these groups? In particular, do you have any information concerning the status of the mediastinum, either determined preoperatively by mediastinoscopy or at the time of surgery?

Dr. Amery: The two treatment groups are comparable from the start except for one parameter, and that is the histology of the tumor. There are more squamous cell carcinoma patients in the levamisole group and there are more adenocarcinoma patients in the placebo group. On the other hand, we do not feel that differences in histology have affected the results. A recent publication in the *Journal of Thoracic and Cardiovascular Surgery* indicated that after surgery the prognosis of the several types of lung cancer is similar except for small cell carcinoma. I don't know what Dr. Cohen thinks about that.

Information on the status of the mediastinum is contained in the disease classification. In Category 1 the tumor is limited to the original site; 1-A is without blood vessel invasion; 1-B is with blood vessel invasion. In Category 2, the patients have regional lymph nodes involved. In Category 3 are patients in whom there is a positive resection margin.

Question: You have correlated activity of levamisole with two factors. One is the weight of the patient and also the weight of the tumor; however, we have learned from Dr. Cohen that patients with larger tumors lose weight. Have you attempted to sort out those problems?

Dr. Amery: Not yet.

Dr. Smith (Richmond): I would like to know about granulocytopenia in your patients since this has been a reported complication of levamisole.

Dr. Amery: This has been a reported side effect, that's true. We have no such patients in this trial, and I should say in general it has occurred far more frequently in rheumatoid arthritis patients, in whom levamisole is also used, than in cancer patients.

There are a few cancer patients in whom this side effect has been seen, but it has not been reported in this study.

Dr. Bolt (New York): You have mentioned the importance of weight in determining the results of levamisole therapy. Are you now using a weight formula for giving levamisole, and could you state how you modify the levamisole dosage for weight?

Dr. Amery: Yes. Not in this trial, because when we detected the effect of the weight there were only 40 patients still to be selected for the study, half of them for placebo and half of them for levamisole. This means 20 levamisole patients, and only half of them would possibly have some benefit of the change of the dosage. So we felt it would be of no use to change the program, because we wouldn't find anything else.

In general, I would recommend a daily dose of about 2.5 mg/kg on the treatment days, or, expressed in square meters of body surface, this would be about 100 mg/m².

Dr. Peto: I just wanted to put in another warning about statistical significance. You have retrospectively separated the patients with respect to weight for purposes of analysis. If you pick subgroups in some arbitrary way, you are quite likely to find that there is an apparent difference between groups. I think one should stick with the overall results as one's real index of success or failure. Although you have a tendency in the overall results, it's not absolutely conclusive. I think that subdividing with respect to rather odd variables is really rather dangerous.

Dr. Amery: I quite agree with that. On the other hand, the purpose of doing clinical trials is to help patients. If there is some evidence in clinical trials that we should change the program, and if we can draw tentative conclusions from that trial, I think there is every reason to change that program so that we can have trials designed with an appropriate dose.

Also, from the animal data there is evidence that levamisole only seems to work in a dose of about 2.5 mg/kg parenterally. So we are now giving a dose of 2.5 mg/kg divided over three doses. Therefore I think there was a reason to do this analysis related to the weight of the patient.

Dr. Hersh: I think it would be most important to come back to this during the discussion. In clinical research it's important to identify subcategories of patients with unique or different responses, either positive or negative, because these are the clinical leads on which we build more effective programs of therapy.

Immunotherapy of Cancer: Present Status of Trials in Man, edited by W. D. Terry and D. Windhorst. Raven Press, New York © 1978.

Survival Study of Immunochemotherapy in Lung Cancer

*Thomas H. M. Stewart, **Ariel C. Hollinshead, *Jules E. Harris, ‡Sankaranarayanan Raman, †Raymond Belanger, †André Crepeau, *Alfred F. Crook, *Wolfgang E. Hirte, †David Hooper, *David J. Klaassen, *Edna F. Rapp, and †Harold J. Sachs

*Departments of *Medicine, †Surgery, ‡Epidemiology, and Community Medicine, University of Ottawa, Canada; and **Division of Hematology and Oncology, Department of Medicine, George Washington University Medical Center, Washington, D.C. 20014*

The surgical treatment of resectable lung cancer gives disappointing results. Recurrence of the disease and death within 3 years may be expected in half of those patients with stage I or II disease at the time of curative surgery (1,2). A number of trials have been conducted to try to improve the prognosis following surgery by means of chemotherapy, given either at the time of surgery (3) or on a long-term basis after surgery (4,5). Such studies have resulted in unacceptable toxicity (3,4) or in diminished survival in the chemotherapy regimens (4,5).

The importance of the patient's capacity to exhibit delayed hypersensitivity reactions (DHR) on skin testing with purified protein derivative (PPD) has been shown by Israel (6) in patients with disseminated disease. Where present, the prognosis was better. In patients who had surgical resection of their tumor, those who had a positive preoperative PPD fared significantly better than those who were negative. Similarly, the capacity of a patient to respond, or not, to 2-4-dinitrochlorobenzene (DNCB) correlated well with the presence or absence of recurrence at 12 months (7). Attempts have been made to improve the lung cancer patient's immune competence in order to improve the prognosis. Thus the nonspecific effect of levamisole (8) or the intrapleural injection of living Bacillus Calmette-Guérin (9) has shown striking promise, with prolongation of the disease-free interval in stage I patients. A more specific approach has been that of Takita (10) who has used autologous tumor cells homogenized with Freund's complete adjuvant (Fca). Survival of stage III patients was improved to correspond to that of stage I patients.

In order to strengthen specific cellular defense mechanisms against residual cancer cells following surgery, we have chosen to use separated soluble allogeneic lung cancer antigens, matched for histology and free of human leukocyte HLA antigens, thoroughly homogenized with Fca, as a specific vaccine. This approach was prompted by the knowledge that specific organ damage can be induced in experimental animals (11), if the animal is inoculated with an homogenate of the target organ antigen and Fca. Similarly derived soluble tumor antigens have been shown effective in immunoprophylaxis in viral- and carcinogen-induced (12,13) animal tumors.

Further, we have chosen to combine the immunization with methotrexate (MTX), a drug that has been shown to act synergistically with the host cellular defensive mechanisms in the effective treatment of malignant disease (14,15) and in advanced lung cancer (16). The schedule of immunization following MTX was chosen so that advantage could be taken of the striking rebound overshoot phenomenon that we and others have described (17,18) in patients following chemotherapy. The choice of high dose MTX followed by citrovorum rescue was made since we hoped that long-term immunosuppression would not be seen and since such a dose regimen has been shown effective in treating some cases of advanced lung cancer (19).

In this chapter we report the preliminary findings on survival experience from our randomized clinical trial of immunotherapy and immunochemotherapy on lung cancer patients of stages I and II following surgical resection of their tumor. In an earlier publication (20) we reported in detail the design and rationale of our clinical trial.

METHOD AND MATERIALS

Patients were drawn from those having surgical removal of their tumor at the Ottawa Civic Hospital, the National Defense Medical Center, and the Ottawa General Hospital. Careful staging for tumor-node-metastases (TNM) (1) was assured by preoperative radiography, scans, mediastinoscopy, and postoperative consideration of the notes of the surgeon and pathologist. From March, 1973 to May, 1976, a total of 64 patients had been evaluated. Forty-eight patients of all three stages were randomized into one of the three arms of the treatment groups. The first group received a high dose of MTX once a month followed by folinic acid rescue, for 3 months. The second group was immunized once a month, with soluble antigen homogenized with Fca, for 3 months. The third group was immunized 7 to 9 days following MTX with folinic acid rescue, once a month for 3 months. We have, in addition, followed the survival experience of 16 concomitant controls in the Ottawa-Carleton area from August, 1972 to May, 1976. These control patients were all of stage I treated by the same surgeons and would have been randomized into the study but were precluded owing to a delay of more than 30 days when they were available for immunization following surgery.

In Table 1 we have summarized all the relevant characteristics of the patients with stage I and II disease. In Tables 2, 3, 4, and 5 full details of all patients are given.

TABLE 1. *Data on the three groups of patients—chemotherapy and concomitant controls, immunotherapy, and immunochemotherapy—all of stages I & II*

		MTX & controls[c]	Immunotherapy	Immunochemotherapy
Total patients		26	16	13[a]
Male		21	11	8
Median age (yr)		54	58.4	56
Age range (yr)		39–73	46–71	45–66
PS at surgery[d]	0	3	5	3
	1	23	11	10
Stage I		24	13	11
Dead		6	—	1
Metastases		2	1	—
Recurrence		—	3	—
Cell Type				
Epidermoid		11	11	7[b]
Adenocarcinoma		11	3	4
Anaplastic (small cell)		1	—	1
(large cell)		3	2	1

PS, performance status.
[a] Includes one patient from phase I trial immunized in 1969 who died after 6 years.
[b] Includes one patient who also had adenocarcinoma.
[c] MTX: 8 male, median age 53, 39–65 range; control: 13 male, median age 53, 45–74 range.
[d] PS: 0, asymptomatic and ambulant; 1, symptomatic and ambulant.

The preparation of soluble allogeneic lung cancer antigens has already been described in detail (20,21), as have their characterization with recognition of oncofetal antigens, tumor-associated antigens, and a herpes simplex virus tumor-associated antigen (22). The mean total quantity of antigen given to patients in the immunotherapy group was 1,495 μg, with a range of 1,125 to 2,200 μg. The mean total quantity of antigen given to the immunochemotherapy group was 1,610 μg with a range of 900 to 3,000 μg. An average of 500 μg of antigen in 0.5 ml was homogenized with an equal volume of Fca H37 Ra (Difco Laboratories, Detroit, Michigan) that contained 10 mg of killed mycobacterium tuberculosis per 10 ml, made up of 8.5 ml Bayol-F (mineral oil) and 1.5 ml Arlacil (mannide manolliate). The homogenate was given intradermally into the deltoid region of the arm, the thigh, and again the arm, at monthly intervals. The details of the care of the ensuing ulcer have already been described (20). MTX (Lederle Laboratories) was given by rapid intravenous infusion; 300 and then 700 mg was infused over 6 hr. A normal creatinine clearance is mandatory, and the urine is alkalinized by giving sodium bicarbonate 1.2 to 2.4 g q6h p. o. starting 24 hr before the infusion and continuing during the folinic acid rescue period of 60 hr. The urine pH is monitored Q6h to ensure that the pH remains above 6. DHRs to allogeneic and occasionally autologous soluble cancer antigen have been tested on subsequent visits of the patients, following the initial 3-month course of treatment. The skin test dose has been 100 μg of antigen, unless dilution, dose responses were measured (20). Induration at 48 hr, measured

TABLE 2. Concomitant controls: stage I

Name	Age	Sex	PS[a]	Date of surgery	Surgery	Stage	Histology	Survival	Status
W.P.	62	M	1	August 27, 1972	P.Pnx.	$T_1N_0M_0$	Epidermoid in situ	48 mo	Free
L.B.	60	M	1	Sept. 5, 1972	R.Pnx.	$T_1N_1M_0$	Epidermoid	48 mo	Free
E.C.	73	F	0	Sept. 8, 1972	R.L.Lx.	$T_1N_1M_0$	Adenocarcinoma, alveolar	30 mo	Dead
H.C.	52	M	1	Dec. 4, 1972	R.L.Lx.	$T_1N_0M_0$	Adenocarcinoma endarteritis obliterans—micro	14 mo	Dead
D.L.	45	F	1	Dec. 14, 1972	L.Pnx.	$T_1N_0M_0$	Anaplastic small cell	44 mo	Free
C.O.[e]	52	M	0	August 20, 1973	L.U.Lx.	$T_2N_0M_0$	Epidermoid poorly differentiated	36 mo	Free
R.P.[e]	48	M	1	Sept. 5, 1973	L.U.Lx.	$T_2N_0M_0$	Epidermoid well & poorly difftd.	36 mo	Free
D.M.[b]	57	F	1	Jan. 7, 1974	L.Pnx.	$T_2N_0M_0$	Adenocarcinoma extends to pleura	8 mo	Dead
S.H.[d]	60	M	1	April 18, 1974	L.U.Lx.	$T_1N_0M_0$	Epidermoid	28 mo	Free
B.M.[e]	50	M	1	July 3, 1974	R.U.Lx.	$T_1N_0M_0$	Adenocarcinoma	26 mo	Free
A.L.[d]	50	M	1	Nov. 27, 1974	R.Pnx.	$T_2N_0M_0$	Anaplastic large cell	21 mo	Alive with metastases at 14 mo
O.B.[d]	74	M	1	March 12, 1975	R.Pnx.	$T_2N_0M_0$	Epidermoid well differentiated	17 mo	Free
I.J.[c]	64	M	1	Dec. 1, 1975	R.U.Lx.	$T_2N_0M_0$	Adenocarcinoma	9 mo	Free
L.R.	67	M	1	March 22, 1976	L.Lx.	$T_2N_0M_0$	Epidermoid	5 mo	Free
C.K.	50	M	1	May 5, 1976	L.Pnx.	$T_1N_1M_0$	Anaplastic large cell	4 mo	Free
E.M.[b]	73	M	1	May 7, 1976	R.U.Lx.	$T_1N_0M_0$	Adenocarcinoma, alveolar	4 mo	Free

L.R. and C.K. were randomized as controls.

[a] Performance status.

[b] Refused protocol.

[c] Could not understand consent form.

[d] Distance from Ottawa precluded protocol.

[e] Absence of investigator caused greater than 30 days' delay. Thus they were not entered into protocol.

R.Pnx = Right pneumonectomy; L.Pnx = Left pneumonectomy; R.M-Lx = Right middle lobectomy; R.L-Lx = Right lower lobectomy; R.U-Lx = Right upper lobectomy; L.L-Lx = Left lower lobectomy; L.U-Lx = Left upper lobectomy.

TABLE 3. *MTX with citrovorum rescue*

Name	Age	Sex	PS[a]	Date of surgery	Surgery	Stage	Histology	Survival	Status
Stage I									
P.L.	39	M	1	March 19, 1973	L.U.Lx.	$T_2N_0M_0$	Adenocarcinoma	41 mo	Free
E.L.	54	M	0	Feb. 1, 1974	R.U.Lx.	$T_1N_0M_0$	Adenocarcinoma, alveolar	22 mo	Dead
W.L.	65	M	1	May 30, 1974	L.U.Lx.	$T_1N_0M_0$	Epidermoid well difftd.	27 mo	Free
D.B.	52	M	1	Sept. 3, 1974	R.U.Lx.	$T_2N_0M_0$	Adenocarcinoma	24 mo	Free
R.L.	65	M	1	Oct. 3, 1974	R.U.Lx.	$T_1N_0M_0$	Epidermoid mod. well difftd.	23 mo	Free
C.M.	50	F	1	May 7, 1974	L.U.Lx.	$T_2N_0M_0$	Adenocarcinoma, alveolar	16 mo	Alive with metastases at 14 mo
Y.H.	52	M	1	June 18, 1975	L.L.Lx.	$T_2N_0M_0$	Epidermoid well difftd.	6 mo	Dead
A.A.	45	M	1	August 14, 1975	R.M.Lx.	$T_1N_0M_0$	Epidermoid	12 mo	Free
Stage II									
E.J.	47	F	1	April 7, 1975	R.Pnx.	$T_2N_1M_0$	Adenocarcinoma	17 mo	Free
M.P.	60	M	1	April 28, 1975	L.Pnx.	$T_2N_1M_0$	Anaplastic large cell	7 mo	Dead
Stage III									
D.W.	41	M	1	April 16, 1973	L.Pnx.	$T_2N_2M_0$	Anaplastic small cell	18 mo	Dead
O.L.	47	M	1	Sept. 4, 1973	L.Pnx.	$T_1N_2M_0$	Epidermoid	10 mo	Dead
P.V.[b]	61	M	1	March 30, 1973	L.Pnx.	$T_3N_0M_0$	Epidermoid	24 mo	Dead

[a] Performance status.

[b] This patient was originally staged as I, but later it was realized he had tumor 1½ cm from the carina and was thus stage III.

R.Pnx = Right pneumonectomy; L.Pnx = Left pneumonectomy; R.M-Lx = Right middle lobectomy; R.L-Lx = Right lower lobectomy; R.U-Lx = Right upper lobectomy; LL-Lx = Left lower lobectomy; L.U-Lx = Left upper lobectomy.

TABLE 4. MTX plus immunization with soluble antigen plus Fca

Name	Age	Sex	PS[a]	Date of surgery	Surgery	Stage	Histology	Survival	Status
Stage I									
O.L.	62	M	1	June 10, 1969	R.U.lx.	$T_1N_1M_0$	Epidermoid mod. difftd.	72 mo	Dead
E.C.	56	F	1	August 3, 1973	R.U.lx. Parietal pleural resection	$T_2N_0M_0$	Epidermoid adenocarcinoma	37 mo	Free
P.McA.	45	M	1	Nov. 29, 1973	R.Pnx.	$T_2N_0M_0$	Adenocarcinoma poorly difftd.	33 mo	Free
L.P.	66	F	1	Nov. 12, 1973	R.L.lx.	$T_2N_0M_0$	Epidermoid poorly difftd. (parietal pleura)	33 mo	Free
O.S.	64	M	0	Nov. 29, 1973	L.lx.	$T_2N_0M_0$	Epidermoid mod. well difftd.	33 mo	Free
C.McC.	45	M	1	March 19, 1974	L.Pnx.	$T_2N_0M_0$	Adenocarcinoma	29 mo	Free
J.F.[b]	45	F	1	May 29, 1974	L.Pnx.	$T_1N_1M_0$	Anaplastic small cell	27 mo	Free
O.L.	54	M	1	April 14, 1975	L.Pnx.	$T_2N_0M_0$	Epidermoid poorly difftd., extends to pleura	14 mo	Dead
F.P.	57	M	1	May 8, 1975	L.Pnx.	$T_1N_0M_0$	Epidermoid well difftd.	16 mo	Free
N.B.	66	M	0	Jan. 28, 1976	L.U.lx.	$T_1N_1M_0$	Adenocarcinoma	7 mo	Free
P.C.	46	M	1	March 19, 1976	L.U.lx.	$T_2N_0M_0$	Epidermoid poorly difftd.	5 mo	Free
Stage II									
F.L.	61	M	0	Oct. 7, 1975	L.U.lx.	$T_2N_1M_0$	Anaplastic large cell	11 mo	Free
R.S.	60	F	1	April 28, 1976	R.M.&L.lx.	$T_2N_1M_0$	Adenocarcinoma	4 mo	Free
Stage III									
R.K.	43	M	1	May 3, 1973	R.Pnx.	$T_3N_0M_0$	Epidermoid poorly difftd.	7 mo	Dead
R.B.	49	M	0	May 29, 1973	L.U.lx.	$T_1N_2M_0$	Adenocarcinoma, alveolar	34 mo	Dead
F.L.	41	M	1	Jan. 31, 1975	R.Pnx.	$T_2N_2M_0$	Anaplastic large cell	9 mo	Dead
M.C.	65	M	1	Oct. 22, 1975	L.Pnx.	$T_2N_2M_0$	Epidermoid poorly difftd.	11 mo	Metastases
S.S.	41	M	1	Feb. 5, 1976	R.U.lx.	$T_3N_0M_0$	Adenocarcinoma moderately well difftd.	7 mo	Metastases in ribs @ 2 mo

[a] Performance status.

[b] Initially staged as III but no mediastinal nodes were involved. Initial pathologist's error.

R.Pnx = Right pneumonectomy; L.Pnx = Left pneumonectomy; R.M-Lx = Right middle lobectomy; R.L-Lx = Right lower lobectomy; R.U-Lx = Right upper lobectomy; L.L-Lx = Left lower lobectomy; L.U-Lx = Left upper lobectomy.

TABLE 5. *Immunized with soluble antigen and Fca*

Name	Age	Sex	PS[a]	Date of surgery	Surgery	Stage	Histology	Survival	Status
Stage I									
L.G.	53	F	1	June 26, 1973 (extra pleural resection) pleural scar	R.Pnx.	$T_2N_0M_0$	Anaplastic large cell	38 mo	Free
L.G.	62	M	0	July 12, 1973 Peripheral tumor —fibrosed pleura	L.U.Lx.	$T_1N_0M_0$	Epidermoid mod. difftd.	38 mo stump recurrence at 34 mo	Well
T.StG.	52	F	1	April 4, 1974	R.U.Lx.	$T_1N_0M_0$	Adenocarcinoma Alveolar	29 mo	Free
K.H.	58	M	1	April 12, 1974	R.U.Lx.	$T_2N_0M_0$	Anaplastic large cell	28 mo	Free
R.W.	59	M	1	June 6, 1974	L.U.Lx. L.L. lobe wedge resection—pleura (extra pleural resection) micro vessel invasion	$T_2N_0M_0$	Epidermoid	27 mo suspicious sputum	Free
A.L.	60	M	0	April 21, 1975	R.U.&M.Lx.	$T_2N_0M_0$	Epidermoid poorly difftd.	16 mo	Free
G.C.	56	M	1	May 6, 1975	L.Pnx.	$T_1N_0M_0$	Epidermoid	16 mo	Free
P.G.	69	M	1	May 20, 1975	R.L.Lx.	$T_1N_0M_0$	Epidermoid (2 primaries)	15 mo recurrence at 12 mo Empyema	Free
S.L.	54	M	0	August 25, 1975	L.U.Lx.	$T_2N_0M_0$	Epidermoid	12 mo	Free
A.T.	71	M	0	Sept. 15, 1975	L.U.Lx.	$T_1N_0M_0$	Adenocarcinoma	12 mo	Free
G.L.	60	M	0	Feb. 18, 1976	L.U.Lx.	$T_1N_0M_0$	Epidermoid	6 mo	Free
A.L.	46	F	1	Feb. 16, 1976	R.M.Lx.	$T_1N_0M_0$	Adenocarcinoma	6 mo	Free
R.S.	62	M	1	May 7, 1976	L.U.Lx.	$T_2N_0M_0$	Epidermoid	4 mo	Free
Stage II									
A.L.	51	M	1	April 23, 1975	L.U.Lx.	$T_2N_1M_0$	Epidermoid in situ at line of resection	16 mo	Metastases at 14 mo
D.L.	61	M	1	July 9, 1975	L.Pnx.	$T_2N_1M_0$	Epidermoid mod. well difftd.	13 mo	Free
J.B.	61	M	1	May 3, 1975	L.U.Lx.	$T_2N_1M_0$	Epidermoid poorly difftd.	4 mo	Free
Stage III									
M.N.	62	F	1	August 27, 1975	R.U.Lx.	$T_3N_0M_0$	Epidermoid poorly difftd.	12 mo metastases	Well

[a] Performance status.

R.Pnx = Right pneumonectomy; L.Pnx = Left pneumonectomy; R.M-lx = Right middle lobectomy; R.L-lx = Right lower lobectomy; R.U-lx = Right upper lobectomy; L.L-Lx = Left lower lobectomy; L.U-Lx = Left upper lobectomy.

by the technique of Sokal (23) was recorded over the two greatest diameters. Results are expressed as the surface area of an ellipse. Readings less than 5 mm in diameter were scored as negative. Biopsies of the test sites have been done, for histologic confirmation of a DHR.

RESULTS

Our nonimmunized group is composed of a total of 26 patients (stage I and II), some of whom received MTX with citrovorum rescue. Sixteen concomitant control patients, all stage I, have been followed up for a mean of 23 months; three have died and a fourth has developed a cranial metastasis proved at 14 months at craniotomy. Ten patients who received MTX (8 stage I, 2 stage II) have been followed for an average of 20 months; of these three have died and one has developed metastases at 14 months in the opposite lung. This report excludes from analysis of the MTX-treated controls one patient (P.V.) who was included in error as stage I in our previous report and who died at 24 months (20).

The immunized group consists of a total of 29 patients, some of whom received MTX with citrovorum rescue. We have 16 patients (13 stage I, 3 stage II) who have been immunized with soluble cancer antigen, followed for a mean of 18 months. All are alive. Two had stump recurrences, received Cobalt, and are well at 38 months (patients L.G. and L.G.). One had local recurrence at 14 months (P.G.); the complete pneumonectomy was followed by a stormy postoperative course complicated by empyema. One stage II patient (A.L.) developed metastases at 13 months and is alive, receiving chemotherapy.

Thirteen patients have received immunochemotherapy (11 stage I, 2 stage II) and have been followed for a mean of 23 months. One patient died at 14 months with a cerebral metastasis from the 9-cm primary, which was a poorly differentiated epidermoid carcinoma. No recurrences or metastases have been seen in the remaining patients.

SURVIVAL

Table 6 summarizes the life table survival experience of the treatment and control groups calculated by the method of Cutler and Ederer (24). The overall probability of no difference between the two groups is 0.0011. In Fig. 1 we have drawn the survival curve for the controls and the immunized group. If one uses death only as an end point, the overall probability of no difference is 0.0025. However we have included metastases, feeling this gives a more realistic picture, although the survival probability for the immunized group at 36 months is 87% whereas using death alone as an end point, it is predicted to be 93%.

We have included in the analysis for the immunochemotherapy group one

TABLE 6. *Life table experience of the treated (immunized and immunochemotherapy) and the controls (chemotherapy and concomitant controls), all of stages I and II*

Duration in months	Number of patients alive		Number dead or with metastases		Number withdrawn in the interval		Probability of surviving till the termination of the interval	
	T	C	T	C	T	C	T	C
0–5	29	26	—	—	4	3	1.0	1.0
6–11	25	23	—	3	6	1	1.0	0.8506
12–17	19	19	2	3	6	2	0.8674	0.6894
18–23	11	14	—	1	—	4	0.8674	0.6221
24–29	11	9	—	—	5	2	0.8674	0.6221
30–35	6	8	—	1	3	1	0.8674	0.517
36–41	3	5	—	—	—	2		0.517
42–47	—	3	—	—	—	—		

T, treated; C, controls.

patient from our phase I trial for toxicity (22). He was the only patient given immunization with a crude antigen and MTX in 1969 (20), and he had a bronchial stump recurrence at 36 months and death from metastases at his sixth anniversary.

Figure 2 shows the results of late testing with soluble cancer antigen for DHRs from 4 to 42 months (mean 18 months) of the 11 patients who were not immunized; almost half were anergic toward cancer antigen. All but one were ambulant and asymptomatic when tested. The 16 patients who were immunized were tested at intervals ranging from 6 to 28 months (mean 18 months); all showed a positive DHR to cancer antigen. The mean intensity of induration with one standard error is shown in the figure separately for the patient groups of nonimmunized, immunized, and immunochemotherapy. Clearly immunization confers a positive reaction that is significantly greater than the nonimmunized—$p < 0.05$ for the immunized group and $p < 0.01$ for the immunochemotherapy group. It was noted that the immunochemo-

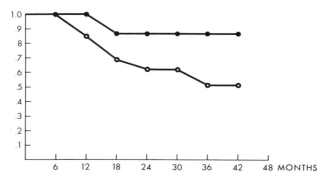

FIG. 1. Life table analysis of survival probability, deaths, and metastases. ●–●–●, Immunized (29 patients); O–O–O, nonimmunized (26 patients). $p = 0.0011$.

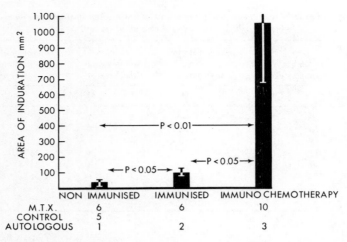

FIG. 2. The intensity of induration at 48 hr on late skin testing with soluble cancer antigen is shown. Autologous testing was done in some patients as indicated. The mean of the greater diameter of induration was 4.8, 11, and 33.4 mm, respectively.

therapy group had a significantly stronger reaction ($p < 0.05$) than the immunized group of patients. Details of autologous testing have already been reported (20), but it should be emphasized that reactivity is retained with as little as 500 ng of autologous antigen. It is of interest that the patient O.L. who was tested at 10 months had a weaker reaction than most who received immunochemotherapy, 11 mm induration, had developed *in vitro* blocking at 4 months (20), and died at 14 months.

DISCUSSION

Immunization with allogeneic soluble lung cancer antigen extends the disease-free interval significantly in stage I and possibly stage II patients who have had surgical resection of their lung tumor.

It appears that stage III lung cancer is less suitable for this approach, probably because the burden of residual tumor cells is too great for cellular defense mechanisms to become effective. Adjuvant MTX alone appears to have no beneficial effect, and conversion to give a positive DHR to cancer antigen was not seen. We have consistently observed conversion of immunized patients. The very strong hypersensitivity response given by those patients who had immunochemotherapy is gratifying, as it justifies the scheduling of immunization following MTX with folinic acid rescue. It is not an invariable phenomenon, however (20). We believe that the enhanced reactivity following immunization is very desirable. The first skin tests in human cancer using autologous cell extracts by Hughes and Lytton (25) were based on the observations of Brent, Brown, and Medawar (26) that guinea pigs actively rejecting foreign skin grafts showed a DHR to an acellular extract of the graft that correlated well with the presence or absence of a graft-rejecting mechanism. In the induction of experimental allergic encephalomyelitis in guinea pigs (27) using a water soluble basic protein derived from brain, a good correlation exists between the onset of paralysis and the appearance of a DHR to the protein. Further examples of such a correlation in experimental autoallergic disease induction in animals are reviewed by Waksman (11). In man the induction of orchitis also correlates well with the presence of a DHR toward testicular antigen (28). Thus we believe that the extension of the disease-free interval, in those patients who were immunized, reflects an heightened cellular defense against microscopic foci of residual disease.

One may speculate on the conditions that exist during the 3 months of immunochemotherapy that are later reflected by the intense skin reactions. A clear understanding of such conditions may allow one to engineer a strong and long-lasting cellular host reaction directed toward cancer antigens. The essential ingredient of the Freund's granuloma is dead tubercle bacilli. Such inflammatory granulomata have been characterized as 'rapid turnover' (29). It is recognized that rapidly dividing cells have a high requirement for folic acid. It has been shown that 25% of the Canadian population have very low folate levels and that a further 35% have low levels (30). Thus one may envisage that the folinic rescue given a total of 6 days in 3 months with high serum levels may encourage optimal instructional function in the Freund's granuloma.

Bain (31) has shown that optimal folate levels for *in vitro* mixed lymphocyte reactivity are 10 times the folic acid levels considered normal in healthy man. Patients with very low folic acid levels and anergy, following treatment with folic acid, have shown conversion to DNCB and rebound overshoot of their lymphocyte performance *in vitro* (32). Thus the contribution of the folinic rescue to the function of the immune system in general and the instructional aspect of the Freund's granuloma in particular may be important. The possibility exists that MTX given before immunization depletes a clone of suppressor cells, upsetting the balance in favor of effector cells in the immunizing schedule. Turk et al. (33) have reviewed control mechanisms in DHRs and point out that depletion of suppressor cells account for strong DHRs in mice where cyclophosphamide has been given 3 days before immunization with antigen with Fca. We planned the immunization to coincide with the period of rebound overshoot hoping to take advantage of the increased reactivity of the patients' lymphocytes. Such rebound has been observed by Turk (34) in mice following cyclophosphamide, which supports the rationale for our treatment schedule.

The use of carefully characterized soluble allogeneic cancer antigens free of HLA has avoided the potential hazard of inducing autoallergic pneumonitis.

The general parameters for phase I, II, and III specific active immunotherapy trials have been documented (22). This small phase II study suggests further problems that have to be solved in future clinical trials. What is the optimal amount of soluble antigen that should be given and what is the frequency? How many cancer cells in man constitute the minimal residual tumor burden amenable to this approach? What are the optimal schedules that may make immunochemotherapy more effective? Answers to these crucial questions are important if the general approach we outline is to be applied to other tumor systems in man.

SUMMARY

A randomized clinical trial of immunization and immunochemotherapy among 55 patients with stage I and II carcinoma of the lung is reported. The survival experience of the treated group is significantly better, $p = 0.0011$, compared to the control nonimmunized patients. The results are discussed in the light of the reactivity of the patients to the specific cancer antigen.

ACKNOWLEDGMENTS

We acknowledge the expert technical help of Peter Jones, Daphne Hyslop, and Katherine Stilwell and the help of Mrs. T. Clayton in the follow-up of patients. This work was supported, in part, by Ontario Cancer Treatment and Research Foundation grants #168 and 292.

REFERENCES

1. Mountain, C. F., Carr, D. T., and Anderson, W. A. D. (1974): A system for the clinical staging of lung cancer. *Am. J. Roentgenol. Radium Ther. Nucl. Med.*, 120:130–138.
2. Israel, L. (1974): Nonspecific immunostimulation in bronchogenic cancer. *Scand. J. Respir. Dis.*, 89:95–105.
3. Slack, N. H. (1970): Bronchogenic carcinoma: Nitrogen mustard as a surgical adjuvant and factors influencing survival. *Cancer*, 25:987–1002.
4. Medical Research Council Study (1971): Study of cytotoxic chemotherapy as an adjuvant to surgery in carcinoma of the bronchus. *Br. Med. J.*, 2:421–428.
5. Brunner, K. W., Marthaler, T. H., and Muller, W. (1971): Unfavourable effects of long-term adjuvant chemotherapy with endoxan in radically operated bronchogenic carcinoma. *Eur. J. Cancer*, 1:285–294.
6. Israel, L. (1973): Cell-mediated immunity in lung cancer patients: data, problems, and propositions. *Cancer Chemother. Rep.*, 4:279–281.
7. Wells, S. A., Burdick, J. F., and Joseph, W. L. (1973): Delayed cutaneous hypersensitivity reactions to tumor cell antigens and to non-specific antigens. Prognostic significance in patients with lung cancer. *J. Thorac. Cardiovasc. Surg.*, 66:557–562.
8. Amery, W. K. (1976): Double blind, placebo controlled clinical trial of levamisole in resectable bronchogenic carcinoma. *Ann. NY Acad. Sci.*, 277:260–268.
9. McKneally, M. F., Maver, C., and Kansel, H. W. (1976): Regional immunotherapy of lung cancer with intrapleural B.C.G. *Lancet*, 1:377–379.
10. Takita, H., Minowada, J., Han, T., Takada, M., and Lane, W. W. (1976): Adjuvant immunotherapy in bronchogenic carcinoma. *Ann. NY Acad. Sci.*, 277:345–354.
11. Waksman, B. (1959): Experimental allergic encephalomyelitis and the "autoallergic" diseases. *Int. Arch. Allergy Appl. Immunol.*, Suppl., 14:1–87.

12. Hollinshead, A. C., McCammon, J. R., and Yohn, D. S. (1972): Immunogenicity of a soluble membrane antigen from adenovirus—12 induced tumour cells demonstrated in inbred hamsters (PD-4). *Can. J. Microbiol.,* 18:1365–1369.
13. Prager, M. D., Hollinshead, A. C., Ribble, R. J., and Derr, I. (1973): Induction of immunity to a mouse lymphoma by multiple methods including vaccination with soluble membrane fractions. *J. Natl. Cancer Inst.,* 51:1603–1607.
14. Burkitt, D. (1967): Chemotherapy of African (Burkitt) lymphoma—clinical evidence suggesting an immunological response. *Br. J. Surg.,* 54:53.
15. Elston, C. W. (1969): Cellular reaction to choriocarcinoma. *J. Pathol.* 2:261–268.
16. Stewart, T. H. M., Klaassen, D., and Crook, A. F. (1969): Methotrexate in the treatment of malignant tumours: Evidence for the possible participation of host defence mechanisms. *Can. Med. Assoc. J.,* 101:191–199.
17. Harris, J. E., Bagai, R. S., and Stewart, T. H. M. (1973): Serial monitoring of immune reactivity in cancer patients receiving chemotherapy as a mean of predicting anti-tumour response. In: *Proc. 7th Leuk. Cult. Conf.,* edited by F. Daguillard, p. 443. Academic Press, New York.
18. Harris, J. E., Sengar, D., Stewart, T. H. M., and Hyslop, D. (1976): The effect of immunosuppressive chemotherapy on immune function in patients with malignant disease. *Cancer,* 37:1058–1069.
19. Djerassi, I., Rominger, J. C., Stewart, T. H. M., and Hyslop, D. (1972): Phase I study of high doses of methotrexate with citrovorum factor in patients with lung cancer. *Cancer,* 30:22–30.
20. Stewart, T. H. M., Hollinshead, A. C., and Harris, J. E. (1970): Immunochemotherapy of lung cancer. *Ann. NY Acad. Sci.,* 277:436–466.
21. Hollinshead, A. C., Stewart, T. H. M., and Herberman, R. B. (1974): Delayed hypersensitivity reactions to soluble membrane antigens of human malignant lung cells. *J. Natl. Cancer Inst.,* 52:327–338.
22. Hollinshead, A. C., and Stewart, T. H. M. (1976): Lung tumour antigens. In: *Proc. 3rd Int. Natl. Symp. Cancer Detection and Prevention, New York,* edited by H. E. Nieburgs. Karger, Basel.
23. Sokal, J. E. (1975): Measurement of delayed skin test responses. *New Engl. J. Med.,* 293:501–502.
24. Cutler, S. J., and Ederer, F. (1958): Maximum utilization of the life table method in analyzing survival. *J. Chronic Dis.,* 8:699–712.
25. Hughes, L. E., and Lytton, B. (1964): Antigenic properties of human tumours: Delayed cutaneous hypersensitivity reactions. *Br. Med. J.,* 1:209–212.
26. Brent, L., Brown, J., and Medawar, P. B. (1958): Skin transplantation immunity in relation to hypersensitivity. *Lancet,* 2:561–564.
27. Shaw, C. M., Alvord, E. C., Kalu, J., and Kies, M. W. (1965): Correlation of experimental allergic encephalomyelitis with delayed type skin sensitivity to specific homologous encephalitogen. *Ann. NY Acad. Sci.,* 122:318–331.
28. Mancini, R. E., Anchada, J. A., Saraceni, D., Bachman, A. E., Lavieri, J. C., and Remirovsky, J. (1965): Immunological and testicular response in man sensitized with human testicular homogenate. *Clin. Endocrinol. Metabol.,* 25:859–875.
29. Papadimitrious, J. M., and Spector, W. G. (1972): The ultrastructure of high-and-low turnover inflammatory granulomata. *J. Pathol.,* 106:37–43.
30. Sabry, Z. I. (1973): *Nutrition Canada. Natl. Survey 1973,* Information Canada, p. 114.
31. Bain, B. (1975): Folate requirement for blast cell transformation in mixed leukocyte cultures. *Cell Immunol.,* 15:237–245.
32. Gross, R. L., Reid, J. V. O., Newberne, P. M., Burgess, B., Marston, R., and Hift, W. (1975): Depressed cell-mediated immunity in megaloblastic anemia due to folic acid deficiency. *Am. J. Clin. Nutr.,* 28:225–232.
33. Turk, J. L., Palack, L., and Parker, D. (1976): Control mechanisms in delayed-type hypersensitivity. *Br. Med. Bull.,* 2:165–170.
34. Turk, J. L., and Poutter, L. W. (1972): Effects of cyclophosphamide on lymphoid tissues labelled with 5-iodo-2-dioxyuridine-125-I and 51 Cr. *Int. Arch. Allergy,* 43:620–629.

Question and Answer Session

Dr. LoBuglio: In the nonimmunized patients, there have been nine out of 26 recurrences, and in the immunized there have been six out of 29 recurrences. Is that right?

Dr. Stewart: We divide our groups into those who have died, those who have metastasized, and those who have recurrence.

There were 7 deaths and 2 metastases in the 26 nonimmunized patients and 2 deaths and 3 recurrences in the immunized group.

Now, the reason we say recurrence, and we don't think it is as sinister as metastases, is that it took three years for our toxic patient to die from recurrence, and we've got another patient with recurrence who received cobalt and is now clear on bronchoscopy a year and a half later. So we don't feel intrathoracic recurrence is quite so sinister as metastases.

Dr. Lobuglio: The disease comes back.

Dr. Stewart: Yes, in one of our patients it came back a year and a half ago. The patient responded to cobalt.

Dr. Fudenberg: I note that you have no control group using complete Freund's adjuvant without antigen. Since Freund's adjuvant administration produces a sizable factor which enhances immunity, unless there is a group receiving Freund's adjuvant alone, it isn't possible to be sure the antigen is doing anything.

Dr. Stewart: Yes, I think we are much wiser now than when we started this trial. We went by the principle of go to the bank because that's where the money is. I think if we are seeing an effect, the analysis of this effect is now open to scrutiny. You are quite right.

Dr. Mathé: I would like to ask whether those patients who died in the nonimmunized group had cancers of other histological types than did the immunized patients. Were they small cell carcinoma?

Dr. Stewart: We have two small cell carcinomas, both doing very well, one control, and one immuno. We have four anaplastic tumors in our immunized group. All are well. We have two patients with anaplastic tumors in our control group. One is dead.

*Immunotherapy of Cancer: Present Status of
Trials in Man,* edited by W. D. Terry and D. Windhorst.
Raven Press, New York © 1978.

Adjuvant Immunotherapy of Stage III Lung Carcinoma

Hiroshi Takita, Mitsuru Takada, Jun Minowada,
Tin Han, and Francis Edgerton

*Department of Thoracic Surgery, Roswell Park Memorial Institute
Buffalo, New York 14263*

The overall cure rate of lung carcinoma is 6 to 8% and the only effective therapy of lung carcinoma remains surgery (6). Neither adjuvant chemotherapy (except for small cell carcinoma) nor radiation therapy (except for a small series in squamous cell carcinoma) is known to improve the patients' survival following lung resection (3–5,8). Therefore, it is imperative to explore new methods of treating lung carcinoma, such as immunotherapy.

The results of surgical treatment of locally far advanced lung carcinoma (stage III) are so poor that surgical resection is usually contraindicated (7,12). For this reason we chose this group of patients to study the effects of adjuvant immunotherapy with tumor vaccine.

PATIENTS AND TREATMENT

Thirty patients with locally far advanced primary lung carcinoma (stage III), having mediastinal node metastasis, direct extension to the mediastinum, chest wall, and/or surgical line of resection were included in this study. The patients underwent radical lung resection in order to remove all visible evidence of tumor. Postoperatively they were randomly assigned into two groups: a control group and a treated group.

In the control group, five patients had lobectomy and 10 pneumonectomy. In the treated group, nine had lobectomy and six pneumonectomy. Histological types of the lung carcinomas in the control group were seven squamous cell, four adenocarcinoma, two large cell, and two mixed squamous adenocarcinoma. In the treated group, there were three squamous cell, 10 adenocarcinoma, one small cell, and one mixed squamous adenocarcinoma. The age of the patients in the control group ranged from 51 to 71, the mean was 60.4, and 14 were males and one was female. In the treated group, the age of the patients ranged from 46 to 76, the mean was 57.5, and 12 were male and three were female.

Postoperatively, the patients in the control group received conventional management: three patients received postoperative radiation therapy, and the rest had no treatment until recurrence of the disease. All the patients in the treated group received autologous tumor cell vaccine. Besides the immunotherapy, one patient received postoperative radiation therapy and another patient, preoperative radiation therapy. When there was recurrence of the disease, the patients in both groups were treated with radiation and/or chemotherapy.

There were 88 patients who underwent lung resection for stage III lung carcinomas at this same Institute during the 10 previous years, and the survival of these patients was compared with that of the study groups as a historical control.

Autologous Tumor Vaccine (Table 1)

The tumor vaccine was prepared from surgically excised autologous tumor cells treated with Concanavalin A and *Vibrio cholera neuraminidase* according to the method developed in our preclinical experimental animal model (1). The lung carcinoma was obtained from surgically removed specimens in

TABLE 1. *Preparation of tumor vaccine*

Fresh autologous tumor cell suspension
↓
Add Concanavalin A 25 µg/ml/10^7 tumor cells
↓
Wash
↓
Add *Vibrio cholerae neuraminidase* 50 U/ml/10^7 tumor cells
↓
Wash
↓
Tumor cells 5 × 10^7/ml + 1 ml complete Freund's adjuvant

aseptic condition. It was first minced in small pieces by scissors and then strained through a stainless steel mesh using a spatula. This tumor cell suspension was washed twice in cold buffered normal saline and counted. Concanavalin A was added at a concentration of 25 µg/ml/10^7 tumor cells and incubated at 37°C for 30 min. After incubation, the cell suspension was again washed in cold buffered saline; *Vibrio cholera neuraminidase* at the concentration of 50 U/ml/10^7 tumor cells was then added and incubated at 37°C for 30 min. The tumor cells were again washed and resuspended in buffered saline to make a cell suspension of 5 × 10^7/ml. One milliliter of this final tumor cell suspension was injected into the patient together with an equal amount of complete Freund's adjuvant (DIFCO Laboratories). The remaining portion of prepared tumor vaccine was stored at −80°C for later use.

Administration of Tumor Vaccine (Table 2)

The first dose of tumor vaccine was given on the day of surgery as soon as the vaccine was prepared. It was usually given to the lateral aspect of

TABLE 2. *Administration of tumor vaccine*

#1　On the day of surgery—two sites, intradermally
then every 2 weeks for 3 to 4 times
then BCG every 1 month $\times$ 12
then BCG every 6 weeks $\times$ 18
then BCG every 2 months

BCG, Bacillus Calmette-Guérin.

both thighs, intradermally. Subsequently the tumor vaccination was repeated at 2-week intervals three times.

One month after surgery, Bacillus Calmette-Guerin (BCG) treatment (BCG vaccine, USP, Glaxo Laboratories) was begun. BCG (0.1 ml) was usually given intradermally to both the deltoid regions, every other week four times initially and subsequently given every month for the first year, every 6 weeks for the second and third year, and every 2 months thereafter.

RESULTS (TABLES 3 AND 4, AND FIG. 1)

Thirty patients have been followed for 5 to 51 months. The therapeutic results were analyzed by the life table analysis and Breslow test of failure rates.

The estimated median survival of the control group is 12.1 months, three of the 15 patients are alive, and the longest survival is 25 months. The estimated median survival of the treated group is 34.8 months, seven of the 15

TABLE 3. *Adjuvant immunotherapy of stage III lung carcinoma, control group*

Patient	Cell type	Staging		Surgery	Survival (months)
F.R.	Large	$T_3N_2M_0$	III	Pneumo	
K.A.	Squamous Adeno	$T_2N_2M_0$	III	Lobe	
O.E.	Squamous	$T_3N_2M_0$	III	Pneumo	
C.E.	Squamous	$T_3N_1M_0$	III	Pneumo	
B.E.	Adeno	$T_3N_0M_1$	III	Lobe	
W.L.	Squamous	$T_3N_0M_0$	III	Pneumo	
W.H.	Large	$T_3N_0M_0$	III	Lobe	
C.C.	Squamous	$T_2N_1M_0$	II	Pneumo	
A.A.	Adeno	$T_3N_1M_0$	III	Lobe	
C.L.	Squamous	$T_3N_2M_0$	III	Pneumo	
S.R.	Adeno	$T_2N_2M_0$	III	Pneumo	
V.A.	Squamous	$T_3N_0M_0$	III	Lobe	
C.J.	Squamous Adeno	$T_2N_2M_0$	III	Pneumo	
U.S.	Squamous	$T_2N_2M_0$	III	Pneumo	
P.E.	Adeno	$T_3N_0M_0$	III	Pneumo	

TABLE 4. *Adjuvant immunotherapy of stage III, treated group*

Patient	Cell type	Staging		Surgery	Survival
P.L.	Squamous	$T_3N_2M_0$	III	Pneumo	
P.C.	Adeno	$T_3N_0M_0$	III	Pneumo	
M.W.	Adeno	$T_2N_2M_0$	III	Lobe	
K.J.	Adeno	$T_2N_2M_0$	III	Lobe	
L.G.	Squamous	$T_2N_2M_0$	III	Lobe	
R.A.	Adeno	$T_1N_2M_0$	III	Lobe	
Z.L.	Adeno	$T_2N_2M_0$	III	Lobe	
W.W.	Small cell	$T_2N_2M_0$	III	Lobe	
R.F.	Squamous Adeno	$T_2N_2M_0$	III	Pneumo	
B.M.	Adeno	$T_3N_0M_0$	III	Pneumo	
N.C.	Adeno	$T_2N_2M_0$	III	Pneumo	
L.J.	Squamous	$T_3N_2M_0$	III	Lobe	
M.G.	Adeno	$T_3N_0M_1$	III	Pneumo	
D.L.	Adeno	$T_1N_2M_0$	III	Lobe	
B.R.	Adeno	$T_2N_2M_0$	III	Lobe	

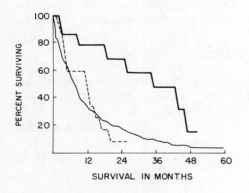

FIG. 1. Adjuvant immunotherapy of stage III lung carcinoma. ——, Tumor vaccine; – – – –, random control; ——, historical control.

patients are alive, and the longest survival is 51 months. The difference in survival between the two groups was significant at $p = 0.05$.

The median survival of the 88 patients with stage III lung carcinoma who had pulmonary resection at the Institute in the past 10 years was 7.3 months. The difference in survival between the randomized control and the historical control was not significant at a $p = 0.05$ level.

SIDE EFFECTS OF TUMOR VACCINATION

Local Reaction

Erythema, measuring 8 to 10 cm in diameter, and edema were noted at the injection site 1 day after the first tumor vaccination. These changes gradually subsided over a period of 4 to 5 days. An induration remained after the initial reaction subsided, and in 7 to 10 days the injection site became ulcerated. Local reaction after the second and subsequent vaccination was usually more intense. At times, moderate erythema and edema were noted simultaneously at the previous vaccination sites. All the vaccination sites eventually became ulcerated and slowly healed in about 2 to 3 months. In no case was growth of tumor at the injection site observed.

Systemic Reaction

Systemic reactions were not common; only in two patients were they noted. One patient had transient malaise and a fever of 103°F, lasting overnight. The other patient had the same symptoms with the addition of nausea and vomiting. There has been no incidence of autoimmune disease.

DISCUSSION

Past studies have shown that the immunological status of lung carcinoma patients was related to the extent of the disease and the prognosis and that the presence of tumor-associated antigen seemed to be specific to each cell type (2,9). Therefore, it would seem more logical to apply tumor-specific immunotherapy to lung carcinoma than to use a nonspecific stimulation such as BCG.

For active immunotherapy to be effective, the patients must maintain their ability to react to the stimulus of immunization. Our previous studies have shown that patients with locally far advanced lung carcinoma usually maintained good immunological status (2). For this reason, this group was selected for our project.

In this study, adjuvant autologous tumor vaccination with radical surgery in conventionally inoperable lung carcinoma significantly improved survival (median survival 34.8 versus 12.1 months). Our laboratory studies found that the treated patients were effectively sensitized to the lung carcinoma when they were monitored by the leukocyte migration inhibition test (11) and the membrane immunofluorescence antibody test (10).

Vincent et al. (12) reported the results of surgical therapy of lung cancer at this same Institute. They found the median survival of 138 stage I patients following surgery was 26.7 months. In this study, when the stage III-treated patients were plotted on the survival curve of the above stage I patients, it appeared that the adjuvant immunotherapy with autologous tumor vaccine converted the prognosis of stage III patients to that of stage I (Fig. 2).

Judging from the therapeutic effectiveness of our adjuvant immunotherapy in stage III patients, a better result may be expected from adjuvant immunotherapy of earlier stages of lung carcinomas (stages I and II). Indeed reports by Stewart et al. (9) of the results of such therapy in stage I and II patients have shown excellent therapeutic effects.

A phase III study to definitely assess the effectiveness of adjuvant immuno-

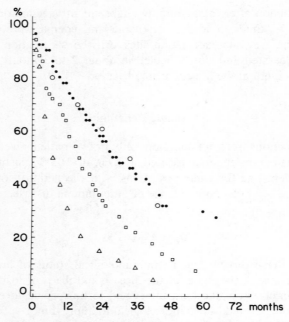

FIG. 2. Carcinoma of lung survival after surgery (RPMI, 1976). ●, Stage I (138); □, stage II (58); △, stage III (88); ○, stage III immunotherapy (15). RPMI, at Roswell Park Memorial Institute, as of 1976.

therapy of lung carcinoma to curative surgery is now under way as a joint project with Stewart et al.

SUMMARY

Thirty patients with locally far advanced lung carcinoma (stage III, conventionally inoperable) had radical lung resection in order to remove all visible evidence of tumor. The patients were postoperatively divided into two equal groups. One group of 15 received adjuvant immunotherapy that consisted of autologous tumor cell vaccine, whereas the control group received conventional management. Seven of the 15 patients in the treated group are alive, and the longest survivor has lived 51 months. The estimated median survival of this group is 34.8 months. In the control group only three of the 15 patients are alive, and the longest survivor has lived 25 months. The estimated median survival of this group is 12.1 months. The difference in the survival between the groups is significant at $p = 0.05$.

ACKNOWLEDGMENT

This investigation was supported by the National Institute of Health Research grant CA-15691.

REFERENCES

1. Brugarolas, A., Takita, H., Han, T., and Shimaoka, K. (1973): Immunotherapeutic effect of syngeneic tumor cells sequentially treated with concanavalin A, and vibrio cholera neuraminidase in mouse. *Proc. Am. Assoc. Cancer Res.,* 14:121.
2. Brugarolas, A., and Takita, H. (1973): Immunologic status in lung cancer. *Chest,* 64:427–430.
3. Higgins, G. A., Humphrey, E. W., Hughes, F. A., and Keehn, R. J. (1969): Cytoxan as an adjuvant to surgery for lung cancer. *J. Surg. Oncol.,* 1:221–228.
4. Piessens, W. F. (1970): Evidence for human cancer immunity. *Cancer,* 26:1212–1220.
5. Shields, T. W., Higgins, G. A., Lawton, R., Heilbrunn, A., and Keehn, R. J. (1970): Preoperative X-ray therapy as an adjuvant in the treatment of bronchogenic carcinoma. *J. Thorac. Cardiovasc. Surg.,* 59:49–61.
6. Shields, T. W. (1972): *General Thoracic Surgery.* Lea & Febiger, Philadelphia.
7. Shields, T. W. (1974): The fate of patients after incomplete resection of bronchial carcinoma. *Surg. Gynecol. Obstet.,* 139:569–572.
8. Slack, N. H. (1970): Bronchogenic carcinoma. Nitrogen mustard as a surgical adjuvant and factors influencing survival. *Cancer,* 25:987–1002.
9. Stewart, T. H. M., Hollinshead, A. G., and Harris, J. E. (1975): Immunochemotherapy of lung cancer. *Proc. NY Acad. Sci. (In press.)*
10. Takada, M., Takita, H., and Marabella, P. C. (1976): Antitumor antibody of lung carcinoma patients. *Proc. Am. Assoc. Cancer Res.,* 17:175.
11. Takita, H., Minowada, J., Han, T., Takada, M., and Lane, W. W. (1975): Adjuvant immunotherapy in bronchogenic carcinoma. *Proc. NY Acad. Sci. (In press.)*
12. Vincent, R. G., Takita, H., Lane, W. W., Gutierez, A. C., and Pickren, J. W. (1976): Surgical therapy of lung cancer. *J. Thorac. Cardiovasc. Surg.,* 71:581–591.

Question and Answer Session

Question: Dr. Takita, your study has 15 patients in each group, and in your illustrations I noticed that there were twice as many pneumonectomies in the control group as there were in the vaccine group. Thus, the type of surgery done in the two groups is quite different, and I wonder if that couldn't go a long way in explaining the significant results.

Dr. Takita: I realize the control group is very small. I think many squamous cell patients require pneumonectomies, because usually the lesions are located proximally. In squamous cell carcinoma, the prognosis is a little better compared to other cell types. And in the treatment group we have more nonsquamous lung cancer. Therefore it might balance off.

Dr. Cohen: What was the surgical mortality you had in the two treatment groups, and how did you handle patients who died?

Dr. Takita: I had two immediate surgical mortalities that were excluded, one from each group.

Immunotherapy of Cancer: Present Status of
Trials in Man, edited by W. D. Terry and D. Windhorst.
Raven Press, New York © 1978.

Adjuvant BCG Immunotherapy in Recurrent Superficial Bladder Cancer

Alvaro Morales, David Eidinger, and Andrew W. Bruce

Department of Urology, Queen's University, Kingston, Ontario, Canada

Superficial bladder cancer (stages $T_0 - T_1$) is an ambivalent disease from the therapeutic point of view; these tumors are easily eliminated by surgical means when they are small and few in number; however, the very high incidence of tumor recurrence following seemingly adequate endoscopic resection or fulguration poses a significant problem for the urologist and a great burden to the patient. The incidence of recurrence in superficial bladder cancer has been estimated to be as high as 70% within 2 years after initial diagnosis and appropriate surgical treatment (1).

The studies of Bubenik et al. (2) and O'Toole et al. (3) as well as the more recent work of Bean and associates (4) have demonstrated the antigenicity of human vesical neoplasms. This would suggest that augmentation of immunity may be useful in the treatment of these tumors and in the prevention of their recurrence. Experimental studies have shown the efficacy of Bacillus Calmette-Guerin (BCG) in inducing tumor regression (5), and in the clinical situation, the intratumoral administration of BCG has been noted to produce a favorable response (6,7). Certain conditions, however, must be met for successful BCG therapy. They have been defined by Bast et al. (8) and include (a) an adequate number of living organisms, (b) direct contact between BCG and tumor cells, (c) a relatively small tumor load, and (d) an ability of the host to respond to mycobacteria antigens. Bladder tumors appear to be a particularly adequate system for BCG treatment. Here we summarize the results obtained in a group of patients with a history of multiple recurrent bladder tumors treated with BCG. Early results have been previously published (9).

PATIENT POPULATION

Twelve male and four female patients entered the study. Their ages ranged from 43 to 88 years (mean 68.8). Transitional cell carcinoma was histologically diagnosed in 12 patients and squamous cell carcinoma in the remaining one. All tumors were staged clinically and histologically and were considered superficial, categories P1S to P1 according to the classification of the Internal Union Against Cancer (10). The initial lesion(s) had been treated surgically and subsequent recurrences by endoscopic resection or fulguration. In addition, intracavitary chemotherapy with thiotepa (triethyleneethiophosphoramide) and/or epodyl (trietilene-glycol diglyceridyl ether) had been previously used without apparent benefit in six patients. In every case two or more recurrences had been documented in the 12-month period immediately prior to entering the study, and most cases had a long history of recurrences dating back several years.

TREATMENT

Within 10 days following cystoscopy and documentation of recurrence, treatment was initiated. One hundred and twenty milligrams of lyophilized BCG (Institute de Microbiologie Armand Frappier, Montreal), reconstituted in 50 ml of normal saline, was forcefully instilled into the bladder via an indwelling urethral catheter. The patients were instructed to retain the suspension for no less than 2 hr. Simultaneous intradermal administration of 5 mg of the vaccine to alternate thighs was accomplished utilizing a multiple puncture apparatus (Heaf gun). These procedures were carried out weekly for a total of 6 consecutive weeks and then terminated.

FOLLOW-UP

Four to 6 weeks after completion of therapy a cystoscopy was performed. Areas of the mucosa suggestive of neoplastic change were biopsied; otherwise multiple random samples were obtained. Follow-up endoscopic examinations were repeated at approximately 3-month intervals thereafter.

RESULTS

Of the 16 patients, the one with squamous cell carcinoma died of unrelated causes 9 months after completion of treatment. Data from the 16 patients are summarized in Table 1.

Recurrence Rate

In those cases with a long history of tumor recurrence, only the 12-month period immediately preceding the onset of BCG administration was tabulated. In the remaining cases the interval between detection of the tumor and entry into the study is as indicated in the table. Before BCG therapy a total of 53 recurrences were found during an interval of 162 patient months. Following completion of BCG therapy these patients yielded a total of six tumors during a period of follow-up of 229 patient months.

Statistical Analysis

For this purpose patients no. 8, 9, and 11 were removed from consideration because of the different biological behavior of their tumors; however, they

TABLE 1. *Effect of BCG on bladder tumor recurrence*

Patient	Age	Sex	Pre-BCG		Post-BCG	
			No. of tumors	Follow-up (months)[c]	No. of tumors	Follow-up (months)
1	68	M	2	12	0	30
2	81	M	5	12	0	24
3	51	M	5	9	0	17
4	57	M	7	12	1	16
5	43	M	6	12	0[a]	16
6	71	F	6	12	0	16
7	64	M	3	9	0	12
8	75	F	CIS[b]	12	CIS	12
9	83	F	CIS	9	CIS	9
10	68	M	3	9	0	20
11	69	M	SqC	12	SqC	9
12	70	M	4	12	0	9
13	67	F	2	9	0	9
14	70	M	3	9	0	9
15	73	M	2	6	0	7
16	66	M	2	6	1	7

[a] Recurrence found in the left ureter.

[b] CIS found in several biopsies.

[c] In cases with long history of tumor recurrence, only the 12-month period preceding BCG treatment is recorded; in remaining cases the time between tumor detection and entry into study is indicated.

CIS, carcinoma *in situ*; SqC, squamous cell carcinoma.

were considered treatment failures. Of the remaining patients, tumor recurrences were detected in three following BCG administration. In all of these patients there were fewer tumors following treatment than before treatment. A statistical test of the efficacy of the treatment was performed, considering

TABLE 2. *Comparison of recurrence rate within identical observation periods*

Patient	Months of observation	Number of tumors	
		Pre-BCG	Post-BCG
1	12	2	0
2	12	5	0
3	9	5	0
4	12	7	1
5	12	6	0[a]
6	12	6	0
7	9	3	0
10	9	3	0
12	9	2	0
13	9	2	0
14	9	3	0
15	6	2	0
16	6	1	1

[a] Recurrence found in the left ureter.

only identical pre-BCG and post-BCG periods (Table 2). The sign test (11) yields a p value of 0.005 for the test of the hypothesis that the patterns of tumor incidence are not changed by BCG treatment. Hence there is evidence that treatment does reduce the incidence of bladder tumor recurrence. This evidence is reinforced by the fact that in most cases the posttreatment observation period was longer than the pretreatment period.

Histological Studies

Biopsies taken from areas corresponding to the location of previous tumors were carried out. Specimens taken within 6 weeks of completion of treatment revealed variable degrees of granulomatous inflammation (Fig. 1). It was noted that the degree of inflammatory response became less marked in subsequent examinations.

Side Effects

Side effects attributable to the regimen of BCG immunizations were minimal, and in every case, of short duration. Four patients reported low grade fever and malaise that subsided within 24 hr after treatment. Seven patients

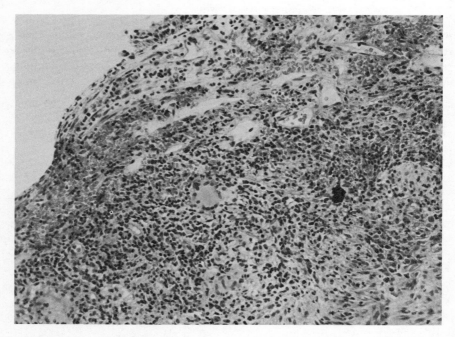

FIG. 1. Biopsy of the bladder taken 6 weeks after completion of treatment and showing the characteristic granulomatous inflammation. H & E. × 220.

developed urinary frequency and urgency. In two of these patients a urinary infection caused by *Escherichia coli* was documented; in the remaining five patients the lower urinary symptoms subsided spontaneously in less than a week. In no case was it necessary to delay or interrupt treatment because of side effects or complications. Two elderly women with a long history of urgency incontinence had difficulty retaining the BCG in the bladder; both had persistent tumor after treatment. All patients showed a circumscribed but strong reaction at the sites of intradermal administration of the vaccine. This healed within 6 weeks of completion of treatment.

DISCUSSION

The finding of a significant decrease in the number of superficial bladder tumor recurrences suggests a beneficial effect induced by BCG administration. In the majority of patients prevention of recurrences was obtained; in the remaining the number of new lesions was decreased. This is in agreement with the findings of Eilber et al. (12) indicating that BCG immunotherapy is not an all-or-nothing phenomenon. In addition, it is conceivable that a longer course of therapy could have prevented the persistence or relapse of tumors in those cases considered treatment failures. Because of this possibility we have modified the protocol and continue the intracavitary and intradermal administration of BCG at monthly intervals for 1 year after the initial period of weekly treatments.

Intracavitary therapy of bladder cancer has attracted considerable interest over the years. The lower urinary tract readily permits the delivery of a high local concentration of therapeutic agents with concomitant low systemic effects, and, in addition, it allows a prompt and objective evaluation of results. Evidently no other tumor, with the general exception of cutaneous malignancy, fulfills the requirements of relatively small tumor load, adequate dose, and close intimate contact between BCG and tumor as does the superficial vesical neoplasm.

The histological picture observed in our patients is very similar to the ones reported in experimental studies in which instillations or intramural injection of BCG in the bladder of cancer-free animals has produced a vigorous and extensive granulomatous reaction (13,14). Active granulomatous inflammation was found in a patient with a vesical melanoma successfully treated by deKernion et al. (15), with a transurethral, intramural injection of BCG.

It has been suggested that the concomitant administration of autologous tumor cells with BCG will give better results than BCG alone, as employed in this study. The concept was advanced by Mathé et al. (16) that the combination of BCG and tumor cells is more effective than either one alone in the treatment of malignancies. This remains an unproven concept in man. Immunotherapy trials for melanoma (12) and lung cancer (17) have failed to show that tumor cells enhance the effect of the vaccine. Furthermore, the number of cells obtainable by endoscopic removal of these generally small tumor recurrences in the bladder is too small for effective immunization.

Local immunotherapy, alone or in combination with other modalities, holds substantial potential in the treatment of superficial bladder cancer. Notwithstanding the short period of follow-up and the limited number of patients, our results provide initial evidence that BCG may favorably alter the natural history of this tumor in man.

ACKNOWLEDGMENTS

Dr. Maxwell Layard, National Institutes of Health, assisted in the statistical analysis.

REFERENCES

1. Greene, L. P., and Yalowitz, P. A. (1972): The advisability of concomitant transurethral excision of vesical neoplasms and prostatic hyperplasia. *J. Urol.,* 107:445–447.
2. Bubenik, J., Perlman, P., Helmstein, K., and Moberger, G. (1970): Cellular and humoral immune responses to urinary bladder carcinomas. *Int. J. Cancer,* 5:310–319.
3. O'Toole, C., Helmstein, K., Perlman, P., and Moberger, G. (1975): Cellular immunity to transitional cell carcinoma of the urinary bladder. III. Effect of hydrostatic pressure therapy. *Int. J. Cancer,* 16:413–425.
4. Bean, M., Pees, H., Fogh, J. E., Grabstald, H., and Oettgen, H. F. (1974): Cytotoxicity of lymphocytes from patients with cancer of the urinary bladder: Detection by ^3H proline microcytotoxicity assay. *Int. J. Cancer,* 14:186–197.
5. Zbar, B., Bernstein, I. D., and Rapp, H. J. (1971): Suppression of tumor growth at the site of infection with living Bacillus Calmette-Guerin. *J. Natl. Cancer Inst.,* 46:831–839.
6. Pinsky, C., Hishaut, Y., and Oettgen, H. (1973): Treatment of malignant melanoma by intratumoral injection of BCG. *Natl. Cancer Inst. Monogr.,* 39:225–228.
7. Nathanson, L. (1973): Regression of intradermal malignant melanoma after intralesional injection of BCG. *Cancer Chemother. Rep.,* 56:659–665.
8. Bast, R. C., Zbar, B., Borsos, T., and Rapp, H. J. (1974): BCG and Cancer. *New Engl. J. Med.,* 290:1413–1420.
9. Morales, A., Eidinger, D., and Bruce A. W. (1976): Intracavitary BCG in the treatment of superficial bladder cancer. *J. Urol.,* 116:180–183.
10. Collins, E. E. (1975): The classification of malignant tumors of the bladder, prostate, testis and kidney. *Can. J. Surg.,* 18:468–475.
11. Armitage, P. (1971): *Statistical Methods in Surgical Research.* Wiley, New York.
12. Eilber, F. R., Morton, D. L., Holmes, E. C., Sparks, F. C., and Ramming, K. P. (1975): Adjuvant immunotherapy with BCG in treatment of regional lymph node metastases from malignant melanoma. *New Engl. J. Med.,* 294:237–240.
13. Bloomberg, S. D., Brosman, S. A., Hausman, M. S., Cohen, A., and Battenberg, J. D. (1975): Effects of BCG on dog bladder. *Invest. Urol.,* 12:423–427.
14. Schellhammer, P. F., Kaplan, M. H., Pinsky, C. M., and Whitmore, W. F. (1975): Study of local and systemic effects of intravesical BCG. *Urology,* 6:562–565.
15. deKernion, J. B., Golub, S. H., Gupta, R. K., Silverstein, M., and Morton, D. L. (1975): Successful transurethral intralesional BCG therapy of a bladder melanoma. *Cancer,* 36:1662–1667.
16. Mathe, G., Pouillart, P., Schwarzenberg, L., Amiel, J. L., Schneider, M., Hayat, M., De Vassal, F., Jasmin, C., Rosenfeld, C., Weiner, R., and Rappaport, H. (1972):

Attempts at immunotherapy of 100 with acute lymphoid leukemia. *Natl. Cancer Inst. Monogr.*, 35:361–365.

17. Oldham, R. K., Weese, J. L., and Herberman, R. B. (1977): Immunological monitoring and immunotherapy in carcinoma of the lung. *Int. J. Cancer (in press.)*

Question and Answer Session

Dr. Russell: Could you just clarify the status of your treated patients at the beginning of the trial? Were all patients free of disease or did some actually have tumors?

Dr. Morales: These patients were free of tumor when we started the BCG immunotherapy. There was no evidence of tumor as detected by cystoscopy.

Dr. David Byar (National Cancer Institute): There is one point which is of utmost importance in clarifying the results of this study. Do you refer to the number of recurrences or to the number of tumors seen at a single examination: If you look in the bladder and you see five tumors and that counts for five, that is quite different from having a patient who recurs five separate times.

Dr. Morales: This refers to the total number of recurrences found in the year before BCG therapy.

It was usually one or two recurrences seen per cystoscopy. The cystoscopies are done every three months. That is the regular schedule for the follow-up of these patients on or off this type of study.

DISCUSSION: LUNG CANCER

Dr. Hersh: The format for this discussion will be to ask each individual to briefly state the overall results of his studies, including the number of patients in the study, the treatment, and the disease-free interval and survival for the control and experimental groups.

Dr. McKneally: In our study in Albany, we treated 95 patients with either intrapleural BCG, followed by isoniazid, or isoniazid alone (Table 1). There were 26 patients in the BCG-treated Stage I group, and 32 in the control Stage I group; 10 in the BCG-treated Stage II group, 9 in the control Stage II group; 11 in the BCG-treated Stage III group, and 7 in the control Stage III group.

There were two recurrences among the 26 BCG-treated patients. The median duration of follow-up was 20 months, and we have not yet reached a median point in terms of recurrence.

There were nine recurrences in the 32 control patients. The median duration of follow-up was also 20 months.

Dr. Hersh: What is your estimate of the current status of lung cancer immunotherapy? Where is your own program going, or where you think the field should go in the future?

TABLE 1. *Lung cancer discussion*

		Stage I		
			Disease Recurrence	
	Route of	Survival	(# Recurrences/# Patients)	
Immunotherapy	Administration	Gain (T/C)	IT Group	Control
BCG	Intrapleural	Yes	2/26	9/32
TAA in Freund's ± MTX	Intradermal	Yes	4/24	7/24
Levamisole	P.O.	No	0/11	4/14
	(Patients weighing less than 70 kg)			
	Stage II			
BCG	Intrapleural	No	5/10	5/9
TAA + Freund's ± MTX	Intradermal	Probably No	1/5	1/2
Levamisole (Stage II & III)	P.O.	Yes	6/19	16/25
	(Patients weighing less than 70 kg)			
	Stage III			
BCG	Intrapleural	No	7/11	2/7
ADR ± *C. parvum*	s.c.	Not significant	12/37	13/29
BCG-CWS	Intralesional	Yes		
	Intradermal ± Tumor Cells	median survival	18 months	7 months
Tumor Cells + Freund's	Intradermal	Yes	6/15	8/15

Dr. McKneally: Well, I think that the principal agencies that are effective against lung cancer are not immunological ones. Prior to these presentations, I would have said the impact of immunological manipulations on lung cancer are extremely small, but I think the fact that there are positive results with immunological manipulation alone (Drs. Yamamura and Takita), was encouraging. Dr. Stewart and I have really only been seeing an effect with our techniques in early stage disease. Dr. Ward Young also uses intra-cutaneous BCG in lung cancer and sees what looks like a positive effect in Stage I.

I think now that there is some promise in more advanced surgical stages for combined modalities. I think it's very unlikely that immunological ma-nipulations alone will be very effective in the bulk of lung cancer patients who are unresectable. My inclination is toward using other agencies, like surgery and X-irradiation and chemotherapy, to get the total amount of tumor down before we start doing things with the immune response. Stimu-lating the immune response during infectious illness really isn't very effective when the organisms are overwhelming the host, and it is reasonable to expect the same to be true of cancer.

As to exactly where we will go in this general direction isn't yet de-termined. Our mission is to finish our study.

Dr. Cohen: Are your Stage I patients completely staged? If they start BCG on day 4 after treatment, presumably you don't have the pathology data back on many patients. Do you have some people included in your results who were thought to be Stage I but after pathologic evaluation of surgical material turned out to be some other stage?

Dr. McKneally: In a certain sense, yes. We do have pathological data back, but it isn't a detailed report, so we use the staging system that I showed on that slide.

If we revise it exactly according to the criteria of Mountain, there are minor changes in T status usually because of the distance of the tumor from the carina, and so on, but none of the patients jumped stages.

Since we leave the patients in the stage that they are assigned to on that day, there is at least one patient who I mentioned who is really a Stage III or IV in Dr. Yamamura's category, in that he had abdominal metastases at the time of the surgery. But we leave them in Stage I.

Dr. Hersh: There has been some concern expressed about possible differences between the relapse rate of the control group at Albany and the control groups seen at places like Roswell Park, Mayo Clinic, et cet. Is that really a significant concern? What is the survival of your concurrent randomized control compared to the historical control experience in your own group?

Dr. McKneally: Dr. Takita illustrated that his immunologically manipulated Stage III patients are just like his Stage I patients, their five-year survival fraction was about 45 percent or 40 percent, and their one-year survival fraction was in the 80's. That's our experience, too, in Stage I. That is, our one-year survival fraction is 87 percent, and our five-year survival fraction is around 45 or 50 percent.

I am happy that we did a randomized simultaneous control series, because this question would be frightening to me, to look at how low the survival rate was in Stage I in our institution. But it's just as low in the randomized simultaneous control group. I think it's the same as the Roswell Park experience. I know the Memorial group and the Mayo group are enjoying a higher surgical survival fraction at one year than we are, in the 90s, 90 percent or 92 percent. But I think those are relatively trivial differences and maybe if we had 100 patients, we'd be two or three points in either direction.

Dr. Hersh: Your plan, then, is to continue the clinical trial as it is designed?

Dr. McKneally: We don't have to go very much further, as Dr. Pinsky said, to prove a negative in Stage III. We're really not getting any place. Any one of the leads that has been mentioned here might be picked up—levamisole or repeated immunization with some BCG-derived product. But I do feel, in addition, we should be doing something to get rid of residual tumor.

Dr. Cohen: Why did you use INH in the control group?

Dr. McKneally: To deal with the question: How do you know it wasn't the INH that caused this favorable effect? I decided to use INH in the BCG group because, unlike scarification or Heaf gun, when you put the BCG into the pleural space, it's all in; that's it. I felt I had to be able to treat the patients with an antituberculous agent and that this treatment should be controlled for in the control group. If I were replicating the study, as some others are doing, I wouldn't give INH to the control patients, because the question has been answered even by the small study. If there is an effect seen here, it's caused by the BCG, and I think that's all that needs to be done in terms of a replication.

In our animal system with intrapulmonary tumors, the combination of BCG and isoniazide is synergistic. BCG alone reduces the number of tumor growths in the lung. Isoniazid alone has no effect. The combination of isoniazid and BCG is significantly better than BCG alone. That is not an original observation of mine. It is an original observation of Dr. Sparks in Dr. Morton's group, and it was also made here at the NIH in Dr. Rapp's lab several years ago.

Dr. Hersh: Dr. Yamamura, would you reiterate in one sentence the overall results of your study?

Dr. Yamamura: We have 157 control patients and 104 BCG-CWS-treated patients. The numbers of patients in each stage are shown in Table 1 of my chapter. In the control groups, 90 percent of Stage I and 80 percent of Stage II patients are still alive. On the other hand, in the CWS-treated patients, all of the patients in Stage I and II are still alive. We intend to continue the repeated intradermal injection of BCG in these patients. For Stage III, 5 percent of the 72 control patients are still alive while 30 percent of the 56 CWS-treated patients are still alive. In Stage IV, all the patients (43 control and 30 treated) have died.

We shall continue the intradermal injection of 200 mg of CWS to these patients who are still alive.

Dr. Hersh: As I understood it from your presentation, a major modality of treatment in the Stage III and Stage IV patients was the intrapleural injection of cell wall skeleton. Is that correct?

Dr. Yamamura: The intrapleural injection is remarkably effective in the treatment of lung cancer in improving the survival rate especially in Stage III patients. There is a lesser effect in Stage IV.

Dr. Cohen: Was there any difference in the surgery performed in Stage III patients between the group of patients that received the cell-wall skeleton versus the control?

Dr. Yamamura: I can't answer your question because we have never checked this.

Dr. Hersh: What are your immediate future plans for your immunotherapy studies in your patient population based on your observations to date?

Dr. Yamamura: Well, as I mentioned in my chapter, I should like to do some trials of the intrapleural injections in patients with cancerous pleuritis. In addition, recently we find that the Nocardia cell wall is much more potent than BCG cell-wall skeleton in the suppression of experimental syngeneic and autochthonous tumors. Nocardia is not pathogenic to the animals and to the human beings and is easily cultivated within three or four days.

We know a great deal about the chemical structure of cell-wall skeleton of BCG. A most important moiety of the cell-wall skeleton is the mucopeptide portion. The mycolic acid is also very important. Based on this information we are trying to synthesize the active subunit of cell-wall skeleton to be available for experimental use.

Dr. Hersh: Dr. Dimitrov, can you summarize your results?

Dr. Dimitrov: Well, we had a problem deciding on what dose of *C. parvum* to use. Everyone treating patients with *C. parvum* has used a dose which nobody knows is the right one, and we did the same thing. It is our impression that with very small doses, much smaller than this one, when injected intradermally or subcutaneously, we may obtain the same results.

The second question, which we have been thinking about is why should we inject *C. parvum* simultaneously with chemotherapy when we are looking for *C. parvum* to protect the bone marrow. The best thing seems to be to give *C. parvum* one week after chemotherapy but before the nadir of the leukopenia.

Dr. Hersh: You demonstrated the bone marrow protective effect. Did the patients receiving *C. parvum* actually receive more adriamycin chemotherapy either at a total dose or at the height of the single dose?

Dr. Dimitrov: They did not. The total drug dose in both groups was the same but for patients treated with chemotherapy alone it was necessary to interrupt therapy until the WBC count returned to 5,000 cells/mm³. For patients treated with chemotherapy plus *C. parvum* it was not necessary to interrupt therapy for low white blood cell counts.

Dr. Amery: Well, regarding future studies, I think that the data are clear enough to try to use these high doses of levamisole in patients with a higher body weight.

Regarding the future use of immunotherapy in lung cancer, I think there are some trends not only in lung cancer but in other cancers which become more and more apparent. First of all, there might be two types of immunotherapeutic approaches. One attempts to increase the immunization status of the patients, for example, by regional or intratumoral application of such substances as BCG or *C. parvum* or antigen. In contrast to that, there are immunotherapies which try to restore the already established but depressed immunity resulting from the presence of the tumor.

In this latter category, we find levamisole and thymosin, and perhaps other substances. If one looks at the animal data there are a few studies in the literature which indicate that if you follow the kinetics of tumor-specific immunity, you first have a phase of building up tumor-specific immunity, and then you reach a certain plateau and it then goes down. So my feeling would be that in this first phase, before you reach the plateau, you should expect benefit from measures which would increase immunity whilst in the later phase, after you are coming down from your plateau again, you should especially expect benefit from the second type of immunotherapy.

The intrapleural application of BCG, and the intra-bladder installations of BCG in patients with small tumors seem to be effective, whilst intrapleural application of BCG in more advanced disease stages seems less effective. We have just the reverse with levamisole. The problem is, of course, you can hardly define the point where you reach the plateau.

So in our current status of knowledge, I would guess that surgery with combination immunotherapy, including the intrapleural administration of a substance which attacks immunocompetent cells, together with systemic treatment with either levamisole or thymosin would be the best approach from a theoretical point of view.

Dr. Stewart: First of all, one wants to know if the results one has achieved are real. Despite one's own prejudice, the only way one can answer that is to see if other people can do it. Is it reproducible? We chose lung cancer, partly because of its very short statistics. That is, one can establish treatment principles in the disease before one goes into diseases such as breast cancer where the natural history of disease is considerably longer.

My first desire, therefore, is to see whether or not we are really seeing an accurate picture, if it is reproducible in other hands, and then will it be applicable to other tumor systems. At the local level we are very interested in the interactions of methotrexate and folic acid on the immune response. We have some preliminary data we are not showing today concerning pulsed folinic acid. It does, in fact, very favorably affect the immune function.

So that is the sophisticated side of things. I think we would much welcome the capacity to have radioimmunoassays of the various antigens we are using. At the moment, we are really uncertain. Radioimmunoassays should be incorporated into any future larger study so we can monitor what we are doing.

Dr. Takita: From our preliminary results adjuvant immunotherapy in Stage III lung cancer appears to be effective. If you apply immunotherapy to earlier stages of lung cancer, like Stage I, Stage II, you should get much better results. Indeed, this was proven by Dr. McKneally and Dr. Stewart.

I think it is important that first we try to improve the particular results in the earlier stages of disease, because even nowadays if you see a patient with far-advanced tuberculosis, you cannot cure it. Now it comes to the problem of tumor-specific immunity. We have started a joint project of immunotherapy with Dr. Stewart and Dr. Hollinshead and we are using the same antigen preparations.

Regarding complete Freund's adjuvant, I think this is the best available adjuvant for active immunotherapy at this moment. Its side effects, however, leave a lot to be desired. But I think I am going to stick to complete Freund's adjuvant until there is evidence that something else is superior.

The next step I am considering is for inoperable lung cancer. Patients would first get chemotherapy. If the tumor is reduced, it should be removed by surgery, followed by immunotherapy. It may be an interesting approach.

Dr. Morales: As far as cancer of the bladder, very little has been done with immunotherapy. Generally, the only studies have been those of Dr. Finch. I want to emphasize that our report is yet a very preliminary trial, and obviously our first job now is to increase the number of patients, and we obviously would like to have a clinical trial with appropriate controls. We suspect that if we prolonged the treatment that we have been giving the BCG for more than the six weeks, the results would be better. Actually, we have had now a number of patients who are being continued on BCG for a whole year. It is also possible that a combination of BCG with effective chemotherapeutic agents such as thiotepa which has been used in this country, and epolium, which is being used in Europe, could offer better results than BCG alone.

Dr. Holland: I would like to return to Dr. Fudenberg's question because it is very relevant. It disturbs me to ascribe the effects Dr. Stewart noted to his tumor-associated antigens alone when he doesn't have an independent Freund's adjuvant control group.

Dr. Stewart: This is a recurrent theme. In planning this study I was influenced by my early training when I touched on the induction of experimental autoallergic diseases. You can't induce any of these diseases with Freund's adjuvant without the organ antigen. I assumed, therefore, that Freund's adjuvant alone would not have an effect on lung cancer.

Now, from Yamamura's data, I think you are absolutely right. I think it would be very important in a prospective study to incorporate this. Also, if one saw a result with Freund's adjuvant alone, wouldn't someone say, "I think you'd better have a series where you just give Tween, and another with oil."

Dr. Holland: Dr. Stewart, your data are beautiful, but I think it's erroneous to ascribe it to the tumor vaccine. I think you should say, "We have used a complex system, and this is what the results are."

Dr. Stewart: My personal prejudice is that it is the tumor antigen, but you are quite right; it is open to question.

Dr. Hersh: It is conceivable biologically that the intense, large inflammatory reaction seen with Freund's could release lymphokines or other agents which would have profound immunotherapeutic effect.

Dr. Stewart: It wouldn't explain our skin test data, Dr. Hersh, absolutely not.

Dr. Hersh: I think it might, because we do see augmentation of skin test reactivity to presumably unrelated antigens when we administer BCG. Furthermore, it is conceivable that there are lung cancer cross-reactive antigens in the microbacterial component.

Dr. Stewart: Dr. Hollinshead, I think, should answer that question. But I might just point out if you review the entire literature, as I have done, on skin tests that one sees without immune stimulation, they are rarely more than 1.5 centimeters. Responses as large as ours have not been seen without significant immune stimulation.

Dr. Hersh: What Dr. Holland is saying, I think, is that at the moment your results are achieved with a mixture of therapies.

Dr. Hollinshead: I think the comment by Fudenberg and Holland is very, very important. I agree pretty much with Dr. Stewart, but I can tell you that Takita has a Freund's adjuvant alone arm on the study we are just starting, and I think that's a very important thing to do.

Now, as to shared antigens. I have been working with Ribi, Hanna, Hersh, Minden and others, looking at the bits and pieces of BCG, cell-wall skeleton, and so forth, and antisera to these, and to cross-reactivity with our tumor antigens and antisera. The study is far too early. There appear to be some types of tumors which do share antigens with bacteria. We are going to look at a lot of bacteria. I think for the future, the study of these shared antigens, the possibility of turning them on, is very, very important. I have no data to answer this question at this moment.

Dr. Cohen: Dr. Stewart, when you report your data, it seems you are lumping the groups that get tumor-associated antigens versus the groups that don't get tumor-associated antigens. Is that because you feel methotrexate is playing no role in your treatment results?

Dr. Stewart: It is a trick to get numbers to work with. We only have about 13, 15, 16 in each subgroup, and you get nothing out of that.

Question: Dr. Yamamura, is the immune competence of any of your patients checked prior to starting immunotherapy and, if so, is survival related to this factor?

Dr. Yamamura: There is no statistical difference whatsoever.

Dr. McKneally: In our hands, there is a statistical correlation between skin tests and survival, but you can't project from individual skin tests what the outcome will be for any single patient. We have been using PHA as an equivalent of DNCB because we don't have enough lead time preoperatively to sensitize and test the patient. PHA, like DNCB, shows a general trend to lower values in Stage III patients and lower values in patients who subsequently are proven to have recurrence. But I wouldn't predict from a positive or negative PHA skin test what the outcome would be for an individual patient.

Question: Dr. Amery, you said that levamisole is not an immunostimulator. Could you comment on that, since two years ago you said it was an immunostimulator.

Also, in your studies is there a correlation between skin tests and clinical results?

Dr. Amery: Your second question is perhaps more easy to answer. The only immunologic evaluation we have is the DNCB and TB skin tests which probably have nothing to do with tumor immunity.

Regarding the statement that levamisole is not an immunostimulant, as far as I remember, I never made the statement that it was an immunostimulator, so probably there is some misunderstanding. We originally thought that levamisole would have some immunostimulating properties, but later it became clear that we cannot stimulate immunity in normal individuals or in normal animals. We can restore the immunity in 40 percent of the subjects when it is deficient.

Dr. Mathé: A lot of animal and human data are published showing levamisole was supposed to be an immunostimulant. As far as immunorestorations, we studied levamisole for these properties and the result was completely negative. So it is not an immunorestorer in all patients.

Dr. Amery: That's right. It might be related to disease. You are speaking of a lymphocytic malignancy. It might have something to do with the stage of the disease. It is perhaps conceivable that in the late stages of cancer the patients are so severely depressed that you cannot restore the immune response. But what is clear is that in a certain percentage of cancer-bearing subjects who have depressed immunity you can restore it, whereas in normal individuals you cannot increase immune reactivity.

Dr. McKhann: Dr. Takita, from your protocol, it is clear that no attempt was made to kill the tumor cells. I was wondering whether you feel that it is important that viable tumor cells be injected and whether you have ever seen any evidence of local growth at the area of injection.

Dr. Takita: So far 60 patients received the tumor vaccine with this type of preparation, and only on one occasion did we see growth of tumor locally. This patient had an incomplete resection at the time of surgery, and died in three months. An autopsy showed local growth, but no metastases from the injection.

Dr. Rosenberg: Earlier, we discussed negative studies. Virtually all of the studies that we have discussed now have claimed to be positive. I would like to direct several questions to different members of the group.

In terms of Dr. Dimitrov's studies, there is in fact no statistical significance, and although there is a trend, statistical significance is not present and we should not consider it a positive study.

In Dr. Amery's study of levamisole, when all the patients are considered, there is no statistical significance. Statistically significant differences have only been detected in that subset of patients that weigh less than 70 kg. It seems likely to me that in analyzing your data you probably examined a large number of subsets of patients differing by variables such as age, sex and other characteristics before you found the difference in the under 70 kg group. If you do this, it becomes statistically more likely that one will find some criterion that will lead to statistical significance. That needs to be taken into account when performing the statistical analysis. I wonder if when that is done, you still find significance for patients less than 70 kg.

Finally, Dr. Takita, in your study the differences between treatment and control are 3 of 15 compared to 7 out of 15. I wonder what kind of statistic is significant at the 0.05 level with those small numbers?

Dr. Dimitrov: We consulted our statistician. His suggestion was that it is a good pilot study and somebody else should confirm it.

Dr. Amery: Regarding the analysis of our study with levamisole, as I already pointed out, there was an indication from the animal studies that dose was important. From that point of view, we looked at our dosage relative to weight, because this was low as compared to the dosage which proved effective in animal models.

The second point is that it has been found that in children with recurrent upper respiratory infection, as reported in *Lancet,* the effective dose seemed to be 2.5 mg/kg as a minimum. That is a bit higher than our dose.

The third point is that we overlooked this point when we did the first analysis, but from the second analysis we recognized that this trend was present. We went back to the data of our first analysis and found it was different at that time. It has remained consistently present since then. This is not to claim that this is now conclusive evidence, but I think it is suggestive enough to look at a higher dosage in future trials.

Dr. Takita: As a clinician, I asked my statistician to analyze the data and give me the results. This was analyzed by life table analysis and the Breslow method of test and failure, and the significance was 0.05.

Dr. Cohen: The major problem that I see in the levamisole study is in the staging system that is used. Patients with a wide variety of prognoses were all lumped together. I wonder whether it would be possible to retrospectively go back and put those patients into a more conventional staging system and to really analyze the effect of levamisole.

Dr. Amery: You have to recognize that we drafted this protocol in the winter of 1972, and at the time the modern staging papers had not been published. So, we had to rely on other systems of looking at the patients.

Dr. Byar: (National Cancer Institute). As far as I can tell from what's been said, the problem raised by both Dr. Peto and Dr. Rosenberg, that the so-called multiple comparison problem or "how many things did you look at before you found one which was significant," was not taken into account in computing the probability level in the levamisole study. It is actually seldom possible in medical trials to take into account all of the things you might have looked at that reduce the probability level proportionately, especially because you don't know how related these different evaluations are. Thus, while the problem is a real one, it is difficult to deal with.

Another pertinent criticism of your trial concerns the questions of whether the patients were comparable in the two groups with respect to prognostic factors when only those under 70 kilos were studied. For example, in your

Table 4, there were twice as many patients with more advanced regional disease in the placebo group than in the treatment group and there were also about twice as many patients in Stage II as compared to Stage I. Since both of these effects go in the same direction against the placebo effect, and could reinforce each other, I would suggest making an adjusted survival analysis before claiming significance in that group.

Dr. Amery: You are speaking about Table 4 in my chapter?

Dr. Byar: Yes, I am.

Dr. Amery: Of course, there is the tendency that there are more advanced cases in the placebo group. But if you make a breakdown, if you make an analysis as you see in Table 4, you find the significant difference just in these more advanced cases and not in the cases with smaller amounts of disease. In other words, if you eliminate the patients with small tumor burdens, you increase the difference between levamisole and placebo.

Dr. LoBuglio: I would like to return to the general statistical question raised by Peto and Rosenberg. This has really become a big problem in the Southwest Group where the computer takes all of our data, and analyzes it by a huge number of variables. For example, in the regimen that Costanzi presented, four different subgroups have highly statistically significant increases in response rates as 'compared to another subgroup.

Should we walk away saying, "If you're between 40 and 50, you're better off to be on BHD, but if your leukocyte count is over 10,000, you're much better off on some other regimen"? How do we evaluate those highly statistically significant results? Before we can consider them valid, do we have to do a new study designed only to ask that single question or is there a valid statistical technique that will permit us to analyze our data in terms of the hundreds of variables that can be looked at in that large group? I think somebody who has some sophistication in this area ought to tell us how much of a problem this is.

Dr. Peto: I think when you have a problem like this, you take an overall look at the data and see if overall you have a statistically significant difference. If you do, then start looking at where the differences are.

But if you don't have an overall significant difference, then you can really get into trouble, because in every single trial that's ever done, if you split the patients up you will always get subgroups where you get an apparent treatment effect because random variation is so large. Thus, when the numbers get small in subgroups, you are bound to get great differences between groups.

If you've got an overall statistically significant difference, then you can reasonably safely look at subgroups. If you don't get overall differences, look at subgroups to get leads into future studies, but don't trust what you find.

Dr. Gehan: I agree with Dr. Peto to a large extent. Thus, if in leukemia, you are looking at age groups or histological types, those are variables that have been established over many studies to be of prognostic significance. And if you are looking at treatment groups within those groups, that is meaningful. I'm not sure we really need any new statistical procedures for handling these data.

In follow-up to what Dr. LoBuglio said, when we do these clinical studies, we test for treatment differences and do it by some regression methods where we include in our regression equation factors that are known to be of prognostic significance. Then we can get a valid test.

In Costanzi's study, we did find certain subgroups where there were differences. I think we have to accept these as leads to be looked at in other studies. Some of these differences are not correlated with factors known to influence clinical course, or to factors related to response in other studies.

Dr. Hersh: Even in regard to conventional therapy, there are small subgroups which would be lost in the overall group, where the subgroup clearly benefits from that conventional therapy. Stage I lung cancer is an example. The long-term survival of all lung cancer patients subjected to surgery is abysmal, but Stage I does very well.

Dr. Peto: I am saying look at subgroups, but you can't trust things which you just noted in one particular subgroup unless there is some *a priori* reason for looking in that particular subgroup for that particular thing. In Stage I lung cancer, there is an *a priori* reason for using the staging characteristics to establish subgroups for data analysis. The 70 kg separation is archetypally the thing which is just plucked out of the air.

Dr. Hersh: Not entirely. I take issue with that, because dose per meter square of body surface area is a well recognized principle of chemotherapy.

Dr. Peto: But it shouldn't go the other way. I mean the thing is actually the other way in the next group. I would like to make a comment about Dr. Yamamura's chapter. Of all the studies presented, his is the most definite. There are reasonably large numbers and the differences are quite striking. The disadvantage is that it wasn't a randomized study, but was based on historical controls.

The pattern of survival observed in the historical control group and in the treated group differs very markedly in the first few months. It doesn't differ in the way that one would expect if immunotherapy were acting in the way that one might expect it to. The data show many deaths in the first month in the controls, and a lot more deaths in the second month. In the treated patients you are getting no deaths in the first month, and no deaths in the second month. If your data are true, this must be saving patients who otherwise were going to die the next day. How exactly did you get your historical control group?

Dr. Yamamura: I have never selected the patients. All the patients admitted to the hospital received BCG-CWS. No selection was made and the results were shown in the figures. I don't know the mechanism, but, by the repeated injections or by the combined therapy with surgery or chemotherapy and treatment, the survival time of the patient was prolonged.

Dr. Hersh: Does anybody wish to respond to Dr. Peto's question?

Dr. Amery: I would like to reply to your remarks with a question. I think you said that if you have a significant difference using the data of the populations, you are allowed to make breakdowns to further define trends in the materials. Now, how do you define this difference which can be present between the two populations or subpopulations?

Dr. Peto: The more significant it is, the more confidant you are in your breakdowns; the less significant, the less confident you are.

Dr. Amery: The only thing I would like to point out is this is detailed analysis and you have to see several papers.

Dr. Powles: I would strongly support the point made concerning the possible weakness of Professor Yamamura's control group being a historical control group, but I think the statisticians and mathematicians have to be very careful. They don't have any right at the moment to tell us exactly what an immunotherapeutic effect should look like on a curve, in view of the fact we have absolutely no idea of what immunotherapy is, whether it exists or not, whether it is specific or not. I think it would be nice to stick to examining the two groups of patients and seeing if there is a difference.

Dr. Woodruff: I would like to return to Dr. McKhann's questions of Dr. Takita. Is there likely to be any advantage in using living cells as against irradiated cells? I don't know how many tumor cells are killed by being emulsified and exposed to neuraminidase. If there are only a few live cells left, I wonder whether there is any advantage or whether they might just as well be radiated?

Dr. Takita: At the beginning of our study we did a comparison of live cells, cultured cells, stored cells, radiated cells, and we found that the fresh live cells were the most immunogenic. After homogenizing with adjuvant and vibrio cholera neuraminidase (VCN), the viability drops to less than 10 percent.

Dr. Hollinshead: I am intrigued by Sir Michael Woodruff's questions about live versus dead, and I think it deserves some thought. In lung cancer, it very much depends on type. I think one of the problems with killed oat cells would be that you'd be releasing inhibitory antigens present on the cell surface. For that reason, killed cells could be bad.

Dr. Woodruff: But if you kill a cell accidentally, I imagine you liberate just the same amount of antigen as if you actually murder it.

Immunotherapy of Cancer: Present Status of Trials in Man, edited by W. D. Terry and D. Windhorst. Raven Press, New York © 1978.

Sarcoma: Natural History and Treatment

Emil Frei III, Ronald Blum, and Norman Jaffe

The Sidney Farber Cancer Institute, Boston, Massachusetts 02115

SOFT TISSUE SARCOMA

Soft tissue sarcomas consist of a heterogenous group of rare mesenchymal tumors. For these and other reasons they present major difficulties with respect to analysis of the natural history, response to treatment, and prognosis. Some of the factors responsible for these difficulties and for the complexities in constructing therapeutic trials are presented in Tables 1 and 2 and in more detail below.

As with other tumors, particularly those wherein progress in treatment is ongoing, histopathologic and other factors important to the selection of treatment and prognosis become increasingly evident. This requires subspecialty pathology analysis and, ideally, a sarcoma pathology repository committee to review slides within and between studies to assure comparability and proper interpretation of data.

The proliferative thrust of the tumor, as evaluated histologically and by volume doubling times, markedly influences the prognosis (Tables 3, 4, and 5) (24,16). Histopathologically, the tumors are divided into three grades on the basis of the number of mitotic figures per 10 high-powered fields. The

TABLE 1. Sarcomas—problems of data collection

1. Lumping of all soft tissue sarcomas
2. Heterogeneity within tumor specimen
3. No standard classification system
4. Failure to classify mitotic index
5. Different histologies at different sites
6. Rare tumors (1% of all cancer)

From Suit et al. ref. 24.

TABLE 2. Sarcoma—prognostic factors

1. Histologic grade
2. Doubling time
3. Tumor size
4. Local invasion, e.g., skin, bone, nodes
5. Histopathologic type

TABLE 3. Sarcoma—definition of histologic grade

Grade 1. One mitotic figure per 10 high-powered fields
Grade 2. One to five mitotic figures per 10 high-powered fields
Grade 3. Five mitotic figures per 10 high-powered fields

From Suit et al., ref. 24.

TABLE 4. Sarcoma—correlation of grade
and > 2-yr disease-free survival

Grade	N	% Disease free
1	23	86[a]
2	53	51
3	24	17[a]

From Suit et al., ref. 24.
[a] $p < 0.05$.

correlation of such grading systems with prognosis is evident in Table 4. Thus, a high percentage of patients with grade 1 tumors are disease free at 2 years. Grade 2 is intermediate, and less than 20% of patients with grade 3 soft tissue sarcoma are disease free at 2 years. This last group has a prognosis not unlike that of osteogenic sarcoma prior to adjuvant chemotherapy. It is emphasized that this grading system has been applied effectively to all forms of sarcoma. In terms of constructing adjuvant chemotherapy studies, such information is highly useful. Thus, patients with grade 3 primary disease have a high risk of having hematogenous microscopic disease and are prime candidates for adjuvant chemotherapy and/or immunotherapy studies. At the other extreme, patients with grade 1 disease have a relatively good prognosis, and it would be extremely difficult to construct an experimental design that would demonstrate quantitatively the benefit of adjuvant chemotherapy. The presence of "markers" of microscopic disease might, of course, change these interpretations. There is a good correlation between the histopathologic thrust as demonstrated in Table 3 and the actual doubling time of the tumor as presented in Table 5. This is not surprising, nor is it surprising that the doubling time correlates directly with the time to the development of recurrence or metastases (Table 5).

TABLE 5. Sarcoma—correlation of doubling time and
mean time to recurrence

Doubling time	N	Mean time
< 20 days	71	4.8 months
21–40 days	17	11.1 months
> 40 days	25	29.5 months

From Jaffe, ref. 12.

TABLE 6. Sarcoma—Joint Committee staging
system, proposal, 1976

T: $T_1 < 5$ cm; $T_2 > 5$ cm; T_3, invasion
N: N_0, no path. nodes; N_1, path. pos. nodes
M: M_0, no mets.; M_1, mets.
G: G_1, well diff.; G_2, mod. well diff.; G_3, poorly

Stage I, A: G_1, T_1, N_0, M_0
         B: G_1, T_2, N_0, M_0

Stage II, A: G_2, T_1, N_0, M_0
          B: G_2, T_2, N_0, M_0

Stage III, A: G_3, T_1, N_0, M_0
           B: G_3, T_2, N_0, M_0
           C: G_{1-3}, T_{1-2}, N_1

Stage IV, A: G_{1-3}, T_3, N_{0-1}, M_0
          B: G_{1-3}, T_{1-3}, N_{0-1}, M_1

G, grade; M, metastases; N, nodes; T, tumor.

The initial extent of the disease in terms of size of primary, nodal involvement, and presence of distal metastases along with the histopathologic grade has been incorporated into a proposed staging system (Table 6). Note that this staging system correlates with prognosis as evident in Fig. 1, and that, again, as in Tables 3 and 4, the histopathologic grading is a significant, if not the major, determinant of prognosis (1).

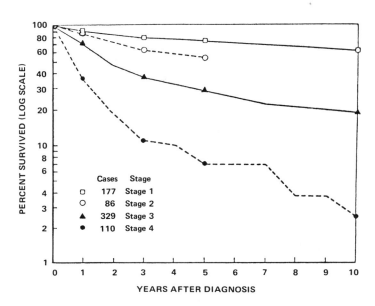

FIG. 1. Survival curves by stage for 702 cases with complete information for staging; 423 cases with and 279 cases without slide review (the curve for stage 2 was not plotted beyond 5 years since at that point the standard error was 5% or higher). (From ref. 1.) ☐, Stage I (177). ○, Stage II (86). ▲, Stage III (329). ●, Stage IV (110).

The above survival figures relate in the main to patients in whom the primary was controlled by surgery and/or radiotherapy and whose relapse was due to hematogenous metastasis.

Although available for certain pediatric soft tissue sarcomas, such as Ewing's and embryonal rhabdomyosarcoma, there was no effective chemotherapy for adults with soft tissue sarcoma prior to five years ago. Since then, dimethyl-imidazole-carboxamide (DIC) has been established to produce tumor regression in 10 to 15% of patients with metastatic soft tissue sarcomas (17). Doxorubicin hydrochloride (adriamycin®) is more effective, producing an objective response rate of approximately 30% (19). Doxorubicin hydrochloride plus DIC is approximately 40% (9,10). A number of combination studies have been employed using doxorubicin hydrochloride and DIC with the addition of vincristine, cyclophosphamide, and in some instances, actinomycin D (Table 7) (2). In a large study in the Southwest Oncology Group, Gottlieb has demonstrated an overall objective response rate of close to 50%, with complete tumor regression occurring in approximately 10% of patients (8). Although the median duration of partial responses has been in the range of 6 months, complete remissions are durable and over 70% of patients who enter complete remission remain so at 30 months (8). This experience further attests to the importance of complete remission in affecting prognosis, and considering the proliferative thrust of this disease it is reasonable to hope that some patients entering complete remission have, in fact, been cured. Accordingly, current protocols and treatment plans often involve multidisciplinary approaches designed to eradicate all clinically evident disease (that is, produce complete remission).

It is of interest (Table 7) that the response rate for this heterogeneous

TABLE 7. Sarcoma studies—doxorubicin hydrochloride alone and in combination[a]

	Evaluable	Complete response	Partial response	Percent response
Angiosarcoma	35	3	17	57
Chondrosarcoma	29	1	4	17
Ewing's sarcoma	15	2	2	27
Fibrosarcoma	90	9	37	51
Leiomyosarcoma	147	14	60	50
Liposarcoma	71	7	28	49
Mesothelioma	36	3	9	33
Neurofibrosarcoma	50	7	15	44
Osteogenic sarcoma	87	5	23	32
Rhabdomyosarcoma	69	13	25	55
Synovial cell sarcoma	25	4	10	56
Undifferentiated sarcoma	76	9	27	47
Total	730	77	257	46
Complete response rate = 11%				

[a] Doxorubicin hydrochloride, DIC, vincristine, cyclophosphamide. From Gottlieb et al., ref. 8.

group of mesenchymal tumors is generally comparable across the given categories. The significantly lower response rate in adults with chondrosarcoma is perhaps related to the fact that such lesions are indolent, well-differentiated, have few mitoses, and might, therefore, be less susceptible to chemotherapy. Also, the comparability of the response rate for a given treatment among the different subcategories would suggest that patients with metastatic soft tissue sarcoma may be pooled in clinical trial analyses.

As in osteogenic sarcoma, the above observations have led to the use of adjuvant chemotherapy programs following control of the primary in patients with high risk of having microscopic hematogenous metastasis (grade 3 disease). Such studies present problems in experimental design for the reasons indicated above. If one may extrapolate from breast cancer, osteogenic sarcoma, Wilm's tumor, etc., it seems probable that combination chemotherapy involving doxorubicin hydrochloride is sufficiently effective in overt metastatic soft tissue sarcoma to be capable of effecting microscopic disease in a significant proportion of patients. Such studies are ongoing (3) and deserve major priority.

OSTEOGENIC SARCOMA

Osteogenic sarcoma occurs during the growth spurt, usually in the extremities, and most commonly in the distal femur. In such circumstances, the primary can generally be controlled by amputation. In spite of this, 80 to 90% of patients developed overt pulmonary metastases and died within 12 to 18 months. In those patients with proximal extremity or axial skeletal lesions, the primary cannot be controlled and curative treatment cannot be delivered. In osteogenic sarcoma secondary to Paget's disease, the primary site is usually in the axial skeleton.

Prognostic variables include the following:

1. *Histopathology*. In classic osteogenic sarcoma, there is involvement of the medullary cavity with extension to the subperiosteum, elevation of the periosteum, and, frequently, invasion of surrounding soft tissue. Such patients almost always have grade 3 disease, in terms of numbers of mitoses per high powered field (Table 3), and have a prognosis as indicated above. Less than 10% of patients have parosteal sarcoma. These lesions generally have fewer mitotic figures and a substantially better prognosis. Thus, in such patients, 50 to 90% will be cured by control of the primary (6). There is frequently evidence of cartilaginous differentiation. In general, the prognosis is determined by the most adverse histopathologic features. Pure chondrosarcomas in adults tend to be more differentiated and have a more favorable prognosis (6). In pediatric patients, they are rare, less differentiated, and have a prognosis approximating that of classic osteogenic sarcoma.

Major emphasis on therapeutic trials in this disease has resulted in an increasing focus on the prognostic implications of the histopathology. As with soft tissue sarcoma, there is a major need for more precise classification, development of subspecialty expertise, and development of an osteogenic sarcoma pathology repository committee to implement the aforementioned and serve as a reviewing body for evaluating prognostic factors and the impact of various forms of therapy.

2. *Size of primary*. The size of the primary and the degree of invasion of the medullary cavity have, in some studies, been negatively correlated with prognosis.

3. *Location of primary*. Primaries located in the proximal extremities or axial skeleton where local control cannot be achieved are associated with a grave prognosis. Otherwise, there is no clear evidence that a primary site on the extremity influences prognosis.

4. *Age of patient*. This does not influence prognosis except insofar as age is correlated with known etiologic factors, such as Paget's disease and X-ray exposure.

In adjuvant chemotherapy studies of osteogenic sarcoma, historical controls have been employed. This is because of (a) the rarity of osteogenic sarcoma, (b) an objective and quantifiable parameter of response (development of pulmonary metastases), (c) the grave prognosis in the absence of adjuvant chemotherapy, and (d) evidence that the prognosis has not changed over the years. This last point is a central issue in the evaluation of adjuvant treatment.

In an earlier study at the Farber Institute, it was demonstrated that the survival curves for patients with osteogenic sarcoma in whom the primary could be controlled had not changed during various time periods in the 20 years preceding the initiation of adjuvant studies (1972) (Fig. 2) (3). It has been reported in very recent years that, at least in one large clinic, the 2-year survival rate in the absence of adjuvant chemotherapy is as high as 40%. Among possible explanations for this is the more routine use of lung tomograms in patients in the initial evaluation. The elimination of such patients could most certainly favorably affect the prognosis in the remaining. However, at the Farber Center an analysis of the prognosis of patients with osteogenic sarcoma in temporal increments between 1965 and 1972 indicates no change in prognosis (Fig. 3). During the past 8 years there were only two of 50 patients who presented with positive tomograms but negative chest films. Other large institutions are currently examining their experience relative to this point.

As is generally the case, the chemotherapy of osteogenic sarcoma was developed and initially evaluated in patients with overt metastatic disease (Table 8). Prior to 1970, chemotherapy was ineffectual aside from isolated reports that certain alkylating agents, such as mitomycin C, had limited activity. Recently, more intensive treatment with the alkylating agent cyclophosphamide has established the fact that certain alkylating agents under proper circumstances have limited activity.

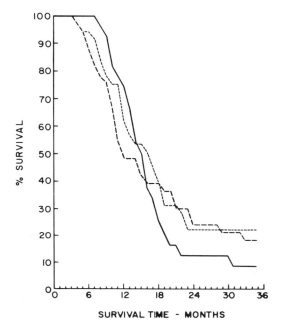

FIG. 2. Survival curves of the historical group in whom diagnosis of osteogenic sarcoma was made over three successive periods. — —, ≤ 1959 (33); - - -, 1960–1964 (28); ———, 1965–1972 (37).

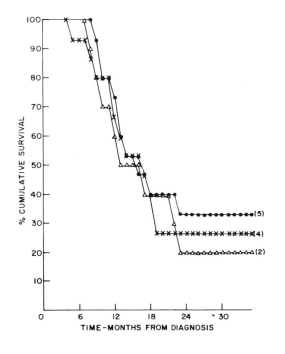

FIG. 3. Osteogenic sarcomas—historic controls. Year of diagnosis: ●—●, 1963–1965 (15); x—x, 1966–1968 (15); 1968–1971 (10).

TABLE 8.

Agent(s)	Objective response[a] (%)
Alkylating agents	20
Doxorubicin hydrochloride	35
MTX-CF q 3 weeks	35
MTX-CF q 1 week	80

[a] > 50% decrease in product of 2 diameters.

In the early 1970s, it was demonstrated that doxorubicin hydrochloride and high dose methotrexate with citrovorum factor rescue (MTX-CF) given every 3 weeks, produced tumor regression in 30 to 40% of patients (Table 8) (5,12). These regressions were usually partial, though occasionally a durable complete remission occurred. The MTX-CF program is complex and has the potential for producing serious and fatal toxicity. However, with proper pharmacologic and toxicologic monitoring, it has been possible to deliver this program safely, effectively, and, in the main, without myelosuppression (20). This last fact has made it possible to deliver MTX-CF at a threefold increase in dose rate, that is weekly, as compared to triweekly. This has resulted in a substantial increase in the objective response rate with approximately half of the patients achieving complete response (Table 8) (14).

The recognition that effective treatment existed for overt metastatic disease led to the use of the above and additional agents immediately following control of the primary in an effort to eradicate micrometastatic disease and to thus increase the cure rate. The first study at the Farber Institute involved MTX-CF every 3 weeks. There were 12 such patients, seven of whom continue free of disease with a minimum follow-up time of 24 months (Table 8) (13). Because adriamycin was effective in overt metastatic disease and also in micrometastatic disease (4) and because MTX-CF was nonmyelosuppressive, doxorubicin hydrochloride was added to the MTX-CF with minimum compromise in the dose rate of each program. Subadditive host toxicity has been the basis for a number of successful combination chemotherapy regimens in man (7). In this program by life table plot, the plateau is currently at 60% (Fig. 4). However, the follow-up is insufficiently long.

The difference between these curves and our historical controls is highly significant. There are four major questions: (a) Are historical controls valid? (See above.) (b) Does the histopathology in these cases match that of the historical controls? (c) Does this group match the historical control group for other variables such as age, sex, size, and site of primary? The answer is that it does, very precisely. (d) Are micrometastases suppressed or eradicated?

There are a number of studies that relate to the above and particularly to the crucial last question. These are summarized in Table 9. The cumulative number of patients in these studies is large. The proportion of patients by life

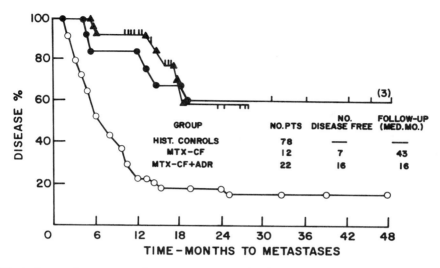

FIG. 4. Osteogenic sarcoma—adjuvant chemotherapy. ○—○, Historical controls; ●—●, MTX-CF; ▲—▲, MTX = CF + ADR.

table plot alive and free of disease at 18 months in all of these studies is in the range of 60%. Importantly, relapse after 18 months, with follow-up at a maximum of 5 years, is rare. This would suggest that those patients who make 18 months free of relapse have, in the main, been definitively treated.

The development of effective systemic treatment has allowed for a re-examination and revision of treatment of the primary. Thus, in several centers, the initial treatment for a patient with osteogenic sarcoma involves in-

TABLE 9. Osteogenic sarcoma—summary of adjuvant studies

Institute (ref. no.)	Study	No. pts. entered	Disease free at 18 mo.[a] (%)	Relapse after 18 mo.	Maximum followup (yrs)
Farber	MTX — CF	12	58	0	5
	MTX — CF + Adr	22	60	0	2
Anderson	CONPADRI — I	43	55	1	6
	CONPADRI — II	58	65	4	3¼
CALGB	Adr	45	65	1	4
St. Judes	MTX — CF + Adr + CPA	24	55	1	4
MSKI	MTX — CF + Adr + CPA	60	63[b]	6	3
Stanford	MTX — CF Adr + CPA	31	34	4	3

[a] From life table plot.
[b] Not extrapolated by life table plot.
These data were updated as of Oct. 15, 1976 (refs. 4, 19–27). Adr, doxorubicin hydrochloride; CALGB, Cancer and Leukemia Group B; CPA, cyclophosphamide; MSKI, Memorial-Sloan Kettering Institute.

tensive chemotherapy, sometimes with radiotherapy, in an effort to maximally reduce the primary. This is followed by a subamputative limb preservation surgical procedure and then adjuvant chemotherapy. Such studies have been successful in the short run, that is, limbs, in fact, have been preserved. Further follow-up will be necessary to determine the magnitude of complications and functional problems (11,22).

At the other end is the patient with overt metastatic osteogenic sarcoma who either presents as such or relapses after adjuvant chemotherapy. In the past, selected patients with late relapse and with one or only a few pulmonary lesions have had durable disease-free states following multiple pulmonary resections (18). More recently, because of the development of effective systemic chemotherapy, a multidisciplinary approach to such patients, designed to produce no clinically evident disease, followed by chemotherapy, to eradicate micrometastases, has been undertaken. In 21 such patients so treated at the Farber Institute, complete remission was achieved in 15, and has been durable in 11, with a maximum follow-up of 28 months (15).

ACKNOWLEDGMENT

These studies were supported in part by research grant 5P30 CA06516–13 from the National Cancer Institute.

REFERENCES

1. American Joint Committee for Cancer Staging, 1976.
2. Blum, R. (1975): An overview of studies with adriamycin. *Cancer Chemother. Rep.,* 6:247.
3. Blum, R. (1974): *Personal communication.*
4. Cortes, E., Holland, J., Wang, J., and Glidewell, O. (1974): Adriamycin and amputation in primary osteogenic sarcoma. *Proc. AACR/ASCO,* (Abstr. 745.), 15:170.
5. Cortes, E., Holland, J., Wang, J., and Sinks, L. (1972): Doxorubicin in disseminated osteosarcoma. *JAMA,* 221:1132.
6. Dahlin, D. C. (1967): *Bone Tumors: General Aspects and Data on 3,987 Cases,* 2nd ed. Charles C Thomas, Springfield, Ill.
7. Frei, E., III (1972): Combination cancer therapy: Presidential address. *Cancer Res.,* 32:2593.
8. Gottlieb, J. A., Baker, L. H., O'Bryan, R. M., Sinkovics, J. F., Hoogstraten, B., Quagliana, J. M., Rivkin, S. E., Bodey, Sr., G. P., Rodriguez, V. T., Blumenschein, G. R., Saiki, J. H., Coltman, Jr., C., Burgess, M. A., Sullivan, P., Thigpen, T., Bottomley, R., Balcerzak, S., Moon, T. E. (1975): Adriamycin used alone and in combination for soft tissue and bony sarcomas. *Cancer Chemother. Rep.,* 6:271.
9. Gottlieb, J. A., Baker, L. H., Quagliana, J. M., Luce, J. K., Whitecar, J. P., Jr., Sinkovics, J. G., Rivkin, S. E., Brownlee, R., Frei, E. III (1972): Chemotherapy of sarcomas with a combination of adriamycin and DIC. *Cancer,* 30:1632.
10. Griswald, D. P., Laster, Jr., W. R., Schabel, Jr., F. M. (1973): Therapeutic potentiation of adriamycin with DIC in B16 melanoma, C3H breast, Lewis lung, and leukemia L1210. *Proc. Am. Assoc. Cancer Research,* 14:15.
11. Jaffe, N. (1975): The potential for an improved prognosis with chemotherapy in osteogenic sarcoma. *Clin. Orthop.,* 113:111.
12. Jaffe, N. (1974): Progress report on high-dose methotrexate (NSC-740) with

citrovorum rescue in the treatment of metastatic bone tumors. *Cancer Chemother. Rep., 58*:275.

13. Jaffe, N., Farber, S., Traggis, D., Geiser, C., Kim, B., Lakshmi, D., Frauenberger, G., Djerassi, I., Cassady, J. R. (1973): Favorable response of osteogenic sarcoma to high-dose methotrexate with citrovorum rescue and radiation therapy. *Cancer, 31*:1367.

14. Jaffe, N., Frei, E. III, Traggis, D., and Watts, H. (1977): Weekly high-dose methotrexate-citrovorum factor in osteogenic sarcoma. *Cancer, 39*:45.

15. Jaffe, N., Traggis, D., Cassady, J. R., Filler, R. M., Watts, H., and Frei, E. III (1976): Multidisciplinary treatment for macrometastatic ostogenic sarcoma. *Br. Med. J., 2*:1039.

16. Joseph, W. (1974): Criteria for resection of sarcoma metastatic to the lung. *Cancer Chemother. Rep., 58*:285.

17. Luce, J., Thurman, N. G., Issacs, B. L., and Talley, R. W. (1970): Clinical trials with DIC. *Cancer Chemother. Rep., 54*:119.

18. Martini, N., Huvos, A., Mike, V., Marcove, R., and Beattie, E., Jr. (1971): Multiple pulmonary resections in the treatment of osteogenic sarcoma. *Ann. Thorac. Surg., 12*:271.

19. O'Bryan, R. M., Luce, J. K., Talley, R. W., Gottlieb, J. A., Baker, L. H., and Bonadonna, G. (1973): Phase II evaluation of adriamycin in human neoplasia. *Cancer, 32*:1.

20. Pitman, S., Parker, L., Tattersall, M., Jaffe, N., and Frei, E., III (1975): Clinical trial of high-dose methotrexate (NSC-740) with citrovorum factor (NSC-3590)—Toxicologic and therapeutic observations. *Cancer Chemother. Rep., 6*:43.

21. Pratt, C., Hustu, H., and Shanks, E. (1974): Cyclic multiple drug adjuvant chemotherapy for osteosarcoma. *Proc. AACR/ASCO.* (Abstr. 76), 15:9.

22. Rosen, G., Murphy, M., Huvos, A., Gutierrez, M., and Marcove, R. (1976): Chemotherapy, *en bloc* resection and prosthetic bone replacement in the treatment of osteogenic sarcoma. *Cancer, 37*:1.

23. Rosen, G., Suwansirikul, S., Kwon, C., Tan, C., Wu, S., Beattie, E., Jr., and Murphy, M. (1974): High-dose methotrexate with citrovorum factor rescue and adriamycin in childhood osteogenic sarcoma. *Cancer, 33*:1151.

24. Suit, H., Russell, W., and Martin, R. (1975): Sarcoma of soft tissue: Clinical and histopathological parameters and response to treatment. *Cancer, 35*:1478.

25. Sutow, W., Sullivan, M., Fernbach, D., Cangir, A., and George, S. (1975): Adjuvant chemotherapy in primary treatment of osteogenic sarcoma. *Cancer, 36*:1598.

26. Sutow, W., Sullivan, M., Fernbach, D., Cangir, A., and George, S. L. (1975): Adjuvant chemotherapy in primary treatment of osteogenic sarcoma—A Southwest Oncology Group Study. *Cancer, 36*:1598.

27. Wilbur, J., Etcubanas, E., Long, T., Glatstein, E., and Leavitt, T. (1974): Drug therapy and irradiation in primary and metastatic osteogenic sarcoma. *Proc. AACR/ASCO,* 15:188 (Abstr.).

Immunotherapy of Cancer: Present Status of Trials in Man, edited by W. D. Terry and D. Windhorst. Raven Press, New York © 1978.

Osteogenic Sarcoma Experience at the Mayo Clinic, 1963–1974

*W. F. Taylor, **J. C. Ivins, †D. C. Dahlin, and **D. J. Pritchard

*Departments of *Medical Research Statistics, **Orthopedic Oncology, †Surgical Pathology, Mayo Clinic, Rochester, Minnesota 55901*

In recent years at the Mayo Clinic considerable attention has been given to planning clinical trials for evaluating treatment of osteogenic sarcoma (OGS). The need for control patients, treated only by surgery, was challenged because of a general belief that the survival of such patients was very poor and had not changed for many years. Widely acknowledged data of Marcove et al. (1) were thought to be decisive, and the length of disease-free intervals among Mayo Clinic patients was believed to be adequately described by the Marcove experience. In spite of this belief the authors felt it would be sensible to confirm with Mayo Clinic data this presumed stability of OGS survival. In 1975 a pilot survey of previous Mayo Clinic OGS cases was done. Both total and metastasis-free survival were measured and related to a few easily determined variables. Suitable records on 133 patients treated from 1963 to 1971 were studied with results as follows—survival free from metastasis (as well as total survival) was longer (a) for females than for males, (b) for lower grades of cell differentiation than for higher grades, (c) for nonosteoblastic OGS than for osteoblastic OGS, (d) for distal primary sites than for proximal sites, and (e) for patients treated recently (1969–1971) than for those treated earlier (1963–1965). No strong differences in survival by age were found.

The indications that recent treatment was better than earlier treatment was particularly intriguing because if a strong improvement in disease-free intervals has occurred over recent years then the practice of using old historical controls for new research is of questionable value. Concurrent, randomly assigned, untreated controls would have to be considered as a part of experimental designs.

Recently, a new, more thorough investigation of all OGS seen at the Mayo Clinic from 1963 to mid-1974 was done. The results, in essence, confirmed the pilot study findings that OGS does indeed show significant improvement in the metastasis-free interval and total survival time since 1963.

METHODS

Studied first were *all* patients with a diagnosis of OGS confirmed histologically by the Mayo pathologist David Dahlin. Both the diagnostic index of the Mayo Clinic record system and Dahlin's exceptionally complete personal files were searched. Since all OGS patients were included, no selection bias existed on the part of the investigators.

For clarity and appropriateness, patients to be studied intensively were limited to those with classic primary OGS who received their first definitive treatment at the Mayo Clinic. In such selection, bias can enter. In order to avoid this, exclusions were made with strict adherence to definitions and in ignorance of outcome.

The definition of classic primary OGS used here implies that osteoid must be produced by malignant cells (2). Some tumors showed marked chondroid or fibromatoid differentiation away from the zones of such osteoid production. Two pathologists knowledgeable in osseous disease, but not at the Mayo Clinic, assessed the microscopic pathology of these study cases. These authorities disagreed with the diagnosis of osteosarcoma in only one case that came from the earliest year of the study; in this one instance, they judged the lesion to be chondrosarcoma rather than chondroblastic osteosarcoma.

For analyzing time to metastasis and time to death, the start of follow-up was dated from the start of first definitive treatment. Usually this was the date of definitive surgery. When preparatory therapy (radiation) to the primary site was part of definitive treatment prior to surgery, the date of start of preparatory therapy was used.

Variables were chosen for study on the basis of experience and because they seemed to show trends over time that might explain trends in survival. A search for "important" variables was made by a discriminatory analysis procedure aimed at distinguishing between patients who were and those who were not metastasis free at 1 year. Variables most highly correlated with metastasis were time, age, and sex, and they are presented separately (Fig. 7).

Median metastasis-free time was chosen as a convenient summary of the first 2 years of survival experience. This enables one to examine complex survival data in a condensed form using only one number. This median time was an estimate based on the assumption that, for the first 2 years, survival was exponentially distributed. The median time Y is given as $Y = \dfrac{t_2}{d_2} \times \ln 2$, where t_2 is the number of person-years lived metastasis free during the first 2 years after treatment, d_2 is the number of cases in which metastasis developed during that period, and $\ln 2 = 0.69315$. This approach is used in Fig. 7.

Sixty-six percent of the study patients received no therapy other than surgery to the primary site. Treatments used in addition to this surgery on the remaining 34% of patients were studied, and their effects evaluated. This evaluation varied from being very good indeed (there was a randomized clinical trial in 1969–1972) to being an unsatisfactory comparison of undoubtedly differing subgroups of patients treated for reasons not apparent in the records.

A particular interest was expressed in possible deleterious effects of using a tourniquet in connection with amputation. This subject was studied separately, particularly in view of a strong decrease in the frequency of tourniquet use in recent years.

RESULTS

Table 1 provides an accounting of the total OGS patient population seen at the Mayo Clinic in 1963–1974, showing reasons for excluding some from this study. Thirty percent had a primary site other than the long bones of the extremities, 15% had tumor types that were not considered classic OGS, 29% did not receive their first definitive treatment at the Mayo Clinic, 17% had already had metastasis when first seen at the Mayo Clinic, and 38% were older than the arbitrary limit of 20 years chosen in this report to agree with the age limits used in the Marcove and associates' study (1).

Table 2 describes the patients included and presents trends with time. These time trends were examined closely in a search of reasons for improvement in OGS survival over time. Some possible reasons appeared. During

TABLE 1. OGS cases excluded from study with reasons for exclusion: Mayo Clinic, January, 1963—June, 1974, total of 363 cases

	Number excluded		Percent of total (363)
Cases excluded from study[a]	214		59
Reasons for exclusion			
Primary site other than bones of extremities	109		30
Head and neck		21	6
Shoulder girdle (scapula and clavicle)		7	2
Spine (including sacrum)		9	2
Pelvic girdle (ileum, ischium, pubis)		33	9
Soft tissue		36	10
Ribs or sternum		2	0.6
Unknown site (pulmonary metastasis, primary site unknown)		1	0.3
Tumor type not classic OGS	55		15
Parosteal		10	3
Periosteal		9	2
Radiation-induced		16	4
OGS arising in Paget's disease		13	4
Type unknown		7	2
First definitive treatment not at Mayo Clinic (Treated elsewhere; palliative only or no treatment at Mayo Clinic)	107		29
OGS already metastasized	63		17
Age greater than 20 years	139		38

[a] Some cases had more than one reason for exclusion. There were 214 patients excluded for 473 reasons.

TABLE 2. *Osteogenic sarcoma cases included in study of extremities only by characteristics of cases and by calendar period: ages restricted to 20 and under*

Characteristics of patients included	Total	Calendar period			
		1963–1965	1966–1968	1969–1971	1972–mid 1974
Total cases recorded	363	73	90	100	100
Cases excluded (including sites on trunk)	214	44	54	57	59
Cases included	149	29	36	43	41
% Included	41	40	40	43	41
Age of patients					
Under 15	80	18	22	19	21
15–20	69	11	14	24	20
% Under 15 (of those included)	54	62	61	44	51
Sex					
Male	83	14	19	25	25
Female	66	15	17	18	16
% Male (of those included)	56	48	53	58	61
Primary site					
Distal to knee or elbow	42	3	12	13	14
Knee to upper femur / Elbow to upper humerus	77	18	17	21	21
Upper femur / Upper humerus	30	8	7	9	6
% Proximal to knee or elbow	72	90	67	70	66
% Upper femur or upper humerus	20	28	19	21	15
Histology					
Osteoblastic	94	22	27	20	25
Chondroblastic	16	4	2	6	4
Fibroblastic	23	3	5	5	10
Unspecified	16	0	2	12	2
% Osteoblastic (of those included)	63	76	75	47	61
Grade					
I, II	3	0	2	0	1
III	50	12	8	17	13
IV	95	17	26	25	27
Unknown	1	0	0	1	0
% Grade 4 (of those known)	64	59	72	60	66
Tumor size					
< 10 cm	64	15	14	14	21
≥ 10 cm	71	14	21	18	18
Unknown	14	0	1	11[a]	2
% ≥ 10 cm (of those known)	53	48	60	56	46
Treatment in addition to surgery					
A. None	98	20	32	17	29
B. Radiation to primary only	10	0	0	6	4
C. Radiation to lungs (prophylactically)	6	0	0	2	4
D. Chemotherapy	15	9	4	0	2
E. Both C and D	20	0	0	18	2
% Treated at least once (of those included)	34	31	11	60	29
Use of tourniquet					
Suitable sites (distal to upper femur or to upper humerus)	119	21	29	34	35
Tourniquet used	74	20	25	22	7
% Tourniquet (of those suitable)	62	95	86	65	20

[a] Use of radiotherapy sometimes prevented reliable measurement of tumor size.

1963–1968 there were slight excesses of high-risk patients compared with 1969–1974; there were relatively more early patients under the age of 15, more with proximal sites of primary tumors, and more with grade IV osteoblastic cell types. On the other hand, there were more males (high risk) in the later years. As a check on selectivity bias, the proportion of patients included from the early years to the later years was found to be always around 40%, indicating no gross trend in selection of patients for this study. There was a big increase in patients receiving treatment other than surgery in 1969–1971. This was due almost entirely to a clinical trial that was carried out during this time and into 1972. Some patients received surgical treatment only, and a roughly equal number received prophylactic radiotherapy to the lungs plus some chemotherapy. Finally, a striking difference is observed (at the bottom of Table 2) in the use of the tourniquet in conjunction with amputation. This change went from a 95% use of tourniquet in the early years to only 20% use in the later years.

Having noted the trends in the nature of the patients, we directed our analytic efforts toward studying changes in survival with time in such a way as to place the patient changes in proper prospective and to see if any unexplained changes still remained.

Figure 1 shows crude survival curves by time. A steady progression toward improved survival occurred from 1963–1965 to 1972–1974.

From the preliminary studies there seemed to be an effect of histology and grade of the tumor (Fig. 2). The worst combination—osteoblastic grade IV tumors—was examined separately from all the others. There was a strong improvement in survival of osteoblastic grade IV patients from the first half of the time period to the second. Similarly, there was an improvement in all

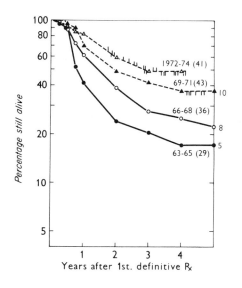

FIGS. 1–6, 8–11. Actuarial estimates of percentage still alive (or still free from metastasis) during first 5 years after first definitive treatment for OGS. The vertical marks along the curves indicate the time at which a patient was last known still alive. Patient was "withdrawn" at that time from the survival analysis. Numbers along right margin indicate numbers of patients withdrawn after 5 years. There were no deaths or metastasis observed after 5 years (time was too short). Total sample sizes are shown in parentheses. FIG. 1. Survival by calendar time in 3-year intervals (the latest, 1972–1974, was only 2½ years).

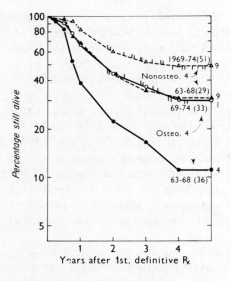

FIG. 2. Survival by histology and grade, by time Patients were classified histologically as having osteoblastic OGS, Broders' grade IV, or not. Other classes were chondroblastic OGS, fibroblastic OGS, and unspecified OGS.

other patients in the same time period. Restricting the study to the highest risk patients (Fig. 3), namely osteoblastic grade IV, examination was made of sex differences. It was found that females consistently did better than males and that for both sexes there was an improvement over time. Figures 4, 5, and 6 illustrate the same sorts of findings with respect to the metastasis-free interval as were found with survival. Here things are not quite as clear-cut; in particular, the metastasis-free interval for 1972–1974 is somewhat shorter after 1 year than for 1969–1971. The two more recent periods combined,

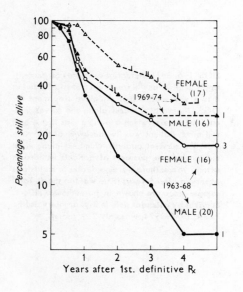

FIG. 3. Survival by calendar time and sex, restricted to the high-risk histologic class—osteoblastic OGS grade IV.

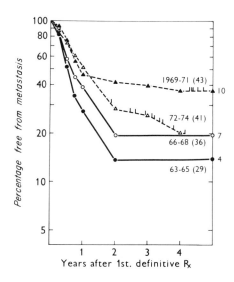

FIGS. 4–6. Analogous to Figs. 1–3. Here metastasis, not death, is the end point. FIG. 4. Metastasis-free survival by calendar time. Attention is drawn to the curve for 1972–1974. This is closely similar to that for 1969–1971 for the first year. The subsequent drop in the 1972–1974 curve seems inconsistent with findings in Fig. 1 for survival. See also Fig. 11, which presents total data for eligible patients.

however, show significantly better metastasis-free intervals than does 1963–1968. Once again (Fig. 5), the high-risk (osteoblastic grade IV) patients did considerably better in later years than in the early years of this period and, similarly, the remaining patients showed an improvement from the first half to the second half of the time period studied. Also, among the highest risk patients (Fig. 6), females did better than males and there was an improving trend for both sexes during the time period.

Figure 7 presents, in summary form, the effects of three variables—calendar time, age, and sex—in terms of the median metastasis-free time. (See the

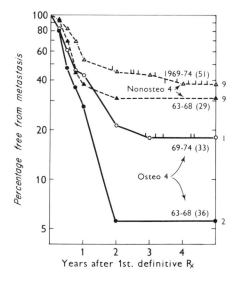

FIG. 5. Metastasis-free survival by calendar time, histology, and grade. See Fig. 2.

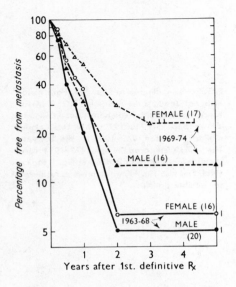

FIG. 6. Metastasis-free survival by calendar time and sex; restricted to osteoblastic grade 4 patients only. See Fig. 3.

methods section for further definition.) The difference between the early years, 1963–1968, and the later ones, 1969–1974, is obvious and is statistically significant at $p < 0.01$. There are apparently strong effects of age and sex that are not statistically significant but that could be considered borderline ($p \sim 0.08$).

Naturally there is a concern about changes in treatment that have occurred over the span of years from 1963 to 1974. Table 2 shows the occurrence of these treatments and the changes in their use over time. There are two gen-

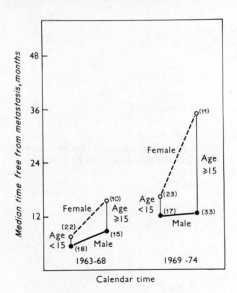

FIG. 7. Median time to metastasis by age, sex, and calendar time. Each point typifies the first 2 years of a survival curve (metastasis free). See methods section for details.

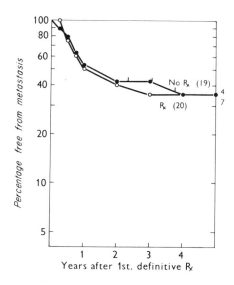

FIG. 8. Metastasis-free survival among patients in a controlled clinical trial of radiotherapy (with chemotherapy) used prophylactically as an adjunct to surgery, 1969–1972. Patients randomly assigned to treatment are compared with untreated patients.

eral classes of treatment. One occurred in uncontrolled trials in which the treatment was assigned for no generally known reason. It was a question of "clinical judgment." The second was the deliberately controlled trial done in the period 1969–1972 in which patients were assigned randomly to receive either no postsurgical treatment or postsurgical prophylactic radiation to the lungs plus actinomycin D. Figure 8 shows some results for the controlled trials. There was no difference in the time to metastasis between the two treatment groups, a result that has been reported elsewhere (3,4). By contrast, Fig. 9 shows some striking findings in uncontrolled trials in which

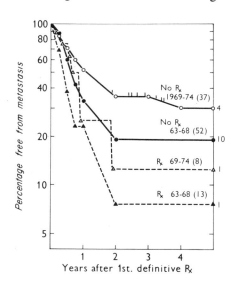

FIG. 9. Metastasis-free survival, by calendar time, among patients receiving or not receiving additional therapy in connection with surgery. Uncontrolled trials: radiotherapy and chemotherapy used at discretion of physician.

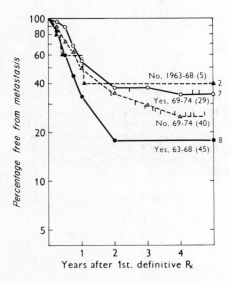

FIG. 10. Metastasis-free survival, by calendar time, among patients whose OGS surgery was done with or without use of a tourniquet. Note trend toward abandoning tourniquets in recent years. Only surgery for primary OGS distal to upper femur or upper humerus was considered.

treated and untreated patients are compared both for the first half and the second half of the time period under study. In both cases, those patients without postsurgical treatment apparently did somewhat better than those with postsurgical treatment. This result is attributed not to ill effects of treatment but to subtle selection processes by the physician who selected patients for treatment on the basis of the characteristics of the patient and the disease—characteristics that, incidentally, were not detectable by a study of the histories. Treated and untreated patients looked very similar when their characteristics were examined with respect to sex, age, grade, site, etc. This example is included here as an illustration of the problems that arise in uncontrolled trials when patient selection is based on unknown or even unknowable factors.

Attention is directed to the effect of the use of the tourniquet in conjunction with amputation. Data were available on patients throughout the time period of the study, some with and some without the use of the tourniquet in their surgical treatment (Fig. 10). There was some indication of improved duration of metastasis-free intervals, but the only finding that might be called statistically significant was that the patients treated with a tourniquet in 1969–1974 did significantly better than those treated with a tourniquet in 1963–1968. Otherwise tourniquet use seems of little effect. (Only patients with primary sites distal to the upper femur or distal to the upper humerus were included here.)

DISCUSSION

That there has been improvement in the survival and the metastasis-free interval of OGS patients at the Mayo Clinic since 1963 seems indisputable.

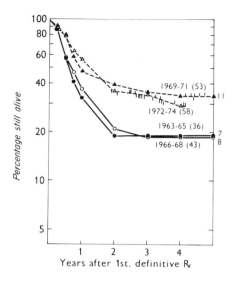

FIG. 11. Metastasis-free survival, by calendar time, for all 191 patients eligible for this study including 25 over age 20, five with primary sites surgically accessible but not in extremities (head and neck excluded throughout), and 12 with both the above characteristics.

The reasons for this improvement remain unclear, although conjectures can be made. One of these is based on the fact that since about 1968 improved radiographic techniques have permitted earlier detection of metastases. Thus some of the recent patients with metastasis would have been rejected from this study whereas before 1968 they would have been included. This could have created an artificial lengthening of recent survival and metastasis-free intervals that might explain the findings of the study. There have been few metastases detected by the new tomography, however, and any bias is considered to be negligible.

OGS is a rare disease, and every eligible case is needed for analysis. In this study 42 cases were eligible in all respects except age and primary site. They were excluded in order to be compatible with the Marcove study. Twenty-five of these were over age 20, five had surgically accessible sites other than the extremities (and other than head or neck), and 12 had both these characteristics. When these 42 cases are included, a total of 191 cases are available. These have been analyzed extensively, but only the metastasis-free intervals are presented here in Fig. 11. The sharp contrast between early and late cases is accentuated in this figure. Similar findings occurred when total survival was considered.

REFERENCES

1. Marcove, R. C., Miké, V., Hajek. J. V., Levin, A. G., and Hutter, R. V. P.(1970): Osteogenic sarcoma under the age of twenty-one: A review of one hundred and forty-five operative cases. *J. Bone Joint Surg.* [*Am.*], 52:411–423.
2. Dahlin, D. C., and Coventry, M. B. (1967): Osteogenic sarcoma: A study of six hundred cases. *J. Bone Joint Surg.* [*Am.*], 49:101–110.
3. Rab, G. T., Ivins, J. C., Childs, D. S., Jr., Cupps, R. E., and Pritchard, D. J. (1976):

Elective whole lung irradiation in the treatment of osteogenic sarcoma. *Cancer,* 38:939–942.
4. Ivins, J. C., and Pritchard, D. J. (1976): Management of osteogenic sarcoma at the Mayo Clinic. *Recent Results Cancer Res.,* 54:221–230.

Question and Answer Session

Dr. LoBuglio: Are there any questions regarding techniques, or design, or analysis of the study?

Dr. Rosenberg: Is there, in fact, an improvement with more recent time that is statistically significant and not explainable on the basis of any non-therapeutic criterion, such as sex, age, or whatever?

Dr. Taylor: Survival can be modified by several factors including treatment after metastasis. But, if you compare the two recent time intervals with the earlier two intervals, there is a statistically significant improvement.

Dr. Rosenberg: Would you comment on the duration of disease-free interval?

Dr. Taylor: Disease-free interval was significantly longer in the period 1969 to 1971.

Dr. Rosenberg: But is there a difference between the results during the period 1972 to 1974 and any of the other groups?

Dr. Taylor: No. That's why I say that this is not a consistent change with time in terms of disease-free interval.

Dr. Frei: One of the things that is evident in Fig. 4 is that in the earlier years you do not see metastases after two years, whereas later you tend to see attrition after that. Is that real?

Dr. Taylor: I don't know. The sample size is pretty small. There are seven people left metastasis-free at five years in one group and four in the other group.

Dr. LoBuglio: Let's just be sure we put the sample size in perspective. The sample size is certainly equivalent to most of the clinical trials at this time.

Dr. Rosenberg: I think it is important to emphasize that when we look at the data we need to look at time free from metastases and not survival, because survival may have changed dramatically due to other measures, such as chemotherapy, laminar-flow rooms, and other supportive care for children.

Dr. Taylor: I have tried to look at this and do not believe that this is the explanation.

Dr. LoBuglio: The question is: Can a lot of this, in terms of the survival data, be due to good chemotherapy prolonging survival after metastases? That certainly has to be looked at to evaluate the survival data.

Dr. Taylor: In response to a suggestion from Dr. Gehan, I looked at survival from metastasis to death, and this has improved strikingly over this same time interval. The latest survival after metastasis is really quite good and significantly better than the earlier survival.

Dr. LoBuglio: Is that true in the 1969 to 1971 time interval, also?

Dr. Taylor: No, only the 1972 to 1974 time interval.

Dr. Byar: I want to ask two specific methodologic questions. When you tried to summarize your regression analysis in those two trapezoids, were the four corners of the trapezoids separate estimates from those data, or were they estimated from the overall regression model?

Dr. Taylor: No, each point was separately estimated from the data.

Dr. Byar: And the second question is, though you tried to look at one variable at a time to see if it had changed over time in a way which might explain these results, was any attempt made to evaluate whether slight changes in alot of them added together might produce the results?

Dr. Taylor: No.

Dr. Blumenschein: I am still not clear concerning the years during which the adjuvant chemotherapy and the adjuvant radiation therapy studies were done.

Dr. Taylor: 1969 and a part of 1972.

Dr. Blumenschein: Could they have possibly influenced the disease-free interval?

Dr. Taylor: Well, that is the reason I presented the data. We could find no difference in the survival or in the disease-free interval for those treated compared with those not treated; therefore, I am assuming the treatment did no good.

Dr. LoBuglio: The point was that the randomized trial had the identical time to recurrence for those not receiving radiation as compared to those that did get radiation.

Dr. Morton: It is my understanding that there was a major change in surgeons and surgical approach to osteogenic sarcoma at the Mayo Clinic from 1970–1971. The new team had a much more direct interest in osteogenic sarcoma. Is this correct, and might it not influence the results?

Dr. Taylor: You are correct. It is my understanding, however, that the basic surgical approach to OGS did not change as a result of this transition.

Immunotherapy of Cancer: Present Status of Trials in Man, edited by W. D. Terry and D. Windhorst. Raven Press, New York © 1978.

Osteosarcoma: The M. D. Anderson Experience, 1950–1974

E. A. Gehan, *W. W. Sutow, †G. Uribe-Botero, **M. Romsdahl, and T. L. Smith

Departments of Biomathematics, *Pediatrics, and **Surgery, The University of Texas System Cancer Center; and †Department of Pathology, Veterans Administration Hospital, Houston, Texas 77011

The purpose of this chapter is to review the experience of patients with osteosarcoma treated at M. D. Anderson Hospital and Tumor Institute from 1950–1974. The specific group of patients consisted of those with primary lesions in the extremities aged 20 years or younger with no evidence of metastases at diagnosis. Most patients received surgery alone as treatment for their disease, whereas others received surgery plus adjuvant chemotherapy.

The analysis of the cases was meant to answer the following questions.

1. Was there any evidence of a trend by calendar time period in time to metastatic disease or survival time after treatment with surgery alone?

2. Were there any characteristics of the patients that were related to time to development of metastases or survival time for patients treated with surgery alone?

3. Has the prognosis for recent patients treated with surgery and adjuvant chemotherapy changed significantly from patients treated with surgery alone?

A review by Friedman and Carter (4) showed that there was a remarkable similarity in the 5-year survival rates of patients with osteogenic sarcoma treated by surgery alone. Among nine studies with 50 cases or more, the percent of patients surviving 5 years varied from 16 to 23% with the overall survival rate in 1,286 cases being 19.7%. At Memorial Sloan-Kettering Cancer Center, a review by Marcove et al. (8) of 145 cases showed 23% of cases disease free at 2 years and 17.4% disease free at 5 years. A current analysis of 133 patients treated from 1963–1974 at the Mayo Clinic reported by Taylor et al. (*This volume*) suggests that survival is improving with time, the 5-year survival being about 18% for 1963–65 and a projected 50% for cases treated in 1972–1974. Results were not as clear-cut for time to metastases, the percent of patients metastasis free at 2 years being about 13% in 1963–1965 and about 30% for 1972–1974.

This chapter examines the time to metastases and survival experience of 89 cases of osteosarcoma admitted to M. D. Anderson Hospital and Tumor

Institute between 1950 and 1974 who had disease in the extremities, no evidence of metastases at diagnosis, and surgery alone for treatment of their disease. Also analyzed were 36 patients meeting the same criteria who received surgery and adjuvant chemotherapy with CONPADRI or COMPADRI at M. D. Anderson Hospital and Tumor Institute between March, 1971 and September, 1974. CONPADRI stands for treatment with a four-drug combination of cyclophosphamide, vincristine, phenylalanine mustard, and doxorubicin hydrochloride and COMPADRI is the same four drugs plus methotrexate with citrovorum factor. Drug dosages and schedules are given in another report (9) along with data from a larger series of patients reporting the effectiveness of multidrug chemotherapy in the primary treatment of osteosarcoma.

MATERIALS AND METHODS

Uribe-Botero et al. (11) gave a report of 243 patients who had pathologically verified primary osteosarcoma of the bone and who were treated at M. D. Anderson Hospital and Tumor Institute between 1950 and 1974. From these cases, a series of 89 have been selected who met the following criteria: (a) the age of the patient was less than or equal to 20 years, (b) primary disease was confined to the extremities (femur, tibia, humerus, fibula, or radius), (c) histological types were osteoblastic, fibroblastic, or chondroblastic, (d) there was no evidence of metastatic disease at time of diagnosis, and (e) patients received surgery alone (amputation, disarticulation, or hemipelvectomy) for treatment of their disease. The data available for each case were age of the patient, sex, race, date of admission to M. D. Anderson Hospital, primary bone site of the tumor, location of the tumor (proximal or distal), histological type, type of surgery, time to evidence of first metastasis (from date of admission), and length of survival or time to last follow-up (both measured from date of admission). Data on size of tumor were considered too sketchy for detailed analysis. Note that time to metastases and survival have both been measured from date of admission rather than from date of surgery. Patients nearly always received operative treatment within 2 weeks of date of admission, so the additional time and effort to obtain the dates of surgery for all cases were not expended.

Survival or time-to-metastases curves have been calculated using the method of Kaplan and Meier (7). Tests of differences between two survival curves were carried out using a generalized Wilcoxon test (see ref. 5); when more than two curves were being compared, Breslow's generalization of the Wilcoxon test for k samples was used (1). Chi square tests were used to test for differences in frequencies of events among groups.

To determine which patient characteristics might be related to time to metastases or survival, Cox's regression model (2) was fitted to the data. The form of this model is as follows:

$$\log_e \left(\frac{\lambda(t)}{\lambda_0(t)}\right) = b_1(x_1 - \bar{x}_1) + \cdots + b_k(x_k - \bar{x}_k)$$

where the b's are regression coefficients that can be fitted using maximum likelihood techniques, the x's are patient characteristics potentially related to prognosis, $\lambda(t)$ is the hazard function (or risk of death per unit time) at time t, and $\lambda_0(t)$ is a standardized hazard function when no patient characteristics are in the model. The model can be fit in stepwise fashion so that the first patient characteristic selected is that most related to survival time, the second is that which, when added to the first, gives the best pair of characteristics related to survival, and so on. The statistical significance level of each variable entering the model can be calculated.

RESULTS

Table 1 gives the distribution of patient characteristics for the 89 patients in this study for three time periods: 1950–1962, 1963–1968, and 1969–1974. A total of 77 cases (87%) were aged 11 or older, with 36% of the cases between ages 16 and 20. When ages of the patients were considered by calendar time period, there was moderate evidence ($p = 0.07$) that the age distribution

TABLE 1. *Distribution of patient characteristics by calendar period*

Patient characteristic		Total patients (%)	Calendar period			p Value[b]
			Pre–1963	1963–68	1969–74	
All cases		89(100)	38(100)	31(100)	20(100)	
Age (yrs)	less than 11	12(13)[a]	2(5)	7(23)	3(15)	
	11–15	45(51)	25(66)	13(42)	7(35)	0.07
	16–20	32(36)	11(29)	11(35)	10(50)	
Sex	Male	57(64)	26(68)	19(61)	12(60)	
	Female	32(36)	12(32)	12(39)	8(40)	0.76
Race	Caucasian	64(72)	30(79)	21(68)	13(65)	
	Black	13(15)	4(11)	6(19)	3(15)	0.69
	Latin	12(13)	4(11)	4(13)	4(20)	
Site	Femur	45(53)	18(50)	13(43)	14(74)	
	Humerus	12(14)	5(14)	5(17)	2(11)	0.33
	Tibia	27(32)	12(33)	12(40)	3(16)	
	Radius	1(1)	1(3)	0(0)	0(0)	
Location	Proximal	48(56)	21(58)	18(60)	9(45)	
	Distal	38(44)	15(42)	12(40)	11(55)	0.53
Histology	Osteoblastic	53(80)	25(76)	14(78)	14(93)	
	Other	13(20)	8(24)	4(22)	1(7)	0.35
Surgery	Amputation	46(53)	19(51)	19(63)	8(40)	
	Disarticulation	36(41)	15(41)	10(33)	11(55)	0.51
	Hemipelvectomy	5(6)	3(8)	1(3)	1(5)	

[a] Numbers in parentheses are percentages of cases with known values of each patient characteristic.
[b] Statistical significance level is p.

differed by time period. The percentage of patients aged 16 to 20 was 29% pre-1963, 35% in 1963–68, and 50% in 1969–74. Younger cases tended to be underrepresented in this series because some pediatric patients began receiving adjuvant chemotherapy treatment in 1963.

More than one-half of the patients were male, the male/female ratio being 1.78. There was no evidence that sex distribution differed by calendar time period ($p = 0.76$).

The most common tumor site was the femur in 45 (53%) cases, which is consistent with other series (8). There was no real statistical evidence that site distribution differed by time period ($p = 0.33$). A preponderance of cases was osteoblastic (80%), and nearly all (94%) cases received amputation or disarticulation as primary treatment of their disease.

Except for age distribution, there was no statistical evidence that the distributions of other patient characteristics were changing with time (Table 1). In Marcove et al. (8), patients aged 11 to 20 years had superior disease-free survival than younger patients; hence, here the possibility of an increasing trend in time to metastatic disease with calendar time period should be considered.

Figure 1 gives time to metastases curves (or disease-free survival curves) for the three calendar periods. Median times to metastases were 6 months for

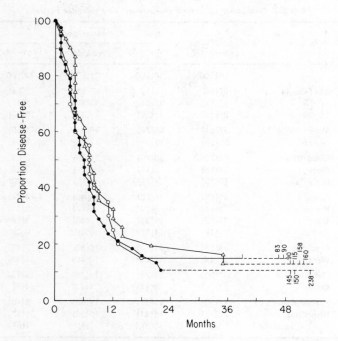

FIG. 1. Time to metastases for osteogenic sarcoma patients by calendar period. ●, Pre-1963 (total 38, recurrence 34); △, 1963–1968 (total 31, recurrence 27); ○, 1969–1974 (total 20, recurrence 17).

cases admitted prior to 1963 and 7 months for cases admitted in 1963–1968 and 1969–1974. There was no statistical evidence that time to metastases differed by calendar period ($p = 0.49$). The percentage of patients disease-free at 2 years was 11% prior to 1963, 19% for 1963–1968, and 15% for cases admitted 1969–1974. The results since 1963 are consistent with other reported series (4,8); the percentage of patients disease free at 2 years has not increased for each calendar period.

Table 2 considers whether there is evidence that pretreatment characteristics are related to time to metastases. The percentage of patients disease free 1 and 2 years after time of admission is given for each patient characteristic. Race was the only patient characteristic even moderately related ($p = 0.12$) to time to metastases. The median time to metastases was 7 months for Caucasians, 4 months for blacks, and 5 months for Latins. There was no statistical evidence of a relationship between time to metastases and age ($p = 0.47$), sex ($p = 0.59$), site of disease ($p = 0.51$), histology ($p = 0.42$), or type of surgery ($p = 0.76$).

Cox's regression model was fitted to the 84 patients for whom data were available on six patient characteristics. Patient characteristics considered were admission year ($0 =$ pre-1963, $1 = 1963$–1968, $2 = 1969$–1974), sex ($1 =$ male, $2 =$ female), race ($1 =$ Caucasian, $2 =$ non-Caucasian), type of surgery ($0 =$ amputation or disarticulation, $1 =$ hemipelvectomy), age

TABLE 2. Percentages of patients disease free at 1 and 2 years after admission—surgery alone treatment

Patient characteristics		No. of patients	No. of metastases	1 yr	2 yr	Significance level
Admission	pre-1963	38	34	22	11	
	1963–1968	31	27	29	18	0.49
	1969–1974	20	17	25	15	
Age (years)	≤10	12	9	25	25	
	11–15	45	42	24	8	0.47
	16–20	32	27	29	18	
Sex	Male	57	51	23	12	
	Female	32	27	31	18	0.59
Race	Caucasian	64	55	31	17	
	Black	13	13	8	0	0.12
	Latin	12	10	17	17	
Site	Femur	45	39	27	17	
	Humerus	12	10	17	17	0.51
	Tibia	27	25	30	7	
Location	Proximal	48	44	23	8	
	Distal	38	32	26	17	0.47
Histology	Osteoblastic	53	48	23	11	
	Nonosteoblastic	13	10	23	23	0.42
Surgery	Amputation	46	41	24	11	
	Disarticulation	36	30	31	21	0.76
	Hemipelvectomy	5	5	6	0	

$(0 = < 14$ years, $1 = 14$ years and over), and location $(1 = $ proximal, $2 = $ distal). The variable for race entered the model first at significance level $p = 0.043$; Caucasian patients tended to have longer times to recurrence than non-Caucasian patients. None of the other patient characteristics, including year of admission, was related in an important way to disease-free survival.

Figure 2 gives survival curves for the three calendar periods. The percentage of patients surviving 2 years or more is 23% for cases admitted pre-1963, and about 40% for patients admitted in either 1963–68 or 1969–74. There is highly significant evidence $(p = 0.01)$ that survival before and after 1963 differed significantly, however, there is no evidence at all of any survival change between 1963–1968 and 1969–1974 $(p = 0.94)$. Since about 1963, intensive multimodal treatment has been used to treat patients developing metastases; this treatment may explain the improved survival subsequent to 1963.

Cox's regression model was fitted to the 84 cases for whom data were available on admission year, sex, race, type of surgery, age, and location. In the preliminary analysis, histology was considered a possible characteristic related to survival, and it was not near statistical significance; it was eliminated from the final analysis for this reason and because 23 patients had unknown histologies. The variables in order of importance that entered the survival model

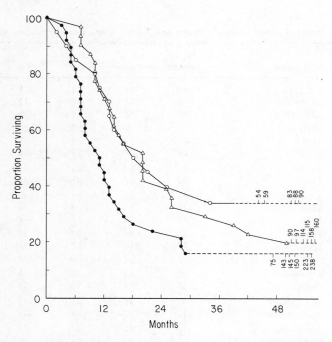

FIG. 2. Survival of osteogenic sarcoma patients by calendar period. ●, Pre-1963 (total 38, deaths 33); △, 1963–1968 (total 31, deaths 25); ○, 1969–1974 (total 20, deaths 13).

were admission year ($p = 0.01$) and race ($p = 0.03$). This analysis suggested that patients entering the study pre-1963 had significantly poorer survival than patients entering post-1963. Also, non-Caucasian patients had poorer survival than Caucasians.

Table 3 gives the estimated percentages of patients surviving 1 and 2 years after admission by patient characteristics. There was slight evidence that females had better survival than males ($p = 0.12$). There was no real statistical evidence of a relationship between survival and age ($p = 0.55$), race ($p = 0.19$), site ($p = 0.44$), location ($p = 0.64$), histology ($p = 0.43$), and surgery ($p = 0.76$). With respect to type of surgery, patients having hemipelvectomy had very poor survival experience; however, since only five patients received this operative procedure, the differences among groups were not near statistical significance.

A total of 36 patients meeting the criteria for this study received surgery and adjuvant chemotherapy with CONPADRI or COMPADRI at M. D. Anderson Hospital between March, 1971 and September, 1974. The distribution of characteristics of these patients is given in Table 4. There is some evidence that these patients are younger ($p = 0.04$) than those in the total series of 89 patients for the reason given previously. Sex, race, and site distribution did not differ between the groups of patients.

Figure 3 gives time to metastases curves for patients receiving surgery plus

TABLE 3. *Percentages of patients surviving at 1 and 2 years after admission—surgery alone treatment*

Patient characteristics		No. of patients	No. of deaths	1 yr	2 yr	Significance level
Admission	pre-1963	38	33	42	23	
	1963–1968	31	25	71	40	0.02
	1969–1974	20	13	73	41	
Age (yrs)	≤10	12	9	62	43	
	11–15	45	38	53	32	0.55
	16–20	32	24	66	30	
Sex	Male	57	48	57	26	
	Female	32	23	66	45	0.12
Race	Caucasian	64	49	63	41	
	Black	13	13	62	3	0.19
	Latin	12	9	47	25	
Site	Femur	45	34	58	35	
	Humerus	12	10	46	24	0.44
	Tibia	27	23	71	35	
Location	Proximal	48	41	58	28	
	Distal	38	28	60	38	0.64
Histology	Osteoblastic	53	45	53	30	
	Nonosteoblastic	13	9	65	31	0.43
Surgery	Amputation	46	37	63	31	
	Disarticulation	36	27	61	40	0.76
	Hemipelvectomy	5	5	36	3	

TABLE 4. *Distribution of patient characteristics for surgery plus adjuvant chemotherapy and surgery alone groups*

Patient characteristics		Surgery plus adjuvant chemotherapy		Surgery alone	
		Number	Percent	Number	Percent
All		36	100	89	100
Age (yrs)	≤10	11	31	12	13
	11–15	18	50	45	51
	16–20	7	19	32	36
Sex	Male	20	56	57	64
	Female	16	44	32	36
Race	Caucasian	27	96	64	72
	NonCaucasian	1	4	25	28
Site	Femur	21	58	45	53
	Humerus	3	8	12	14
	Tibia	10	28	27	32
	Other	2	6	1	1

adjuvant chemotherapy versus surgery alone. Patients receiving CONPADRI and COMPADRI were combined in this analysis, since a previous analysis (9) had not demonstrated any significant differences between them. There was a marked difference in the percentage of patients having metastases at 2

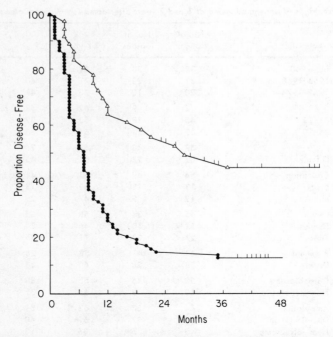

FIG. 3. Time to metastases for surgery plus adjuvant chemotherapy and surgery alone groups. ●, Surgery alone (total 89, recurrence 78); △, surgery plus adjuvant chemotherapy (total 36, recurrence 19).

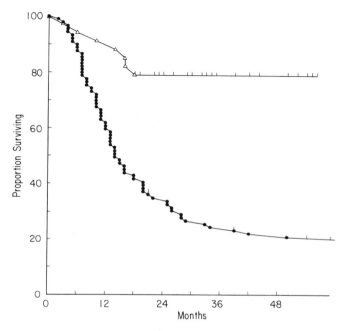

FIG. 4. Survival curves for surgery plus adjuvant chemotherapy and surgery alone groups. ●, Surgery alone (total 89, deaths 71); △, surgery plus adjuvant chemotherapy (total 36, deaths 7).

years between groups; 54% of patients receiving surgery and adjuvant chemotherapy are disease free at 2 years compared with 15% for patients receiving surgery alone. The difference between curves is highly statistically significant ($p < 0.01$). Patients in the adjuvant chemotherapy group tended to be younger than those in the surgery alone group, which might suggest less favorable prognosis; however results here are significantly better.

Figure 4 gives survival curves for patients in the surgery plus chemotherapy group compared to controls. The percentage of patients surviving at 2 years is estimated to be 79% for patients receiving adjuvant chemotherapy and only 34% for patients in the control group. The difference between survival curves was highly statistically significant ($p < 0.001$).

DISCUSSION

The data from 89 patients with osteosarcoma treated with surgery alone show no evidence of a trend in time to metastases with calendar period; overall, 15% of patients were disease free at 2 years, and this is consistent with data reported from other series (4,8). Surgery plus adjuvant chemotherapy has increased the percentage disease free at 2 years to 54%, and other series of cases (3,6) with adjuvant chemotherapy have reported 60% or higher disease-free survival at 2 years. The use of 2 years as the time interval of disease-free follow-up for analytical purposes may be too short since "late" metastases have been reported in osteosarcoma (10).

The data reported by Taylor et al. (*this volume*) from the Mayo Clinic show a disease-free survival at 2 years of 13% for 1963–1965, 20% for 1966–1968, 42% for 1969–1971, and 30% for 1972–1974. The trend in disease-free survival, the most meaningful measure of response to treatment, is not consistent among all calendar periods. The best 2-year disease-free survival is for 1969–1971 and was obtained when 42% (18/43) of patients were treated with chemotherapy. This is still substantially less than results with adjuvant chemotherapy at M. D. Anderson. Rather than suggesting "concurrent, randomly assigned untreated controls" (Taylor et al., *this volume*) to evaluate new treatments, it would appear more ethical and fruitful to treat patients with programs involving combination chemotherapy to confirm and extend the superior results obtained with COMPADRI, CONPADRI, and other combination treatments (3,6).

A trend in survival has been observed among cases treated at M. D. Anderson by surgery alone from 1950–1974; post-1963 cases have 40% surviving 2 years or longer compared with 23% for cases prior to 1963. However, results with adjuvant chemotherapy have 79% surviving at 2 years. The Mayo Clinic data demonstrate consistent improvement with calendar period, the best 2-year survival being 60% for 1972–1974. One explanation of improved survival at M. D. Anderson among cases treated by surgery alone is the better use of aggressive and intensive multidisciplinary programs for the treatment of metastatic disease. This may also be an explanation of improved survival for the Mayo Clinic cases. One test of this hypothesis would be to examine the Mayo Clinic data for possible trends with calendar period of survival subsequent to occurrence of metastatic disease. Consistently better survival could be explained by the better treatments for metastatic disease.

The advantage in survival of cases treated by adjuvant chemotherapy at M. D. Anderson over cases treated by surgery alone seems directly attributable to the adjuvant chemotherapy program. Similar results have been obtained by two adjuvant chemotherapy programs (9), and the percentage surviving disease free at 2 years was similar to that observed by Cortes et al. (3) and Jaffe et al. (6) who also utilized adjuvant chemotherapy programs. The survival curve for the patients receiving adjuvant chemotherapy reflects the influence of several factors. First, these patients were followed closely, and metastases were noted while the lesions were small. It is possible that the results of treatment for metastatic disease are better when the lesions are small. Secondly, intensive multimodal therapy was given postmetastases. Many underwent thoracotomy (some more than once), and all received radiation therapy and chemotherapy. The same cannot be said of the control group. Third, there is good evidence (Fig. 3) that time to metastasis is delayed by adjuvant chemotherapy; survival is lengthened automatically in this group. Fourth, the curve does not distinguish between those living with or without disease; if chemotherapy given postmetastasis increased subsequent survival, then the survival curve for the adjuvant chemotherapy group would still be improved.

The data from cases treated by surgery alone at M. D. Anderson do not suggest any patient characteristics strongly related to time to metastases. Overall, the race of the patient showed a slight relationship to time to metastases; the small number of cases (5) treated with hemipelvectomy had very short times to metastatic disease. For survival, sex and race of the patient were the only variables even slightly related; there was some tendency for females to have better survival than males, and for Caucasians to have better survival than non-Caucasians.

SUMMARY

This chapter reviews the experience of 89 patients with osteosarcoma treated by surgery alone at M. D. Anderson Hospital and Tumor Institute between 1950 and 1974. The patients all had primary lesions in extremities, were 20 years or younger at time of admission, and had nonmetastatic disease. There was no evidence of an improving trend in disease-free survival by calendar period; the percentage disease free at 2 years for all groups combined was 15%. There was evidence of an improvement in survival with time period, the percentage surviving at 2 years being 23% prior to 1963 and 40% subsequent to 1963.

There were 36 patients with osteosarcoma meeting the same criteria who received surgery and adjuvant multidrug chemotherapy with CONPADRI or COMPADRI between March, 1971 and September, 1974. The estimated percentage disease free at 2 years was 54%, and the percentage surviving at 2 years was 79%; both of these figures are significantly superior ($p < 0.01$) to the 18% of patients disease free and 34% surviving at 2 years for patients treated by surgery alone. These data suggest that future studies should be directed toward confirming and extending the results obtained with surgery and adjuvant chemotherapy.

ACKNOWLEDGMENTS

E. A. Gehan wishes to acknowledge support from National Cancer Institute grant CA-12014 and NIH grant CA-11430 in the preparation of this report. W. W. Sutow wishes to acknowledge support from HEW grants CA2501 and CA3713.

REFERENCES

1. Breslow, N. J. (1970): A generalized Kruskal-Wallis test for comparing k samples subject to unequal patterns of censorship. *Biometrika*, 57:579–594.
2. Cox, D. R. (1972): Regression models and life tables. *J. R. Stat. Soc. (B)*, 34:187–220.

3. Cortes, E. T., Holland, J. S., Wang, J. J., Sinks, L. F., Blom, J., Senn, H., Banks, A., and Glidewell, O. (1974): Amputation and adriamycin in primary osteosarcoma. *New Engl. J. Med.*, 291:998–1000.
4. Friedman, M. A., and Carter, S. K. (1972): The therapy of osteogenic sarcoma: Current status and thoughts for the future. *J. Surg. Oncology*, 4:482–510.
5. Gehan, E. A. (1965): A generalized Wilcoxon test for comparing arbitrarily singly-censored samples. *Biometrika*, 52:203–223.
6. Jaffe, N., Frei, E., III, Traggis, D., and Bishop, Y., (1974): Adjuvant methotrexate and citrovorum-factor treatment of sarcoma. *New Engl. J. Med.*, 291:994–997.
7. Kaplan, E. L., and Meier, P. (1958): Nonparametric estimation from incomplete observations. *JASA*, 53:457–481.
8. Marcove, R. C., Miké, V., Hajek, J. V., Levin, A. C., and Hutter, R. V. P. (1970): Osteogenic sarcoma under the age of 21. *J. Bone Joint Surg.*, 52-A:411–423.
9. Sutow, W. W., Gehan, E. A., Vietti, T. J., Frias, A. E., and Dyment, P. G. (1976): Multidrug chemotherapy in primary treatment of osteosarcoma. *J. Bone Joint Surg.*, 58-A, 5:629–633.
10. Sutow, W. W. (1976): Late metastases in osteosarcoma. *Lancet*, 1:856.
11. Uribe-Botero, G., Russell, W. O., Sutow, W. W., and Martin, R. G. (1977): Primary osteosarcoma of bone: A clinicopathologic investigation of 243 cases with necropsy studies in 54. *Am. J. Clinical Pathol. (In press.)*

Question and Answer Session

Dr. Pinsky: In the years 1971 to 1974, some patients had surgery alone, and some had surgery plus chemotherapy. How were they selected for one treatment or the other?

Dr. Sutow: The pediatric patients received chemotherapy for some years before adults began to receive chemotherapy, and that is the reason that the number of younger children in the surgery alone group is small compared to the number of adults in later years.

Dr. Frei: Dr. Gehan, in your disease-free curve, there seem to be several relapses after a two-year interval.

Dr. Gehan: There were three. One relapse occurred right at about two years. There were two other relapses, one at about twenty-six months and one at about thirty-six months.

Dr. Frei: When was chemotherapy stopped? How long after surgery?

Dr. Sutow: Fifteen to eighteen months.

Question: In trying to explain some of the differences, we have focused on possible treatment. Both groups have utilized patients with no evidence of metastasis. However, we have developed different methods of diagnosis of metastatic disease during this time period, such as tomography of the lung.

Have either of the studies looked at differences in survival in relation to accurate selection of patients without metastatic diseases?

Dr. Gehan: We haven't looked at that.

Dr. William F. Taylor: We have worried about it, but we haven't looked yet.

Dr. Frei: Dr. Jaffe at Boston Children's Hospital has looked at this, and in the last 55 patients there were two who, on the basis of tomography, were excluded because of pulmonary metastases.

Immunotherapy of Cancer: Present Status of Trials in Man, edited by W. D. Terry and D. Windhorst. Raven Press, New York © 1978.

Osteogenic Sarcoma Under the Age of 21: Experience at Memorial Sloan-Kettering Cancer Center

Valerie Miké and Ralph C. Marcove

Biostatistics Laboratory and Department of Surgery, Memorial Sloan-Kettering Cancer Center, New York, New York 10021

The original series published by Marcove et al. (6,7) on childhood osteogenic sarcoma included 145 consecutive cases diagnosed at Memorial Sloan-Kettering Cancer Center from January, 1949 through December, 1965. Patients under the age of 21 with central type osteogenic sarcoma of the extremities were included in this study. All these patients had ablative surgery of their primary tumor, no evidence of metastases at the time of diagnosis, and no subsequent local recurrence in the area of amputation. This series was analyzed to serve as historical control for a trial of adjuvant therapy with an autogenous tumor vaccine that was begun in 1966 and has since been used by other investigators as a control in the evaluation of new modalities of therapy.

It was recently called to our attention that an increased rate of disease-free survival has been observed for osteogenic sarcoma at the Mayo Clinic during the last few years (Taylor et al., *this volume*). If in effect there has been a change in the natural history of the disease, then our published series is clearly no longer a valid base-line criterion and, as suggested by the Mayo Clinic, randomized clinical trials with concurrent controls are necessary to demonstrate the efficacy of new treatments.

In order to answer this question, the decision was made to update our own series, and the following is a preliminary report. No mention is made of results pertaining to our experience with chemotherapy as an adjunct to surgery (12), since our main purpose here was to analyze additional data that might serve as control.

MATERIALS AND METHODS

A total of 210 patients were available for study, including the 145 in our published series who had been diagnosed from 1949 to 1965. Between 1966 and 1974 an additional 65 patients in this category were seen who did not receive chemotherapy prior to the onset of pulmonary metastases. Nineteen received no adjuvant therapy of any kind. The other 46 were given one of two types of autogenous tumor vaccine; 33 an ultraviolet (UV)-irradiated lysed cell vaccine and 13 a γ-irradiated whole cell vaccine. These vaccine trials have been reported previously (9) and are included here for completeness.

In addition to date of surgery and length of disease-free survival, age, sex, and site of primary tumor were recorded for each patient.

The statistical analysis was by means of actuarial curves for disease-free survival of the various subgroups of patients. Since most of the patients had some form of therapy after the onset of pulmonary metastases (2,10,11), length of disease-free survival after ablative surgery was used as our sole response criterion for this preliminary report.

The difference between two groups was tested for statistical significance by the Wilcoxon-Gehan statistic (5) and between several groups by the k-sample generalized Wilcoxon test (3).

In view of the fact that an analysis of disease-free survival rate as a function of calendar time was the main reason for the study, this aspect of the data was examined in still another way. Since all the patients had been followed for at least 2 years and since this is the crucial postsurgery interval for osteogenic sarcoma, a special technique was applied to examine the 2-year disease-free survival rate over time (Fig. 5). The patients were ordered according to date of surgery, and the 2-year rate was computed using a moving block of size 50. The rate was obtained for the first 50 patients (first point), then five were dropped and five new patients added (second point), etc. This procedure resulted in a sequence of 33 rate estimates. The year shown along the X-axis is the median year of surgery for each block of 50 (shown only when different from the preceding one). This approach provides a method of smoothing the data for the detection of any trends.

The question of course is whether the observed fluctuations can be expected to occur by chance. A 95% control band based on the binomial distribution (valid for individual points) has been added here. The process was also simulated by computer; the purpose was to estimate the joint probability of such a correlated time series exceeding the given limits.

This smoothing technique was subsequently applied to studying the variation of sex, age, and site over time.

Finally, a method used in the Mayo Clinic report for simultaneously showing the relationship of age, sex, and calendar time to median time to metastasis was applied to the corresponding subsets of our data (Fig. 7). The median time was estimated from data for the first 2 years, under the assumption of exponential disease-free survival times during this interval.

RESULTS

A breakdown of the total sample analyzed is shown in Table 1, according to the categories that may be relevant for prognosis. The first column refers to our published series, the second column to the additional 19 patients who

TABLE 1. Osteogenic sarcoma under the age of 21

		Control I 1949–65	Control II 1966–74	Vaccine I (Lysed cell)	Vaccine II (Whole cell)	Total
No. patients		145	19	33	13	210
Sex:	Male	82	11	21	4	118
	%	57	58	64	31	56
Age:	<15 yrs.	90	10	15	7	122
	%	62	53	45	54	58
Site:	Femur	84	13	9	6	112
	%	58	68	27	46	53
	Tibia	32	4	13	5	54
	Humerus	22	2	8	1	33
	Other	7	0	3	1	11

had received no adjuvant therapy, and the last two to the two vaccine series, respectively. The distribution by sex and age was similar in the four groups, discounting the low proportion of males in the small vaccine II group. Fifty-six percent of the total number were male, and 58% were under age 15. This subdivision for age was used to match the Mayo Clinic study. The primary

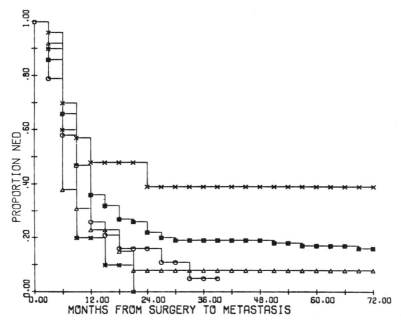

FIG. 1. Osteogenic sarcoma under the age of 21. Disease-free survival curves for the four groups of patients included in the study. The vaccine I (lysed cell) series has been divided into group A, patients treated and followed by one of us (RCM), and group B (see text). ■, Original series 1949–65 (145 patients); O, new series 1966–74 (19 patients); △, whole cell vaccine (13 patients); x, lysed cell vaccine IA (25 patients); *, lysed cell vaccine IB (8 patients).

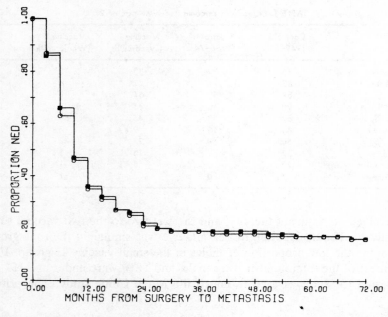

FIG. 2. Osteogenic sarcoma under the age of 21. Disease-free survival curves for the original and updated series. ■, Original series 1949–65 (145 patients); ○, updated series 1949–74 (210 patients).

tumor was in the femur in 53% of the cases; this site was somewhat under-represented in the vaccine series, especially series I.

The disease-free survival curves for the four groups of patients are shown in Fig. 1. The lysed cell vaccine group has been further subdivided since not all patients were treated in the same way or completed what was considered an adequate course of therapy. The 25 patients in group A were personally treated and followed by one of us (RCM); the remaining eight patients, who received partial or possibly inadequate therapy, constitute group B. Lysed cell group A has been doing consistently better than the control series but not at the level of statistical significance. For purposes of this report we are considering all groups as part of one general series.

Figure 2 shows the disease-free survival curve for the original series of 145 patients together with that for the updated series of all 210 patients. The agreement is overwhelming.

A breakdown of the entire series by sex revealed no difference in length of disease-free survival and neither did the breakdown by age (< 15 years versus ≥ 15 years). Grouping the patients by site of primary tumor (femur versus other sites) resulted in the curves shown in Fig. 3. The difference between these groups is statistically significant, with $p < 0.02$. Since there were comparatively few cases of femur in the lysed cell series, these two groups were also examined by site (femur versus other sites). There was, however,

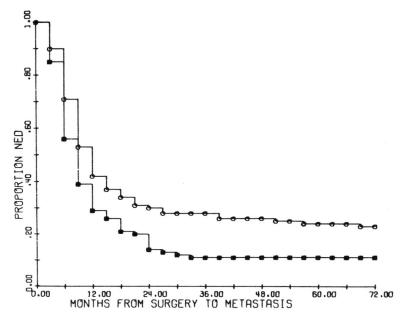

FIG. 3. Osteogenic sarcoma under the age of 21. Disease-free survival by site. ■, Femur (112 patients); ○, site other than femur (98 patients).

no essential difference in 2-year disease-free survival rates or median disease-free survival times in either of the groups. In other words, the relatively good performance of lysed cell group A cannot be attributed to the shortage of femur cases.

An analysis of disease-free survival by year of surgery, in five categories, is shown in Fig. 4. The observed 2-year disease-free survival rate ranged from 10 to 28%, but in no particular order. The two lowest were for 1958–1962 and 1969–1974, respectively. None of these rates is unusually high, and the curves seem to fall in a cluster. The overall significance test for a difference between these groups yielded $p < 0.04$. This in itself is not a very meaningful result, because the ordering of groups appears random.

A further analysis of the trend in disease-free survival rates as a function of calendar time is shown in Fig. 5. The overall 2-year rate was 21%, and the smoothed series exhibits fluctuation about this point. There was a trough around 1961 and again at 1971 and a peak around 1966; this corresponds to what was observed in the survival curves. None of the points fell outside the 95% control band. From our Monte Carlo study, based on 50,000 simulations of this process, the probability of at least one point falling above or below the control band was estimated to be about 0.25 each. In other words, what we have observed is well within what could be expected by random fluctuation.

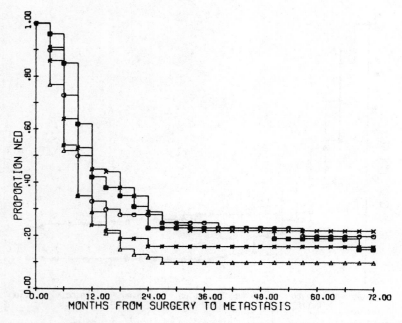

FIG. 4. Osteogenic sarcoma under the age of 21. Disease-free survival by year of surgery. ■, year of surgery 1949–52 (26 patients); ○, surgery 1953–57 (40 patients); △, surgery 1958–62 (52 patients); x, surgery 1963–68 (55 patients); *, surgery 1969–74 (37 patients).

A closer look at this graph suggests a reason for the statistically significant difference between the curves in Fig. 4. It so happened that in partitioning the data into time periods, we assigned troughs and peaks into different groups. This is one way to generate significant results even from a random set of data.

Since site was found to be significantly related to prognosis, tumors in the femur being associated with a lower disease-free survival rate, it was of interest also to examine the incidence of femur as a function of calendar time, as shown in Fig. 6. We do see a sort of peak corresponding to the trough in

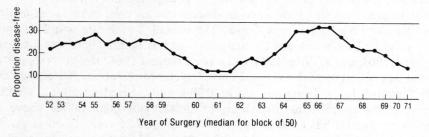

FIG. 5. Osteogenic sarcoma under the age of 21. Disease-free survival rate at 2 years versus year of surgery. Smoothing obtained by using moving block of size 50, with 95% control band. N = 210.

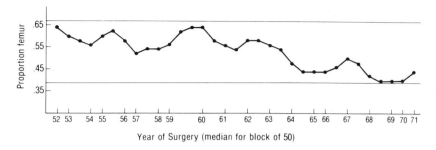

FIG. 6. Osteogenic sarcoma under the age of 21. Proportion of patients with tumor in the femur versus year of surgery. Smoothing obtained by using moving block of size 50, with 95% control band. N = 210.

Fig. 5 from about 1959 to 1963, and a trough corresponding to the peak from 1964 to 1967. The low proportion of femur cases during the most recent period would suggest a correspondingly higher disease-free survival rate. But this in effect was not observed.

The same procedure was carried out for sex (proportion male) versus year of surgery, and for average age versus year of surgery. A slight upward trend in average age was revealed, but both processes were within expected limits.

Figure 7 is a duplication of a figure from the Mayo Clinic report, using our data. The figure was designed to show the relationship of age, sex, and

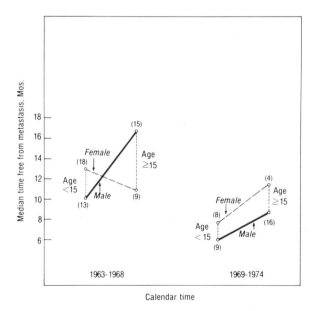

FIG. 7. Osteogenic sarcoma under the age of 21. Median disease-free survival time by age, sex, and calendar period.

calendar time to median disease-free survival time. A higher median was found by the Mayo Clinic for the period 1969–1974 as compared to 1963–1968 (the balance of the period studied), for female patients, and for patients aged $\geqq$ 15 years. Except for a slight advantage of the older age group during these periods, the pattern observed at the Mayo Clinic was not confirmed here.

DISCUSSION

Thus nothing essentially new emerged from our updated analysis. Why the difference between our results and those observed at the Mayo Clinic? A few tentative suggestions may be in order.

There may be a discrepancy in our histologic diagnoses of what constitutes central type osteogenic sarcoma. Our definition specifies a fully malignant spindle cell tumor beginning within the bone, with a significant proportion of malignant cells elaborating tumor membrane bone (or osteoid). Cartilage is occasionally present and forms endochondral bone, usually at the peripheral region of a cartilage lobule. However, the presence of endochondral type of bone, often with its central cartilage core still visible in the osteoid, does not justify inclusion of a tumor as osteogenic sarcoma. Such a tumor, composed primarily of lobules of malignant cartilage cells without significant areas of malignant spindle cells forming membrane bone, is diagnosed as chondrosarcoma, which has a higher cure rate for grade I and II tumors (8). Fibrosarcoma similarly has been shown to have better prognosis (4).

The 2-year disease-free survival rates observed at the Mayo Clinic were approximately 17% for 1963–1968 and 36% for 1969–1974. It is possible that our definition of central type osteogenic sarcoma is most closely approximated by what at the Mayo Clinic is called osteoblastic grade IV osteogenic sarcoma. In this category, the Mayo Clinic observed a 2-year disease-free survival rate of 21% for the period 1969–1974, in agreement with the overall Memorial experience. During the earlier period the corresponding rate was only 6%. Could this be due to a difference in surgical procedures? In our original series of 74 cases involving a tumor in the lower femur, 22 had subtrochanteric amputation, whereas 52 were treated by hip joint disarticulation. The resulting 2-year disease-free survival rates were 4 and 18%, respectively (7). Although this difference is not statistically significant, the point may be relevant. Subtrochanteric amputations were discontinued at Memorial Hospital in 1960.

Finally, the prognosis for low grade parosteal or juxtacortical osteogenic sarcoma is considerably better (1). In the Mayo Clinic series, 3% of the sample were excluded as parosteal osteogenic sarcoma. At Memorial Hospital the corresponding incidence is estimated to be about 10%. Could this again be due to a discrepancy in definitions? Certainly a juxtacortical lesion can invade secondarily into the bone marrow.

An exchange of slides and X-rays between the two institutions on all patients being included in these studies may be one way of attempting to resolve this problem.

SUMMARY

A review of a consecutive series of 145 cases of operative central type osteogenic sarcoma of the extremities, diagnosed in patients under the age of 21 from January, 1949 through December, 1965, was reported by Marcove et al. in 1970. This series has been used by other investigators as a historical control in the study of different types of adjuvant therapy following ablative surgery. Between 1966 and 1974 an additional 65 patients in this category were seen. Nineteen of these patients received no adjuvant therapy; the other 46 were given one of two types of autogenous tumor vaccine. An updated analysis of the complete series of 210 patients has been carried out, with emphasis on evaluating any change in disease-free survival rate as a function of calendar time. This study was motivated by the fact that a substantially increased rate of disease-free survival has been observed for osteogenic sarcoma at the Mayo Clinic during the last few years. Our own results, however, indicate no change in the course of the disease, with the updated estimate of 2-year disease-free survival rate of 21% matching that of the first series.

ACKNOWLEDGMENTS

The authors are grateful to members of the Biostatistics Laboratory who were instrumental in the completion of this study: Sharon Passe, Pat Middleman, and Cynthia Kosloff assisted in the collection and analysis of the data; the computer simulation was the work of Dr. David W. Braun, Jr.

This research was supported in part by National Cancer Institute grant CA-08748.

REFERENCES

1. Ahuja, S. C., Villacin, A. B., Smith, J., Bullough, P. G., Huvos, A. G., and Marcove, R. C. (1977): Juxtacortical (parosteal) osteogenic sarcoma. Histological grading, radiographic findings, prognosis and management. *J. Bone Joint Surg. (in press)*.
2. Beattie, E. J., Jr., Martini, N., and Rosen, G. (1975): The management of pulmonary metastases in children with osteogenic sarcoma with surgical resection combined with chemotherapy. *Cancer,* 35:618–621.
3. Breslow, N. (1970): A generalized Kruskal-Wallis test for comparing k samples subject to unequal patterns of censorship. *Biometrika,* 57:579–594.
4. Cunningham, M. P., and Arlen, M. (1968): Medullary fibrosarcoma of bone. *Cancer,* 21:31–37.
5. Gehan, E. A. (1965): A generalized Wilcoxon test for comparing arbitrarily singly-censored samples. *Biometrika,* 52:203–223.
6. Marcove, R. C., Miké, V., Hajek, J. V., Levin, A. G., and Hutter, R. V. P. (1970): Osteogenic sarcoma under the age of twenty-one. A review of 145 operative cases. *J. Bone Joint Surg.,* 52-A:411–423.

7. Marcove, R. C., Miké, V., Hajek, J. V., Levin, A. G., and Hutter, R. V. P. (1971): Osteogenic sarcoma in childhood. *NY State J. Med.*, 71:855–859.
8. Marcove, R. C., Miké, V. Hutter, R. V. P., Huvos, A. G., Shoji, H., Miller, T. R., and Kosloff, R. (1972): Chondrosarcoma of the pelvis and upper end of the femur. An analysis of factors influencing survival time in 113 cases. *J. Bone Joint Surg.*, 54-A:561–572.
9. Marcove, R. C., Miké, V., Huvos, A. G., Southam, C. M., and Levin, A. G. (1973): Vaccine trials for osteogenic sarcoma. A preliminary report. *Cancer*, 23:74–80.
10. Marcove, R. C., Martini, N., and Rosen, G. (1975): The treatment of pulmonary metastasis in osteogenic sarcoma. *Clin. Orthop.*, 3:65–70.
11. Martini, N., Huvos, A. G., Miké, V., Marcove, R. C., and Beattie, E. J., Jr. (1971): Multiple pulmonary resections in the treatment of osteogenic sarcoma. *Ann. Thorac. Surg.*, 12:271–280.
12. Rosen, G., Murphy, M. L., Huvos, A. G., Gutierrez, M., and Marcove, R. C. (1976): Chemotherapy, *en bloc* resection, and prosthetic bone replacement in the treatment of osteogenic sarcoma. *Cancer*, 37:1–11.

Question and Answer Session

Dr. Presant: Were the patients in this study randomized to be treated with various types of lysed cells or whole cells?

Dr. Miké: No, that is a very important point. They were not randomized studies. All of Dr. Marcove's patients from 1966 to 1972 received the vaccine.

Dr. Presant: Have you looked at the cases that were treated by vaccines versus those treated by just surgery alone to see if various prognostic factors varied in those groups?

Dr. Miké: Yes. Several published reports address the comparability of groups.

Dr. Morton: Your data indicate that the patients that received the lysed-cell vaccine had a lower incidence of femur lesions—only 20 percent as compared to 58 or 57 percent in your controls. In addition, the patients who had osteosarcomas in locations other than in the femur appeared to do about 20 percent better than the patients that had femur lesions. Can these differences in site explain the differences between the lysed-cell vaccine and the surgery-alone group?

Dr. Miké: Yes, possibly.

*Immunotherapy of Cancer: Present Status of
Trials in Man,* edited by W. D. Terry and D. Windhorst.
Raven Press, New York © 1978.

Transfer Factor Versus Combination Chemotherapy: An Interim Report of a Randomized Postsurgical Adjuvant Study in Osteogenic Sarcoma

Roy E. Ritts, Jr., *Douglas J. Pritchard, **Gerald S. Gilchrist,
*John C. Ivins, and †William F. Taylor

*Department of Microbiology; *Section of Orthopedic Oncology, Department of
Orthopedics; **Section of Pediatric Oncology, Department of Pediatrics;
and †Section of Medical Research Statistics, Department of Medical
Statistics and Epidemiology, Mayo Clinic and Mayo Foundation,
Rochester, Minnesota 55901*

The details of this postsurgical adjuvant study comparing the effects of transfer factor (TF) and methotrexate, doxorubicin hydrochloride (Adriamycin®), and vincristine (Concovin®) have been presented by Ivins et al. (1). In summary, all patients with primary, classic, and histologically confirmed osteogenic sarcoma seen between July 1, 1974 and December 30, 1975 were eligible and randomized to receive either TF or combination chemotherapy (MAO). TF was prepared by the dialysis method of Lawrence and Al-Askari (2) from long-term (> 5 years) survivors of osteogenic sarcoma. On the 10th postoperative day not more than three successive 0.1-ml doses of TF (equivalent to 1 unit contained in 10^9 lymphocytes) were given subcutaneously to effect a systemic transfer of a skin delayed type hypersensitivity reaction to a specific microbial antigen-induced reaction present in the donor greater than 20 mm of induration and observed to be absent in the recipient. If transfer was not achieved, the patient was immediately crossed over to the MAO arm of the protocol. This combination chemotherapy was started on the 15th postoperative day and consisted of intravenous vincristine 1.4 mg/m², followed by methotrexate 2,500 mg/m² as a 4-hr infusion, followed within 30 min of its completion by infusion with calcium citrovorum (Leucovorin®), 15 mg. Thereafter calcium citrovorum is given intravenously or intramuscularly 12 mg every 6 hr for 12 doses. Doxorubicin 40 mg/m² is given intravenously at 24 hr. This sequence of drugs is repeated every 4 weeks for a total of 12 treatments. Depending upon the toxicity observed, the dose of doxorubicin is increased or decreased by 10 mg/m².

Failure of either treatment occurs with evidence of recurrence or metastasis, removing such patients from the protocol. All failures are considered for further treatment. Resectable lesions are removed surgically, TF failures receive the noted combination chemotherapy, and MAO failures are entered on other chemotherapy.

INTERIM RESULTS AND COMMENT

To date 18 patients have been entered on each arm of the protocol. As noted in Table 1, five of the TF recipients failed to demonstrate systemic reactivity after the third dose of TF and were crossed over to the chemotherapy arm. They have fared about the same as the group receiving MAO alone, their death rate being slightly less. Another four patients failing to demonstrate systemic transfer refused chemotherapy. Although these observations are little more than anecdotal given the few patients and present duration of study, it is of interest that these patients had a marked increase in metastasis and death rates.

If failure to effect a systemic transfer under the given conditions can be interpreted as an explicit deficit in cellular immunity, then such patients appear to be at special risk without further therapy. Their cohorts who received MAO appeared to respond to chemotherapy as well as other patients who were not anergic. However, we have not had occasion to observe the other obvious permutation, the TF responders who are given chemotherapy and who might have had an even better response.

Table 2 illustrates the interim results on those remaining nine patients who received only TF compared to the 18 patients receiving MAO. Similarly combined data are presented on these 18 patients plus the five nonresponding TF recipients. There are no significant differences to be observed in these re-

TABLE 1.

	TF (all entered)	MAO	TF to MAO	TF only (excluded)
No. entered	18	18	5	4
Metastasis	9	9	2	3
Patient days	4,351	3,882	1,223	529
Rate (100 patient month)	6.3	7.2	5.0	17.2
Death, OGS	6	4	1	3
Patient days survived	6,229	5,120	1,343	995
Rate (100 patient month)	2.9	2.4	2.3	9.2
Death, all cases	6	7	1	3
Patient days survived	6,229	5,120	1,343	995
Rate (100 patient month)	2.9	4.2	2.3	9.2
Alive, no recurrence	9	6	3	1
Recurrence	3	5	1	0
OGS removed	1	1	0	0
Present	2	4	1	0
Dead, OGS	6	4	1	3
Other cause	0	3	0	0

OGS, osteogenic sarcoma.

TABLE 2.

	TF only (in study)	MAO + TF to MAO	MAO	
No. entered	9	23	18	
Metastasis	4	11	9	
Patient days	2,599	5,105	3,882	
Rate (100 patient month)	4.7	6.6	7.2	
Death, OGS	2	5	4	
Patient days survived	3,891	6,463	5,120	
Rate (100 patient month)	1.6	2.4	2.4	
Death, all cases	2	8	7	
Patient days survived	3,891	6,463	5,120	
Rate (100 patient month)	1.6	3.8	4.2	
Alive, no recurrence		5	9	6
Recurrence		2	6	5
OGS removed		1	1	1
Present		1	5	4
Dead, OGS		2	5	4
Other cause		0	3	3

OGS, osteogenic sarcoma.

sults to date although both the disease-free interval and death rate appear to be marginally better in the group receiving TF.

Figure 1 illustrates the interim disease-free intervals in the perspective of both historical and contemporary controls referred to earlier by Taylor et al. (*this volume.*) At 18 months our TF group is comparable with the contemporary control group who received no adjuvant therapy (~55%), but the MAO group is lower (~32%) and comparable to those historical controls reputed by Marcove et al. (3) as well as observed at the Mayo Clinic from 1963–1968.

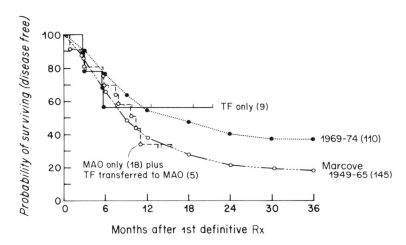

FIG. 1. Osteosarcoma—disease-free survival.

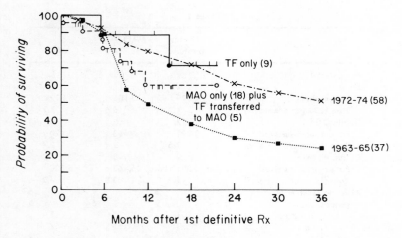

FIG. 2. Osteosarcoma—survival.

Figure 2 compares the survival curves of the two treatment groups again in the perspective of historical and contemporary controls. At 18 months it is evident that neither group has a better survival than comparable contemporary controls who received no adjuvant therapy. However, in the light of historic control data, both groups are seen to have a markedly improved survival.

As noted in our previous report (1) and worthy of reemphasis, we have no evidence that the TF possessed any immunological specificity for this tumor. Indeed, with Stephen Elliott, we have been unable to demonstrate any significant alteration in TF recipients' leukocyte adherence inhibition with osteogenic sarcoma extracts. However, it has been observed that when systemic transfer has been specifically effected to a given microbial antigen, there has been a general, nonspecific enhancement of all other delayed-type hypersensitivity (DTH) responses even though the donor may have not had even a minute skin reaction to the antigens evoking them. This is in contrast to our observations using methanol extracted residue of BCG (MER) (4) in advanced carcinoma where no enhancement of any measure of cellular-mediated immunity was seen.

DISCUSSION

Although 18 months is generally considered a pivotal time in the course of a patient with osteogenic sarcoma, the few patients in this series preclude any definitive conclusion. As we interpret the interim data, there appears to be no significant improvement in the disease-free interval or survival in either the TF- or MAO-treated patients compared to contemporary controls who received no adjuvant therapy following amputation.

Great care has been taken in these analyses to exclude the high percentage of surgically curable osteogenic sarcomas of the parosteal type, of the jaw, of low grade central type, or of periosteal variety. Similarly, extramural reviewers have confirmed classic osteogenic sarcoma in all but one of the 192 cases. The one case in dispute was excluded from the statistical analysis. The details of these analyses are presented elsewhere in this volume by Taylor et al.

We believe that it is essential for all to reach agreement on clinical and pathological criteria of osteogenic sarcoma before including patients on experimental protocols or comparing the results of such investigations with historical or contemporary control material that may be based on a different data base. Alternatively, the histological types of tumor, the sites of the lesions, and pertinent clinical information should be presented to make relevant comparisons between institutions and between treatment groups and controls in the same institution.

Thus, if the clinical and pathological features of our patients as reported earlier (1) and herein are comparable to the reports of others, we can make the preliminary interim judgment that the patients in both treatment arms have a significantly improved disease-free interval compared to the historical controls of Marcove et al. but that neither the TF nor the MAO arm has given as good a result as those high-dose methotrexate regimens reported by Frei et al. (5) and Jaffe et al. (6) although the amount of drugs, duration of administration, and timing are greater than used by us in this study.

ACKNOWLEDGMENT

This investigation was supported in part by research grant CA-11911 from the National Cancer Institute. This study was approved by the Mayo Clinic Human Studies Committee.

REFERENCES

1. Ivins, J. C., Ritts, R. E., Pritchard, D. J., Gilchrist, G. S., Miller, G. C., and Taylor, W. F. (1976): Transfer factor versus combination chemotherapy: A preliminary report of a randomized postsurgical adjuvant treatment study in osteogenic sarcoma. *Ann. NY Acad. Sci.,* 277:558–574.
2. Lawrence, H. S., and Al-Askari, S. (1971): The preparation and purification of transfer factor. In: *In Vitro Methods in Cell-Mediated Immunity,* edited by B. R. Bloom and P. R. Glade, pp. 542–545. Academic Press, New York.
3. Marcove, R. C., Miké, V., Hajek, J. V., Levin, A. G., and Hutter, R. V. P. (1970): Osteogenic sarcoma under the age of twenty-one: A review of one hundred and forty-five operative cases. *J. Bone Joint Surg. [Am.],* 52:411–423.
4. O'Connell, M. J., Ritts, R. E., Jr. and Moertel, C. G. (1976): Immunological assessment of MER and placebo in advanced cancer: A double blind study. *Proc. Am. Assoc. Cancer Res./Am. Soc. Clin. Oncol.,* 17:214 (Abstr. #854).
5. Frei, E., III, Jaffe, N., Tattersall, M. H. N., Pitman, S., and Parker, L. (1975): New approaches to cancer chemotherapy with methotreaxte. *N. Engl. J. Med.,* 292:846–851.

6. Jaffe, N., Frei, E., III, Traggis, D., and Bishop, Y. (1974): Adjuvant methotrexate and citrovorum-factor treatment of osteogenic sarcoma. *N. Engl. J. Med.*, 291:994–997.

Question and Answer Session

Dr. LoBuglio: I guess the prior discussion about the right control or untreated natural history of the disease isn't relevant to your study. Clearly, the current Mayo experience is the appropriate control group for comparison with your treatment limbs. If there is a problem with pathology or surgery, et cetera, this should be consistent within your institution.

Dr. Bornstein: Have there been any recurrences in your transfer factor donors?

Dr. Ritts: No.

Dr. Frei: As I recall, your tumor-free survival on chemotherapy had an 18-patient denominator at the beginning and had dropped off to about 30 percent, which is not different from the control group. But you have three deaths in complete remission which were drug related.

Dr. Ritts: Yes.

Dr. Frei: Now, in a life table plot of a year with that fall-off, that would make a 20 or 30 percent difference. And you could censor those toxic deaths if you wanted to plot time to metastases. I take it they were included as relapses.

Dr. Ritts: Yes.

Dr. Fudenberg: In our series if patients survive five years without evidence of disease, they just don't have positive assays of specific tumor immunity. This also holds true for autoimmune disease. Three years after the antigen is eliminated, the immunologic system no longer retains sufficient memory to provide transfer factor with specificity for the original disease. This has an important bearing on selection of donors for transfer factor.

Immunotherapy of Cancer: Present Status of Trials in Man, edited by W. D. Terry and D. Windhorst. Raven Press, New York © 1978.

Adjuvant Immunotherapy of Osteosarcoma with BCG and Allogeneic Tumor Cells

Frederick R. Eilber, Courtney M. Townsend, and Donald L. Morton

Division of Oncology, Department of Surgery, UCLA Medical School, Los Angeles, California 90024; and Department of Surgical Services, Sepulveda Veterans Administration Hospital, Sepulveda, California 91343

At the time of initiation of this study, the treatment of patients with osteosarcoma by surgical resection resulted in few cures. Even though local control was achieved in all patients, metastatic disease was evident within 12 months of surgical resection. Therefore, it was apparent that some method of systematically active adjuvant therapy had to be devised for these patients.

RATIONALE

The rationale for immunotherapy of osteosarcoma comes from several sources. In 1968 Morton and Malmgren (15) demonstrated the tumor-associated antigens of osteosarcoma cells. They indicated that there was some evidence of the presence of a common cross-reacting tumor antigen in sarcomas of the same as well as different histologic types (16). Additional evidence comes from the identification of complement fixing (4,5) and cytotoxic antibodies (1,2,23) against these sarcoma-associated antigens. The immunologic materials used in these assays were obtained entirely from sarcoma specimens, and, therefore, it seemed evident that sarcoma patients generated an *in vivo* immune response against these sarcoma antigens (8,9,14). Evidence from investigations of animal sarcomatous neoplasms indicated that Bacillus Calmette-Guerin (BCG) was an effective immunologic adjuvant and therapeutic agent specifically for osteosarcomas (6,22).

At the initiation of the study there were no active chemotherapeutic agents that appeared to be effective against osteosarcoma, and, therefore, this study was designed as a phase I trial to evaluate the toxicity and possible therapeutic benefits of the administration of active immunotherapy following surgical resection of both primary osteosarcomas and pulmonary metastases for metastatic disease.

MATERIALS AND METHODS

Twenty-nine patients with osteosarcoma were seen by the Division of Surgical Oncology, UCLA, from January, 1972 to August, 1974. Fourteen patients had stage I osteosarcoma, and 15 had stage III disease with evidence of pulmonary metastases. Of the 29 patients, 17 patients had operative procedures to remove all gross tumor, followed by a program of immunotherapy 2 to 8 weeks later. Nine patients had stage I disease, and eight patients, receiving adjuvant immunotherapy after surgical resection for pulmonary metastases had stage III disease. (17). A nonrandomized series of 12 patients who elected surgical resection alone or who had chemotherapy for nonresectable pulmonary metastases served as controls.

The immunotherapeutic agents used were BCG combined with an allogeneic sarcoma tumor tissue culture cell vaccine. The BCG (Tice strain, Chicago Research) was given intradermally by the tine technique in both axillas and groins every week, one ampule per treatment. Allogeneic sarcoma cell vaccine at a dose of 1×10^7 tissue cultured cells was injected at separate sites into each axilla and each groin. These cells were obtained from a single tissue cultured cell line, SA-2, derived from a malignant osteosarcoma (16). Immunotherapy was administered once every week for 3 months, and then once every other week for 2 years or until a recurrence was noted.

RESULTS

Analysis of treatment results for all patients seen during this interval is given in Table 1. Of 15 patients with stage I sarcoma, i.e., disease confined to the primary site, none remained free of recurrence following surgical resection whether or not they received adjuvant immunotherapy. All died from their disease. One patient remains alive and free from disease following resection of osteosarcoma of the mandible plus adjuvant immunotherapy. However, because the natural history of disease in this location differs from osteosarcoma in the extremities, this patient was not included in the analysis.

Eight patients with stage III disease had pulmonary resection for metastatic disease. Two remain alive free of disease at 22 and 42 months, postoperatively. Six died of progressive pulmonary metastases despite immunotherapy.

Seven patients with nonresectable stage III osteosarcoma who did not undergo operative resection for their metastases were treated with chemotherapy alone without evidence of their disease, and all expired.

TABLE 1. *Results of treatment—osteosarcoma*

Stage	Treatment	No. patients	NED	Alive
I	Surgery + Immunotherapy	9	0/9	0/9
	Surgery	5	0/5	0/5
III	Surgery + Immunotherapy	8	2/8[a]	2/8
	Chemotherapy	7	0/7	0/7

NED, no evidence of disease.
[a] Follow-up 22 and 36 months.

TABLE 2. *Interval between treatment and recurrence*

Stage	Treatment	No. patients	Time to recurrence (months)	
			Range	Median
I	Surgery + immunotherapy	9	(1–32)	8.5
	Surgery alone	5	(1–13)	3.1
III	Surgery + immunotherapy	6[a]	(2–4)	3.0
	Chemotherapy	5		

[a] Only includes those who recurred; two patients remain free of disease.

Toxicity in patients treated with postoperative immunotherapy was minimal. No systemic BCG infections were noted, and no patients developed granulomatous hepatitis (16). Mild itching and pustule formation at the immunization sites were noted, and a mild temperature elevation to 101°F was noted in 75% of the patients. Fifty percent of these patients had generalized malaise for 24 hr following vaccination. No tumor growth occurred from the allogeneic cell vaccine at the sites of vaccination.

An additional analysis was done to determine if immunotherapy delayed the time to recurrence in patients who recurred. These results are shown in Table 2. No statistical differences were found in the time from diagnosis to recurrence, regardless of initial clinical stage or whether or not patients were receiving immunotherapy. Seventy-five percent (6/8) patients with stage I disease who received immunotherapy developed recurrences within 3 months. The median time to recurrence was 8.1 months compared to 3.1 months in patients treated by amputation alone. These differences are not statistically significant. In the stage III patients who had recurrence, the time from surgical resection to evidence of recurrent disease occurred at a median of 3.0 months. However, it must be pointed out that two of these patients are alive and free of disease, one at 4 years following surgical resection.

DISCUSSION

Results of this study indicate that there is little apparent benefit from adjuvant immunotherapy with BCG and allogeneic tissue culture cell vaccine for patients with osteosarcoma. The poor clinical results were observed even though tumor-associated antigens were demonstrated in the sarcoma cell vaccine as well as tumor-associated antibodies in patient sera. There are numerous reasons for treatment failure in this group of patients, although the most striking one is the rapidity of the occurrence of pulmonary metastases (median time of 3 months). This failure might be explained by the delay of 6 weeks before the immunotherapy was started following the surgical resections. It is very possible that the residual tumor burden was too great for treatment with immunotherapy (14). Although all of these patients had extensive preoperative evaluation, including whole chest tomography, it is apparent that they had residual disease at the time of initiation of immunotherapy.

Another possibility for failure concerns the combination of BCG and tumor cell vaccine. This combination may not have been the optimal antigenic stimulant. The immunizing tissue culture cell line was an osteosarcoma and, although serologic cross-reactivity with the other osteogenic sarcoma antigen was evident, it is possible that both quantitative and qualitative differences existed between these antigens (10,15,18). Since the toxicity levels were very acceptable in this group of patients, it appears that toxicity from immunotherapy was not an adverse factor in contributing to the patients' course.

Since the initiation of these studies, it has become evident that there are at least two highly effective chemotherapeutic agents for treatment of patients with osteosarcoma—doxorubicin hydrochloride (Adriamycin®) and high-dose methotrexate. Most reported trials using these agents have been limited to 6 months treatment with doxorubicin hydrochloride, and 1 year total treatment with high-dose methotrexate (3,7,11–13). Although the results of these studies are very impressive, in that at least 50% of the patients remain free of recurrence for at least 2 years, it is clear that recurrence continues to occur in patients treated with chemotherapy alone (19,21).

Therefore, on the basis of our study plus a review of the current chemotherapeutic results, we advocate treatment with an active chemotherapeutic regimen immediately following surgical resection of primary sarcoma to further reduce the tumor cell burden or subclinical disease. When tumor burden is reduced, a long-term immunotherapeutic regimen should be integrated into the treatment schedule. To this end we have initiated an adjuvant study employing operation, combination chemotherapy of doxorubicin hydrochloride and high-dose methotrexate, and immunotherapy. In an effort to improve the immunogenic potential of the vaccine we have included two additional tissue culture cell lines to the SA-2 cell line. Hopefully, this multidisciplinary approach will result in an increased disease-free interval, and ultimately a greater percentage of cure for patients with osteosarcomas.

ACKNOWLEDGMENTS

These investigations were supported by grant CA-12582 from the National Cancer Institute of the Department of Health, Education and Welfare and Medical Research Service of the Veterans Administration.

REFERENCES

1. Cohen, A. M., Ketcham, A. S., and Morton, D. L. (1972): Cellular immunity to a common human sarcoma antigen and its specific inhibition by sera from patients with growing sarcomas. *Surgery,* 72:560.

2. Cohen, A. M., Ketcham, A. S., and Morton, D. L. (1973): Tumor-specific cellular cytotoxicity to human sarcomas: Evidence for a cell-mediated host immune response to a common sarcoma cell-surface antigen. *J. Natl. Cancer Inst.*, 50:585.
3. Cortes, E. P., Holland, J. F., Wang, J. J., Sinks, L. F., Blom, J., Senn, H., Bank, A., and Glidwell, O. (1974): Amputation and adriamycin in primary osteosarcoma. *N. Engl. J. Med.*, 291:998.
4. Eilber, F. R. (1970): Sarcoma specific antigens: Detection by complement fixation with serum from sarcoma patients. *J. Natl. Cancer Inst.*, 44:651.
5. Eilber, F. R., Morton, D. L., and Malmgren, R. A. (1970): Immunologic factors in malignant melanomas, skeletal and soft tissue sarcomas of man. *Oncology*, 1:242.
6. Eilber, F. R., Holmes, E. C., and Morton, D. L. (1971): Immunotherapy experiments with a methyl-cholanthrene induced guinea pig liposarcoma. *J. Natl. Cancer Inst.*, 46:803.
7. Gottlieb, T. A., Baker, L. H., Quagliana, T. M., Luce, J. K., Whitecar, J. P., Senkovics, J. G., Rivken, P. E., Brownlee, R., and Frei, E. III (1972): Chemotherapy of sarcomas with a combination of adriamycin and dimethyltriazenoimidazol carboxamide. *Cancer*, 30:1632.
8. Hellström, I., Hellström, K. E., Evans, C. A., Hepper, G. H., Pierce, G. E., and Yang, J. P. S. (1969): Serum-mediated protection of neoplastic cells from inhibition by lymphocytes immune to their tumor-specific antigens. *Proc. Natl. Acad. Sci. USA*, 62:362.
9. Hellström, I., Sjögren, H. O., Warner, G., and Hellström, K. E. (1971): Blocking of cell-mediated tumor immunity by sera from patients with growing neoplasms. *Int. J. Cancer*, 7:226.
10. Holmes, E. C., Kahan, B. D., and Morton, D. L. (1970): Soluble tumor-specific transplantation antigens from methylcholanthrene induced guinea pig sarcomas. *Cancer*, 25:373.
11. Jaffe, N. (1972): Recent advances in the chemotherapy of metastatic osteosarcoma. *Cancer*, 30:1627.
12. Jaffe, N., Farber, S., Traggis, D., Geiser, C., Kim, B. S., Das, L., Frauenberger, G., Djerassi, I., and Cassady, J. R. (1973): Favorable response of metastatic osteosarcoma to pulse-high-dose methotrexate with citrovorum rescue and radiation therapy. *Cancer*, 31:1367.
13. Jaffe, N., Frei, E., Traggis, D., and Bishop, Y. (1974): Adjuvant methotrexate and citrovorum factor treatment of osteogenic sarcoma. *N. Engl. J. Med.*, 291:994.
14. Morton, D. L. (1973): Horizons in tumor immunology. *Surgery*, 74:69.
15. Morton, D. L., and Malmgren, R. A. (1967): Human osteosarcomas: Immunologic evidence suggesting an associated infectious agent. *Science*, 162:1279.
16. Morton, D. L., Malmgren, R. A., and Hall, W. T. (1969): Immunologic and virus studies with human sarcomas. *Surgery*, 66:152.
17. Morton, D. L., Joseph, W. L., Ketcham, A. S., Geelhoed, G. W., and Adkins, P. C. (1973): Surgical resection and adjunctive immunotherapy for selected patients with multiple pulmonary metastases. *Ann. Surg.*, 178:360.
18. Priori, E. S., Wilbur, J. H., and Dmochowski, L. (1971): Immunofluorescence tests on sera of patients with osteosarcoma. *J. Natl. Cancer Inst.*, 46:1299.
19. Rosen, G., Suwansirikul, S., Kwon, C., Tan, C., Wu, S. J., Beattie, E. J., and Murphy, M. L. (1974): High dose methotrexate with citrovorum factor rescue and adriamycin in childhood osteosarcoma. *Cancer*, 33:1151.
20. Sparks, F. C., Silverstein, M. J., Hunt, J. S., and Morton, D. L. (1973): Complication of BCG immunotherapy in patients with cancer. *N. Engl. J. Med.*, 289:827.
21. Sutow, W. W., Sullivan, M. P., and Fernbach, D. J. (1974): Adjuvant chemotherapy in primary treatment of osteosarcoma. *Proc. Am. Assoc. Cancer Res.*, 15:20.
22. Wepsic, H. T., Kronman, B. S., Borsos, T., Zbar, B., and Rapp, H. J. (1970): Immunotherapy of an intramuscular tumor in strain-2 guinea pigs. *J. Natl. Cancer Inst.*, 45:377.
23. Wood, W. C., and Morton, D. L. (1970): Microcytotoxicity tests: Detection of antibody in sarcoma patients cytotoxic to human sarcoma cells. *Science*, 170:1318.

DISCUSSION: OSTEOGENIC SARCOMA

Dr. LoBuglio: Dr. Taylor, it would be useful if you would comment in response to some of the chapters regarding explanations for your data.

Dr. Taylor: The problem in my mind is: Who do you study? In an institution which is using a lot of chemotherapy, those patients receiving surgery only represent a highly selected population.

I would recommend a task force type of approach to osteosarcoma in which pathologists, surgeons, and statisticians get together and standardize the definitions. This disease hasn't been properly studied at our place, and I suggest it hasn't been properly studied anywhere.

Dr. Gehan: I'd like to add a comment. The major issue here was: How should we proceed in future studies of osteogenic sarcoma? Should we be concerned about a trend for improved disease-free survival or overall survival and thus require a randomized group of patients to protect against just pure changes in trend, or should we try to do the best we can with the cases that are available with osteosarcoma in a nonrandomized series?

I do not know why the Mayo Clinic has observed an improving trend, but in any case, their results with surgery alone are not as good as that reported at M.D. Anderson Hospital with adjuvant chemotherapy or that reported in a number of other chemotherapy adjuvant series. Hence, it seems to me that one should take as a baseline, 60 percent disease-free at two years, and to try to find a series of cases that do significantly better than that.

Dr. LoBuglio: That's a very important point, because I think that is a question that's being asked nationally. Should we require a concurrent non-treated control in osteosarcoma? That's a difficult decision to consider when you look at the numbers, especially in regard to time to relapse, and even when you look at the numbers in terms of time to death of patients treated with adjuvant chemotherapy.

Dr. Eilber: I think the idea of concomitant controls is unrealistic in centers that are getting good results with adjuvant treatment.

Dr. Ritts: It's clear that the pathologists who are recognized to be expert in the area of bone tumors must develop a sense of agreement about what constitutes osteogenic sarcoma. These should be subjected to a panel examination to see what kind of reproducibility they have. We have done this with lung cancer with some very interesting and productive and occasionally shocking results.

There are other data on osteosarcoma from around the world, in Sweden, and in Gainesville, that show a time trend with improved disease-free intervals and survivals. We have to have some baselines to know what the benchmark is against which to measure the results of many of these studies. At the Mayo Clinic we are persuaded that the problem is not settled, and we are still disposed to think that contemporary controls are worthwhile.

Dr. LoBuglio: It's important to mention that this isn't a problem unique to osteogenic sarcoma. Unfortunately, as more work is done with adjuvant chemotherapy, the same questions are going to come up in regard to melanoma regarding definition of bad-prognosis groups. The same things are already happening in breast carcinoma. There are a tremendous number of therapeutic decisions being made and interpretations of clinical trials that will be markedly affected by this variability in pathologic criteria and interpretation.

Dr. Miké: I'd like to emphasize some of the points that have been made. It was just pointed out that until we can get together, we should have controlled studies. But which takes less time? Wouldn't the most important thing be to get together with all the pathologists who are actually reporting on the large series from the major centers before we introduce more and more confusion into the issue? Shouldn't that be done before carrying out more controlled studies which take several years at best? I would also like to point out that newer techniques for the application of covariant analysis prospectively and retrospectively to clinical trials are developing rapidly. If we could develop a computerized registry of all of these cases that all the major investigators at these institutions agree on, very powerful statistical techniques could be applied.

Dr. Frei: There is a major perturbation that's coming in from several centers and I think is going to make large-scale trials more difficult or make the interpretation of some of the osteosarcoma data even more complex. This relates to the limb-preservation surgical approach, prior to the introduction of adjuvant chemotherapy. This is being introduced at our institution, at Memorial, and I believe at M.D. Anderson.

In the limb-preservation approach, the primary tumor remains in place for a period of four to eight weeks. It is being reduced in size as a result of chemotherapy, but one worries whether the sensitive cells aren't being eliminated, and perhaps resistant cells are cut loose. That is a very big factor in affecting the natural history and potentially affecting the response to adjuvant treatment.

At the other end are the patients who develop pulmonary metastases, and I think Dr. Eilber's study and some of the others are very excellent ones. Dr. Jaffe has done a study of such patients. He decided to use the best of chemotherapy, the best of surgery, and the best of radiotherapy in an effort to create complete remissions in patients with metastatic disease. In the past 24 months, he has studied 21 patients, and in 15, he has eliminated all evident disease. He has continued, then, with adjuvant chemotherapy designed to eradicate microscopic metastases, and 12 of 15 remain disease-free. How that curve will go, I'm not sure, but it certainly has markedly affected the overall survival.

Dr. LoBuglio: Dr. Ritts, there is a study presently accruing patients in Texas where they are using combination chemotherapy with or without transfer factor. As an immunologist looking at this problem, would you envision this being the kind of approach that ought to be taken? Dr. Eilber has obviously made that decision because their group is using chemotherapy as the base treatment, and then half the patients are randomized to immunotherapy. Do you feel comfortable with that approach?

Dr. Ritts: Moderately. With transfer factor, as Hugh Fudenberg was implying, it would certainly be necessary to demonstrate some immunologic specificity. That is rather difficult to do *in vitro,* although one perhaps would be able to do it *in vivo.* We have not been able to do that, but we understand that Dr. Vera Byers has been able to, and we hope to attempt that. So we are attracted to the idea of immunotherapy in an adjunctive role, certainly, with minimal disease, and perhaps with appropriate timing with chemotherapy.

Dr. Spitler: I'd like to take up something that was implicit in the statement of Dr. Ritts about specificity of transfer factor. It has been assumed that transfer factor has to be specific, although a review of the literature shows that the evidence for specificity is very weak. It really hinges on the experiments of Lawrence with the transfer of homograft sensitivity in man, which has not been reproduced or attempted in any other laboratories. On the other hand, the evidence for nonspecificity is just overwhelming. Increased PHA response has been reported in many papers, as has increased mixed leukocyte activity, increased chemotaxis, nonspecific increase in skin-test reactivity, etc. I think it's really time we stop thinking that transfer factor has to be specific, and maybe we should look at it in another light.

Dr. Pinsky: I wish to support Dr. Spitler's comments. The evidence is overwhelming that transfer factor can act by nonspecific immunostimulation. What's more, it has virtually no toxicity. I think to exclude transfer factor from consideration in a combination therapy program on the basis that it doesn't demonstrate tumor-specificity seems to me to not have any good basis. I don't know why we continue to include or exclude transfer factor on such a basis.

Dr. LoBuglio: You notice Dr. Ritts did not.

Dr. Frei: I think one has to consider the evidence that most of the adjuvant studies are holding at about 60 percent disease-free survival with relatively little attrition between two and five years. That could mean cure, but it is too early to use that term. The background cure rate is 20 percent. Anyone considering a nonchemotherapy adjuvant control group must confront these facts.

Immunotherapy of Cancer: Present Status of Trials in Man, edited by W. D. Terry and D. Windhorst. Raven Press, New York © 1978.

Manifestations and Prognostic Features of Acute Myelocytic Leukemia

Rose Ruth Ellison

Department of Medicine, School of Medicine, State University of New York at Buffalo, Buffalo, New York 14263

Acute myelocytic leukemia (AML) is a heterogenous disease or group of diseases occurring primarily in adults, characterized by replacement of normal marrow elements by immature cells. A number of morphologic variants of acute leukemia have been included in discussions and descriptions of AML with the subdivisions based on the preponderant cell seen, i.e., myeloblastic, promyelocytic, myelocytic (or granulocytic), myelomonocytic (Naegeli type), and erythroleukemia. Monocytic leukemia (Schilling type) is often included in discussions of AML despite the feeling that a different cell of origin is involved. Morphologic subclassifications depend on the use of a Romanowsky stain supplemented by a variety of cytochemical procedures. Generally, the bulk of cases in any large series are those categorized as acute myeloblastic leukemia, with approximately a third of the cases falling into the category of acute myelomonocytic leukemia. A lesser number, usually in the range of 5%, are characterized as acute promyelocytic leukemia with about the same number diagnosed as erythroleukemia. A small number of patients have a marrow that is not predominantly blastic but may have from a quarter to a half of the cells appearing as myeloblasts. These patients often have morphologic abnormalities of the more mature granulocytic elements, suggesting that these too are leukemic cells. Such patients may be called AML by some and subacute leukemia by others. It is not clear that this is a prognostically separate group. Some of these patients are diagnosed as having leukemia after a long period of hematologic abnormalities not definitely diagnosable as leukemia. Patients may be labeled "preleukemic" retrospectively, after a florid picture of acute leukemia evolves. It would thus appear that subsumed under the term AML may be a disease with explosive onset or one with a very long prodrome, slowly evolving manifestations, and a course smoldering over many years.

AML is seen at all ages. Of 2,172 patients with AML registered by the Acute Leukemia Group B (ALGB) from its inception in 1956 through June, 1970, 17% were less than 20 years old at the time of diagnosis (4). The median age for those with AML was 49. No specific age peak is seen in absolute numbers but age analysis, based on the annual death rate per

100,000 at each age, indicates a rising incidence of AML with increasing age. No significant variation is seen in the month of diagnosis. In a number of series there has been a slightly greater incidence of male than female patients with AML.

AML is a disease in which the clinical manifestations are related primarily to the quantitative abnormalities of the marrow (decreased hematopoiesis) and to organ involvement by leukemic tissue with consequent functional abnormality. There are also, in some instances, qualitative changes in the function and behavior of various marrow elements. Anemia is a major abnormality in the course of the disease, although it is not necessarily present at the outset. Whereas 20% of patients with AML have hemoglobin concentrations of less than 7 g/100 ml at diagnosis, another 20% have more than 11 g/100 ml. There is great variability in the circulating leukocyte level and in the percentage of abnormal cells. Half of the patients with AML in one series had fewer than 15,000 white blood cell count/mm^3, and one-quarter had less than 5,000/mm^3. Very high white counts, more than 100,000/mm^3, occurred in less than 20% of those with AML. Those with more than 75% leukemic cells in the marrow generally had a higher white count than did those with lesser marrow infiltration. When the leukocyte level is elevated, the circulating cells are predominantly leukemic. In those patients with leukopenia, the circulating cells are predominantly lymphocytes. Circulating granulocytes may still be present, however, although the functional status of such cells may be questioned as well as their derivation from normal or leukemic stem cells.

The occurrence of quantitative or qualitative platelet abnormalities is the major cause of hemorrhage. Twenty-five percent of patients with AML have been found to have platelet counts of 25,000/mm^3 or lower at the time of diagnosis, with another 25% having platelet counts greater than 100,000/mm^3. Other coagulation abnormalities, particularly hypofibrinogenemia and disseminated intravascular coagulation, are seen predominantly in acute promyelocytic leukemia, although these abnormalities have been reported also in myeloblastic, monoblastic, and myelomonocytic leukemia.

Fever with or without obvious infection is frequently present at the time of diagnosis of AML. The presence of infection has been related primarily to the degree of neutropenia, but immune factors play a role. Impairment of cell-mediated immunity has been reported in some patients with AML, as judged by *in vivo* delayed hypersensitivity to skin testing and *in vitro* lymphocyte blastogenic responses to mitogens (12).

Leukemic infiltrates can occur in any and all parts of the body. Detectable hepatosplenomegaly or lymphadenopathy is present in 40 to 50% of patients with AML at the time of diagnosis. Splenomegaly is minimal in 20% but is marked (6 cm or more) in 10%. The degree of splenomegaly usually correlates well with the degree of hepatomegaly and lymphadenopathy. Massive lymphadenopathy, however, is not usual in AML. The degree of such organ involvement does not necessarily correlate with the number of circulating leukemic cells. Gingival swelling, due to infiltration by leukemic cells, is seen in any of the morphologic variations of AML but is more common in the myelomonocytic and monocytic varieties, as is infiltration of the skin by leukemic cells. Clinical meningeal involvement in AML is unusual early in the disease and develops in fewer than 10% of those with AML.

In the absence of the production of remission or after relapse from a hematologic remission, any of the previously described abnormalities can become manifest and proceed to the point of death. Although hemorrhage contributes significantly to the cause of death, infections are by far the most frequent cause. The disease is uniformly fatal at the present time, except, possibly, in rare patients who have survived for long periods without relapse. The median survival from the time of diagnosis was 2 to 3 months before effective agents for treatment were found. The median survival remained at 2 to 3 months even after drugs that produced remission were developed. Remissions are now in the 50% range in many series (5) with a variety of drug combinations (but always requiring intensive chemotherapy). The median survival in the best regimen of a recent ALGB study for patients with AML is now in the range of 1 year for those under 60, and 7 months for those over 60. Those patients who achieve a complete remission survive considerably longer than those who do not respond or have a partial remission.

Projection of survival for an individual is difficult. A workshop on prognostic factors in human acute leukemia (1) yielded relatively few criteria that were generally agreed on as being of prognostic value in AML. A recent review (17) again surveys this field. Many of the data analyzed in both reviews, however, represent series of patients in which the complete remission rate was in the 40% range for all with AML but was considerably lower in older adults. Currently used more intensive early therapy that aims at producing early aplasia of the leukemic marrow results in an overall remission rate of 50 to 60%, with response rates of 40 to 45% even among those over 60. It may be that further analysis of such cases will yield information relevant to prognostic features.

It is generally accepted that the gender of the patient with AML does not affect the outcome with regard to either the production of remission or the survival of the patient from the time of diagnosis. That age does affect the prognosis is also accepted by almost all investigators (6–8,11). The younger the patient with AML the better the prognosis for response rate and survival. It is possible that problems in older patients, particularly those over 60, are related to their inability to resist infection at the time of marrow suppression related to chemotherapy. Those under 40 do better than those ranging from 40 to 60 and, in turn, those 40 to 60 do better than those over 60. The choice of prognostic "cut-off" age varies with different investigators.

Type of leukemia seems to make much less difference, and in many series makes no difference at all. It has been said that patients with promyelocytic leukemia have a distinctly worse prognosis, presumably because of the special hemorrhagic problems (11). With the advent of more intensive therapy, particularly treatment with daunorubicin or doxorubicin hydrochloride (Adriamycin®), responses are probably seen equally in patients with promyelocytic leukemia, and it is not clear that patients with this disease fare any worse than do others. Erythroleukemia has been thought to be worse by some and to have a better prognosis by others. Some of the problems in judging this may be related to a prolonged period of preleukemia in some of the patients with this type of AML, leading to variability in the time of diagnosis. Myelomonocytic leukemia has been found by most to have a response rate and survival identical to that of typical myeloblastic leukemia (6,11).

Categorization by means of cytomorphology, cytochemistry, cytogenetics, and cytokinetics has lead to varied reports. Thus, Auer rods have been reported to be prognostically favorable by Levin and by Henderson (11). A relationship to various cytochemical staining reactions has been reported by Shaw (18) but has not been seen by Bennett and Reed (2). Analysis of chromosomes has indicated to Hart et al. (10) and Biran et al. (3) that those patients who are hypodiploid have a worse prognosis than others. Sandberg and Sakuri have found, however, that any type of aneuploidy is worse than the presence of a diploid marrow (14–16). Hart et al. (9) reported that a labeling index greater than 9% in the marrow cells gives a better chance of production of complete remission but does not favorably affect the median length of this remission. A correlation between the degree of maturation of marrow cells and the survival of patients has been found by some but not by others.

Freireich et al. (7,8) demonstrated that the presence of infection (defined as a fever of greater than 101°F) at the time of diagnosis was correlated with a significant decrease in complete remission and survival time. Analyzing a group of 424 patients (including 301 with AML), they found a complete remission rate of 53%, with a 44 week median survival in the 338 patients with temperatures lower than 101°F, but a complete remission rate of only 27% with a 9-week median survival in the 99 patients with a fever of 101°F or greater.

There have been many contradictory reports about the influence of the initial degree of leukemic involvement. Analysis by Freireich et al. (7) and subsequently by Gehan et al. (8) of the leukocyte level at the time of diagnosis in patients treated at M.D. Anderson Hospital for acute leukemia showed no influence of this parameter. Analysis of a group of 517 patients with AML treated in the ALGB indicated a wide range of survival when groups were divided on the basis of the initial leukocyte level (6). The best survival was seen in those with a white count ranging from 10,000 to 19,900/mm³. The worst survival rates were in those with either 50,000 to 99,900 leukocytes/mm³ or 0 to 1,900/mm³. These findings correlated with the response rates in the same group. Further analysis, looking at survival in groups defined both by leukocyte level and by age, showed that survival was affected adversely by a leukocyte level of 50,000/mm^3 or greater in those who were younger than 59, but no such variation was seen in those aged 60 and over, where all groups did poorly despite pretreatment white count. Analysis with these characteristics in mind has not yet been done in patients treated more recently with the intensive therapy that produces a higher remission rate in the elderly.

Analysis of the absolute number of circulating leukemic cells was not found by Freireich and Gehan to be predictive (7,8), although the presence of 50,000/mm^3 or more circulating leukemic cells gave the poorest survival in the ALGB series (6). There was no consistent variation with smaller numbers of circulating leukemic cells. Analysis of the percent of leukemic cells in the marrow in two groups of patients treated by the ALGB indicated a slight advantage in median survival for those with fewer than 75% leukemic cells in the marrow at the time of diagnosis, but this was not a major difference (6). Similar predictive value was not found by Freireich and Gehan (7,8), looking either at the percent of marrow infiltration or at a figure resulting from multiplication of a number representing the cellularity of the marrow by the percent of blastic cells.

The degree of organomegaly appeared to be of prognostic significance in some series, not in others. Henderson et al. (11), reporting on a group of patients treated at Roswell Park Memorial Institute, noted a decrease in survival for those patients with a liver palpable to 4 cm or more below the costal margin, and a lesser correlation between survival and splenomegaly. Gehan et al. (8) reported that patients with enlarged livers had shortened survival times and patients with enlarged nodes tended to have longer survival times. This group, however, contained individuals with both acute lymphoblastic leukemia (ALL) and AML, which raises a question about the significance of this observation for AML. Analysis of the ALGB data does not indicate such a correlation (6).

The hematologic changes that accompany the marrow involvement by leukemia do not appear to be of major prognostic significance. A slightly better survival curve was found in the ALGB patients for those with at least 100,000 platelets/mm^3 or 7 g/100 ml hemoglobin before treatment (6). Similar results were seen in the M. D. Anderson series for those with the same platelet level or with 12 g/100 ml hemoglobin before treatment (8). Other reports are not consistent. Surprisingly, there was no evidence of an orderly or rational variation in analyses of survival related to the absolute number of circulating granulocytes in the ALGB patients, although lower response rates and shorter median survival times were seen in those patients at M. D. Anderson with fewer than 300 or greater than 4,500 polymorphonuclear leukocytes/mm^3 (8). The latter finding does not fit with the clinical impression that patients who have problems with infection are primarily those with marked granulocytopenia.

Several studies have indicated a poor prognosis related to the presence of hemorrhagic tendencies. The stepwise logistic regression analysis conducted by Gehan et al. on the M. D. Anderson data (8) did not find this characteristic to be of major significance. Performance status has been found to be of prognostic value in several series. This has been shown specifically in the ALGB patients with regard to both the response rate and the survival time of the patients (6). A graded variation was seen in the survival, with the poorest occurring in those with severe or life-threatening symptoms and with major impairment of performance at the time of diagnosis. A poor performance rating is, admittedly, a rough value judgement that results from an aggregation of clinical phenomena that are the essence of the abnormalities resulting from acute leukemia. It may result from the presence of incapacitating sepsis, hemorrhage, anemia, or a combination of any or all of these.

Immunocapability of patients has been reported by Hersh et al. (12) to be decreased in a number of patients with AML. About a third have been found to be anergic. Those who are not anergic have fewer positive reactions to recall antigens than normal and may have decreased reactivity where any reaction is seen. The level of immunosuppression appears to be related inversely to the probability of production of complete remission (12,13).

A variety of other points have been reported to have some prognostic significance. Wiernik and Serpick found that obese patients had a poor prognosis (19). Others have reported a relationship between the period from first symptoms to diagnosis and the subsequent behavior of the disease, but these reports have not been consistent. Henderson et al. reported a variety of biochemical abnormalities that were of prognostic significance (11). A poor prognosis was associated with any of the following: an LDH above 500 units%, blood urea nitrogen greater than 30 mg%, serum uric acid greater than 12 mg%, any elevation of fasting blood sugar, and a serum calcium level of less than 9 mg%. Analysis of the rate and pattern of growth of leukemic cells in various types of *in vitro* cultures has provided contradictory answers. Biochemical characteristics of the leukemic cells have also not contributed to clinical prognostication in AML.

The major factor in prolonging survival in AML is the production of a complete remission, with a somewhat lesser prolongation of survival resulting from the production of a partial remission. This effect is seen at all ages studied. Production of these responses requires adequate treatment with an effective agent. Such treatment in almost all instances necessitates the production of marrow aplasia, preferably early. Specific analysis has not been made of the relationship between remission duration and presumptive prognostic factors. It is less clearly evident in AML than in ALL that the duration of the remission, once produced, is related to the intensity and frequency of maintenance treatment, but there are suggestions that this is so.

Finally, supportive therapy throughout the intensive treatment required for induction is essential. Changes in the availability of such supportive treatment over the years may result in changes in the percent of complete remission and therefore in the survival of patients regardless of any inherent variations in the patients that may be of prognostic significance. Thus, there is a major need for concurrent controls at this stage in the study of AML.

ACKNOWLEDGMENT

This work was supported in part by Grant CA16451 from the National Cancer Institute.

REFERENCES

1. Fliedner, T. M., and Perry, S. (editors) (1975): *Advances in the Biosciences, Vol. 14: Workshop on Prognostic Factors in Human Acute Leukemia.* Pergamon Press, Oxford.
2. Bennett, J. M., and Reed, C. E. (1975): Acute leukemia cytochemical profile: Diagnostic and clinical implications. *Blood Cells,* 1:101–108.
3. Biran, H., Hart, J. S., Trujillo, J. M., Freireich, E. J., and Liau, M. C. (1975): Pre-treatment (PreR) cytogenetic evaluation versus response and patient characteristics in Adult Acute Leukemia (ALL). *Proc. Am. Assoc. Cancer Res.,* 16:184.
4. Ellison, R. R. (1973): Acute myelocytic leukemia, In: *Cancer Medicine,* edited by J. Holland and E. Frei, pp. 1199–1234. Lea Febiger, Philadelphia.
5. Ellison, R. R. (1975): Management of acute leukemia in adults. *Med. Ped. Oncol.,* 1:149–158.
6. Ellison, R. R., Wallace, H. J., Hoagland, H. C., Woolford, D. C., and Glidewell, O. J. (1975): Prognostic parameters in acute myelocytic leukemia as seen in the Acute Leukemia Group B. In: *Advances in Biosciences, Vol. 14: Workshop on Prognostic Factors in Human Acute Leukemia,* edited by T. M. Fliedner and S. Perry, pp. 51–69. Pergamon Press, Oxford.
7. Freireich, E. J., Gehan, E. A., Speer, J. F., Heilbrun, L., Smith, T., Bodey, G. P., McCredie, K. B., Rodriguez, V., Hart, J. S., and Burgess, M. A. (1975): The usefulness of multiple pretreatment patient characteristics for prediction of response and survival in patients with adult acute leukemia. In: *Advances in Biosciences, Vol. 14: Workshop on Prognostic Factors in Human Acute Leukemia,* edited by T. M. Fliedner and S. Perry, pp. 131–144. Pergamon Press, Oxford.
8. Gehan, E. A., Smith, T. L., Freireich, E. J., Bodey, G., Rodriguez, J., Speer, J., and McCredie, K. (1976): Prognostic factors in acute Leukemia. In: *Seminars in Oncology, Vol. 3, No. 3: Prognostic Factors in Acute Leukemia,* edited by J. W. Yarbro, pp. 271–282. Grune & Stratton, New York.
9. Hart, J. S., Livingston, R. B., Murphy, W. I. C., Barlogie, B., Gehan, E. A., and Bodey, G. P. (1976): Neoplasia, kinetics, and chemotherapy. In: *Seminars in Oncology, Vol. 3, No. 3: Prognostic Factors in Acute Leukemia,* edited by J. W. Yarbro, pp. 259–270. Grune & Stratton, New York.
10. Hart, J. S., Trujillo, J. M., Freireich, E. J., George, S. L., and Frei, E., III. (1971): Cytogenetic studies and their clinical correlates in adults with acute leukemia. *Ann. Intern. Med.,* 75:353–360.
11. Henderson, E. S., Wallace, H. J., Yates, J., Scharlau, C., Rakowski, I., Ellison, R. R., and Holland, J. F. (1975): Factors influencing prognosis in acute myelocytic leukemia. In: *Advances in Biosciences, Vol. 14: Workshop on Prognostic Factors in Human Acute Leukemia,* edited by T. M. Fliedner and S. Perry, pp. 71–82. Pergamon Press, Oxford.
12. Hersh, E. M., Whitecar, J. P., Jr., McCredie, K. B., Bodey, G. P., Sr., and Freireich, E. J. (1971): Chemotherapy, immunocompetence, immunosuppression, and prognosis in acute leukemia. *N. Engl. J. Med.,* 285:1211–1216.

13. Konior, G. S., and Leventhal, B. G. (1976): Immunocompetence and prognosis in acute leukemia. In: *Seminars in Oncology, Vol. 3, No. 3: Prognostic Factors in Acute Leukemia,* edited by J. W. Yarbro, pp. 283–288. Grune & Stratton, New York.
14. Sakurai, M., and Sandberg, A. A. (1974): Chromosomes and causation of human cancer and leukemia. IX. Prognostic and therapeutic value of chromosomal findings in acute myeloblastic leukemia. *Cancer,* 33:1548–1557.
15. Sakurai, M., and Sandberg, A. A. (1973): Prognosis of acute myeloblastic leukemia —Chromosomal correlation. *Blood,* 41:93–104.
16. Sandberg, A. A., and Sakurai, M. (1975): The crucial role of karyotypes in the diagnosis and therapy of AML. *Proc. Am. Assoc. Cancer Res.* 16:185.
17. J. W. Yarbro (editor) (1976): *Seminars in Oncology, Vol. 3, No. 3: Prognostic Factors in Acute Leukemia.* Grune & Stratton, New York.
18. Shaw, M. T. (1976): The cytochemistry of acute leukemia: A diagnostic and prognostic evaluation. In: *Seminars in Oncology, Vol. 3, No. 3: Prognostic Factors in Acute Leukemia,* edited by J. W. Yarbro, pp. 219–228. Grune & Stratton, New York.
19. Wiernik, P., and Serpick, A. (1970): Factors affecting remission and survival in adult non-lymphocytic leukemia. *Medicine (Baltimore),* 49:505–513.

*Immunotherapy of Cancer: Present Status of
Trials in Man,* edited by W. D. Terry and D. Windhorst.
Raven Press, New York © 1978.

Immunotherapy for Acute Myelogenous Leukemia: Analysis of a Controlled Clinical Study 2½ Years After Entry of the Last Patient*

*R. L. Powles, *J. Russell, **T. A. Lister, **T. Oliver,
**J. M. A. Whitehouse,[1] **J. Malpas, *B. Chapuis,
**D. Crowther,[2] and *P. Alexander

*Divisions of Tumor Immunology and Medicine, Institute of Cancer Research, The Royal
Marsden Hospital, Sutton, Surrey; **the ICRF Department of Medical Oncology,
St. Bartholomew's Hospital, London, E.C.I., England*

In August, 1970 a study was initiated to determine if Bacillus Calmette-Guérin (BCG) and leukemia cells could be used for the treatment of patients with acute myelogenous leukemia (AML) during the remission phase of their disease. The first analysis of the results of this trial was published in 1973 (8) shortly before the last patient had been admitted to the study. It was found that the patients who had received immunotherapy plus intermittent chemotherapy during remission lived significantly longer than those who had received the same chemotherapy alone. Moreover, at that time, life table analysis indicated that immunotherapy produced a survival curve that had a tail indicating that some of these patients might be expected to have a very prolonged survival. The data available in 1973 also showed that the median length of the first remission for patients receiving immunotherapy was prolonged by 66%, but because of the variations in the remission length within the two groups the overall difference was not statistically significant at the 5% level. In this chapter we report the outcome of the follow-up of this trial for a further period of 2½ years. Since the trial was closed toward the end of 1973, this means that all the patients have been followed for at least 2 years. The historical background and scientific basis for this study has already been described (8).

TREATMENT PROTOCOLS

Patient Selection

All patients with AML who were first seen at St. Bartholomew's Hospital between August 10, 1970 and December 31, 1973 were included in the

---

* Reprinted from Powles et al. (1977): *Br. J. Cancer,* 35:265.
[1] Present address: CRC Medical Professorial Oncology Unit, Southampton University, Southampton, England.
[2] Present address: CRC Medical Professorial Oncology Unit, The Christie Hospital, Manchester, England.

study. Analysis was made of the data completed to August 7, 1975. Before any treatment was given to induce remission, all patients were allocated into one of two groups on an alternate basis to determine whether they would receive immunotherapy if they achieved remission. The total entry of new patients was 139. One hundred seven of these were included in the series described by Powles et al. (8), and the rest represent patients seen subsequently. The final allocation of patients who attained full remission was 22 to chemotherapy only and 31 to chemotherapy plus immunotherapy. These two groups do not have equal numbers because they were allocated when they first entered the hospital and the number in each group that attained remission happened not to be the same. Of the 31 patients allocated to immunotherapy, three have not been included in the analysis. One of these patients died of infection after attaining full remission but before immunotherapy was given, one patient was 74 years old and could not tolerate the repeated journey to and from the hospital, and the third patient only passed into remission while receiving the immunotherapy so it was felt she was not representative of the rest of the group.

Induction Treatment

The induction protocol of drugs (for details see ref. 8) consists of daunorubicin and cytosine arabinoside given in slightly modified ways (studies 2, 3, 4A, and 4B) (2,2a) Fifty-three patients passed into full remission so that the overall remisison rate during the trial period now stands at 38%. All patients in remission in studies 2, 3, and 4A received the identical maintenance chemotherapy described by Powles et al. (8), consisting of 5-day courses of cytosine arabinoside and daunorubicin alternating with 5 days of cytosine arabinoside and 6-thioguanine. Between every 5 days of treatment there was a 23-day gap, and it was during this period that patients received immunotherapy. The patients in study 4B were all aged over 60 years, and their maintenance chemotherapy consisted of 3-day courses every 2 weeks. All patients stopped maintenance chemotherapy after 1 year (12 courses); thereafter the immunotherapy patients received only immunotherapy and the chemotherapy patients received no further treatment.

Immunotherapy

Whenever possible immunotherapy was started just before complete remission at a time when the marrow was hypoplastic. In all instances subsequent marrow biopsies confirmed that these patients had achieved a full remission. The immunotherapy described in detail previously (8) consisted of weekly Glaxo BCG and 1×10^9 irradiated allogeneic myeloblastic leukemia cells given i.d. and s.c. and timed to avoid the 5-day courses of chemotherapy. All four limbs received the BCG in turn, one weekly, and the cells were injected into the other three limbs. The cells were collected in a manner described previously (10) using an NCI/IBM Blood Cell Separator and preserved in a viable state at $-179°C$ in the presence of DMSO (9). Individual patients received cells from the same donor for as long as possible.

Treatment After Relapse

When patients relapsed the initial induction treatment with daunorubicin and cytosine arabinoside was repeated whenever possible. If no regression of leukemia was seen, the treatment was usually changed to a combination of cyclophosphamide and 6-thioguanine. If remission occurred, then the maintenance treatment was modified to a single injection of daunorubicin and 3 days of cytosine arabinoside, followed 11 days later by 3 days of oral cyclophosphamide and 6-thioguanine. After another 11-day gap, the whole cycle was repeated with maintenance chemotherapy for 3 days every fortnight. Those patients who previously received immunotherapy were given further treatment with BCG and a different population of irradiated AML cells.

RESULTS

Tables 1 and 2 give the clinical details at presentation, the remission lengths, and the survival time for each of the patients in the two arms of the trial. At this time—August, 1975—five of the 28 patients in the immunotherapy arm remain alive although four of these have relapsed. Two of the 22 patients who received only chemotherapy are alive, both still in their first remission. The actuarial analysis of the duration of survival of these patients after attaining remission is given in Fig. 1. The median duration of survival of the chemotherapy group is 270 days and for the immunotherapy group 510 days. Statistical analysis of survival data calculated by the "log rank" nonparametric method (11) gives an overall Chi squared for the differences between these two groups of 4.48 and a p value equal to 0.03. One of the three immunotherapy patients excluded from the analysis died in remission at day 0, prior to immunotherapy, and the other two patients remained alive at the time of analysis at 465 and 655 days. Their exclusion therefore does not materially affect the analysis.

Figure 2 shows the actuarial analysis for the length of first remission, the median durations being 305 days for the chemotherapy plus immunotherapy group and 191 days for the chemotherapy only group. However, the overall difference between the two groups was not statistically significant at the 5% level.

The actuarial analysis of the length of survival after relapse for the two

TABLE 1. Clinical details of immunotherapy plus chemotherapy patients

Patient	Sex	Age	△	Presenting WBC × 109/1	Remission length	Days Survived from 1st remission	Survived after relapse
1	F	52	AML	1,100	313	546	233
2	M	49	AML	1,300	+1,648	+1,648	—
3	F	29	AMML	1,000	209	300	91
4	M	14	AMML	68,000	374	533	159
5	F	44	APML	29,000	417	462	45
6	F	52	AML	25,000	914	1,165	251
7	F	50	AMML	25,000	539	932	393
8	M	34	AML	1,900	622	952	330
9	F	23	AML	38,000	646	833	187
10	F	39	AMML	4,000	106	235	129
11	M	23	AML	23,000	253	687	434
12	M	55	AML	1,600	172	378	206
13	M	52	AMML	3,800	305	401	96
14	F	58	AMML	2,400	495	515	20
15	M	42	AML	8,100	84	168	84
16	M	37	AML	500	737	807	70
17	M	26	AML	7,200	43	251	208
18	M	25	AML	8,400	144	204	60
19	M	56	AMML	9,500	573	+911	+338
20	M	20	AML	1,400	80	124	44
21	M	59	AMML	95,400	116	280	164
22	M	23	AML	2,900	253	619	366
23	M	57	AML	1,700	666	+752	+86
24	F	30	AML	5,100	759	+787	+28
25	M	23	AMML	77,600	370	+821	+451
26	M	68	AML	27,500	91	300	209
27	M	61	EL	2,800	82	116	34
28	F	66	AML	11,100	229	270	41

AML, Acute myeloblastic leukemia; AMML, Acute myelomonocytic leukemia; APML, Acute promyclocytic leukemia; EL, Erythro-leukemia; WBC, White blood cell count.

groups of patients is shown in Fig. 3. The median values are 75 days for the chemotherapy patients and 165 days for the immunotherapy patients, and the difference between the two groups has a very high statistical significance (overall Chi square = 12.24; p value 0.0005). One-third of the patients in the chemotherapy plus immunotherapy group achieved a second remission, and those who did not had a prolonged survival when compared with chemotherapy controls.

DISCUSSION

Values and Limitations of Actuarial Analysis of an On-going Trial

The data from this study were analyzed at six month intervals starting in May, 1972 (i.e., 18 months after the trial was initiated); the survival of the

TABLE 2. Clinical details of chemotherapy alone patients

Patient	Sex	Age	△	Presenting WBC × 109/1	Days Remission length	Survived from 1st remission	Survived after relapse
1	M	49	AML	3,000	348	528	180
2	F	67	AML	4,500	119	194	75
3	F	45	EL	1,800	188	252	64
4	M	44	AML	1,800	217	403	186
5	M	63	AML	14,000	326	376	50
6	F	63	AMML	28,000	377	491	114
7	M	22	AMML	8,800	211	293	82
8	M	16	AMML	52,000	180	312	132
9	F	28	AML	800	129	304	175
10	M	19	AML	1,300	81	161	80
11	M	33	AML	133,000	76	129	53
12	M	42	AML	800	143	143	0
13	F	55	AMML	31,800	+1,019	+1,019	—
14	F	59	AML	1,100	468	497	29
15	M	65	AML	1,700	659	807	148
16	M	37	AML	84,000	191	219	28
17	M	26	AML	10,900	72	162	90
18	M	26	AML	32,000	48	161	113
19	M	58	AML	94,000	+885	+885	—
20	F	64	AML	2,200	209	261	52
21	M	64	AML	1,500	237	273	36
22	M	61	AML	1,500	55	93	38

AMML, Acute myelomonocytic leukemia; EL, Erythro-leukemia; WBC, White blood cell count.

immunotherapy group was plotted as raw data without actuarial correction (i.e., fixed interval) in Fig. 4 and after actuarial correction in Fig. 5. Only the actuarial method predicted the median survival. Thus, 6 months before the trial was completed (curve 2, Fig. 5) at a time when 80% of the patients were still alive and new patients were still being admitted, the median was accurately predicted. However, it required another 1 year after completion of the study (curve 5, Fig. 5) before it became certain, even with actuarial analysis, that the inclusion of immunotherapy in the treatment regimen did not lead to a significant deviation of the survival curves from the constant risk pattern in which all patients ultimately die of their disease, i.e., the treatment had not given rise to a subpopulation of patients who had become long-term survivors. Initially, the actuarially corrected curves indicated a tail and the possibility of long survivors (curves 3 and 4, Fig. 5); as time went on, it became clear that the fraction of patients in the tail progressively decreased (curves 6 to 8, Fig. 5). We must now conclude that although immunotherapy increases the median length of survival by approximately 90%, it does not change the shape of the survival curve, which is the same for both treatment methods and indicates that fewer than 5% of patients with AML treated by either of the two procedures in this trial are going to be long-term

SURVIVAL

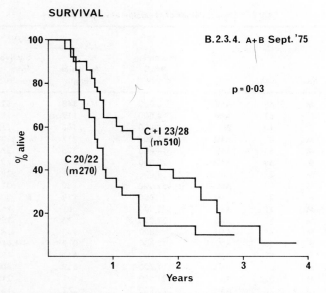

FIG. 1. Survival following remission of two groups of patients with AML (Bart's 2, 3, 4A, and 4B) allocated at presentation, one group receiving maintenance chemotherapy alone (C), the other group chemotherapy plus immunotherapy (C + I). The percentage surviving at different times has been calculated by standard actuarial methods. The vertical drops show the times at which individual patients died. Twenty of the 22 chemotherapy-alone patients and 23 of the 28 chemotherapy-plus-immunotherapy patients have died. Analysis of follow-up to August 7, 1975.

survivors. Currently (July, 1976) only one immunotherapy and two chemotherapy patients remain alive. Thus, although actuarial analysis reliably predicted the median duration of survival, it did not show whether or not long-term survival was probable for a subpopulation until long after the study was completed.

Mechanisms of Prolongation of Life by Immunotherapy

There is a high probability that adding immunotherapy to the intermittent chemotherapy given as a maintenance treatment during remission extended the length of survival of patients in our study. Two distinct components can contribute to this effect: (a) prolongation of the length of the first remission, and (b) extension of the length of survival after relapse. The present study did not allow us to decide if the length of the first remission was extended by the immunotherapy because the differences in the median of 60% were not statistically secure. The inability to resolve this aspect in this trial was due to the wide variation in remission lengths within each group, and thus the observed difference may have arisen by chance in view of the small number of patients in each group. It is, therefore, fruitless to speculate on whether the administration of BCG and leukemic cells during remission has produced in

REMISSION DURATION

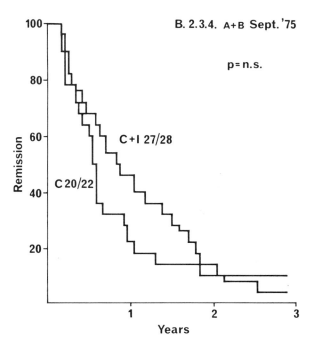

FIG. 2. Analysis similar to Fig. 1 of the duration of first remission of the same patients shown in Fig. 1. Two of the 22 chemotherapy-alone patients and one of the 28 chemotherapy-plus-immunotherapy patients remain in first remission.

patients with AML an effect like that seen in experimental animals, where similar therapies heightened the capacity of the host to contain residual malignant cells.

It is unlikely the prolongation of survival after relapse was caused by the immunotherapy increasing the immune reaction of the host against leukemia-specific antigens; it seems more probable that this effect was produced by stimulation of the bone marrow that permitted patients who had received immunotherapy and who had then relapsed to tolerate the high doses of cytotoxic chemotherapy necessary to constrain the disease. Such an effect has been seen in animal systems (3,14) and could be of importance because patients who relapse usually die from bone marrow failure. In this sense the outcome of our study was disappointing since we cannot tell if we achieved an effect of specific active immunotherapy. Furthermore, the chemotherapy regime used for this study was devised 6 years ago, and it is possible that current studies using chemotherapy alone may produce better survival results than our control arm and not differ significantly from our chemoimmunotherapy results.

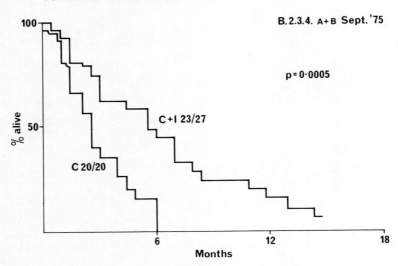

FIG. 3. Analysis similar to Fig. 1 of the duration of survival after relapse of the relapse patients shown in Fig. 2.

A group in Manchester (4) followed the same immunotherapy protocol used here, and although they did not carry out a controlled clinical trial they commented on the ease with which patients who had received immunotherapy but no maintenance chemotherapy achieved a second remission and also noted the long period of survival after relapse in this group.

Relative Contribution of Leukemia Cells and of BCG in Extending Life After Relapse

In many animal systems the immunotherapeutic effect achieved by systemic administration of BCG is much inferior to that produced by inoculation of killed tumor cells at multiple sites (6,7). However, the two procedures given simultaneously were found in some animal situations to act synergistically, hence we introduced this combined treatment of BCG and cells in this trial of immunotherapy. In view of the animal data, we did not feel justified in having an arm of treatment that contained only BCG. Unexpectedly, the treatment given as potential immunotherapy prolonged life after relapse, and we cannot resolve the question about the relative contribution of BCG and irradiated cells in bringing about this effect. It is possible that both components may contribute.

Vogler and Chan (13) gave a preliminary report of a trial in patients with AML, in whom they noted a prolongation of remission length with immunotherapy. However, a follow-up does not appear to have been published, and

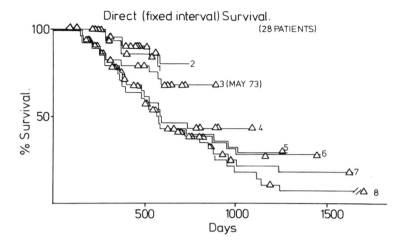

FIG. 4. Sequential six month analysis of the duration of survival (from diagnosis) of the 28 patients receiving chemotherapy plus immunotherapy in Bart's 2, 3, 4A, and 4B studies. The first analysis (curve 1)
was in May, 1972, curve 3 (May, 1973) corresponds to the entry of the last patient in the group, and
curves 4 to 8 are analyses at six monthly intervals thereafter. Triangles denote patients remaining alive,
and the curves drop each time a patient dies by an amount proportional to the total number of patients
in the study.

no data are available concerning the length of survival of patients who have
received BCG in remission in this study. Another investigation involving the
use of BCG in AML that was essentially similar to the trial reported by Vogler and Chan has been carried out by the Houston group (5). Although they

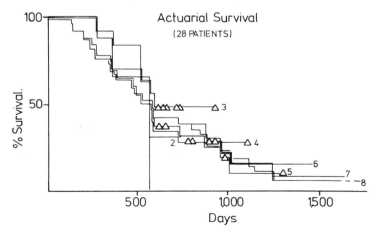

FIG. 5. The same patients have been analysed in the same way as in Fig. 4 except the standard actuaria
method of analysis has been used. Each time a patient dies the curve drops by an amount proportional
to the number of patients who have reached and had the chance to die at that moment in time.

claim a distinct benefit from the use of BCG in maintaining AML patients in remission, criticism of the statistical analysis and data in this study (12) must lead to reservations concerning the significance of these conclusions. More recently a controlled study by leukemia Group B in the United States (1) has claimed that neuraminidase-treated AML cells (with or without an extract of tubercle bacillus—MER), given to patients receiving chemotherapy has had a highly significant effect in prolonging remission when compared with patients treated with chemotherapy alone. Time must elapse before the significance of these three studies can be fully appreciated, particularly concerning the possibility of a group of patients becoming long-term survivors.

CONCLUSION

It is obvious that this trial has raised more questions than it has answered. From a clinical point of view, it is useful in that it has shown that a relatively atraumatic type of maintenance treatment, i.e., BCG and irradiated leukemia cells, extends the life of patients with AML, but without curing a significant number of these. To progress further in the treatment of AML by methods other than the use of cytotoxic chemotherapeutic agents requires that the nature of the reaction (if any) of the host against his tumor must be measured so that it can be determined if immunotherapy has a place for this aspect of the disease. The first requirement for such studies is to establish whether patients with AML are capable of reacting to a macromolecule in the membrane of their leukemia cells.

SUMMARY

One hundred thirty-nine untreated patients with AML were admitted between August, 1970 and December, 1973 and allocated into two remission treatment regimens; one to receive chemotherapy alone and the other chemotherapy with immunotherapy. Of the patients who attained remission, 22 were in the chemotherapy only group and in September, 1975 two remained alive, the median survival being 270 days and survival after relapse 75 days. Twenty-eight patients received immunotherapy during remission in addition to chemotherapy, and five remained alive; the median survival of the group is 510 days and the duration of survival after relapse 165 days. Ongoing actuarial analysis precisely predicted early in the study the median survival of the two groups, but it took a 2-year follow-up after entry of the last patient before it became clear that there were very few long-term survivors. The increase in survival length produced by the immunotherapy is apparently made up of two components—prolongation of the first remission and the length of survival after the first relapse. But it must be noted that the chemotherapy for this study was devised 6 years ago, and the results of the control arm (chemotherapy alone), may be poorer than those obtained in contemporary studies being conducted.

ACKNOWLEDGMENTS

We are indebted for support for this study to the Leukemia Research Fund, The Imperial Cancer Research Fund, the Joseph Frazer Strong Trust, and the Medical Research Council. We gratefully acknowledge that the late Professor G. Hamilton-Fairley initiated this study. The statistical analysis of this study was performed by Dr. Richard Peto of the D.H.S.S. Cancer Epidemiology and Clinical Trials Unit, Department of the Regius Professor of Medicine, University of Oxford, and we gratefully acknowledge his help throughout the study and with the preparation of this manuscript.

NOTE ADDED IN PROOF

The Medical Research Council of Great Britain has confirmed the results of the Barts Marsden study. The results will be published.

REFERENCES

1. Bekesi, G. J., Roboz, J. P., and Holland, J. F. (1976): Therapeutic effectiveness of neuraminidase treated tumor cells as immunogen in man and experimental animals with leukaemia. *Proc. Natl. Acad. Sci. USA. (In press.)*
2. Crowther, D., Bateman, C. J. T., Vartan, C. P., Whitehouse, J. M. A., Malpas, J. S., Hamilton-Fairley, G., and Bodley-Scott, R. (1970): Combination chemotherapy using L-asparaginase, daunorubicin and cytosine arabinoside in adults with acute myelogenous leukaemia. *Br. Med. J.,* iv:513.
2a. Crowther, D., Powles, R. L., Bateman, C. J. T., Beard, M. E. J., Ganci, C. L., Wrigley, R. F. M., Malpas, J. S., Hamilton-Fairley, G., and Bodley-Scott, R. (1973): Management of Adult Acute Myelogenous Leukemia. *Br. Med. J.,* i:131.
3. Dimitrov, N. V., Andre, S., Eliopoulos, G., and Halpern, B. (1975): Effect of Cornebacterium parvum on bone marrow cultures. *Proc. Soc. Exp. Biol. Med.,* 148:440.
4. Freeman, C. B., Harris, R., Geary, C. G., Leyland, M. J., MacIver, J. E., and Delamore, I. W. (1973): Active immunotherapy used alone for maintenance of patients with acute myeloid leukaemia. *Br. Med. J.,* iv:571.
5. Gutterman, J. U., Hersh, E. M., Rodriguez, V., McCredie, K. B., Mavlight, G., Reed, R., Burgess, M. A., Smith, T., Gehan, E., Bodey, G. P., and Freiriech, E. J. (1974): Chemotherapy of adult acute leukaemia. Prolongation of remission in myeloblastic leukaemia with BCG. *Lancet,* ii:1405.
6. Haddow, A., and Alexander, P. (1964): An immunological method of increasing the sensitivity of primary sarcomas to local irradiation with X-rays. *Lancet,* i:452.
7. Parr, I. (1972): Response of syngeneic murine lymphomata to immunotherapy in relation to the antigenicity of the tumour. *Br. J. Cancer,* 26:174.
8. Powles, R. L., Crowther, D., Bateman, C. J. T., Beard, M. E. J., McElwain, T. J., Russell, J., Lister, T. A., Whitehouse, J. M. A., Wrigley, P. F. M., Pike, M., Alexander, P., and Hamilton-Fairley, G. (1973): Immunotherapy for acute myelogenous leukaemia. *Br. J. Cancer,* 28:365.
9. Powles, R. L., Balchin, L. A., Smith, C., and Grant, C. K. (1973): Some properties of cryopreserved acute leukaemia cells. *Cryobiology,* 10:282–289.
10. Powles, R. L., Lister, T. A., Oliver, R. T. D., Russell, J., Smith, C., Kay, H. E. M., McElwain, T. J., and Hamilton Fairley, G. (1974): Safe method of collecting leukaemia cells from patients with acute leukaemia for use as immunotherapy. *Br. Med. J.,* 4:375–379.

11. Peto, R., and Pike, M. (1973): Conservation of the approximation $\Sigma(O - E)^2/E$ in the Logrank Test for survival data or tumour incidence data. *Biometrics,* 29:579.
12. Peto, R., and Galton, D. A. G. (1975): Chemoimmunotherapy of adult leukaemia. *Lancet,* i:454.
13. Vogler, W. R., and Chan, Y.-K. (1974): Prolonging remission in myeloblastic leukaemia by Tice-strain bacillus Callmette-Guérin. *Lancet,* ii:128.
14. Wolmark, N., Levine, M., and Fisher, B. (1974): The effect of a single and repeated administration of Corynebacterium parvum on bone marrow macrophage colony production in normal mice. *J. Reticuloendothel. Soc.,* 16:252.

Question and Answer Session

Dr. Terry: Could you tell us the actual median duration of survival and of survival after relapse?

Dr. Powles: Chemotherapy: 22 patients; two alive; median survival, 270 days; median survival after relapse, 75 days. Chemotherapy plus immunotherapy: 28 patients; five alive; median survival, 510 days; median survival after relapse, 165 days.

I don't think it's meaningful to give you the median remission lengths of those two groups, because we have to bear in mind it was a controlled trial and it was not statistically different.

Dr. Terry: Those numbers might be interesting to look at, though, relative to other studies to be presented.

Dr. Powles: For immunotherapy, 305 days; and 191 days for the chemotherapy. That's about a 60 percent increase.

Dr. Frei: Could you be a little more specific on the evidence that bone marrow function is better preserved in patients relapsing after immunotherapy?

Dr. Powles: No, the only evidence I can present is the hypothetical explanation for the difference between those two groups. In fact, from a scientific point of view, it has been rather disappointing.

I will give you two examples. One, there is certainly no difference in the blood counts of the patients in those two groups; and secondly, the animal model work of Nick Blackett. We gave mice 37 rads every day, to achieve a steady state where the animal in fact has normal blood counts, but its number of colony-forming cells, both committed and uncommitted, is about 10 percent of normal. When those animals were immunized with BCG, the number of committed and noncommitted colonies doubled. However, when we then challenged those animals with an LD-50 dose of either radiation or chemotherapy, there was no protection. So, as it stands at the moment, there is not a scrap of experimental evidence that supports the concept that immunotherapy is effective in protecting the bone marrow.

Dr. Holland: How do you count your survival? From the onset of chemotherapy? From the onset of diagnosis?

Dr. Powles: This is from the onset of remission. But, in fact, if analyzed from diagnosis it makes no difference. On an average patients required about 2½ to 3 months to go into remission.

Dr. Peto: Although I accept your conclusion that there is a difference in what happens after relapse, the group given only chemotherapy did worse than they ought to, didn't they?

Dr. Powles: There is some confusion here because, in fact, if you are looking at the medians—which is what we are interested in as far as survival after relapse is concerned—then the Barts 1 chemotherapy study was exactly identical to the Barts 2, 3, and 4 chemotherapy study. And the reason we were criticized when we presented these data in Paris was that we lumped together chemotherapy 1 with chemotherapy 2, 3, and a bit of 4. I do not think this is justified. In fact, I would say that as far as our studies are concerned, our chemotherapy arms have been remarkably consistent. These programs were designed six, seven, or eight years ago, and it may be that subsequent chemotherapy programs are better—this may mask an effect of an immunotherapy-plus-chemotherapy arm.

Immunotherapy of Cancer: Present Status of Trials in Man, edited by W. D. Terry and D. Windhorst. Raven Press, New York © 1978.

Effect of Immunotherapy on Survival and Remission Duration in Acute Nonlymphatic Leukemia

*P. Reizenstein, †G. Brenning, ***L. Engstedt, *S. Franzén, ††G. Gahrton, *B. Gullbring, †††G. Holm, §P. Höcker, *S. Höglund, ††P. Hörnsten, ‡S. Jameson, *A. Killander, D. Killander, **E. Klein, *B. Lantz, ***Ch. Lindemalm, ††D. Lockner, ‡B. Lönnqvist, †††H. Mellstedt, ***J. Palmblad, *C. Pauli, *K. O. Skärberg, ***A-M. Udén, **F. Vànky, and §B. Wadman

*Division of Hematology, Department of Medicine and Radiumhemmet, Karolinska Hospital, Stockholm; **Department of Tumor Biology, Karolinska Institute, Stockholm; Departments of Medicine, ***Södersjukhuset, ‡Huddinge Hospital and †††Serafimer Hospital, Stockholm; †Departments of Medicine, Akademiska Hospital, Uppsala; ‡Regional Hospital Örebro, Sweden; and §Ludwig Boltzmann Institute for Leukemia Research, Hanusch Hospital, Vienna*

In several experimental systems prophylactic immunization leads to marked resistance to tumor cell grafts. Once the tumor is established, however, efficient immunotherapy can rarely be achieved, although this is reported in the AKR leukemia system (1).

In man, several preliminary studies (3,4,7,14,23,24,28) suggest a positive effect. So do some more definite properly randomized studies (8,18). On the other hand, it has been reported preliminarily that no significant effect is being found so far in the randomized study conducted by the British Medical Research Council (13). There is thus a need for further properly randomized studies of the effect of immunotherapy on acute leukemia in man.

MATERIAL

Randomized Group

Six hospitals in the central part of Sweden participated in the study. Virtually all patients diagnosed as acute leukemia from this area of 1.9 million inhabitants are referred to one of these hospitals. Immediately after a confirmed bone marrow diagnosis, all patients under 70 years of age who had acute nonlymphatic leukemia reported to the randomizing secretary. Randomization, however, was performed only when remission had been achieved.

TABLE 1. *Subjects excluded prior to randomization*

No.	Initials	Sex	Age (yrs)	Reason for exclusion
1	E.M.	F	67	Glandular tbc
2	N.L.	F	36	Diagnosis based on peripheral blood alone, bone marrow samples lost.
3	G.P.	F	41	Left for Spain
4	W.P.	M	62	Distance to treating hospital
5	Ö.M.	F	56	Distance to treating hospital
6	H.I.	F	33	Diabetes, pulmonary insufficiency with respirator treatment
7	W.K.G.	M	66	Atrial fibrillation, rubidomycin discontinued, other chemotherapy.
8	L.F.	M	64	Distance to treating hospital
9	N.B.	F	66	Refused immunotherapy
10	E.M.	F	58	Distance and refusal
11	A.G.	F	58	Refused immunotherapy
12	A.T.	M	56	Distance to treating hospital

tbc, tuberculosis.

A total of 88 patients were registered; 42 remissions were obtained. However, only 30 of these patients were randomized to chemotherapy plus immunotherapy (CT + IT) or chemotherapy alone (CT). Twelve of the 42 patients could not be included for reasons separately described in Table 1. The CT + IT group contained nine men and seven women with a mean age of 49 years. The corresponding figures in the CT only group were seven, seven, and 49.

Nonrandomized Groups

As a first step a nonrandomized *pilot group* of nine patients (two men, seven women, mean age 54 years) was started on immunotherapy 6 to 224 days after remission had been induced in order to test feasibility, side effects, etc.

At the Ludwig Boltzmann Institut für Leukämie-Forschung at the Hanusch Krankenhaus in Vienna, 27 patients with acute nonleukemia (*Vienna group*) received the same chemotherapy, and in six instances, immunotherapy as described above (five men and one woman with a mean age of 33 years). Procedures were closely coordinated through repeated personal visits. Since randomization in Vienna was independent and based on the patient's birth date and since supportive therapy during relapse may have been different, these patients are considered in a separate group.

Partial Remission Group

Partial remission was defined as normal blood values and over 5% myeloblasts in the marrow. All patients in the randomized group were judged quantitatively, by the referring hospital, to be in complete remission. Later, marrows were reexamined with differential marrow counts. Complete remission was defined as less than 5% marrow myeloblasts. On reexamination three patients in the CT + IT group were found to have 5.2, 6.2, and 12% marrow myeloblasts, respectively, and were classified as partial remissions. Since they had been randomized as complete remissions, however, these three patients were not excluded from the complete remission group. In addition, they are included in a separate partial remission immunotherapy group. Six of the patients in the pilot group were in partial remission at the start of immunotherapy with 6.2, 6.2, 7.6, 7.8, 8.0, and 14.0% myeloblasts in the marrow, respectively, but it was not felt to be justified to exclude them from the pilot group. In addition, these patients are included in the partial remission group.

One later patient was not allowed to enter the randomized study since he was obviously not in complete remission. He had received all available chemotherapy, and was given immunotherapy despite incomplete remission.

In order to study possible prognostic differences between complete and partial remission, these 10 patients were thus examined separately in a partial remission group given immunotherapy. Five patients in the CT only group had 5.4, 6.0, 6.4, 7.6, and 8.6% myeloblasts and were classified as partial remissions. They were *not* excluded from the control group. The frequency of partial remissions was thus of the same order of magnitude in the CT only group (5/15), the randomized CT + IT group (5/14), and the total CT + IT group (9/30).

METHODS

Chemotherapy

Remission was induced in all patients with 5- to 7-day courses of treatment with rubidomycin (Cerubidine®, 1.5 to 4.5 mg/kg/course) and cytosine arabinoside (Cytarabin®, 10 mg/kg/course). If no complete remission was obtained with 4 to 6 courses of treatment, other cytostatic combinations were given. Supportive treatment during relapse has been described separately (9–11,15,16).

Remission was maintained in all patients with alternating monthly 5-day courses of rubidomycin (dose as above) and cytosine arabinoside (5 mg/kg/course) or cytosine arabinoside (dose as above) and thioguanine (10 mg/kg/course). A minimum of 4 days was allowed to pass after each chemotherapy course before any immunotherapy was given, and 14 days before any immunologic tests (17,20,21,26) were performed. During the week of chemotherapy, no immunotherapy was given.

Immunotherapy

Immunotherapy was given weekly as described (7,20) with 10^9 nonirradiated, viable, allogeneic myeloblasts thawed immediately before sub- or intracutaneous injection into three limbs and 10^6 Bacillus Calmette-Guérin (BCG, Glaxo) given intracutaneously with a multiple puncture technique into one of these limbs. This method is the same as that used by Powles et al. (18) in 1973 with two modifications: (a) viable, nonirradiated cells are used, and (b) cells and BCG are injected into the same limb.

Methods of leukemic cell harvesting and conservation are described elsewhere (17,26).

Actuarial median survival times and remission durations and Chi square tests for statistical significances were calculated by S. Ekblom, Statistical Research Group, University of Stockholm.

RESULTS

Randomized Group

In the randomized group, median survival, 20 months, was significantly longer in the CT + IT group than the corresponding value, 10 months, in the CT only group (Figs. 1 and 2, Table 2).

The statistical chance to stay alive was about 70% after 20 months in the CT + IT groups as compared to 0% in the CT group.

Ten of the 15 patients in the CT + IT group were alive at the time of evaluation (April, 1976) compared to only three of 15 in the CT group (Figs. 1 to 3).

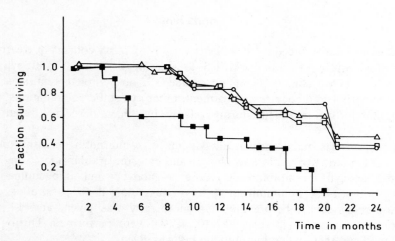

FIG. 1. Survival in randomized (O), randomized + pilot (□), and randomized + pilot + Vienna groups (△). ■, CT only.

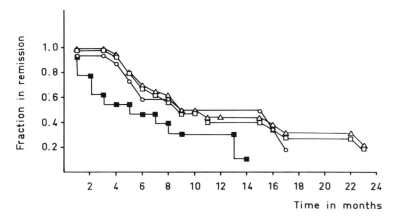

FIG. 2. Duration of first remission in randomized (○), randomized + pilot (□), and randomized + pilot + Vienna groups (△). ■, CT only.

TABLE 2. *Survival and remission duration—statistical significances between groups*

	CT + IT			CT only group (14 patients)
	Randomized group (16 patients)	Randomized and pilot groups (25 patients)	Randomized, pilot, and Vienna groups (31 patients)	
Approximate median survival, months	20–21	20–21	20–21	10–11
Degree of statistical significance of difference to CT group; $p <$	0.05 after 6–19 0.01 after 20 months	0.05 after 5 and 7–20 months 0.01 after 6 months	0.05 after 5 and 7–20 months 0.01 after 6 months	–
Approximate median remission duration, months	8–9	8–9	8–9	5–6
Degree of statistical significance of difference to CT group; $p <$	NS	0.05 after 3–4 months	0.05 after 14 months 0.01 after 3–4 months	—

NS, not significant.

Nonrandomized Groups

The median survival found in the randomized CT + IT group could be confirmed in two nonrandomized groups (Fig. 1). Good agreement was also found between the median duration of the first remission (8 months) in the randomized CT + IT group and the corresponding durations in the two nonrandomized groups (Fig. 2). This time (8 months) differs only numerically from the corresponding time in the randomized patients. If it is con-

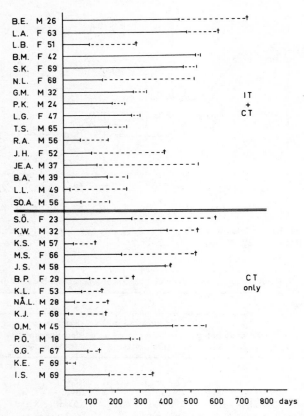

FIG. 3. Individual patient remission duration (—) and survival (----) in randomized CT + IT (*top*) and CT only (*bottom*) patients.

sidered justifiable to include the nonrandomized patients the difference becomes statistically significant (Table 2).

Partial Remission Group

Median remission duration and median survival were appreciably shorter numerically in the partial remission group, but these differences were not statistically significant (Fig. 4).

Complete Remission Group

When partial remissions were excluded from both CT alone and CT + IT subgroups in the randomized material, only 12 patients remained in the CT + IT group, and nine in the CT alone group, and the difference between

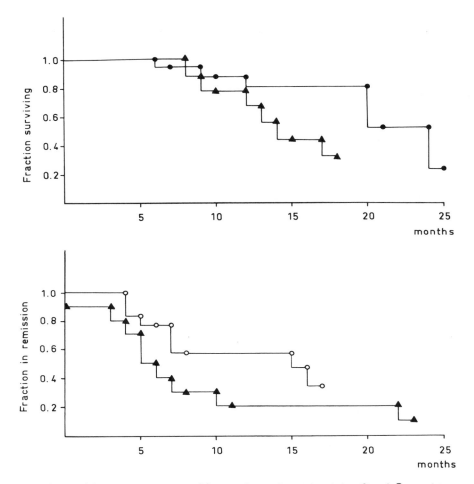

FIG. 4. Survival (A) and remission duration (B) in complete and partial remission. ● and ○, complete remission; ▶, partial remission.

the groups is no longer significant. However, even in these reduced groups, the numerical difference was fairly impressive (Table 3). In the CT alone group seven of the nine patients had died, whereas only four of the 12 given immunotherapy had died.

Side Effects and Quality of Life

A total of 30 patients (Table 2) have been given weekly immunotherapy; some patients up to 150 times. One patient developed a rash after a BCG injection, refused immunotherapy for 18 months, and remains well. Another showed anaphylactic symptoms after the cell injection, was given BCG alone

TABLE 3. *Comparison between patients in complete and partial remission given immunotherapy (randomized, pilot, and Vienna groups)[a]*

	Complete remission (19 patients)	Partial remission (11 patients)
Approximate median survival, months	24	14
Approximate median remission duration, months	15	6

[a] No statistically significant differences were found.

for 4 months, and remains well. For the rest, side effects, including short time local reactions, were surprisingly negligible or absent. No other patient raised the question of interrupting treatment.

Since viable cells were given immediately after thawing they were not washed, and the DMSO used for cell conservation was injected together with the cells. Possible DMSO side effects were followed, and they were virtually absent (12).

During the period of remission and immunotherapy, travel to the hospital where immunotherapy was given seemed to affect the quality of life far more than the treatment itself. Patients remained in their usual activities during treatment.

DISCUSSION

When immunotherapy was started, there was no firm evidence of the presence of antigens on the leukemic cells (19). Possible adverse effects of immunotherapy were feared because of the occurrence and perhaps over-emphasized role of immunologic enhancement. Immunotherapy was therefore started, with greater hesitations than expectations, chiefly because no alternative addition to conventional chemotherapy consolidation treatments was available that could perhaps prolong remission.

Our results confirm the beneficial effects previously reported in randomized (2,18,24) and nonrandomized studies (5,8,28). If one accepts that this justifies immunotherapy for patients with acute myeloblastic leukemia, it becomes necessary to consider the strategy of immunotherapy in order to make it available, under controlled conditions, to as many patients as possible. To do so, the mechanism of the effect of immunotherapy has to be examined (22). It is the preparation of cells that is most laborious. Some studies report appreciable effects of nonspecific immunization without cells (8,24,28), but contradictory reports exist (2). Some studies (2,24) use about monthly intervals between injections, whereas others use weekly intervals (18). It should be studied whether immunotherapy could be limited to only nonspecific stimulation and/or to monthly injections.

One of the differences between the present study and that by Powles et al.

(18) in the immunotherapeutic method was the use of viable, nonirradiated leukemic blasts. Irradiation and the preparatory work associated with it is a time-consuming procedure, and there is no evidence that patients given irradiated cells do better than the present group given viable cells. Another reason to select unirradiated cells in the present study was reports by Sjögren that irradiated polyoma cells failed to induce resistance. In a methyl-cholanthrene system, E. Klein found better immunization with viable than irradiated cells.

Do the present results really demonstrate an effect of immunotherapy on the course of the disease? A possible weakness in the design of the study is the difference between IT + CT and CT subgroups in the frequency of hospital visits during remission. The CT + IT patients were seen weekly, the CT patients less often. Conceivably this could facilitate the early detection of relapse and consequently the median life span, but it could hardly explain the difference in duration of the first remission.

Twelve patients were excluded from randomization. It is unlikely that these, who were fairly evenly distributed among the participating hospitals, could affect results. If they had been randomized, they would probably have been evenly distributed between the CT + IT groups.

An earlier group of leukemia patients treated by us had a median duration of the first remission and a median survival slightly longer than the present CT alone group (7,25). On the other hand, the present remission frequency (48%) is higher than the earlier one (39%) (6). This suggests that in the present remission group some initially weak and seriously affected patients are included, in which remission could not be achieved in the earlier studies. The present remission durations after CT alone agree better with published data than our earlier groups. The present median remission duration and median survival are longer in the IT + CT patients than in the previous groups (7).

ACKNOWLEDGMENT

This study was supported by the Swedish Cancer Society, grant no. 699–B76–04XA.

REFERENCES

1. Bekesi, G. J., and Holland, J. (1974): Combined chemotherapy and immunotherapy of transplantable and spontaneous murine leukemia in DBA/2 and AKR mice. In: *Recent Results in Cancer Research,* edited by Mathé, G., and Weiner, P., p. 357. Springer, New York.
2. Bekesi, G. J., and Holland, J. (1976): Immunotherapy with neuraimmunodase treated leukemic cells. *Proc. Am. Assoc. Cancer Res.,* 17:184.
3. Brenning, G. (1975): For Leukemia Group of Central Sweden. Chemoimmunotherapy in acute nonlymphatic leukemia in adults (in Swedish). *Sw. Physicans Natl. Conf. Stockholm,* p. 116 (Abstr.) Svenska Läkarsallskapet, Stockholm.

4. Engstedt, L. (1976): For Leukemia Group of Central Sweden. Immunostimulation treatment in acute myeloid leukemia. BCG + unirradiated myeloblasts (in Swedish). *7th Scand. Congr. Hematol.* Stanley Nielsen, Aarhus.
5. Freeman, C. B., Taylor, G. M., Harris, R., Geary, C. G., McIver, J. E., and Delamore, B. (1975): Maintenance of acute myeloid leukemia patients with irradiated allogenic leukemia cells and BCG. *3rd Congr. Haematol., Eur. Afr. Div., London,* p. 10:21 (Abstr.) Kent, London.
6. Gahrton, G., Engstedt, L., Franzén, S., Gullbring, B., Holm, G., Höglund, S., Killander, A., Killander, D., Lockner, D., Mellstedt, H., Palmblad, J., Reizenstein, P., Skårberg, K-O., Swedberg, B., and Udén, A-M. (1974): Induction of remission with L-asparaginase, cyclophosphamide, cytosine arabinoside, and prednisolone in adult patients with acute leukemia. *Cancer,* 34:427–479.
7. Gahrton, G. (1977): For Leukemia Group of Central Sweden: Maintenance therapy of acute leukemia in adults (in Swedish). *Finn. J. Med. Assoc. (In press.)*
8. Gutterman, J. U., Hersh, E. M., Rodriguez, V., McCredie, K. G., Mavligit, G., Reed, R., Burgess, M. A., Smith, T., Gehan, E., Bodey, G. P., and Freireich, E. J. (1974): Chemoimmunotherapy of adult acute leukemia with BCG. *Lancet,* 2:1405–1409.
9. Höcker, P., and Reizenstein, P. (1974): Calcium and potassium disturbances in acute leukemia. *Blut,* 29:398–406.
10. Höcker, P., and Reizenstein, P. (1975): Effect on platelet counts and fever of platelet transfusions in leukemia. *Blut,* 31:143–148.
11. Lantz, B., and Reizenstein, P. (1977): Management of septicemia in acute leukemia. *Acta Med. Scand. (In press).*
12. Lindemalm, C. (1976): Mild toxic effects of systematic DMSO in man. *Int. Res. Comm. Serov. Hematol. (To be published.)*
13. Lowenthal, R. M. (1976): Discussion. In: *Erkrankungen der Myelopoiese,* edited by A. Stacher and P. Höcker, p. 532. Urban & Schwarzenberg, Munich.
14. Mathé, G., Pouillard, P., and Laphyrague, F. (1969): Active immunotherapy of L₁₂₁₀ leukemia applied after the graft of tumor cells. *Br. J. Cancer,* 23:814–824.
15. Palmblad, J. (1972): Septicemia in acute leukemia (in Swedish). *Läkartidningen,* 69:4395.
16. Palmblad, J., and Wretlind, B. (1976): Fever and bacterial infections in acute leukemia. *Opusc. Med.,* 21:20.
17. Pauli, C. (1976): For Leukemia Group of Central Sweden. Lymphocyte stimulation with autologous myeloblasts in leukemia patients given or not given immunotherapy (in Swedish). *7th Scand. Congr. Hematol.* Stanley Nielsen, Aarhus.
18. Powles, R., Crowther, D., Bateman, C. J. T., Beard, M. E. J., McElwain, T. J., Russel, J., Lister, T. A., Whitehouse, J. M. A., Wrigley, P. F. M., Pike, M., Alexander, P., and Hamilton-Fairley, G. (1973): Immunotherapy for acute meylogenous leukemia given immunotherapy. *Eur. J. Cancer,* 13:3060.
19. Rapp, J. (1972): Immunotherapy of cancer. In: *Current Research in Oncology,* edited by C. B. Arhusen. Academic Press, New York.
20. Reizenstein, P. (1974): For Leukemia Group of Central Sweden: Immunotherapy, an attempt in acute myelogenous leukemia (in Swedish). *Sw. Physicians Natl. Conf., Stockholm,* p. 120 (Abstr.) Svenska Läkarsallskapet, Stockholm.
21. Reizenstein, P., Höglund, S., Lindemalm, C., Pauli, C., Lehtinen, T., and Sjögren, A-M. (1975): Lymphocyte recognition of myeloblasts and survival in myeloblastic leukemia given immunotherapy. *Eur. J. Cancer,* 13:3060.
22. Reizenstein, P., Lindemalm, C., Pauli, C., Udén, A-M., and Vanky, F. (1976): Lymphocyte recognition of blasts in myeloblastic leukemia. (Preliminary results on the frequency of spontaneous and immunotherapy induced reactions.) In: *Erkrankungen der Myelopoiese,* edited by A. Stacher and P. Höcker, p. 534. Urban & Schwarzenberg, Munich.
23. Skurkovich, S. V., Makhonova, L. A., and Reznichenko, F. M. (1969): Treatment of children with acute leukemia by passive cyclic immunization with autoplasma and autoleukocytes operated during the remission periods. *Blood,* 33:186–197.
24. Stupp, Y., Manny, N., Weiss, D. V., and Izak, G. (1975): Correlation between immunological capacity and clinical status; and combined treatment with MER and

chemotherapy. *3rd Congr. Haematol. Eur. Afr. Div., London,* 4:21 (Abstr.) Kent, London.

25. Udén, A-M., Brenning, G., Engstedt, L., Franzén, S., Gahrton, G., Gullberg, B., Holm, G., Höglund, S., Jameson, S., Killander, A., Killander, D., Lockner, D., Mellstedt, H., Palmblad, J., Reizenstein, P., Skärberg, K-O., Swedberg, B., Wadman, B., and Wide, L. (1975): L-asparaginase and prednisolone pretreatment followed by rubidomycin and cytosine arabinoside reinduction of remission in adult patients with acute myeloblastic leukaemia. *Scand. J. Haematol.,* 15:72–80.
26. Udén, A-M., (1976): For Leukemia Group of Central Sweden. Effects of immunotherapy and chemotherapy on immunocompetence. A study of patients with acute myeloblastic leukemia in remission. *7th Scand. Congr. Hematol., Aarhus.*
27. Visa, D. (1972): Immunological aspects of human leukemia. *Ser. Haematol.,* 87:108.
28. Whiteside, M. G., Cauchi, M. N., Paton, C. M., Foy, A., and Stone, J. M. (1974): Immunotherapy in the maintenance period of acute nonlymphatic leukemia. *XV Congr. Int. Soc. Hematol., Jerusalem,* p. 295 (Abstr.) Kenes, Jerusalem.

Question and Answer Session

Dr. Fudenberg: Have any laboratory parameters of immunologic status been measured to see if those with the increase in remission or survival have a rise in one or another aspect of macrophage function, B- or T-cell function, or something, which eventually wears out from being overstimulated?

Dr. Reizenstein: We have done a lot of tests and it's difficult to summarize them. I can say that by immunizing the patients with allogeneic cells, we have not been able to increase their immunity to autologous cells, nor have we been able to find any differences in the immunotherapy patients between those who have lymphocytes recognizing their autologous cells and those who don't. The difference between the immunotherapy and the chemotherapy groups is that spontaneous DNA synthesis in lymphocytes and T cells is higher in the immunotherapy group, and that the slight immunodepression caused by chemotherapy is not found in the immunotherapy group.

Dr. Powles: Following my thesis, would you speculate that you have seen the same pattern of response we have seen in our study, namely, that by far the most significant effect is survival after relapse? And, if so, could you give us some details about that?

Dr. Reizenstein: I would speculate that this is the case. I think our results confirm very neatly your results, but I don't want to speculate about the details at this time.

Immunotherapy of Cancer: Present Status of Trials in Man, edited by W. D. Terry and D. Windhorst. Raven Press, New York © 1978.

Immunotherapy of Acute Myeloid Leukemia

Richard Peto

Oxford University, Oxford OX1 3UD England

In 1973, a group of workers from St. Bartholomew's Hospital, London (Barts), reported that if acute myeloid leukemia (AML) patients already in remission were given chemotherapy plus immunotherapy, remission and survival were longer than had the same chemotherapy been given alone (1). However, the trial was small (44 patients, only half of whom had relapsed), the differences were only just statistically significant, and, although it is not clear whether any bias arose from this, the patients were allocated by *alternation* at first presentation and inclusion in the published trial only took place if and when remission was considered achieved. Even then, a few patients were excluded who had achieved remission but who were old or who died so quickly after remission induction that postremission treatment was never instituted. It was clearly necessary to duplicate the Barts trial on a larger scale, separating the patients by randomization only when remission was achieved and then following all randomized patients without exception. The British Medical Research Council (MRC) attempted to do so in a collaborative trial, and this chapter reports our results.

Details of remission induction, maintenance chemotherapy, and immunotherapy may be found in Powles et al. (1); the MRC trial attempted, with advice from Barts, to follow these exactly.

We referred to the chemotherapy used to maintain remission as B3 chemotherapy; it was straightforward, but the immunotherapy, which consisted of Bacillus Calmette-Guerin (BCG) and irradiated allogeneic blast cells, was technically difficult. Only three of the centers (Oxford, Hammersmith, and Birmingham) wishing to collaborate with this MRC trial had the technical facilities needed to obtain and irradiate the blast cells. Only the 71 patients achieving remission at these three centers could be randomized between B3 chemotherapy alone and B3 cheromtherapy plus immunotherapy. The AML patients presenting at the other centers who would normally be part of MRC collaborative trial could not be thus randomized, and so we have failed to achieve our primary objective of a large-scale randomized repetition of the Barts trial.

Some limited use may be made of the patients treated at the other centers, however, for in previous trials we have found that the prognosis of those AML patients who achieve remission is on average the same at the other centers as at the three "immunotherapy" centers and is not strongly correlated with age or with any presenting features of the disease that we have measured. Patients achieving remission at the other centers during 1973–1974 were randomized between B3 and another form of chemotherapy for remission maintenance, whereas those during 1974–1975 have all been given B3 chemotherapy in remission. The other centers, therefore, do provide us with a group of AML patients treated in remission by B3. This group of patients is of *some* interest, even though it was not separated from the immunotherapy group by randomization, because our randomized control series was very small.

PATIENTS AND METHODS

Our trial, therefore, consists of:

1. Seventy-one AML patients achieving remission at Oxford, Hammersmith, or Birmingham, randomized between B3 alone (24 patients) and B3 + I (47 patients), "I" being weekly immunotherapy continued indefinitely with BCG and irradiated allogeneic blast cells. These patients have been followed up to September, 1976; 57 have relapsed.

2. Seventy-three patients in remission at other centers, given B3. These patients have been followed up to January, 1976; by coincidence, 57 have relapsed.

I shall refer to these groups as randomized B3, randomized B3 + I, and nonrandomized B3. Unbalanced randomization, in which patients were twice as likely to be randomized to B3 + I as to B3 alone, was deliberate. Formal statistical comparison of two randomized groups is almost as powerful if a two-to-one imbalance exists as if equal balance exists, whereas informal comparison of the B3 + I group with other series is more reliable if the B3 + I group is larger. The statistical methods used are those described in the Medical Research Council's Report (4).

RESULTS

Because follow-up is not yet complete, in that some patients remain alive perhaps even in their first remission, the full number of relapses and deaths that will occur within, for example, 1 year of entry is still not known. Because of this, simple tabulation of the numbers of deaths or of relapses by time from entry might underestimate the percentages that will eventually prove to fail by those times, and in order to avoid this bias Kaplan-Meier actuarial estimates of these percentages must, therefore, be used instead of simple percentages. The tables (Tables 1–3) cite these estimated percentages for (a) the randomized B3 + I group (originally of 47 patients), (b) the randomized

TABLE 1. *Duration of first remission*

Days from randomization (i.e., from remission)	Estimated percentage still alive and in first remission[a]			Number still in first remission and still being followed up		
	(a) Imm.	(b) Chem.	(c) Chem.	(a) Imm.	(b) Chem.	(c) Chem.
0	100	100	100	47	24	73
100	77	75	77	36	19	57
200	53	50	62	26	12	46
300	47	33	47	22	9	36
400	40	33	44	17	7	32
500	29	29	34	10	6	22

Imm., immunotherapy; chem, chemotherapy.
[a] Kaplan-Meier actuarial estimate.

Logrank test comparing the two randomized groups (a) and (b) with each other:

Group	Observed number of patients who have suffered relapse*	Extent of exposure to risk of relapse*
(a) Immunotherapy	36	38.38
(b) Chemotherapy	21	18.62

Continuity-corrected Chi square $= 0.29$, $p = 0.59$.

* Or death during first remission.

B3 group (originally of 24 patients), and (c) the nonrandomized B3 group (originally of 73 patients).

The results presented in the three tables indicate that whichever index of failure is studied (duration of first remission, duration of overall survival, or

TABLE 2. *Duration of survival from randomization*

Days from randomization (i.e., from remission)	Estimated percentage still alive[a]			Number still alive and still being followed up		
	(a) Imm.	(b) Chem.	(c) Chem.	(a) Imm.	(b) Chem.	(c) Chem.
0	100	100	100	47	24	71
100	94	96	89	44	23	66
200	81	78	71	39	18	53
300	68	70	56	32	16	42
400	58	40	49	24	7	35
500	47	40	41	17	7	27
600	37	33	37	10	6	18

Imm., immunotherapy; chem., chemotherapy.
[a] Kaplan-Meier actuarial estimate.

Logrank test comparing the two randomized groups, (a) and (b), with each other:

Group	Observed number of deaths	Extent of exposure to risk of death
(a) Immunotherapy	28	30.10
(b) Chemotherapy	16	13.90

Continuity-corrected Chi square $= 0.27$, $p = 0.60$.

TABLE 3. *Duration of survival after first relapse*

Days from first relapse	Relapsed patients: Estimated percentage still alive[a]			Relapsed patients: Number still alive and still being followed up		
	(a) Imm.	(b) Chem.	(c) Chem.	(a) Imm.	(b) Chem.	(c) Chem.
0	100	100	100	34[b]	21	44
100	60	46	39	19	8	15
200	36	22	24	9	3	8

Imm., immunotherapy; chem., chemotherapy.
[a] Kaplan-Meier actuarial estimate.
[b] Two died while still in first remission.

Logrank test comparing the two randomized groups, (a) and (b), with each other:

Group	Observed number of deaths after relapse	Extent of exposure to risk of death after relapse
(a) Immunotherapy	26	29.25
(b) Chemotherapy	16	12.75

Continuity-corrected Chi square $= 0.87$, $p = 0.35$.

duration of survival among those who relapse) there is no substantial difference between the immunotherapy group and the other two groups. Moreover, comparison of the immunotherapy group with the randomized control group by a logrank[1] test (2,4) indicates that the slight differences actually seen could easily have arisen by chance.

DISCUSSION

No clear benefit attributable to immunotherapy has emerged from this trial, and unfortunately, although larger than the original Barts immunotherapy trial of which it is a rerun, this trial is not large enough for the nonsignificant results it obtains to be clearly interpreted. Although one could easily obtain such results if immunotherapy were without any effect, one could also obtain such results if, for example, immunotherapy doubled the duration of first remission. The apparent difference in the duration of survival after relapse is intriguing, but this too could be a chance finding.

It is noteworthy that the duration of first remission and of survival in both randomized arms of our trial and in the nonrandomized chemotherapy group of 73 patients is the same as among the immunotherapy patients in the original Barts trial and the same as for patients treated at Barts since the original trial was reported in 1973, all of whom have received immunotherapy.

The only group whose remission and survival experience differs from this

---

[1] If there is any real benefit from this form of immunotherapy, then a statistically significant difference between the survival times in the two randomized groups is more likely to be found if the logrank test is used than if any other statistical test is used.

common pattern is the small control group of chemotherapy in the original Barts trial. These 18 control patients fared much worse than all the other (larger) groups, either the chemotherapy- or the immunotherapy-treated patients. The outcome in the original control group led to the original report (1) that the immunotherapy-treated patients fared better. Although comparison of different series of patients is an extremely uncertain practice, such comparison does suggest that our finding of no difference may be nearer the truth than the original Barts finding of a substantial difference. However, larger randomized studies involving hundreds of patients are needed to discover whether any difference really exists, and these may never be done as the forms of immunotherapy involved are no longer the latest thing.

TOXICITY

Three BCG-treated patients have developed progressive infection. In each case, this was successfully controlled by isoniazid.

SUMMARY

The British MRC has duplicated the original trial of the immunotherapy of AML with BCG and irradiated blasts on a slightly larger scale, but failed to discover any significant benefit of such immunotherapy.

Seventy-one patients in whom remission from AML had first been achieved were randomized between chemotherapy alone and the same chemotherapy plus BCG and irradiated allogeneic blast cells. They have been followed for 1 to 3 years; 57 have relapsed, but no material or significant difference in the duration of first remission or survival has emerged.

ACKNOWLEDGMENTS

All MRC trials are achieved only by the collaboration of many centers and of the staff of the Trials Office.

NOTE ADDED IN PROOF

On follow-up experiments the differences in duration of first remission and of survival remained nonsignificant, but the difference in duration of survival after first relapse became statistically significant in favor of immunotherapy. This will be reported in greater detail in 1978.

REFERENCES

1. Powles, R. L., Crowther, D., Bateman, C. J. T., Beard, M. E. J., McElwain, T. J., Russell, J., Lister, T. A., Whitehouse, J. M. A., Wrigley, P. F. M., Pike, M.,

Alexander, P., and Hamilton-Fairley, G. (1973): Immunotherapy for acute myelogenous leukemia. *Br. J. Cancer,* 28 (Suppl. 1):365–376.

2. Peto, R., and Pike, M. C. (1973): Conservatism of the approximation $\Sigma(O\text{-}E)^2$ in the logrank test for survival data or tumor incidence data. *Biometrics,* 29:579–584.

3. Kaplan, G. L., and Meier, P. (1958): Nonparametric estimation from incomplete observations. *J. Am. Stat. Assoc.,* 53:457–481.

4. Medical Research Council (1977): The design and analysis of randomized clinical trials which require prolonged observation of each patient. Part III: Analysis. *Br. J. Cancer,* 35:1–39.

Question and Answer Session

Dr. Fahey: The results in a number of studies seem to be in a positive direction, but the difference is not significant. If you took all the studies, couldn't biostatisticians use the studies themselves as units of measurement, provided all studies were available for assessment?

Dr. Peto: You can do that as long as you combine the trials in some way that gives due weight to the larger trials. You can't just average out the *p*-values.

Dr. Powles: To confirm what Dr. Peto said in his chapter, I was on the Medical Research Committee all the way through the conduct of the trial, and there was no obvious deviation from the study compared to ours. I think that adds value to that study, but I would quarrel with the statement that in recent studies in chemotherapy one is getting a one-year survival of 53 percent, and that, therefore, adding immunotherapy is not realistic or fair. That study was done in 1969 and 1971. Those thirty-seven patients had a survival, as he pointed out, of 34 percent at one year. But the previous twenty-two patients in the Barts 1 study had an absolutely identical survival. If you look at the MRC chemotherapy study for that time, it is the same. So the benefit observed in our trial was certainly not due to the chemotherapy. It was the immunotherapy.

Dr. Mathé: Have you checked all the blood smears from all the centers? The heterogeneity of diagnosis is stronger than you may think.

Second, are the results the same in all centers as your overall results? When we examined the individual results in the big centers, we found differences between the centers which were larger than the differences of the therapeutic arms in some trials. This is the so-called dilution phenomenon in trials.

Dr. Peto: We get big differences between different centers in the number of patients who achieve remission, but once they've gone into remission we don't find differences between the centers. On the question of looking at the slides, yes, we did and they seemed to be comparable in distribution.

Immunotherapy of Cancer: Present Status of
Trials in Man, edited by W. D. Terry and D. Windhorst.
Raven Press, New York © 1978.

Comparison of Chemotherapy with Chemotherapy Plus VCN-Treated Cells in Acute Myelocytic Leukemia

James F. Holland and J. George Bekesi

Department of Neoplastic Diseases, Mount Sinai School of Medicine,
New York, New York 10029

Our work derives from that of Sanford (1), Lindeman and Klein (2), and Currie and Bagshawe (3). We have reported, as did they, that neuraminidase treatment of tumor cells serves as a technique of increasing their immunogenicity.

We have demonstrated this by resistance to challenge with viable leukemic cells after immunization against L1210 leukemia cells in DBA$_2$ mice (4). Delay in onset of spontaneous AKR leukemia was observed after immunization with neuraminidase treated AKR leukemic cells (5). We have also been able to accomplish chemoimmunotherapy in animals with established transplanted or spontaneous leukemia. In the murine system chemoimmunotherapy can lead to cures in as high as 90 percent of animals with L1210 leukemia compared to 20 percent with identical chemotherapy alone (1).

Based upon the discovery of reverse transcriptase in our acute myelocytic leukemia patients (7), suggesting the possibility that they might have a common surface viral antigen, we undertook to use allogeneic myeloblasts from patients with acute myelocytic leukemia in the immunotherapy of other patients with the same disease.

Our immunotherapy differs substantially from that of others who have described their activities herein. The eligibility requirements for donors with AML for the collection and storage of leukemic cells stipulated that the donor be previously untreated. Leukemic cells are harvested by continuous flow or batch centrifugation, and are free of greater than 5% granulocytes. An aliquot is analyzed for sialic acid content. The cells are subjected to programmed freezing, a decrease of 1°C per min until −30°C and then stored in the vapor above liquid nitrogen. Just prior to use they are thawed at 37°C, washed and purified by a modification of the technique of Wepsic on a 22 percent human albumin cushion. The nonviable cells are spun to the bottom and viable myeloblasts that exclude trypan blue remain floating. These myeloblasts are then incubated in neuraminidase, washed, and are used immediately for immunization.

In contrast to Simmons (9), our incubation is carried out for one hour at pH 5.6, which is the optimum for the enzyme. In the murine system, leukemic

347

cells are nonleukemogenic after they are incubated in neuraminidase. In no instance involving several thousand immunization sites in man have neuraminidase-incubated leukemic cells caused any evidence of tumefaction.

Patients are induced into remission with 7 days of continuous infusion of cytosine arabinoside, 100 mg/m^2/day, and 3 days of daunorubicin at 45 mg/m^2/day by rapid injection on days 1, 2, and 3 (8). Sometimes a second course of five days of ara C and two days of daunorubicin is required. After the first maintenance course of chemotherapy, which is ara C and 6-thioguanine, patients are skin tested for delayed cutaneous hypersensitivity to several common recall antigens, their lymphocytes are tested for mitogenic response to several stimuli, and then they are randomly allocated to continuing chemotherapy or to chemoimmunotherapy.

The immunotherapy consists of neuraminidase treated cells administered intradermally in multiple sites to provide readily accessible antigen. The antigenic load is at least tenfold more per month than that reported by other investigators. A random subset of the treated population also received cells plus MER.

A typical immunization pattern includes supraclavicular and infraclavicular sites, parasternal interspaces, lateral chest, suprainguinal and anterior thigh regions, chosen because these areas drain to different lymph node bearing sites. Originally, we chose the juxtaclavicular areas hoping we would find lymphadenopathy in the neck that would allow us to sample the node response by needle aspiration. The total intradermal dose is 10^{10} myeloblasts, split into about 50 sites of 2.0–2.5 × 10^8 cells each given every month midway between chemotherapy courses. Forty-eight hours after immunization, delayed cutaneous hypersensitivity is present. This may persist, as nonulcerative infiltrative lesions, for as long as several weeks. Microscopically, mononuclear, and lymphoblastoid infiltration of pyroninophilic cells is seen. We have not been able to identify the injected leukemic cells in these lesions (10).

Immunization with myeloblasts incubated in neuraminidase at pH 5.6 after thawing (our technique) and at pH 7 before storing in liquid N$_2$ (a technique used by others for other types of cells) shows a major difference in trial runs we have made. There is a deficit in delayed cutaneous hypersensitivity from the pH 7 cells, presumptively because of elution of antigen during preparation. Indeed, wash solutions have been able to stimulate lymphocytes *in vitro*. We conclude that optimal use of neuraminidase requires individual incubations at pH 5.6 after cell storage in the native state.

MER was given in a dose of 100 to 200 mcg in each of 5 to 10 sites. Reductions of that dose in patients who were substantially hypersensitive to it were made in arithmetic dilutions to a half dose or a quarter dose. Perloff et al. have reported a technique of MER dilution in nonleukemic patients, where reduction in MER dose by several log orders has been carried out, which we have subsequently adopted (11).

The protocol was originally designed for patients under the age of 60. Additional rigorous criteria were also stipulated. The results of the completely qualified group are shown in Fig. 1. Patients were all induced with exactly the same chemotherapy. The abscissa is in months. Curves are plotted from the beginning of immunotherapy, or from an equal time point for control patients. Immunotherapy began 2 weeks after the first maintenance chemotherapy course. Chemotherapy is administered as a maintenance course once a month, as twice daily injections of cytosine arabinoside for 5 days plus either thioguanine for five days, or cyclophosphamide in a single dose or a single dose of CCNU (in recent cases only) and then around the cycle again with ara C plus daunorubicin. Thirty-one additional patients have minor infractions, such as age over 60, failure to follow exact procedures for frequency of bone marrow examination and similar phenomena. Their remission data are shown in Fig. 2. Since the "disqualified" patients are not significantly different in outcome, the groups of patients are combined in Fig. 3 to illustrate all treated patients. In Figs. 1 and 3, the graphs show a line derived from the other centers of the Cancer and Leukemia Group B identical in induction and maintenance chemotherapy to the most recent subset. They are plotted in exactly the same fashion and represent the maintenance arm in the Group, and hence a contemporaneous population control. The subset of patients who received neuraminidase treated cells plus MER is also shown.

The characteristics of patients in terms of the initial leukemic marrow cells, the proportion over age 60, the median age, the percent who are males, the initial hemoglobin less than 8 g/dl, the initial platelets less than 50,000/ul, initial white count greater than 50,000/ul, percentage of circulating blasts greater than 75, and the percent of patients who responded to a single induc-

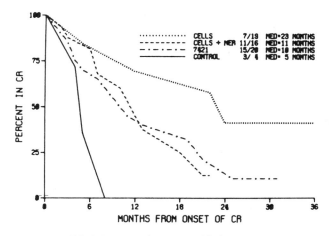

FIG. 1. Remission duration, qualified patients.

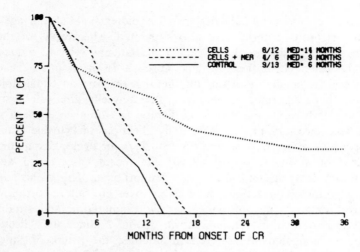

FIG. 2. Remission duration, disqualified patients.

tion course showed no major differences across the entire spectrum, demonstrating that patients were distributed quite evenly at random.

We were, of course, extraordinarily concerned about the MER patients who appeared to be less responsive than those with neuraminidase treated cells alone. Preliminary immunological data may help provide an explanation of the phenomenon. The delayed cutaneous hypersensitivity responses to PPD, mumps, candida, varidase and dermatophytin show little difference after five cycles of chemotherapy in the patients who received chemotherapy alone. Those who were immunized with neuraminidase treated cells showed an increase. Those immunized with cells and MER also show an increase.

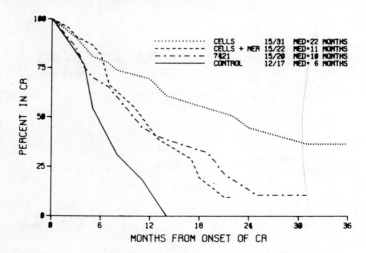

FIG. 3. Remission duration, all treated patients.

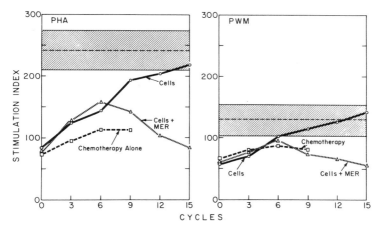

FIG. 4. AML: Lymphoblastogenesis from PHA and PWM mitogens.

Figure 4 is a composite of several patients at the different points. Of those who received chemotherapy alone, only a few remained for study after more than 6 months of chemotherapy. The PHA stimulation index rose slightly during the 6-cycle course of chemotherapy. Those who received chemotherapy plus neuraminidase treated cells are stimulated more persistently up to and including the 12th cycle of chemotherapy.

Those who received cells plus MER showed an early rise in PHA mitogenesis but subsequent decline, perhaps because we didn't change the dose of MER. In Fig. 5, a single patient is shown who is not included in any of the previous graphs. This particular man has completed more than 3 years of re-

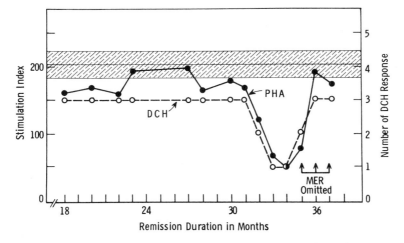

FIG. 5. Change of blastogenesis and DCH in patients who received cells + MER.

mission with cycles of chemotherapy and immunotherapy with neuraminidase treated cells plus MER. At about the 25th cycle, a substantial decrease in his stimulation index occurred; omission of MER rapidly brought this back to the original plateau. This can be interpreted in terms of MER also eliciting suppressor cell activity when given in excess dose.

In summary, we have developed a practicable method of harvesting, storing and using allogeneic myeloblasts. This involves incubation in vibrio cholerae neuraminidase under specific conditions. Immunization at monthly intervals with a large antigenic dose (10^{10} cells) in multiple intradermal loci (approximately 50) together with an interrupted regimen of chemotherapy led to significantly prolonged complete remission duration in controlled clinical trial. Addition of MER to the neuraminidase treated cell arm has not yet been advantageous.

ACKNOWLEDGMENTS

These studies were supported in part by NC1-NO1-CB43879, CA15936-04, and The T. J. Martell Memorial Fund.

REFERENCES

1. Sanford, B. H. (1967): An alteration in tumor histocompatibility induced by neuraminidase. *Transplantation,* 5:1273–1279.
2. Lindenmann, J., and Klein, P. A. (1967): Immunological aspects of viral oncolysis. Springer-Verlag, Berlin, pp. 63–66.
3. Bagshawe, K. D., and Currie, G. A. (1968): Immunogenicity of L1210 murine leukemia cells after treatment with neuraminidase. *Nature (Lond.),* 218:1254–1255.
4. Bekesi, J. G., St. Arneault, G., and Holland, J. F. (1971): Increase of leukemia L1210 immunogenicity by Vibrio cholerae neuraminidase treatment. *Cancer Res.,* 31:2130–2132.
5. Bekesi, J. G., and Holland, J. F. (1974): Combined chemotherapy and immuno-therapy of transplantable and spontaneous murine leukemia in DBA/2 and AKR mice. In: *Recent Results in Cancer Res., Vol. 4,* edited by G. Mathé, p. 357. Springer-Verlag, Berlin.
6. Bekesi, J. G., Roboz, J. P., and Holland, F. J. (1976): Immunotherapy with neuraminidase-treated murine leukemia cells after cytoreductive therapy in leukemic mice. *J. Natl. Cancer Institute,* #31.
7. Baxt, W., Yates, J. W., Wallace, H. J., Holland, J. F., and Spiegelman, S. (1973): A study of leukemia specific DNA sequences in the white blood cells of identical twins. *Proc. Natl. Acad. Sci. USA,* 70:2629–2632.
8. Yates, J. W., Wallace, H. J., Jr., Ellison, R. R., and Holland, J. F. (1973): Cytosine arabinoside and daunorubicin therapy in acute myelocytic leukemia. *Cancer Chemother. Rep.,* 57:485–488.
9. Simmons, R. L., Rios, A., and Lundgren, G., et al (1971): Immunospecific regression of methylcholanthrene fibrosarcoma with the use of neuraminidase. *Surgery,* 70:32–46.
10. Holland, J. F., and Bekesi, J. G. (1976): Immunotherapy of human leukemia with neuraminidase-modified cells. Symposium on Immunotherapy in Malignant Diseases. *Med. Clin. of N. Amer.* 60 (No. 3).
11. Perloff, M., Holland, J. F., Lumb, G. J., and Bekesi, J. G. (1977): Effect of methanol extraction residue of bacillus Calmette-Guérin in humans. *Cancer Res.,* 37:1191–1196.

Question and Answer Session

Dr. Terry: In your study, the median remission of the group receiving chemotherapy alone is rather short when compared to the results in other trials presented.

Dr. Holland: You must realize, though, this is expressed from the mid-point after the first chemotherapy maintenance course, which is probably 60 to 75 days from the initiation of chemotherapy for induction. The latter is the standard point of measurement, from the onset of induction therapy.

Dr. Terry: During the discussion, would it be possible to obtain remission and survival data tabulated from a common starting point for each of the studies? The question that Dr. Peto asked about whether or not we're looking at a particularly bad experience in a chemotherapeutic arm as opposed to a real improvement in an immunotherapy arm is quite germane to the discussion.

*Immunotherapy of Cancer: Present Status of
Trials in Man*, edited by W. D. Terry and D. Windhorst.
Raven Press, New York © 1978.

Viral Oncolysis: Its Application in Maintenance Treatment of Acute Myelogenous Leukemia

Chr. Sauter, *F. Cavalli, **J. Lindenmann, ***J. P. Gmür, †W. Berchtold,
††P. Alberto, †††P. Obrecht, and ††††H. J. Senn

*Division of Oncology, Department of Medicine, University of Zürich; *Division of
Oncology, University of Bern; **Division of Experimental Microbiology, Institute of
Medical Microbiology, University of Zürich; ***Division of Hematology, Department of
Medicine, University of Zürich; †Department of Biometry and Population Genetics, Swiss
Federal Institute of Technology, Zürich; ††Division of Oncology, University
of Genève; †††Division of Oncology, University of Basel; and
††††Division of Oncology, Department of Medicine, St. Gallen, Switzerland*

Augmentation of the immunogenicity of tumor-associated antigens (TAA) by infection with viruses has been shown in several systems (1–3,11,12). Enveloped viruses, mostly influenza viruses, were used for this purpose since the association of viral and host antigens at membrane sites is apparently important for the augmentation of tumor cell immunogenicity (10).

For the use of viruses as immunological potentiators in the immunotherapy of human neoplasms, the virus has to replicate in the tumor cells with the TAA in question. An avian influenza A virus (FPV) has been adapted to several types of human tumor cells including human leukemic myeloblasts (6,7,14,15).

Patients suffering from acute myelogenous leukemia (AML) seem, as soon as they have achieved complete remission by cytoreductive chemotherapy, an ideal population for immunotherapeutic trials—for three reasons.

1. Only a minimal residual tumor mass is left after the induction treatment.
2. TAA are reportedly present in AML (5,13).
3. By today's maintenance chemotherapy the median remission time is less than 1 year. Consequently results of additional treatments are seen within a short period of time.

The present randomized clinical trial was undertaken by the Swiss group for clinical cancer research to examine the effect of immunization by viral oncolysate (FPV-infected leukemic myeloblasts) in AML patients in remission.

PATIENTS

Patients suffering from AML treated in one of the clinics belonging to the Swiss group for clinical cancer resarch (oncological divisions of the clinics of Basel, Bern, Genève, Luzern, St. Gallen, Winterthur, and Zürich) entered the study for induction treatment. The patients achieving complete remission were randomized in two groups—group A and group A + IT.

1. Group A was treated with monthly chemotherapy alone.
2. Group A + IT was treated with the identical monthly chemotherapy plus immunization with viral oncolysate.

Table 1 shows the relevant facts of the patient population studied.

TABLE 1. *Characteristics of the 44 patients who entered maintenance treatment*

Group		A		A + IT
Number of patients		22		22
Mean age (years)		36.8		38.9
		(2–76)		(17–56)
Sex	F	5	F	15
	M	17	M	7
Average follow up per patient (months)		13.9		13.6

Group A was treated with monthly chemotherapy alone. Group A + IT was treated with the same monthly chemotherapy plus immunization with viral oncolysate. See text for further details.

TREATMENT

Induction Treatment

The induction treatment (done as part of a CALGB protocol) consisted of cytosine arabinoside continuously administered intravenously for 7 days at 100 mg/m^2 daily and daunorubicin at a dose of 45 mg/m^2 by direct injection on days 1, 2, and 3 as described by Yates et al. (17). If complete remission as defined by Ellison et al. (4) was achieved, the patients were randomized in one of the two regimens of the so-called Swiss maintenance therapy described below. If complete remission was not achieved, a second course of induction treatment reduced to 5 days' cytosine arabinoside and 2 days' daunorubicin was given. Those patients achieving complete remission now entered the maintenance protocol as well.

Maintenance Treatment

Patients in complete remission (4) were randomized in one of the two maintenance regimens—regimen A or regimen A + IT. Regimen A consisted of chemotherapy alone, whereas regimen A + IT consisted of chemotherapy (identical to that in regimen A) plus immunization with viral oncolysate.

Chemotherapy

Chemotherapy consisted of 5-day courses every 4 weeks of cytosine arabinoside 100 mg/m^2 every 12 hr. In each course one of the following four drugs was added—6-thioguanine (200 mg/m^2 daily for 5 days), cyclophosphamide (1,000 mg/m^2), 1,(2-chloroethyl)3-cyclohexyl-1-nitrosourea (CCNU) (75 mg/m^2), or daunorubicin (45 mg/m^2 daily for 2 days). This 4-month cycle was repeated until the end of the study.

Immunization with Viral Oncolysate

In addition to the maintenance chemotherapy described above the patients in group A + IT received, on day 15 of each 4-week cycle, 1.0 ml of viral oncolysate (0.2 ml i.c. and 0.8 ml s.c.), each month in another limb (counterclockwise starting at the right thigh). Allogeneic material was always given. One milliliter viral oncolysate was prepared from 10^9 leukemic myeloblasts as described (16). Briefly, leukemic myeloblasts were collected in an AMINCO cell separator (8) from untreated AML patients fulfilling the following criteria: (a) leukocyte count higher than 20,000/mm^3 with more than 70% leukemic myeloblasts, (b) platelets above 20,000/mm^3, and (c) no signs of infection. After dextran sedimentation the blasts were washed twice with Earle's balanced salt solution and adjusted to a concentration of 7 to 10 × 10^6/ml in Eagle's minimum essential medium. The leukemia cells were then infected with the leukemia-adapted myxovirus (7,15) (FPV: A/Turkey/ England/63/Hav 1/ Nav 3 /Langham strain) and incubated in roller bottles at 36°C for 48 to 72 hr. During this incubation period virus replication took place in the leukemia cells as checked by hemagglutinin and infectivity determinations (15). After inactivation of the virus by formaldehyde (0.02%) at 36°C for 15 hr, the viral oncolysate (cell debris plus FPV) was centrifuged for 30 min at 1,800 × g and for 60 min at 50,000 × g. The pellets were resuspended in phosphate buffered saline, 1.0 ml containing the viral oncolysate from 10^9 leukemic myeloblasts. The hemagglutination titer (as determined by World Health Organization standard procedure) of the final oncolysate was always between 10,000 and 20,000 hemagglutinating units per ml.

STATISTICAL ANALYSIS

Analysis of the remission duration and survival of patients was made by the method of Kaplan and Meier (9).

RESULTS

Induction Treatment

The results of the induction treatment are shown in Table 2.

TABLE 2. *Results of induction treatment of patients suffering from AML (August, 1974 to September 1, 1976)*

Patients entered	78
Patients achieving complete remission	44
Rate of complete remission	56%

Maintenance Treatment

The results of the maintenance treatment are presented in Figs. 1 and 2. After an average follow up period of 13.5 months, there is no significant difference between the groups A and A + IT with respect to the probabilities of staying in remission or staying alive. The calculated median remission time (9) is for both groups around 6.5 months. The calculated median survival time (9) is for both groups around 12 months.

Antibodies Against FPV

From the patients in group A + IT (receiving viral oncolysate) serum was taken every 4 weeks (just prior to the start of the next chemotherapy course) for determination of antibodies directed against FPV. The results are shown in Table 3.

Delayed type hypersensitivity skin reactions were observed in most patients already at the first injection of viral oncolysate.

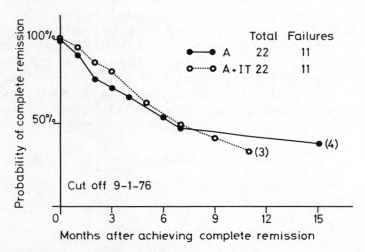

FIG. 1. Probability of complete remission of patients with AML (9). Numbers in brackets indicate number of patients in remission beyond the last failure—for A: 23, 23, 19, and 16 months of continuing remission; for A + IT: 22, 19, and 15 months of continuing remission. ●—●, group A (22 total, 11 failures); O---O, group A + IT (22 total, 11 failures).

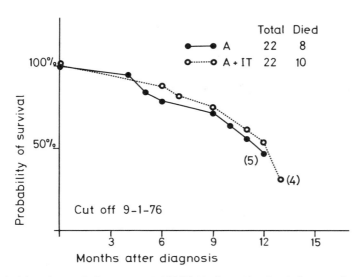

FIG. 2. Probability of survival of patients with AML (9). Numbers in brackets indicate number of patients alive beyond the last failure—for A: 24, 24, 23, 18, and 16 months; for A + IT: 24, 20, 14, and 13 months. ●—●, group A (22 total, 8 died); O----O, group A + IT (22 total, 10 died).

TABLE 3. *Antibodies directed against FPV in sera of patients receiving viral oncolysate (group A + IT)*

| Patient | Months in remission[a] | First serum with antibody | | Highest antibody titer[b] | Antibody titer of relapse[b] |
		Month	Titer		
BT	22+	3	40	640	
CE	19+	3	40	640	
MG	15+	2	20	160	
WH	11+	3	40	640	
BH	11	2	20	10,240	2,560
LA	9+	2	20	160	
GH	9	2	320	2,560	2,560
HJ	7	1	80	640	40
GM	7	2	20	1,280	1,280
BM	5+	3	160	160	
JW	5	3	40	40	40
MR	5	3	80	160	160
GM	5	3	40	160	160
BE	4+	3	40	40	
BB	3+	none			
AA	3+	none			
WH	3	none			none
WW	2+	none			
BH	2+	none			
HH	2	2	80	80	80
BK	2	1	20	20	none
CM	1	none			none

[a] +, Remission continues.
[b] Antibody titers are expressed as hemagglutination inhibition titers—highest serum dilution that inhibits hemagglutination of chicken erythrocytes by FPV.

SIDE EFFECTS OF VIRAL ONCOLYSATE

No side effects besides the local skin reactions were observed.

DISCUSSION AND CONCLUSION

This clinical study, which for the first time took advantage of the immuno-potentiating effect of myxoviruses in a randomized trial, did not show until now any beneficial effect of the immunization by viral oncolysates. On the other hand leukemia enhancement could not be observed either.

As with all immunotherapeutic trials two main questions have to be asked.

1. Were the patients immunocompetent?
2. Were there TAA present in the immunizing material?

The answer to the first question is certainly, Yes, since delayed skin reactions and antiviral antibodies (see Table 3) could be observed. The immunization with respect to viral antigens was successful at least after a few injections in most patients.

The answer to the second question might be, No. In animal experiments antiviral antibodies parallel tumor immunity (12), which apparently was not the case in the present study. This could mean that there were no TAA in the allogeneic immunizing material. TAA might therefore be specific—if present at all—for each individual AML patient .We plan therefore a pilot study where only autologous viral oncolysate will be applied.

SUMMARY

The present clinical trial was designed to study the effect of immunization by viral oncolysate (avian myxovirus-infected leukemic myeloblasts) in patients suffering from AML. From August, 1974 to September 1, 1976, 78 patients entered the study, which was conducted by the Swiss group for clinical cancer research in collaboration with the CALGB. Forty-four patients (56%) achieved complete remission by an induction treatment of cytosine arabinoside and daunorubicin. These 44 patients were randomized in two maintenance treatment groups—22 patients receiving monthly chemotherapy and 22 patients receiving monthly chemotherapy plus viral oncolysate. The viral oncolysate was prepared by infecting leukemic myeloblasts with a leukemia-adapted avian myxovirus (influenza A). Allogeneic material was used in all patients. After an average follow-up period of 13.5 months, there is no difference between the two groups with respect to the probabilities of staying in remission or staying alive. The calculated (Kaplan-Meier method) median remission time is for both groups around 6.5 months; the calculated median survival time is for both groups around 12 months. In a next trial viral oncolysate from autologous leukemic myeloblasts will be taken.

ACKNOWLEDGMENTS

This work was supported by the Ludwig Institute for Cancer Research, Zürich branch, the Universe Tankship, Inc., Zürich, the Hans Gröber Stiftung, Vaduz, and the Swiss National Foundation.

We thank C. Wolfensberger, E. Reinhardt, and R. Leemann for excellent assistance.

REFERENCES

1. Boone, C., and Blackman, K. (1972): Augmented immunogenicity of tumor cell homogenates infected with influenza virus. *Cancer Res.,* 32:1018–1022.
2. Boone, C., Paranjpe, M., Orme, T., and Gillette, R. (1974): Virus-augmented tumor transplantation antigens: Evidence for a helper antigen mechanism. *Int. J. Cancer,* 13:543–551.
3. Eaton, M. D., Heller, J. A., and Scala, A. R. (1973): Enhancement of lymphoma cell immunogenicity by infection with non oncogenic virus. *Cancer Res.,* 33:3293–3298.
4. Ellison, R. R., Holland, J. F., Weil, M., Jacquillat, C., Boiron, M., Bernard, J., Sawitsky, A., Rosner, F., Gussoff, B., Silver, R. T., Karanas, A., Cuttner, J., Spurr, C. L., Hayes, D. M., Blom, J., Leone, L. A., Haurani, F., Kyle, R., Hutchison, J. L., Forcier, R. J., and Moon, J. H. (1968): Arabinosyl cytosine: A useful agent in the treatment of acute leukemia in adults. *Blood,* 32:507–523.
5. Gallagher, R. E., and Gallo, R. C. (1975): Type C RNA tumor virus isolated from cultured human acute myelogenous leukemia cells. *Science,* 187:350–352.
6. Gerber, A., Sauter, C., and Lindenmann, J. (1973): Fowl plague virus adapted to human epithelial tumor cells and human myeloblasts in vitro. I. Characteristics and replication in monolayer cultures. *Arch. Gesamte Virusforsch.,* 40:137–151.
7. Gerber, A., Sauter, C., and Lindenmann, J. (1973): Fowl plague virus adapted to human epithelial tumor cells and human myeloblasts in vitro. II. Replication in human leukemic myeloblast cultures. *Arch. Gesamte Virusforsch.,* 40:255–264.
8. Gmür, J., Deluigi, G., and Straub, P. W. (1975): Improved granulocyte collection from normal donors by combination of continuous-flow centrifugation and filtration leukapheresis. *Transfusion,* 15:565–569.
9. Kaplan, E. L., and Meier, P. (1958): Nonparametric estimation from incomplete observations. *Am. Stat. Assoc. J.,* 53:457–481.
10. Lindenmann, J. (1974): Viruses as immunological adjuvants in cancer. *Biochim. Biophys. Acta,* 355:49–75.
11. Lindenmann, J., and Klein, P. A. (1967): Viral oncolysis: Increased immunogenicity of host cell antigen associated with influenza virus. *J. Exp. Med.,* 126:93–108.
12. Lindenmann, J., and Klein, P. A. (1967): Immunological aspects of viral oncolysis. *Recent Results Cancer Res.,* 9:1–75.
13. Powles, R. L. (1974): Tumour-associated antigens in acute leukemia. In: *Advances in Acute Leukemia,* edited by F. J. Cleton, D. Crowther, and J. S. Malpas. North-Holland, Amsterdam.
14. Sauter, C., Bächi, T., and Lindenmann, J. (1975): Human mammary carcinoma cell line: Infection by an avian myxovirus as a prerequisite for immunopotentiation. *Eur. J. Cancer,* 11:59–63.
15. Sauter, C., Baumberger, U., Ekenbark, S., and Lindenmann, J. (1973): Replication

of an avian myxovirus in primary cultures of human leukemic cells. *Cancer Res.,* 33:3002–3007.

16. Sauter, C., and Lindenmann, J. (1976): Virusassistierte Immunotherapie bei der akuten myeloischen Leukämie. In: *Erkrankungen der Myelopoiese,* edited by A. Stacher and P. Höcker, pp. 280–281. Urban & Schwarzenberg, Munich.
17. Yates, J. W., Wallace, H. J., Ellison, R. R., and Holland, J. F. (1973): Cytosine arabinoside and daunorubicine therapy in acute nonlymphocytic leukemia. *Cancer Chemother. Rep.,* 57:81–84.

Question and Answer Session

Dr. Sinkovics: We are doing similar studies with melanoma patients (M. D. Anderson Staging III and IV) and sarcomas. We use cultured allogeneic cells to make the viral oncolysate, and the PR-8-A influenza virus to infect the cells.

In a group of melanoma patients, who received chemotherapy and BCG, six of twelve progressed to death. Another group of 27 patients received the same chemotherapy, BCG and melanoma cell viral oncolysate. In this group, seven, or 26%, have progressed.

In the sarcoma group, 32 of 48 or 66 percent of the control patients have progressed to death. Another control group of metastatic sarcoma patients received chemotherapy and BCG, and four of the ten patients (or 40%) progressed to death. Fourteen patients with metastatic sarcoma received the same chemotherapy, plus BCG and viral oncolysates of sarcoma cells. In this group, two patients or 14 percent have progressed to death so far. This is a one and one-and-a-half year study.

Dr. Fahey: Would you like to comment from your experience on the report that has just been made?

Dr. Sinkovics: One dose of our oncolysate is made from at least ten million cells. We do not use purified virus obtained from the oncolysate; therefore, our preparation contains large amounts of cell fragments. We inactivate it with ultraviolet irradiation, rather than formaldehyde, and we use it more frequently, specifically on day 17 and day 24, in between 5-day courses of chemotherapy. Our program is more intensive.

Dr. Cavalli: We are not using purified virus either. We are using oncolysates, but we are treating them with formalin. After discussions three years ago with Professor Mathé, we felt that although this virus is not pathogenic for man, we did not know how patients with diminished immunoresistance would respond to such a virus, so we felt it was better to treat the oncolysates with formalin.

Dr. Boone: Picking up from the studies of Lindenmann and Cline on the increased immunogenicity of tumor cell membrane preparations from cultures that are infected with influenza or vesicular stomatitis virus, we confirmed the findings in a number of animal systems. But we also found that formalin fixation completely abrogates the immunogenic effect, whereas UV inactivation does not.

Dr. Cavalli: Professor Lindenmann did not find any difference with formalin.

Dr. Kay: When giving lymphoblasts, it is important to know how many sources the blasts come from. It may be that a fraction of cases of AML have an associated virus, which may be considered as a possible causative agent. Given that possibility, it is very important to know from how many different donors the blasts are drawn. Also, regarding statistical analysis, if there is reason to think only a proportion of cases will benefit, then very much larger numbers of cases must be evaluated in order to detect an effect.

Immunotherapy of Cancer: Present Status of Trials in Man, edited by W. D. Terry and D. Windhorst. Raven Press, New York © 1978.

A Randomized Clinical Trial of BCG in Myeloblastic Leukemia

William R. Vogler, Alfred A. Bartolucci, *George A. Omura, **Donald Miller, †Richard V. Smalley, ††William H. Knospe, and Alice S. Goldsmith

*Division of Hematology and Medical Oncology, Department of Medicine and Department of Biometry, Emory University School of Medicine, Atlanta, Georgia 30322; *Division of Hematology, University of Alabama School of Medicine, Birmingham, Alabama 35294; **Department of Medicine, Duke University School of Medicine, Durham, North Carolina 27710; †Department of Medicine, Temple University School of Medicine, Philadelphia, Pennsylvania 19140; and ††Section of Hematology, Rush-Presbyterian-St. Luke's Medical Center, Chicago, Illinois 60612*

In 1969 Mathé et al. (6) reported the success of immunotherapy in prolonging remission duration in acute lymphoblastic leukemia. Earlier these workers had demonstrated that in order for immunotherapy to be effective, the tumor burden must be low (7). In 1970 the Southeastern Cancer Study Group planned a protocol to determine if nonspecific immunotherapy with Bacillus Calmette-Guerin (BCG) given by the tine technique at a time when the tumor burden was low would be effective in prolonging the duration of remissions in patients with myeloblastic leukemia.

PATIENTS

Criteria for Patient Selection

Newly diagnosed patients over the age of 15 with acute myeloblastic leukemia (AML) and all variants thereof, and the blastic phase of chronic granulocytic leukemia (CGL) were eligible for study. The diagnosis was made from bone marrow aspirates by the investigator of each institution.

Criteria for Response

Patients were judged to be in complete remission or partial remission as previously reported (9).

For the Southeastern Cancer Study Group

TREATMENT SCHEDULES

The protocol consisted of three parts: induction, consolidation, and maintenance. Each part had two arms, and patients were randomly assigned as they entered each part of the study.

Induction Program

Schedules A and B

Schedule A consisted of a combination of cytosine arabinoside, 100 mg/m² by rapid intravenous injection and 6-thioguanine, 100 mg/m² by mouth. Both drugs were given every 12 hr for 10 doses. Schedule B consisted of the same two drugs as schedule A plus the addition of daunorubicin 10 mg/m² daily for 5 days intravenously once every 24 hr. Courses of treatment were repeated every 10 to 14 days if peripheral blood counts permitted. Courses were continued at these intervals as long as blasts persisted in the peripheral blood, however, if the white count fell below 1,000/cm and no blasts were present, a bone marrow was performed. If blasts persisted in the marrow, another course was given. If remission was not achieved after two courses of marrow hypoplasia, patients were switched to schedule D (see below). Those patients achieving complete remission were consolidated by one of two schedules.

Consolidation Program

Schedule C

The induction program was continued except that cytosine arabinoside and 6-thioguanine were given every 24 hr. Courses were repeated at intervals of every 3 weeks for six courses.

Schedule D

Patients were given vincristine, 1.4 mg/m², and cyclophosphamide, 600 mg/m² intravenously once, and methotrexate (MTX) 2.5 mg every 6 hr by mouth for 12 doses. Six courses were given at 2-week intervals. Patients relapsing on schedule C were switched to schedule D. Patients relapsing on schedule D were switched to the original induction program. If complete remissions were obtained in either of these categories, patients were placed on the maintenance program without further consolidation.

Maintenance Program

Patients remaining in documented marrow remission following consolidation were randomized between the following schedules.

Schedule E

Tice-strain BCG (Research Foundation, Chicago, Illinois) was given by the tine technique twice weekly for 4 weeks. The dose, approximately 3×10^8 viable organisms was administered via 288 puncture sites (72 per extremity). Two weeks following the last dose of BCG, patients were skin tested with purified protein derivative (PPD) and started on MTX 30 mg/m^2 twice weekly as a single dose by mouth.

Schedule F

Patients were given MTX 30 mg/m^2 by mouth twice weekly. Appropriate dose adjustments of MTX were made in each group depending on toxicity. All patients were followed to determine the duration of remission and survival.

STATISTICAL ANALYSIS

A Chi square test of proportions was used to determine the difference between remission rates for the induction arms. The generalized Wilcoxon test (2) was used for comparing duration of remission and survival curves. A p value of 0.05 or less was considered significant.

All cases were reviewed by the investigator and at least two members of the Southeastern Cancer Study Group for final classification of response.

RESULTS

From July of 1971 to April, 1974, 351 patients with AML and 21 patients with blastic phase of CGL were entered on this study. Of these 295 were judged evaluable, 284 with AML and 11 with blast phase of CGL. The total experience is given in Table 1. None of the patients with blast phase of CGL responded to treatment, and the protocol was closed to the entry of these patients after the first year. The remaining data are concerned solely with patients with AML. On schedule A, 37% of patients achieved complete

TABLE 1. *Total experience July, 1971 to April, 1974*

Number of patients entered on protocol	372
No data available	1
Not eligible	15
Protocol violations	42
Refused further treatment	10
Early deaths due to other diseases	9
Evaluable patients	295
AML	284
Blast crisis CGL	11

TABLE 2. *Results of induction program in AML*

	Schedule A		Schedule B	
	N	%	N	%
Entered	136	—	148	—
Complete remission	50	37	60	41
Partial remission	9	7	13	9

remission, and on schedule B, 41% achieved complete remission. These results are given in Table 2. Those achieving complete remission were entered on the consolidation program and were randomized to one of the two arms. There was no difference in relapse rates in the two arms. Fifty of 125 patients who were entered into the consolidation program remained in complete remission throughout six courses of chemotherapy. In addition, eight patients who either failed the initial induction schedule or relapsed during consolidation and were switched either to schedule D or back to the initial induction schedule achieved complete remission. These 58 patients were then entered on the maintenance program and were randomized to schedule E or F. As shown in Table 3 the distribution by prior schedules was comparable. The two groups were comparable by the time of onset of remission, sex, and age distribution. The median ages were 39 on schedule E and 32 on schedule F. Table 4 shows a median duration of response. The median duration of remission from the onset of the maintenance program was 24.9 weeks for sched-

TABLE 3. *Maintenance program—distribution by prior schedules*

Prior schedules		Maintenance schedules	
Induction	Consolidation	E	F
A	C	4	6
	C–D	0	1
	D	8	9
B	C	6	8
	D	7	7
	D–B	0	2
Total		25	33

TABLE 4. *Median durations (weeks)*

	Schedule E	Schedule F	p
Remission from onset	40.9	33.5	NS
Remission from maintenance	24.9	13.3	<0.05
Survival from diagnosis	93.2	78.1	NS

NS, not significant.

ule E and 13.3 weeks for schedule F. These differences are statistically significant ($p < 0.05$). The median duration of total remission was 40.9 weeks on schedule E and 33.5 weeks on schedule F. The differences are not significant ($p < 0.10$).

Survival

Table 4 also gives the median duration of survival in the two groups of patients. Those of schedule E survive 93.2 weeks and those on schedule F, 78.1 weeks. This difference in median survival is not significant. However, two patients initially treated on schedule F achieved complete remissions with reinduction therapy and were then placed on BCG treatment. If these patients are eliminated, the median survival on schedule E was 97.7 weeks and schedule F, 71.7 weeks, and this difference is statistically significant ($p < 0.05$).

It should be noted that the difference in remission duration between schedule E and F was 11 weeks, but the difference in survival was 26 weeks. In each group 12 patients obtained subsequent remission under various treatment programs. The median duration of subsequent remission on schedule E was 36.2 weeks and on schedule F was 22.1 weeks, a difference of 14.1 weeks. Thus it would appear that 1 month of BCG prolongs duration of subsequent remission, and this may possibly account for the prolongation in survival.

The actuarial plots of remission duration and survival are illustrated in Figs. 1, 2, and 3. Although the total curves reveal no significant differences between the two groups, if the curves are analyzed according to the time frames designated in the figures, significant differences do occur, and these appear

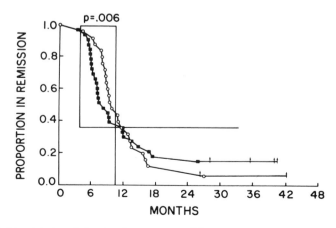

FIG. 1. Life table plot of remission duration as measured from onset of remission. The effect of BCG is noted in the first part of the curves. ○—○, BCG-MTX; ■—■, MTX.

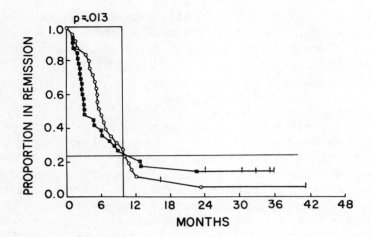

FIG. 2. Life table plot of remission duration as measured from the onset of the maintenance phase. The transient, but significant, effect of BCG is observed in the first part of the curves. O—O, BCG-MTX; ■—■, MTX.

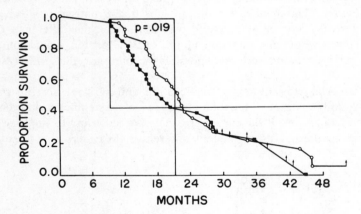

FIG. 3. Survival of those patients entering the maintenance program. The transient effect of BCG is observed in the first part of the curves. O—O, BCG-MTX; ■—■, MTX.

to be related to the time of BCG administration. One month of BCG therapy shifts the curve to the right, but this effect is transient.

TOXICITY

BCG administration produced granulomatous lesions at sites of inoculations. The major complaint of patients is that these were often quite painful, particularly those on the legs. In three instances, severe ulcerations occurred. One became infected with *Staphylococcus aureus* and required antibiotic therapy. Adenitis was observed in three patients. Local reactions were the only findings in 14 patients. Three complained of malaise, four had fever up to 101°F, and two had fever greater than 101°F within 24 hr after receiving BCG. Abnormal liver function tests were noted in two patients, and one developed jaundice, but it was doubtful that these were related to BCG. Liver biopsies done at a later date were inconclusive. Stomatitis occurred in 60% of patients receiving MTX and was judged moderate in 27% and severe in 2% of these patients.

Skin Test Conversion

Seven of eight patients tested converted PPD skin test from negative to positive following immunotherapy.

DISCUSSION

Immunotherapy appears to represent a significant advance in the management of patients with AML. The number of controlled clinical trials are few, but all evidence points toward immunotherapy being a useful treatment in AML (1,8). This is in contrast to the results of lymphoblastic leukemia (4,5). In a study reported by Gutterman et al., using historical controls, immunotherapy combined with chemotherapy in adult acute leukemia significantly prolongs survival (3). Powles et al. (8) induced remission with daunorubicin and cytosine arabinoside, and during remission patients were treated with alternating courses of daunorubicin and cytosine arabinoside and thioguanine and cytosine arabinoside every 28 days. Half of these patients received immunotherapy consisting of Glaxo BCG 1×10^6 viable organisms plus irradiated leukemic cells weekly. Their results showed remission duration of 27 weeks with the chemotherapy group and a median survival of 43 weeks. In contrast 23 patients receiving immunotherapy had remission duration of 45 weeks and survival of 68 weeks. These differences were highly significant. Our data indicate that 1 month of BCG therapy prolongs remission duration approximately 10 to 12 weeks. Obviously this is unsatisfactory in treating acute leukemia. Considerable questions arise as to proper scheduling. The use of allogeneic leukemic cells with or without neuraminidase treatment and the use of different preparation of BCG or extracts of BCG (MER[1]) are being investigated. It is through planned, controlled, clinical trials that further advances can be anticipated in immunotherapy of leukemia.

SUMMARY

Sixteen institutions of the Southeastern Cancer Study Group participated in a randomized trial of Tice strain BCG administered by the tine technique

---

[1] Methanol extractable residue.

to adults with AML in remission. At diagnosis patients were randomly assigned to receive 5-day courses of cytosine arabinoside and 6-thioguanine or the same drugs plus the addition of daunorubicin. Those achieving remissions were rerandomized to receive six courses of consolidation, either with the same drugs or three different drugs—vincristine, MTX, and cyclophosphamide. Those completing consolidation and still in remission were randomized to receive either BCG twice weekly for 4 weeks, followed by MTX maintenance therapy (25 evaluable patients) or MTX alone (33 evaluable patients). The median duration of remission from onset of the maintenance phase was 24.9 weeks in the BCG-MTX group and 13.3 weeks in the MTX group ($p < 0.05$). The median duration of survival was 93.2 weeks in the BCG-MTX group and 78.1 weeks in the MTX group ($p < 0.10$). Although the 4-year survival curves were similar, when analyzed for the first 20 months of the study, a significantly greater proportion ($p < 0.05$) survived in the BCG-MTX group.

The results indicate that a short course of BCG prolongs remission duration and survival in myeloblastic leukemia.

ACKNOWLEDGMENTS

This investigation was supported by the following grant numbers awarded by the National Cancer Institute, Department of Health, Education and Welfare, to the following institutions: CA-03013 to University of Alabama School of Medicine, Birmingham, Alabama; CA-03177 to Duke University School of Medicine, Durham, North Carolina; CA-03227 and CA-11263 to Emory University School of Medicine, Atlanta, Georgia; CA-05641 to University of Miami School of Medicine, Miami, Florida; CA-12639 to Presbyterian University of Pennsylvania Medical Center, Philadelphia, Pennsylvania; CA-06807 to Medical College of Georgia, Augusta, Georgia; CA-07961 to Temple University School of Medicine, Philadelphia, Pennsylvania; CA-03376 to Washington University School of Medicine, St. Louis, Missouri; CA-12223 to University of Puerto Rico School of Medicine, San Juan, Puerto Rico; CA-12640 to Rush-Presbyterian-St. Luke's Medical Center, Chicago, Illinois; CA-13237 to University of Tennessee Memorial Research Center, Knoxville, Tennessee; CA-13249 to New Orleans Veterans Administration Hospital, New Orleans, Louisiana; CA-15584 to Case Western Reserve University School of Medicine, Cleveland, Ohio; CA-15578 to Ochsner Clinic, New Orleans, Louisiana; CA-17027 to University of Tennessee School of Medicine, Memphis, Tennessee; and CA-17214 to St. Louis University School of Medicine, St. Louis, Missouri.

Daunorubicin and MTX (50-mg tablets) were supplied by Cancer Therapy Evaluation, Division of Cancer Treatment, National Cancer Institute.

BCG vaccine (Tice strain) was supplied by Research Foundation, Chicago, Illinois.

REFERENCES

1. Bekesi, J. G., Holland, J. F., Cuttner, J., Silver, R., Coleman, M., Janowski, C., and Vincequerra, V. (1976): Immunotherapy in acute myeloblastic leukemia with neuraminidase treated allogeneic myeloblasts with or without MER. *Proc Am. Assoc. Cancer Res.,* 17:184.
2. Gehan, E. A. (1965): A generalized Wilcoxon Test for comparing arbitrarily singly-censored samples. *Biometrika,* 52:203–223.
3. Gutterman, J. U., Hersh, E. M., Rodriquex, V., Mavligit, G., Burges, M. A.,eTr3Mif Gehan, E., McCredie, K. B., Reed, R., Smith, T., Bodey, F. P., Sr., and Freireich, E. J. (1974): Chemoimmunotherapy of adult acute leukemia. Prolongation of remission in myeloblastic leukaemia with BCG. Lancet, II: 1405–1409.
4. Heyn, R. M., Joo, P., Karon, M., Nesbit, M., Shore, N., Breslow, N., Weiner, J., Reed, A., and Hammond, D. (1975): BCG in the treatment of acute lymphocytic leukemia. *Blood,* 46:431–442.
5. Leukaemia Committee and the Working Party on Leukaemia in Childhood. (1971): Treatment of acute lymphoblastic leukaemia. *Br. Med. J.,* 4:189–194.
6. Mathé, G., Amiel, J. L., Schwarzenberg, L., Schneider, M., Cattan, A., Schlumberger, J. R., Hayat, M., and de Vassal, F. (1969): Active immunotherapy for acute lymphoblastic leukemia. Lancet, I: 697–699.
7. Mathé, G., Pouillart, P., and Lopeyraque, F. (1969): Active Immunotherapy of L1210 leukemia applied after the graft of tumor cells. *Br. J. Cancer,* 23:814–824.
8. Powles, R. L., Crowther, D., Bateman, C. J. T., Beard, M. E. J., McElwain, T. J., Russell, J., Lister, T. A., Whitehouse, J. M. A., Wrigley, P. F. M., Pike, M., Alexander, P., and Hamilton-Fairley, G. (1973): Immunotherapy for acute myelogenous leukemia. *Br. J. Cancer,* 28:365–376.
9. Vogler, W. R., Huguley, C. M., and Rundles, R. W. (1967): Comparison of Methotrexate with 6-mercaptopurine-predisone in treatment of acute leukemia in adults. *Cancer,* 20:1221–1226.

Immunotherapy of Cancer: Present Status of
Trials in Man, edited by W. D. Terry and D. Windhorst.
Raven Press, New York © 1978.

Chemoimmunotherapy of Acute Myeloblastic Leukemia: 4-Year Follow-Up with BCG

Jordan U. Gutterman, Victorio Rodriguez, Kenneth B. McCredie,
Jeanne P. Hester, Gerald P. Bodey, Emil J. Freireich,
and Evan M. Hersh

Department of Developmental Therapeutics, The University of Texas System Cancer Center, M. D. Anderson Hospital and Tumor Institute, Houston, Texas 77030

Despite the major advances achieved in the chemotherapy of acute myeloblastic leukemia (AML), the majority of patients achieving complete remission continue to relapse and die. Thus, additional therapeutic modalities appeared to be indicated in early 1972 when we designed our first trial with chemoimmunotherapy in adult acute leukemia. Our initial report stimulated by Mathé's results in childhood acute lymphocytic leukemia (ALL) was published 3 years ago (9) and demonstrated a statistically significant prolongation of complete remission among patients with acute myelogenous leukemia who were maintained with BCG plus chemotherapy compared to chemotherapy alone. No benefit was measured for patients with adult lymphoblastic leukemia (8).

This report details the follow-up 4-year analysis of our initial trial of chemoimmunotherapy in acute leukemia. Since the publication of our initial paper several studies have demonstrated a significant advantage for AML patients treated with nonspecific as well as specific immunotherapy. The results described in this chapter illustrate continued prolongation of remission and survival among AML patients who achieved a complete remission.

MATERIALS AND METHODS

Remission Induction

Fourteen consecutive patients with AML, who achieved complete remission entered the trial between August 15, 1972 and June 15, 1973. All remissions had been induced by the OAP chemotherapy combination, namely, cytarabine, 200 mg/m², intravenously on days 1 to 5; vincristine, 2 mg intravenously on day 1; and prednisone, 200 mg on days 1 to 5 by mouth. The daily cytarabine dose was given every 8 hr by intravenous push. One patient received daunorubicin in addition to OAP (DOAP), and one patient received cyclophosphamide in addition to OAP (COAP) during remission induction (13). Cycles were repeated every 14 to 21 days (see ref. 8). After remission was induced and consolidated with chemotherapy (13), Bacillus Calmette-Guerin) (BCG) was added to the maintenance chemotherapy regimen at the time of discharge from the hospital.

Before the addition of immunotherapy, complete remission was confirmed by examination of the bone marrow using our previously described criteria (16). Informed consent was obtained from all patients.

Chemoimmunotherapy

During maintenance therapy, OAP chemotherapy was administered as described above for remission induction except that the 5-day courses were repeated every 24 to 48 days. Cytarabine (100 to 200 mg/m^2) was administered subcutaneously divided into four daily doses over 5 days. The maximum tolerated dose of cytarabine was given with each course in an attempt to induce myelosuppression (3). On days 7, 14, and 21 of each monthly cycle, fresh liquid Pasteur strain BCG was given in a dose of 6×10^8 viable units (150 mg).

The BCG was flown weekly from the Pasteur Institute to our institution, stored at 4°C, and used within 10 days. The BCG was administered by scarification in a rotating fashion on the upper arms and upper thighs (8). The total number of viable units administered was calculated from the number of viable units per vial as estimated by the manufacturers at the time of shipment.

The dose of BCG was lowered to 6×10^7 viable units only if inflammatory reactivity at the scarification site was associated with persistently active draining lesions or a severe local reaction extending 5 cm beyond the scarification margins.

Follow-Up

Complete blood counts were repeated weekly. Physical examination and bone marrow aspiration studies were done once a month.

Control Group

Remission in patients receiving chemoimmunotherapy was compared to that for a group of AML patients who were maintained on OAP alone (see ref. 8). All of these patients had been treated during remission induction (from February 1, 1971 to July 31, 1972) with cytarabine, vincristine, and prednisone. In addition, a third had also received cyclophosphamide during induction (COAP) and a third had received daunorubicin (DOAP) (13). After remission induction and consolidation, all were then treated with OAP maintenance alone, and therefore, served as suitable historical controls. The

TABLE 1. Prognostic factors for patients with AML

Patient characteristics	OAP + BCG		OAP	
Age				
35	6	(43%)	11	(46%)
35–49	5	(36%)	5	(21%)
≥50	3	(21%)	8	(33%)
Laboratory values				
Hgb (gm%)	9.7	(4.6–12.6)	9.0	(1.2–12.8)
Platelet count (per mm³)	70.0	(10–156)	35.0	(12–200)
WBC (per mm³)	24.7	(0.80–124)	17.0	(1.0–130)
Absolute blast count (per mm³)	15.3	(0–110.58)	7.0	(0.2–110.6)
% Blasts in bone marrow	64	(25–97)	68	(30–99)

Range in parentheses. Hgb, hemoglobin; WBC, white blood cell count.

durations of remission were equivalent for all three groups, regardless of the induction regimen, and the data were pooled. Three of the patients in the initial group who were unclassified had AML and are included in the control group.

The two groups were analyzed for those factors known to affect prognosis in adult leukemia (6). These factors included histological diagnosis and age, as well as initial hemoglobin level, platelet count, absolute peripheral blood blast count, and the percentage of blasts in the bone marrow. As shown in Table 1, the two groups of patients were comparable with regard to all these factors. Therefore, the control group served as an adequate and comparable historical control.

The statistical methods used included the generalized Wilcoxon test with a one-tailed analysis test for evaluating differences between remission and survival curves (7) and the method of Kaplan and Meier for calculating and plotting remission and survival curves (10).

RESULTS

The duration of remission for the 24 OAP control patients and 14 OAP-plus-BCG patients is shown in Fig. 1. With a maximum of 4 and ½ years of follow-up, 16 of the 24 OAP control patients have relapsed. The median duration of remission for OAP alone was 52 weeks, which is comparable to the best chemotherapy control group reported in the literature. Eight of the 14 AML patients treated with OAP-BCG have relapsed. The median duration of complete remission is 85 weeks. All six patients who remained in remission have been followed now more than 165 weeks. These differences are statistically suggestive ($p = 0.08$).

Figure 2 illustrates the survival among the complete responders with AML. Fifteen of the 24 OAP control patients have died. The median survival among the OAP complete responders was 96 weeks. Seven of the patients with OAP

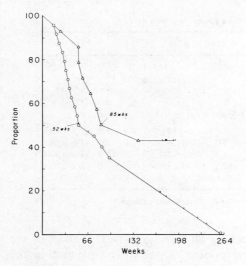

FIG. 1. Chemoimmunotherapy of AML. Duration of remission for OAP control patients (○) and OAP + BCG patients (△). Relapses were 16/24 and 8/14, respectively. (p = 0.08.)

alone are alive at 165 weeks or greater. Only 6 of the 14 OAP-BCG patients have died. Eight of the patients are alive and in remission at 145 weeks or greater. Despite this excellent result with chemotherapy alone, the group of patients treated with OAP-BCG have had a statistically significant prolongation of survival (*p* = 0.05).

In contrast to the beneficial effects among AML patients, there was no benefit for the very small group of patients with adult acute lymphoblastic leukemia (8). All six patients on OAP-BCG relapsed. The median duration of complete remission was 48 weeks for the OAP and OAP-BCG patients. The survival for these two groups of patients was nearly identical.

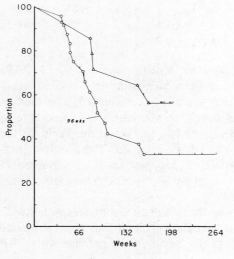

FIG. 2. Chemoimmunotherapy of AML. Survival of complete responders in OAP control group (○) and OAP + BCG group (△). Deaths were 15/24 and 6/14, respectively. (p = 0.05.)

DISCUSSION

Our data, first reported in 1974, continue to suggest that nonspecific immunotherapy with BCG added to chemotherapy after induction of remission favorably prolongs remission and particularly survival among AML patients.

Since our original publication there is an increasing body of literature that supports the benefit of BCG and other forms of active immunotherapy among patients with AML. Thus, intradermal or intravenous BCG (ref. 14 and Whittaker and Slater, *this volume*), intradermal methanol extraction residue of BCG (MER) (5,15), pseudomonas vaccine (4), as well as tumor cell vaccine (12,17) have been reported to prolong chemotherapy-induced complete remissions and/or survival among AML patients.

Some trials have been reported that fail to confirm efficacy of immunotherapy in AML (Hewlett et al., and Peto, *this volume*). For example, a trial using the lyophilized Pasteur strain BCG carried out by the Southwestern Oncology Group failed to show any benefit for immunotherapy. The reasons for these negative results are not clear. From Mathé's experimental screening system, there is a good possibility that the lyophilized Pasteur BCG may not be as effective as the fresh Pasteur BCG that was used in our own trials. Trials failing to show benefit with tumor cell vaccines must take into account the decreased immunogenicity that can develop following storage (1). In general, however, AML is a disease responsive to immunotherapy and appears to be an immunosensitive tumor. This is not surprising considering the strong suggestion that leukemic myeloblasts express neoantigens (9).

In contrast to the beneficial effects in AML, we have found no therapeutic advantage with BCG among adults with acute lymphoblastic leukemia. We have repeatedly showed that the leukemic lymphoblasts from adult patients express low antigenicity that may account for the lack of effect among ALL patients (9). These patients may resemble that subgroup of childhood acute lymphocytic leukemias found not to benefit from BCG by Mathé et al (11). However, other forms of immunotherapy need to be investigated in ALL.

The mechanisms of action for BCG in AML are not entirely known. Mycobacteria are potent immunomodulators and have pronounced amplification effects on antibody and cellular immunological reactions. BCG is a potent stimulator of the reticuloendothelial system (RES) and may affect bone marrow recovery from chemotherapy. Recently there has been a suggestion that BCG shares antigens with leukemic myeloblasts but not with leukemic lymphoblasts (P. Minden, J. U. Gutterman, and E. M. Hersh, *unpublished data*). This may in part account for the failure of patients with ALL to respond or benefit from BCG in comparison to patients with AML.

Although some have suggested that the benefit from immunotherapy in acute leukemia is due to a higher incidence of second remissions, our data do not support this contention since the first remissions with BCG have been prolonged.

We are very encouraged that there appears to be a plateau or tail on the survival curve for the AML patients. Thus, a significant fraction of these patients may be cured by chemoimmunotherapy. However, despite the positive results reported in this and other trials, patients continue to relapse and die of their disease. Thus, the current therapeutic program is far from optimal. Further research on improving maintenance chemotherapy as well as immunotherapy is needed.

However, the current status in 1976 would strongly suggest that immunotherapy is indicated in patients with AML. With improved methods of immunotherapy, chemotherapy, immunological monitoring, as well as immunodiagnosis, further progress in the control of these diseases is anticipated over the next several years.

ACKNOWLEDGMENTS

This work has been supported by contract NO1-CB-33888 from the National Cancer Institute, Bethesda, Maryland 20014. Dr. Gutterman is the recipient of a career development award (CA 71007–03) from the National Cancer Institute.

REFERENCES

1. Bartlett, G., Katsilas, D., Kreider, M., and Purnell, D. M. (1977): Immunogenicity of "viable" tumor cells after storage in liquid nitrogen. *Cancer Immunol. Immunother. (In press.)*
2. Bekesi, J. G., Roboz, J. P., and Holland, J. G. (1976): Therapeutic effectiveness of neuraminadase-treated tumor cells as an immunogen in man and experimental animals with leukemia. *NY Acad. Sci.,* 277:313.
3. Bodey, G. P., Coltman, C. A., Freireich, E. J, Bonnet, J. D., Gehan, E. A., Hout, A. B., Hewlett, J. S., McCredie, K. B., Saiki, J. H., and Wilson, H. E. (1974): Chemotherapy of acute leukemia in adults: Comparison between arabinosyl cytosine alone and in combination with vincristine, prednisone and cyclophosphamide, *Arch. Intern. Med.,* 133:260.
4. Clarkson, B. D., Dowling, M. D., Gee, T. S., Cunningham, I. B., and Burchenal, J. H. (1975): Treatment of acute leukemia in adults. *Cancer,* 36:775.
5. Cuttner, J., Bekesi, J. G., and Holland, J. G. (1967): Chemoimmunotherapy of acute leukemia using MER. *Proc. Am. Assoc. Cancer Res.,* 16:196 (Abstr. #782.)
6. Freireich, E. J., Gehan, E. A., Speer, J. F., Heilbrun, L., Smith, T., Bodey, G. P., McCredie, K. B., Rodriguez, V., Hart, J. S., and Burgess, M. A. (1973): Proceedings of the Reisenburg Workshop on prognostic factors in human acute leukemia. *Adv. Biosciences,* 14:131–144.
7. Gehan, E. A. (1965): A generalized Wilcoxon test for comparing arbitrarily singly-censored samples. *Biometrika,* 52:203.
8. Gutterman, J. U., Hersh, E. M., Rodriguez, V., McCredie, K. B., Mavligit, G., Reed, R., Burgess, M. A., Smith, T., Gehan, E. A., Bodie, G. P. Sr., and Freireich, E. J. (1974): Chemoimmunotherapy of adult acute leukemia prolongation. *Lancet,* II:1405.
9. Gutterman, J. U., Rossen, R. D., Butler, W. T., McCredie, K. B., Bodey, G. P., Sr., Freireich, E. J., and Hersh, E. M. (1973): Immunoglobulin on tumor cells and tumor-induced lymphocyte blastogenesis in human acute leukemia. *N. Engl. J. Med.,* 288:169.

10. Kaplan, E. L., and Meier, P. (1958): Nonparametric estimation from incomplete observations. *J. Am. Stat. Assoc.,* 53:457.
11. Mathé, G., Pouillart, P., Schwarzenberg, L., Amiel, J., Schneider, M., Hayat, M., De Vassal, F., Jasmin, C., Rosenfeld, C., Weiner, R., and Rappaport, H. (1972): Attempts at immunotherapy of 100 patients with acute lymphoid leukemia: Some factors influencing results. *Natl. Cancer Inst. Monogr.,* 35:361.
12. Powles, R. L., Crowther, D., Bateman, C. J. T., Beard, M. E. J., McElwain, T. J., Russell, J., Lister, T. A., Whitehouse, M. A., Wrigley, P. F. M., Alexander, P., and Hamilton-Fairley, G. (1973): Immunotherapy for acute myelogenous leukemia. *Br. J. Cancer,* 28:365.
13. Rodriguez, V., Bodey, G. P., Gutterman, J. U., McCredie, K. B., and Freireich, E. J (1976): Combination chemotherapy of adult acute leukemia for remission induction and maintenance. In: *Therapy of Acute Leukemias,* edited by F. Mandelli, S. Amadori, and G. Mariani, p. 569. Centro Minerva Medica Publishers, Rome.
14. Vogler, W. R., and Chan, Y-K (1974): Prolonging remission in myeloblastic leukemia by Tice strain Bacillus Calmette-Guerin. *Lancet,* II:128.
15. Weiss, D. W., Stupp, Y., and Izak, G. (1974): Treatment of acute myelocytic leukemia patients with the MER tubercle bacillus fraction. *Proc. XV Congr. Int. Soc. Hematol., Jerusalem.* Part II:74 (Abstr.)
16. Whitecar, J. P., Jr., Bodey, G. P., McCredie, K. B., Hart, J. S., and Freireich, E. J. (1972): Cyclophosphamide, vincristine, arabinosyl cytosine and prednisone (COAP) combination chemotherapy for adult acute leukemia. *Cancer Chemother. Rep.,* 56:543.
17. Whiteside, M. G., Cauchi, M. N., Paton, C., and Stone, J. (1976): Chemoimmunotherapy for maintenance in acute myeloblastic leukemia. *Cancer,* 38:1581.

Question and Answer Session

Dr. Powles: In the first paper your group published about 18 months ago, the significance level, if I remember correctly, was something like 0.04 for remission. If that has now fallen off such that the remission duration is not significant, and survival is only just significant at the 5 percent level, can you give us any explanation of what might have happened in the interim?

Dr. Hersh: I don't think I can give you an explanation. That is just how the data stands now.

Dr. Powles: Are you worried now about the present study that you just presented, saying actually that the estimated survivals are greater than 180 weeks?

Dr. Hersh: That estimate is based on the fact that the patient who has been followed for the shortest duration of time is at 180 weeks. Survival therefore can't be any worse than that. How much better it will be, I have no idea. These estimates do change somewhat with time. On the other hand, the trends observed, I think, stand up very well.

The problem with a number of the studies is the small numbers involved. The objective, however, is to try to move ahead as rapidly as possible, and therefore one has to design studies for patient populations who have very poor prognoses rather than doing fewer studies with very large numbers of patients, where you may be relegating large numbers of patients to what may be soon estimated to be suboptimal treatment. That is the philosophy behind the changes that have taken place in our study.

*Immunotherapy of Cancer: Present Status of
Trials in Man,* edited by W. D. Terry and D. Windhorst.
Raven Press, New York © 1978.

Remission Maintenance In Adult Acute Leukemia With and Without BCG. A Southwest Oncology Group Study

*James S. Hewlett, **Stanley Balcerzak, ***Jordon U. Gutterman,
***Emil J. Freireich, ***Edmund A. Gehan,
and ***Anne Kennedy

*Cleveland Clinic, Cleveland, Ohio 44106; **Ohio State University Hospital, Columbus,
Ohio 43210; ***University of Texas, M.D. Anderson Hospital and Tumor Institute,
Houston, Texas 77030*

Animal data have indicated that mice grafted with 10^4 living leukemic cells and treated with Bacillus Calmette-Guérin (BCG) applied after the graft show a delayed and reduced mortality (1). However, such immunotherapy can only affect host survival if less than 10^5 tumor cells are grafted (1). In clinical experiments Mathé has shown that BCG alone can effectively prolong complete remission in acute lymphocytic leukemia (ALL) when administered during remission maintenance when the tumor load is maximally reduced (1). In a previous Southwest Oncology Group study, the combination of vincristine (Oncovin®), cytosine arabinoside (Ara-c), and prednisone had been effective in remission maintenance in adult acute leukemia. In 1973 the Southwest Oncology Group initiated a randomized study to test the value of combination chemotherapy (OAP) with active immunotherapy (BCG) in maintaining complete remission and prolonging survival in adult acute leukemia. This was the first Southwest Group protocol in which immunotherapy was used.

PATIENTS

Patients with acute leukemia who had received no prior therapy and who had more than 30% blasts and/or promyelocytes in the bone marrow were eligible for entry into the induction phase of the study. Patients with chronic granulocytic leukemic blast transformation were included and analyzed separately. Only adult patients 16 years and older were eligible.

TREATMENT

The treatment plan consisted of three phases: remission induction, consolidation, and maintenance (Table 1). All patients were induced with a similar

TABLE 1. *Adult acute leukemia—schemata of 10-day OAP administration*

	Induction		Consolidation		Maintenance

Adult acute leukemia → 10 day OAP[a] (2 courses) → (CR) → 5 day OAP[b] (3 courses) → R A N D O M I Z E → 5 day OAP[b] / 5 day OAP + BCG[c]

(No prior therapy)

No response Off study

Southwest oncology group 7315/16 (7/9/73–1/6/75). CR, complete remission.
[a] Vincristine 2 mg i.v. day 1; Ara-C 100 mg/m² /day, 24 hr i.v. drip, days 1 thru 10; prednisone 100 mg p.o. days 1 thru 5.
[b] Ara-C 100 mg/m²/day, s.c. injection, q 6 hr × 20 doses.
[c] Pasteur BCG (freeze dried) 3 ampules, approx. 2 × 10⁸ viable units (scarification).

regimen that consisted of one to two courses of 10-day OAP (vincristine 2 mg i.v. on day 1, Ara-c 100 mg/m² per day by 24-hr infusion on days 1 through 10, and prednisone 100 mg p.o. days 1 through 5). Patients achieving a complete remission were given three consolidation courses at 14- to 21-day intervals. For consolidation, the Ara-c was administered s.c. 100 mg/m² per day in four divided doses every 6 hr for 5 days, vincristine 1 mg i.v. was given on day 1, and prednisone 100 mg p.o. daily for 5 days. Patients who remained in complete remission after finishing the three consolidation courses were then randomized to one of two maintenance arms: 5-day OAP alone or 5-day OAP plus BCG. The OAP chemotherapy was given every 28 days and was similar to that used in consolidation. Lyophilized Pasteur BCG was used for this study and applied by scarification in a dose of approximately 2 × 10⁸ viable organisms on days 7, 14, and 21 of each maintenance chemotherapy course. The scarification technique used 20 scratches, each 5 cm long, arranged in a square. The site of scarification was rotated with each administration, utilizing both upper and lower extremities. After 1 year, the frequency of BCG was reduced to days 7 and 21 of each course. BCG was to be continued for 1 year after completion of the maintenance chemotherapy the duration of which was left up to the discretion of the investigator.

STATISTICAL ANALYSIS

The test of differences between two survivor curves was carried out using the generalized Wilcoxon test (2). The Chi square test was used to test differences in rates or frequency of occurrence. *p* Values of 0.05 or less were considered significant.

RESULTS

A total of 207 patients have been entered in the induction phase of the study and 56 patients in the maintenance phase since it was opened July 9, 1973. Ten additional patients were entered with a diagnosis of chronic myelogenous leukemia (CML) blast transformation. The distribution of patients according to eligibility and the evaluability status is given in Table 2. In the induction phase 198 patients are eligible. Three of these are too early to evaluate, 23 are partially evaluable (20 due to early deaths and three who refused further treatment), and 19 are not evaluable. Thus, 152 patients in the induction phase are fully evaluable. The complete response rate is 54% (94/175) for all patients including the partially evaluable patients and 62% (94/152) for the fully evaluable patients only. This response rate is 11% higher than for the 5-day OAP used in the previous Southwest Oncology Group study. The advantage in complete remission rate for the 10-day OAP over the 5-day OAP is nearly statistically significant ($p = 0.07$).

Of the 94 patients who had complete response, 86 were in remission for at least 8 weeks and hence were eligible for randomization to maintenance therapy. However, only 56 of these (67%) have been randomized, 33 to OAP and 23 to OAP plus BCG (Table 2). Forty-seven of the 56 randomized patients are fully evaluable, and two additional patients are partially evaluable. Of the 49 fully and partially evaluable patients, 27 received OAP alone and 22 received OAP plus BCG. The relapse rate in the OAP maintenance arm is 56% (15/27) compared to 64% (14/22) in the OAP plus BCG arm. There is not a statistically significant difference in the length of the response between the two maintenance treatments ($p = 0.47$). The median length of response was 55 weeks in the OAP alone group and 54 weeks in the OAP plus BCG group.

TABLE 2. *Adult acute leukemia—patient entries and validity*
(10-day OAP)

	Induction	Maintenance
Number entered	207	56
Eligible	198	54
Too early	3	1
Evaluable	152	47
Partially evaluable	23	2
Early death	20	0
Lost to follow-up	0	1
Refused further Rx	3	1
Not evaluable	19	4
Major protocol violation	9	2
Inadequate data	5	0
Other reasons	5	2

Southwest oncology group 7315/7316 (7/9/73–1/6/75).

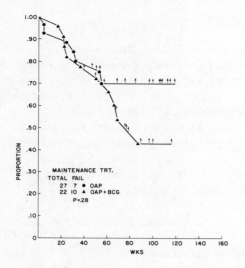

FIG. 1. Survival curves from randomization for all patients on maintenance therapy (OAP or OAP + BCG). Acute leukemia SWOG 7315/16.

Figure 1 shows the survival curves of patients by maintenance treatment. Seven (27%) in the OAP maintenance arm have died, whereas 10 (45%) in the OAP plus BCG maintenance arm have died. The median length of survival from randomization is 55+ weeks for the OAP patients and 75 weeks for the OAP plus BCG patients. There is no real difference between the survival curves ($p = 0.28$).

Figure 2 shows the remission curves of the patients divided into groups by maintenance treatment and cell types. Only four patients with ALL were registered and were evaluable in the maintenance study. Two of these were randomized to OAP and two to OAP plus BCG. The median length of response of acute myelogenous leukemia (AML) patients treated with OAP plus BCG was 59 weeks and for AML patients treated with OAP alone

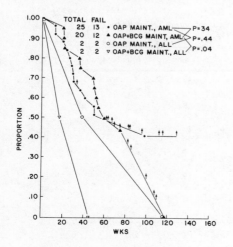

FIG. 2. Remission curves from start of complete remission divided by treatment groups (OAP or OAP + BCG) and cell type (AML or ALL). Acute leukemia SWOG 7315/16.

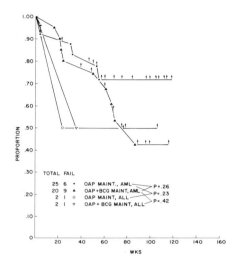

FIG. 3. Survival curves from randomization divided by treatment group (OAP or OAP + BCG) and cell type (AML or ALL). Acute leukemia SWOG 7315/16.

was 55 weeks. There was no difference in the length of response between AML patients treated with OAP alone and those treated with OAP plus BCG ($p = 0.34$). Although there were only two ALL patients in each maintenance treatment arm, there was a statistically significant difference ($p = 0.04$) in the length of response between the AML and ALL patients who received OAP plus BCG. There was no difference ($p = 0.44$) in the length of response between AML and ALL patients who received OAP alone.

Survival curves for the randomized patients divided by treatment group and cell type are given in Fig. 3. Nine of the 20 (45%) AML patients treated with OAP plus BCG have died with the median survival time from randomization being 74 weeks, whereas six of 25 (24%) AML patients treated with OAP alone have died with the median survival time of 55+ weeks. There is no real difference between the two survival curves ($p = 0.26$). One of the two ALL patients in each treatment arm has died. There is no difference in survival between the AML and ALL patients treated with OAP plus BCG ($p = 0.42$).

In conclusion, there is no advantage in terms of either increased length of a response or survival for AML patients receiving BCG. Since there are only four randomized ALL patients, the effect of the addition of BCG in maintenance for ALL patients cannot be evaluated.

SIDE EFFECTS OF TREATMENT

All patients developed a skin reaction at the site of scarification. In seven instances, the local reaction was severe and required reduction in the dose of BCG. One patient developed a *Staphlococcus aureus* infection of the BCG site.

Three patients developed a transient skin rash, and two noted a flare at other scarification sites following the vaccination. No patients developed abnormal liver function tests while receiving BCG, and none showed evidence of systemic BCG disease. Eleven patients had purified protein derivative (PPD) skin tests done before starting BCG, and nine were negative. Six of the nine negative reactors converted to positive after BCG treatments.

DISCUSSION

Immunotherapy for acute leukemia with BCG vaccine was first reported by Mathé and co-workers (1) in 1969. They demonstrated in children with ALL that BCG was effective in prolonging remission duration and survival. Fresh Pasteur strain BCG vaccine was administered by dermal scarification. Since Mathé's report, several negative studies of BCG therapy in childhood acute leukemia have been reported (3–5). Therefore, the effectiveness of immunotherapy in ALL has not been confirmed. On the other hand, a number of groups have demonstrated the efficacy of BCG vaccine alone or in combination with tumor cells in AML. Powles (6) and co-workers demonstrated an increased remission duration and survival compared to chemotherapy alone when BCG vaccine plus allogeneic irradiated leukemic cells were administered weekly between courses of maintenance chemotherapy. Approximately 1×10^6 viable organisms were delivered with each dose. Vogler (7) and members of the Southeast Cooperative Chemotherapy Group used Tice BCG vaccine given in four weekly doses of 3×10^8 organisms by multipuncture technique following consolidation chemotherapy and before remission maintenance chemotherapy began. With this program patients receiving immunotherapy plus chemotherapy had a statistically significant improvement in survival compared to patients receiving chemotherapy alone. Gutterman and associates (8) have recently demonstrated that fresh Pasteur strain BCG vaccine in a dose of 6×10^8 viable units administered by scarification weekly during remission maintenance chemotherapy significantly prolonged remission duration and survival compared to chemotherapy alone.

The present study reported from the Southwest Oncology Group did not show any significant difference between the group receiving maintenance chemotherapy plus BCG and the control group receiving chemotherapy alone. In view of the several positive reports suggesting that BCG is effective in prolonging remissions and survival in patients with AML, the reasons for this present negative study are not readily apparent. It is not possible to discern if the lack of response to BCG noted in our study is related to the form of induction chemotherapy used, the type of BCG vaccine, or the dose, route, schedule, or timing of the BCG administration relative to other therapy. The induction 10-day OAP program appeared to be an effective one producing a 54% complete remission rate in adult acute leukemia. This was the best response rate obtained up to that time by the Southwest Oncology Group. The

BCG dose of 2×10^8 originally planned was not achieved at the onset of the study because of the low potency of the Pasteur strain available at that time and only approximately 10^7 viable organisms were given during part of the study. The higher potency Pasteur strain was used eventually when it became available. This dose still exceeds that used in other studies where BCG appeared effective in AML. The route, schedule, and timing of the administration of the BCG was essentially that used by Gutterman et al. (8) in their positive studies.

In a cooperative group study such as this the question arises whether all patients received the BCG on schedule, and whether it was properly administered. This was the first protocol involving immunotherapy conducted by the Southwest Oncology Group. We checked with each investigator using BCG and confirmed that all patients received the vaccine approximately as scheduled and by the scarification method as outlined in the protocol. All patients started on BCG vaccine who have not died or relapsed are still receiving BCG according to protocol with two exceptions. One patient requested it be stopped after 2 years because of severe reactions, and in another patient the BCG was discontinued after a year and a half because she developed a sterile abscess in the flank and severe reactions to the drug. Both patients remain in complete remission. Thus all patients did receive an adequate amount of BCG and over a sufficiently long period of time when compared to other studies.

In conclusion, this study by the Southwest Oncology Group did not show any advantage for maintenance chemotherapy plus BCG over maintenance chemotherapy alone in adult acute leukemia.

SUMMARY

Patients with adult acute leukemia were induced with a combination of vincristine, Ara-C, and prednisone (10-day OAP). Those achieving complete remission were given three consolidation courses of 5-day OAP then randomized to either chemotherapy alone or chemotherapy plus BCG (lyophilized Pasteur strain). The BCG was given by the scarification method each week between courses of chemotherapy. The planned BCG dose was 2×10^8 viable organisms. Fifty-six patients were randomized, and 49 were partially or fully evaluable. Twenty-seven received OAP alone, and 22 received OAP plus BCG. The median length of response for all patients to OAP was 55 weeks and to OAP plus BCG 54 weeks ($p = 0.47$). The median length of response of AML patients treated with OAP plus BCG was 59 weeks and with OAP alone 55 weeks ($p = 0.34$). The median survival time for AML patients treated with OAP alone was 74 weeks and with OAP plus BCG 55+ weeks ($p = 0.26$). There was no advantage in remission length or survival for AML patients receiving BCG. Fifteen institutions in the Southwest Oncology Group participated in the study.

ACKNOWLEDGMENTS

This investigation was supported by grants awarded by the DHEW: CA-04919, CA-04920, CA-10376, CA-12014, and CA-16943.

REFERENCES

1. Mathé, G., Amiel, J. S., Schwarzenberg, L., Schneider, M., Cattan, A., Schlumberger, J. R., Hayat, M., DeVassal, F. (1969): Active immunotherapy for acute lymphoblastic leukemia. *Lancet,* 1:697–699.
2. Gehan, E. A. (1965): A generalized Wilcoxon test for comparing arbitrarity singly-censored samples. *Biometrika,* 52:203–223.
3. Leventhal, B. G., LePourhiet, A., Halterman, R. H., Henderson, E. S., Herberman, R. B. (1973): Immunotherapy in previously treated acute lymphatic leukemia. *Natl. Cancer Inst. Monogr.,* 39:177–187.
4. Leukemia Committee and the Working Party on Leukemia in Childhood (1971): Report on the treatment of acute lymphoblastic leukemia. *Br. Med. J.,* 4:189–194.
5. Heyn, R., Joo, P., Karon, M., Nesbit, M., Share, N., Buslow, N., Weiner, J., Reed, A., and Hammond, D. (1975): BCG in the treatment of acute lymphocytic leukemia. *Blood,* 46:431–442.
6. Powles, R. L., Crowther, D., Bateman, C. J. T., Beard, M. E. J., McElwain, T. J., Russell, J., Lister, T. A., Whitehouse, J. M. A., Wrigley, P. F. M., Pike, M., Alexander, P., and Hamilton-Fairley, G. (1973): Immunotherapy for acute myelogenous leukemia. *Br. J. Cancer,* 28:365–376.
7. Vogler, W. R., Chan, Y. K. (1974): Prolonging remission in myeloblastic leukemia by Tice strain Bacillus Calmette-Guerin. *Lancet,* 2:128–131.
8. Gutterman, J. U., Rodriguez, V., Mavligit, G. M., Burgess, M. A., Gehan, E., Hersh, E. M., McCredie, K. B., Reed, R., Smith, T., Bodey Sr., G. P., and Freireich, E. J. (1974): Chemoimmunotherapy of adult acute leukemia. Prolongation of remission in myeloblastic leukemia with BCG. *Lancet,* 2:128–131.

Question and Answer Session

Dr. Mathé: It is interesting to see that the same author, Doctor Gutterman, is associated with a positive result in favor of BCG in his own chapter, but here a negative result is described by a cooperative group of which he is a member.

I will ask the same question: Do you have in some centers which co-operate with this group results which are different from the global result? Isn't your negative result possibly due to what I describe as the dilution syndrome?

Dr. Hewlett: I'm not able to say that, Professor Mathé.

Dr. Hersh: At least a part of the difference between the M. D. Anderson result and the group result may relate to BCG dose. We're not 100 percent sure that the dose of BCG is important, but there is some experimental and some clinical evidence that that is true. While this may not even be true in every disease category, I would like to point out to you that in this trial the dose of BCG was certainly no more than one-third and sometimes, in most of the patients, as I recall, one-tenth of the dose of BCG that was used in the M. D. Anderson trial. Now, I think that a competent chemotherapist like Dr.

Holland, for example, would rise in wrath if somebody presented a study with adriamycin in which doses of 20 mg/m² were used rather than 60 mg/m².

It is important that we keep in mind variables such as disease, dose of BCG, and schedule of administration. I don't think that the Southwest Oncology Group Study, which was excellently conducted, either supports or refutes any observations that have been made, negative or positive, in the other chapters reported here, because the trials are just not the same.

Dr. Fahey: Do you think there would be physician or patient resistance to a tenfold increase in dose in BCG in the next study that you undertake?

Dr. Hewlett: We do have another study underway, which is comparable to the present study, and patients are again being randomized to OAP and to OAP plus a larger dose of BCG.

Immunotherapy of Cancer: Present Status of Trials in Man, edited by W. D. Terry and D. Windhorst. Raven Press, New York © 1978.

Immunotherapy of Acute Myelogenous Leukemia Using Intravenous BCG

J. A. Whittaker and A. J. Slater

Department of Hematology, University Hospital of Wales and Welsh National School of Medicine, Heath Park, Cardiff, CF4 4XW, England

Advances in the chemotherapy of acute myelogenous leukemia (AML) in recent years have led to an improved prognosis, and cytarabine used alone or in combination with daunorubicin (DNR) has given complete remission rates of 50 to 70% (5,6,27). However, attainment of complete remission is related to age (1,17), and it is unlikely that higher remission rates will be achieved in unselected series when currently available chemotherapy is used alone. Furthermore, duration of remission is short and does not usually exceed 12 months (5,6,17,27). A considerable effort is being made to prolong remission duration, and promising initial results have been reported using Bacillus Calmette-Guérin (BCG) administered by the intradermal route alone (11,26) or in combination with irradiated tumor cells (24). The mechanism of tumor suppression by BCG is not fully understood, but intimate contact with the tumor cells is important in some animal tumors (2,4,30). Pulmonary metastases of a transplanted rat sarcoma are suppressed by intravenous BCG, and when BCG is mixed with the sarcoma cells prior to transplantation, the subcutaneous primary is suppressed (3). Intravenous BCG also protects against the growth of transplanted sarcomas and carcinomas in various strains of mice (19). These reports encouraged us to examine the use of the intravenous route of administration in patients with AML, and a small pilot study (29) suggested that intravenous BCG could be used in man without serious toxicity. We have recently extended our study in a strictly controlled trial to determine if a combination of BCG with intermittent maintenance chemotherapy prolongs remission and survival in adult AML.

PATIENTS AND METHODS

Diagnosis

Eighty-one unselected adult patients aged 18 to 85 years presenting at the University Hospital of Wales between January 1, 1973 and September 1,

1975 had a diagnosis of acute myeloblastic leukemia or its variant, acute myelomonocytic leukemia, made by previously defined criteria (17).

Remission Induction

All patients were treated with DNR, 1.5 mg/kg by intravenous infusion into a fast-running saline drip, followed by cytarabine, 1.0 mg/kg by intravenous injection every 12 hr for 5 days. Patients received five to nine treatments (mean 6.2) with intervals of 5 to 7 days between courses. Hemoglobin concentration was maintained above 8.0 g/dl at all times by blood transfusion as required, infusions of platelet concentrate were given to all patients with clinical evidence of bleeding, antibiotics were used to treat clinical infection, and prophylactic antifungal mouth care was given to all patients.

Thirty-seven of the 81 patients entered complete remission as previously defined (16), and these patients were randomly allocated to one of two maintenance treatments.

Maintenance Chemotherapy

Maintenance chemotherapy on one day of each month was given in identical manner to all patients (Table 1). The dosage and administration of DNR were the same as during remission induction, but when a total dose of 600 mg was reached doxorubicin hydrochloride (Adriamycin®, ADR), 1.0 mg/kg, was substituted to reduce the incidence of DNR cardiomyopathy. On completion of DNR/ADR therapy, cytarabine, 1.0 mg/kg, was given as an 8-hr intravenous infusion in saline. Two patients (case 3 and case 27, Table 3) developed a cardiomyopathy after a total DNR/ADR dose of 1,120 and 1,170 mg necessitating withdrawal of both drugs, and one patient (case 9, Table 3) would not tolerate repeated intravenous drips. Cytarabine, 100 mg/m² every 12 hr intravenously × 4, and thioguanine, 75 mg/m² 12 hourly × 4 by mouth, were substituted at week 32 of the patient's remission.

Immunotherapy

Patients randomized to intravenous BCG therapy (group B, Table 1) were given freeze-dried BCG (Glaxo, Ltd.) containing 4 to 9 × 10⁶ organisms/ml as shown in Table 2. The BCG dilutions were made with sterile distilled water, patients were kept at rest in the hospital, and hourly recordings of oral temperature were made throughout. When sustained pyrexia (38°C for two successive readings) occurred, further increase in BCG dosage was withheld. Seventeen patients required undiluted BCG before pyrexia was produced, and one patient developed pyrexia with the 1:10 dilution. Once the

TABLE 1. *Treatment schedules*

Remission induction	All patients	DNR 1.5 mg/kg i.v. × 1
		Cytarabine 1.0 mg/kg. i.v. 12 hourly × 10
		(Five to nine treatments with intervals of 5 to 7 days between)
Maintenance treatment	Group A	DNR 1.5 mg/kg i.v. × 1 (or ADR 1.0 mg/kg)
		Cytarabine 1.0 mg/kg: 8 hr i.v. infusion in saline
	Group B	(Given once each month)
		Maintenance treatment A
		plus i.v. BCG at day 14

TABLE 2. *BCG treatment schedule used to establish the dilution required to produce pyrexia*

Day	Treatment
1	1 ml freeze-dried BCG (4 to 9 × 10^6 organisms/ml) diluted 1:100,000 with saline
	0.1 ml given in fast-running i.v. saline drip
2	0.1 ml 1:10,000 i.v.
3	0.1 ml 1:1,000 i.v.
4	0.1 ml 1:100 i.v.
5	0.1 ml 1:10 i.v.
6	0.1 ml i.v.

pyrexia producing dose of BCG was established, the patient was given this dose as an outpatient once monthly. BCG was given 14 days after each course of maintenance chemotherapy, so that any immunosuppressive effect of chemotherapy would be unlikely to interfere with the effects of BCG. Initially, BCG was given by intravenous injection, but following the development of a skin granuloma (case 9, Table 3), BCG has been given into an intravenous saline infusion.

Since November, 1974, all patients have received chlorpheniramine maleate, 10 mg intravenously, immediately prior to any intravenous injection of BCG. Hydrocortisone for intravenous injection and adrenaline for subcutaneous use is always immediately available when giving BCG intravenously.

Skin Testing

Before immunotherapy, intradermal skin testing was performed with *Candida* antigen and 1:1,000 purified protein derivative (PPD). A positive reaction was defined as induration exceeding 3 mm diameter at 48 hr. Skin testing was repeated every 3 months.

Other Investigations

During remission, hemoglobin concentration, total and differential white cell counts, and platelet counts were measured every 2 weeks, and marrow aspirates and trephines were examined every 3 months or whenever the blood count was abnormal. Liver biopsies were obtained ante-mortem from seven patients in the immunotherapy group and a lung biopsy from one patient. Full postmortem examination was performed in two of the four BCG-treated patients who died with relapsed AML.

Statistical Analysis

Statistical methods used to examine differences in remission and survival durations included the 'exact logrank' nonparametric analysis (23).

RESULTS

Eighteen of 37 patients entering complete remission were randomized to treatment with BCG and chemotherapy. The diagnosis, duration of first remission, and total survival of these patients and of 19 patients randomized to treatment with chemotherapy alone are shown in Table 3. Figure 1 shows the survival times and Fig. 2 the remission duration for both groups of patients. Eight of the 18 patients treated with BCG remain alive, five of them in their first remission. Five of the 19 patients maintained with chemotherapy alone are alive, and all five are in remission. At present, median remission duration is 27 weeks for the chemotherapy maintenance group and 34 weeks for the BCG group. Using the logrank test, there is no significant difference between these two groups. The median survival is 50 weeks for the chemotherapy group and 69 weeks for the BCG group. This difference is statistically significant ($p < 0.02$) and is not related to sex or age in the two patient groups.

A second remission was obtained in five patients in the BCG-treated group using identical therapy to that used to obtain the first remission, and two of these patients (case 1 and case 3, Table 3) achieved a third remission. The same treatment was given to 10 of 12 patients who relapsed in the non-BCG-treated group, but only one of these patients entered a second remission (case 27, Table 3).

The results of skin testing are shown in Table 4. No clear pattern has yet emerged from the studies, but it is interesting to note that the four patients who had the longest remissions (cases 4,6,8, and 10 in Table 4) and seven patients who survived for 75 weeks or more (cases 2, 3, 4, 6, 8, 10, and 13 in Table 4) either had a positive PPD skin test initially or converted from negative to positive after treatment with intravenous BCG.

Side Effects of Treatment

Immunotherapy with intravenous BCG has generally been well tolerated. Pyrexia of 38 to 39°C occurring 6 to 12 hr after injection and lasting 12 to

TABLE 3. Lengths of remission and survival in 37 adults
with AML in complete remission

Patient number	Length of 1st remission (weeks)	Length of 2nd remission (weeks)	Length of survival (weeks)
Chemotherapy plus BCG			
1	24	12	69
2	30	18	76
3	30	28	125
4	142*		162**
5	12	0	33
6	125*		131**
7	21	11	64
8	74	30*	155**
9	51	0	65
10	80	0	96
11	25	0	36
12	13	0	27
13	68*		93**
14	50		64**
15	16	0	38
16	31		69**
17	41*		60**
18	38*		48**
Chemotherapy			
19	13	0	26
20	5	0	40
21	12	0	44
22	29	0	63
23	20	NG	57
24	19	NG	44
25	96*		100**
26	42	0	60
27	24	10	65
28	88*		110**
29	18	0	31
30	63*		72**
31	60*		72**
32	37		53
33	12	0	34
34	56	0	64
35	6	0	30
36	40*		61**
37	13	0	39

Difference in survival length for the two groups is significant; p < 0.02. *, still in remission; **, alive; NG, adequate chemotherapy not given.

72 hr is a normal response to intravenous BCG. The 18 BCG group patients have each received between four and 26 intravenous BCG injections, totaling 268 separate intravenous treatments. In addition to pyrexia, three patients had headaches and muscular pains (Table 5), and in the majority of patients,

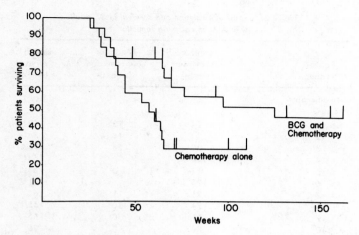

FIG. 1. Length of survival for AML patients treated with chemotherapy (19 patients) and with chemo-therapy-intravenous BCG (18 patients). Vertical lines indicate patients still alive. Difference in survival $p < 0.02$.

the pyrexia has increased in magnitude or duration as the number of BCG injections has increased. For this reason, the dose of BCG was reduced in two patients (cases 3 and 4), and this resulted in a reduction in pyrexia and the disappearance of severe muscular pains. Two patients (cases 8 and 9) had anaphylactic reactions immediately following the second full dose of intra-venous BCG. Both were successfully treated with intravenous hydrocortisone, and the reactions did not recur when the BCG was reduced to one-tenth of

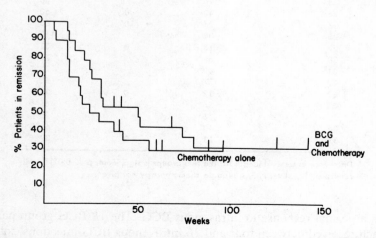

FIG. 2. Remission duration for AML patients treated with chemotherapy (19 patients) and with chemo-therapy-intravenous BCG (18 patients). Vertical lines indicate patients still in complete remission. Difference in remission is not statistically significant.

TABLE 4. *Skin testing before and after BCG treatment in adults with AML in complete remission (16 of 18 patients)*

Patient	Diagnosis	Pretreatment		Posttreatment		1st Remission duration (weeks)	Survival (weeks)
		Mantoux	Candida	Mantoux	Candida		
1	AML	—	—	—	—	24	69
2	AUL	+	—	ND	ND	30	76
3	AML	+	—	+	—	30	125
4	AML	++	++	++	++	142*	162*
5	AML	—	+	—	++	12	33
6	AMMoL	—	—	+	—	125*	131*
7	AML	—	—	—	—	21	64
8	AML	+	—	+	—	74	155*
9	ProML	—	—	ND	ND	51	65
10	AMMoL	—	—	++	+	80	96
11	AML	—	—	ND	ND	25	36
13	AErL	—	—	+	—	68*	93*
14	AMMoL	+	—	++	—	50	64*
16	AML	—	—	+	—	31	69*
17	AML	—	—	+	+	41*	60*
18	AML	+	—	+	—	38*	48*

+, Positive; ++, strongly positive; ND, not done; *, remission (or survival) continues.
AML, acute myeloblastic leukemia; AUL, acute undifferentiated leukemia; AMMoL, acute myelomonocytic leukemia; ProML, acute promyelocytic leukemia; AErl, acute erythro-leukemia.

its original dosage and readministered 1 month later. One of these patients has suffered from recurrent attacks of asthma for over 40 years. He has recently developed an illness characterized by cough, sputum, and pyrexia, and an organism with the characteristics of *M. tuberculosis* has been isolated from his sputum. The organism was sensitive to a range of antituberculous drugs including pyrazinamide and produced tuberculous lesions in the guinea pig.

One patient (case 1) developed a transient urticarial skin rash following her third full dose of BCG. The reaction did not recur, and skin rashes have not been seen in the other patients.

TABLE 5. *Complications of intravenous BCG in adults with AML*

Anaphylactic	2	
Headaches and muscle pains	3	
Transient jaundice	2	
Unexplained splenomegaly	2	
Transient urticarial skin rash	1	
Epithelioid granulomas: Marrow	14	(18)
Liver	9	(10)
Lung	5	(6)
Spleen	2	(4)

Figures in brackets equal total patients where biopsy or postmortem material available.

Two patients (cases 3 and 11) had persistent unexplained splenomegaly, and two patients (cases 2 and 7) had transient jaundice. In one patient (case 7) the jaundice disappeared when an estrogen-containing contraceptive pill was discontinued. Epithelioid noncaseating granulomas (Table 5) occurred in the bone marrow of 14 of the 18 BCG-treated patients, in all six antemortem liver biopsies, in one antemortem lung biopsy, and in the skin at the injection site in one patient. Postmortem granulomas were found, particularly in the liver and lung and also in the spleen. A full report of these findings has been published (28).

DISCUSSION

The use of BCG given by the intravenous route resulted in significant prolongation of survival for adult patients with AML. No prolongation of first remission was demonstrated when the BCG-treated group was compared with a control group of patients treated with identical chemotherapy but without BCG, and it seems likely that the increased survival of BCG-treated patients reflects several second remissions similar to those previously reported in patients treated with irradiated allogeneic acute myeloid leukemia cells and BCG (8).

Other authors (11,26) have reported a prolongation of remission duration in patients with AML given BCG by the intradermal route. Our series differs from that of Gutterman et al. (11), which was not a controlled trial, and that of Vogler and Chan (26), which was performed at 16 different institutions. Although we cannot yet show a statistical difference in the length of first remission, several BCG-treated patients remain in complete remission with survival times of almost 3 years.

A study of immunotherapy in acute lymphoblastic leukemia (ALL) in children (15) indicated that freeze-dried BCG (Glaxo) was ineffective, and many subsequent studies have used Pasteur BCG containing a higher number of viable organisms. However, Pasteur BCG has since proved ineffective in the treatment of ALL in adults (11), and it is likely that the disease being treated is more important than the type of BCG used. Trials in which intradermal BCG has been administered in association with tumor cells (13,24) or in which patients with lymphoblastic leukemia have been studied (13,15) are not comparable with this and other studies (11,26) of BCG in the treatment of AML.

The timing of immunotherapy in relation to chemotherapy is important in animal models, and both *C. parvum* (7) and BCG (22) have a maximum effect when given 12 days after treatment. In a murine lymphoid leukemia, combination of chemotherapy and immunotherapy was more effective than either alone (21) and most effective when the immunotherapy was given early in remission. We attempted to incorporate these animal data into our immunotherapy schedule; intravenous administration was prompted by the effectiveness of BCG on a variety of animal tumors when given by this route (2–4,19,20,30) and by the painful reactions and skin ulcers that occur when BCG is given by intradermal injection (24,26).

In general, intravenous BCG was well tolerated. Patients felt unwell for up to 72 hr after BCG injection, usually in association with pyrexia and sometimes headaches and muscle pains. Similar reactions have been reported after the use of BCG intradermally (11,26). Because two patients had anaphylactic reactions following a second intravenous injection, we agree that BCG should be used intravenously with great caution (18). Similar reactions have been reported when BCG has been injected directly into solid tumors (14) and, for the present, intravenous BCG should not be used except in carefully controlled trials and should be preceded by antihistamine prophylaxis. Although disagreement exists about the effectiveness of these drugs (18,20), we have not seen anaphylactic reactions in a period of 18 months while using intravenous chlorpheniramine maleate prior to intravenous BCG. It is critically important that hydrocortisone is immediately available to treat anaphylactic reactions.

The isolation of *M. tuberculosis* from the sputum of one of our patients was almost certainly the result of a reactivation of an old tuberculous infection by leukemia or by immunosuppressive chemotherapy. The organism differed from BCG in that it produced tuberculous lesions in the guinea pig and was sensitive to pyrazinamide. Unlike others (14), we have been unable to culture BCG organisms from blood and have not observed illness that might have been caused by disseminated BCG (25). We have also been unable to culture BCG organisms from marrow, liver, and lung biopsies taken antemortem from some of these patients (28).

Granulomas similar to those reported by others (9,10,12,25) have occurred in either the liver or the lung of all patients where needle biopsy or postmortem material has been examined (28), and the persistent unexplained splenomegaly detected in two patients is likely to be secondary to granuloma formation. Because one patient developed a granuloma in the skin at the site of intravenous injection, we now give BCG by intravenous saline infusion. It is our opinion that these granulomata are produced by the intravenous administration of BCG, but it is reassuring to note that these lesions appear innocuous despite their widespread distribution. To our knowledge, no *in vivo* study of tissue biopsies in patients receiving BCG by the cutaneous route has been performed, but the demonstration of epithelioid granulomas (10), in the liver, lungs, spleen, and kidneys in 13 of 20 asymptomatic patients dying from a variety of causes 6 weeks to 40 months after BCG vaccination makes it seem likely that BCG administration is also associated with granuloma formation when given by the intradermal route.

Skin testing prior to immunotherapy and at intervals during therapy in our patients has suggested that it may be possible to define a group of patients who do less well. These patients are initially anergic to hypersensitivity skin test antigens and remain so after BCG treatment. These preliminary findings are in keeping with the studies of Gutterman et al. (11), who found that patients who were anergic initially but converted after treatment with BCG subcutaneously survived in remission for longer than 60 weeks. In addition, in a small number of patients, they were able to predict relapse when patients became anergic once more.

Additional controlled trials of chemoimmunotherapy are indicated in the treatment of adult AML, and our findings suggest that BCG can be given intravenously without undue toxicity and without the significant local complications of the intradermal route. Its use warrants further close study.

SUMMARY

In a 2-year period, 37 of 81 adults with AML achieved complete remission after repeated courses of DNR and cytosine arabinoside (ARAC). They were randomized to maintenance treatment with monthly DNR/ARAC or to identical chemotherapy plus intravenous BCG. Eighteen BCG-treated patients had significantly longer survival times than 19 patients treated with chemotherapy only, although no statistically significant difference can be seen in the remission duration of the two groups. Thirteen patients in the BCG-treated group who have relapsed have received DNR/ARAC reinduction, and six second and two third remissions have been obtained. Thirteen control group patients have relapsed, and 11 have received further reinduction treatment with DNR/ARAC, but only one patient has entered a complete remission. Seven patients in the BCG-treated group who survived for 75 weeks or more (76, 93, 96, 125, 131, 155, and 162 weeks) either were PPD positive before treatment or converted to PPD positivity after BCG treatment. Using a battery of skin tests it may be possible to define a good prognostic group of patients and design future treatment accordingly.

The BCG group had a total of 268 intravenous treatments. All patients had pyrexia 6 to 12 hr after injection lasting 12 to 72 hr and occasionally headaches and muscle pains. Two patients had nonfatal anaphylactic reactions that did not recur when BCG was subsequently readministered. Other complications of BCG therapy were not a problem, and we have not needed to withdraw treatment for any patient.

ACKNOWLEDGMENTS

We thank Dr. J. Marks, Director, Tuberculosis Reference Laboratory, for helpful advice, Dr. I. Cavill and Janet Fisher for statistical analysis, and our colleagues in South Wales for referring their patients.

REFERENCES

1. Ansari, B. M., Thompson, E., and Whittaker, J. A. (1975): A comparative study of acute myeloblastic leukaemia in children and adults. *Br. J. Haematol.*, 31:269.

2. Baldwin, R. W., and Pimm, M. V. (1971): Influence of BCG infection on growth of 3-methylcholanthrene-induced rat sarcomas. *Eur. J. Clin. Biol. Res.,* 16:875.
3. Baldwin, R. W., and Pimm, M. V. (1973): BCG immunotherapy of pulmonary growths from intravenously transferred rat tumor cells. *Br. J. Cancer,* 27:48.
4. Bartlett, G. L. (1971): The effect of living BCG on tumor growth in mice. *Proc. Am. Assoc. Cancer Res.,* 12:41.
5. Bodey, G. P., Freireich, E. J., Monto, R. W., and Hewlett, J. S. (1969): Cytosine arabinoside therapy for acute leukaemia in adults. *Cancer Chemother. Rep.,* 53:59.
6. Crowther, D., Bateman, C. J. T., Vartan, C. P., Whitehouse, J. M. A., Malpas, J. S., Hamilton-Fairley, G., and Scott, R. B. (1970): Combination chemotherapy using L-asparaginase, daunorubicin and cytosine arabinoside in adults with acute myelogenous leukaemia *Br. Med. J.,* iv:513.
7. Currie, G. A., and Bagshawe, K. D. (1970): Active immunotherapy with corynebacterium parvum and chemotherapy in murine fibrosarcomas. *Br. Med. J.,* i:541.
8. Freeman, C. B., Harris, R., Geary, C. G., Leyland, M. J., McIver, J. E., and Delamore, I. W. (1973): Active immunotherapy used alone for maintenance of patients with acute myeloid leukaemia. *Br. Med. J.,* iv:571.
9. Freundlich, E., and Suprun, H. (1969): Tuberculoid granulomata in the liver after BCG vaccination. *Isr. J. Med. Sci.,* 5:108.
10. Gormsen, H. (1955): On the occurrence of epitheloid cell granulomas in the organs of BCG vaccinated human beings. *Acta Pathol. Scand. [Suppl.],* 111:117.
11. Gutterman, J. U., Hersh, E. M., Rodriguez, V., McCredie, K. B., Mavligit, G., Reed, R., Burgess, M. A., Smith, T., Gehan, E., Bodey, G. P., and Freireich, E. J. (1974): Chemoimmunotherapy of adult acute leukaemia. Prolongation of remission in myeloblastic leukaemia with BCG. *Lancet,* ii:1405.
12. Hunt, J. S., Silverstein, M. J., Sparks, F. C., Haskell, C. M., Pilch, Y. H., and Morton, D. L. (1973): Granulomatous hepatitis: A complication of BCG therapy. *Lancet,* ii:820.
13. Mathé, G. (1969): Approaches to the immunological treatment of cancer in man. *Br. Med. J.,* iv:7.
14. Morton, D. L., Holmes, E. C., Eilber, F. R., and Wood, W. C. (1971): Immunological aspects of neoplasia: A rational basis for immunotherapy. *Ann. Intern. Med.,* 74:587.
15. Medical Research Council Leukaemia Committee and Working Party on Leukaemia in Childhood. (1971): Treatment of acute lymphoblastic leukaemia. *Br. Med. J.,* iv:189.
16. Medical Research Council Working Party on the Evaluation of Different Methods of Therapy in Leukaemia (1963): Treatment of acute leukaemia in adults: Comparison of steroid therapy at high and low dosage in conjunction with 6-mercaptopurine. *Br. Med. J.,* iv:7.
17. Medical Research Council Working Party on Leukaemia in Adults (1974): Treatment of acute myeloid leukaemia with daunorubicin, cytosine arabinoside, mercaptopurine, L-asparaginase, predisone and thioguanine: Results of treatment with five multiple-drug schedules. *Br. J. Haematol.,* 27:373.
18. Muggleton, P. W., Prince, G. H., and Hilton, M. L. (1975): Effect of intravenous BCG in guinea pigs and pertinence to cancer immunotherapy in man. *Lancet,* i:1353.
19. Old, L. J., Clarke, D. A., and Benacerraf, B. (1959): Effect of Bacillus Calmette-Guerin infection on transplanted tumours in the mouse. *Nature,* 184:291.
20. Owen, L. N., and Bostock, D. E. (1974): Effects of intravenous BCG in normal dogs and in dogs with spontaneous osteosarcoma. *Eur. J. Cancer,* 10:775.
21. Pearson, J. W., Chaparas, S. D., and Chirigos, M. A. (1973): Effect of dose and route of Bacillus Calmette-Guerin in chemoimmunostimulation therapy of a murine leukaemia. *Cancer Res.,* 33:1845.
22. Pearson, J. W., Pearson, G. R., Ginson, W. T., Cherman, J. C., and Chirigos, M. A. (1972): Combined chemoimmunostimulation therapy against murine leukaemia. *Cancer Res.,* 32:904.
23. Peto, R., and Pike, M. C. (1973): Conservatism of the approximation $\Sigma(O-E)^2/E$ in the logrank test for survival data or tumor incidence data. *Biometrics,* 29:579.

24. Powles, R. L., Crowther, D., Bateman, C. J. T., Beard, M. E. J., McElwain, T. J., Russell, J., Lister, T. A., Whitehouse, J. M. A., Wrigley, P. F. M., Pike, M., Alexander, P., and Fairley, G. H. (1973): Immunotherapy for acute myelogenous leukaemia. *Br. J. Cancer,* 28:365.
25. Sparks, F. C., Silverstein, M. J., Hunt, J. S., Haskell, C. M., Pilch, Y. H., and Morton, D. L. (1973): Complications of BCG immunotherapy in patients with cancer. *N. Engl. J. Med.,* 289:827.
26. Vogler, W. R., and Chan, Y-K. (1974): Prolonging remission in myeloblastic leukaemia by Tice-strain Bacillus Calmette-Guerin. *Lancet,* ii:128.
27. Whitecar, J. P., Bodey, G. P., McCredie, K. B., Hart, J. S., and Freireich, E. J. (1972): Cyclophosphamide (NSC-26271), vincristine (NSC-67574), cytosine-arabinoside (NSC-63878) and prednisone (NSC-10023) (COAT) combination chemotherapy for acute leukaemia in adults, 1, 2, 3. *Cancer Chemother. Rep.,* 56:543.
28. Whittaker, J. A., Bentley, P., Melville-Jones, G. R., and Slater, A. J. (1976): Granuloma formation in patients receiving BCG immunotherapy. *J. Clin. Pathol.,* 29:693.
29. Whittaker, J. A., Lilleyman, J. S., Jacobs, A., and Balfour, I. (1973): Immunotherapy with intravenous BCG. *Lancet,* ii:1454.
30. Zbar, B., Bernstein, I. D., and Rapp, H. J. (1971): Suppression of tumor growth at the site of infection with living Bacillus Calmette-Guerin. *J. Natl. Cancer Inst.,* 46:831.

Question and Answer Session

Dr. Rosenberg: Would you clarify the number of viable BCG organisms that your patients received? Did all of the patients go through that sequential increasing concentration of BCG?

Dr. Whittaker: The increasing concentration schedule was given as the initial therapy. Once the dose was established, which in every case was 0.1 ml of the preparation, containing between four and nine times 10^6 organisms, each patient received that dosage every second week.

Dr. Fahey: Do you know of other centers with experience in intravenous BCG? Have they encountered any problems?

Dr. Whittaker: I don't think there is any other controlled trial but Professor Mathé has experience with intravenous BCG.

Dr. Mathé: We have conducted a Phase I trial with fresh French Pasteur BCG using 10^6 and 10^7 organisms given IV and we had no serious toxicity. It was well tolerated, but we got immunodepression in most patients. I think there is a difference between lyophilized Glaxo BCG IV, which is well tolerated and efficient, and the fresh Pasteur IV, which may be too strong or too rich in living organisms, and thus induce immunodepression.

Dr. Whittaker: Could I ask Professor Mathé for clarification of that, because I know he has published a paper about the use of intravenous BCG in melanoma.

Dr. Mathé: We published reports on melanoma and other patients in the first studies, but we got the same immunodepression.

*Immunotherapy of Cancer: Present Status of
Trials in Man,* edited by W. D. Terry and D. Windhorst.
Raven Press, New York © 1978.

Chemoimmunotherapy of Acute Myelocytic Leukemia with MER

Janet Cuttner, Oliver Glidewell, James F. Holland, and J. G. Bekesi

Division of Hematology, Mount Sinai School of Medicine of the City University of New York, New York, New York 10029

INDUCTION

During the last several years there has been a significant improvement in the treatment of acute myelocytic leukemia (AML) (1–6). Cytosine arabinoside (AraC) has been found to be effective in all studies. In a pilot study by Yates et al. the use of a 7-day continuous infusion of AraC plus daunorubicin for 3 days (7 + 3) produced a remission rate of 80% in patients under 60 years of age (7). The Cancer and Leukemia Group B (CALGB) has recently conducted a randomized study, chaired by Kanti Rai (protocol #7421) comparing this induction arm with three others. It was found in this multiinstitutional study that the 7 + 3 arm produced 57% complete remission and 73% complete and partial remissions in patients under 60 years of age. The patients were maintained on monthly 5-day courses of AraC with thioguanine, cyclophosphamide, CCNU, and daunorubicin in successive months. The AraC in maintenance was given either intravenously or subcutaneously, and the subcutaneous administration of AraC was found to be significantly superior to an equivalent dose of drug administered intravenously.

A pilot study was undertaken by Cuttner et al. (2) to test the effectiveness of immunotherapy with methanol extraction residue of BCG organisms (MER) in AML. Twenty-one patients with AML under 60 years of age were treated with AraC 100 mg/m² in a continuous intravenous infusion for 7 days plus daunorubicin 45 mg/m² on days 1, 2, and 3 as a direct intravenous injection. Complete remissions were produced in 15, or 71%. The maintenance chemotherapy was identical to protocol #7421 except that all patients received AraC in maintenance intravenously. When MER became available, seven of the last 10 who achieved complete remission were selected to receive MER based solely on ease of commutation. The remission duration for those receiving chemotherapy alone was 3½ months compared to 15½ months for the chemoimmunotherapy group. This difference was significant ($p = 0.005$). The median survival of patients on chemotherapy alone was 9½

For the Cancer and Leukemia Group B (CALGB).

months. The median survival of patients on chemoimmunotherapy was 21
months. These promising results led to the current controlled clinical trial
protocol #7521.

PATIENTS

All patients with AML (acute myeloblastic, acute myelomonocytic, promyelocytic, erythroleukemia, or acute monocytic) are eligible for this study,
irrespective of age, provided that the following conditions are fulfilled.

1. They have never received any of the drugs prescribed in this study.
2. They have had no more than 1 weeks' therapy with corticosteroids.
3. There are no systemic signs of infection. Patients with proven systemic
infection are not eligible for leukemia chemotherapy until measures designed
to control infections (e.g., performance of appropriate diagnostic studies,
hydration, and administration of antimicrobial therapy) have been initiated.
Such patients become eligible for this study after these measures have brought
infection under control or when the investigator judges that the systemic signs
should not be ascribed to life-threatening infection.
4. Blood urea nitrogen is 30 mg% or lower or creatinine 1.5 mg% or
lower. Patients with uric acid nephropathy are eligible for study after treatment has restored the urine flow and has lowered the blood urea nitrogen
levels below 30 mg%.
5. A written informed consent is obtained from the patients and/or legal
guardian prior to institution of the study.

TREATMENT

In induction patients are randomly allocated to receive chemotherapy with
AraC and daunorubicin with or without MER as follows.

AraC	100 mg/m² daily by continuous i.v. infusion from day 1 through 7
plus	
Daunorubicin	45 mg/m² daily by rapid i.v. injection on days 1, 2, and 3

If the patient does not go into remission on the first course, the second
course of chemotherapy is given as follows.

AraC	100 mg/m² daily by continuous i.v. infusion for *5 days*
plus	
Daunorubicin	45 mg/m² daily by rapid i.v. injection on days 1 and 2 of second course

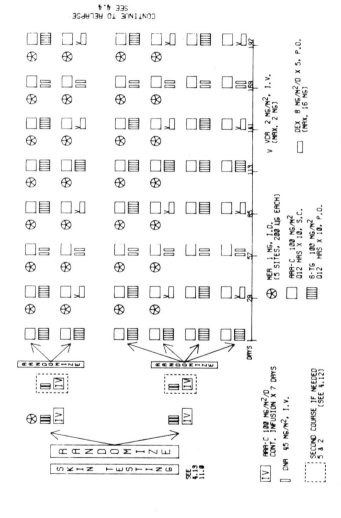

FIG. 1. Study design for protocol #7521, untreated AML.

If the patient has been randomized to receive immunotherapy at induction, he begins chemotherapy and immunotherapy on the same day. The immunotherapy is given in a dose of 1.0 mg, divided into five intradermal sites. Sites used are the anterior thighs, abdominal wall, the dorsal surface of the upper arms, and the lower thorax in the mid axillary line. Two hundred micrograms of MER are given in each of five intradermal sites in 0.2 ml each for a total dose of 1 mg (See Fig. 1). If randomized not to receive MER, he gets another random chance after induction to receive MER only in maintenance.

MAINTENANCE

Patients are randomly allocated to receive one of four maintenance treatments as follows.

In *regimen A* 5-day courses of AraC + thioguanine (TG) are repeated every 4 weeks. AraC given s.c.

In *regimen B* the monthly courses of AraC + TG are alternated with AraC, vincristine, and dexamethasone. In both regimens the third, seventh, and 11th courses are substituted by AraC and daunorubicin.

The other two regimens are chemotherapy identical to regimen A and regimen B, but in addition the patient receives immunotherapy with MER in a dose identical to that of induction.

STATISTICAL ANALYSIS

All clinical data are recorded on standard CALGB flow sheets and summary sheets and are collected centrally with copies maintained at the originating institution, by the study chairman, and the central office. Data to be analyzed are abstracted from these records by the study chairman with sample cases abstracted independently by the CALGB committee chairman for reliability analysis. The criteria used for a complete evaluation are those developed by the CALGB. Patients whose bone marrow qualify for an M^0 or M^1 must have normal erythropoiesis, granulopoiesis, and megakaryopoiesis (except for drug-induced changes such as megaloblastosis, macrocytosis, and/or reactive erythroid hyperplasia). Such marrows must have at least 2+ cellularity. The primary analyses of results were performed using Breslow's modified Wilcoxon test for censored observations, with separate tests for the competing causes of failure—death from leukemia, death with no leukemia, recurrent leukemia in the central nervous system, and recurrent leukemia in the marrow.

RESULTS

As of the last cut-off date of May 14, 1976, 369 patients had been entered on study, of which 255 were evaluable at the time of analysis. In this study

TABLE 1. *Response to induction therapy by age and treatment*

Age	ARA-C + DNR + MER						ARA-C + DNR					
	Eval.	CR	PR	NR	Died	% CR	Eval.	CR	PR	NR	Died	% CR
0–29	18	12	2	2	2	67	58	28	7	9	14	48
30–49	7	4	0	0	3	57	35	19	2	1	13	54
50–59	8	6	0	1	1	75	39	20	5	4	10	51
60+	18	5	1	2	10	28	72	26	2	8	36	36
Total	51	27	3	5	16	53	204	93	16	22	73	46
Age standardized % CR						53						45

CR, complete remission; DNR daunorubicin; NR, no response; PR, partial remission.

TABLE 2. *Response by induction therapy by course and treatment*

Treatment	Course 1					Course 2				
	Eval.	CR	PR	Off	% CR	Eval.	CR	PR	Off	% CR
Ara-C + DNR + MER	50	25	2	14	50	9	2	1	6	22
Ara-C + DNR	197	66	8	46	34	77	24	8	45	31
Totals	247	91	10	60	37	86	26	9	51	30

CR, complete remission; DNR, daunorubicin; PR, partial remission, Off, off study.

25% of the patients received MER in induction. The early results of this protocol show that 66% of patients under 60 years of age who were given 7 + 3 plus MER obtain a complete remission compared to 51% of patients receiving induction chemotherapy alone (Table 1). The age-standardized complete remission rate for chemoimmunotherapy is 53% compared to 45% of patients receiving chemotherapy alone. Table 2 shows response to induction therapy by course of treatment. An interesting finding was that 49% of

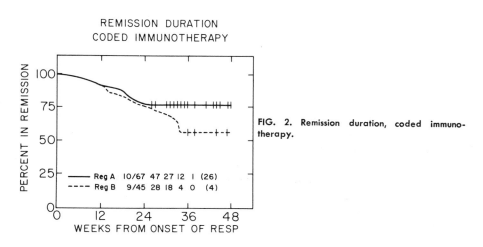

FIG. 2. Remission duration, coded immunotherapy.

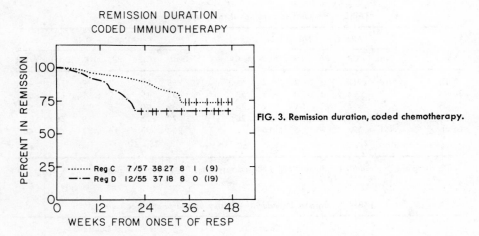

FIG. 3. Remission duration, coded chemotherapy.

patients receiving AraC, daunorubicin plus MER in induction went into complete remission on the *first* course of chemotherapy as compared to only 34% of patients who received chemotherapy alone. Figure 2 shows the survival by induction treatment for the total patients. There appears to be a beginning trend of improvement in patients receiving immunotherapy compared to patients receiving chemotherapy alone (Fig. 3). The results of maintenance therapy must be considered preliminary at this time. However, there do seem to be differences emerging between the chemotherapy and chemoimmunotherapy group.

SIDE EFFECTS OF TREATMENT

The commonest toxicity in induction was bleeding and infection. The MER toxicity in induction was chills, fever, and ulcerations. In maintenance the toxicity of MER was chills, fever, ulcerations, and pain at the site of injection.

DISCUSSION

AML may be more responsive to immunotherapy than ALL, originally pioneered by Mathé. This may be attributable to the detection of leukemia associated antigens on the surface of myeloblasts (8,10). MER has certain advantages over BCG from which it is derived, as originally pointed out by Weiss (11). MER is nonviable, stable, and subject to precise measurement in dose. BCG is living, perishable, and not subject to precise dosing because of its variable multiplication in the host. Treatment with MER can prevent or correct states of immunodepression and facilitate immunoresponse to otherwise nonimmunogenic antigens.

The early results of induction therapy in protocol #7521 have shown that

66% of patients under 60 years of age who were given chemoimmunotherapy in induction obtain a complete remission as compared to 51% of patients receiving chemotherapy alone. The majority of patients receiving chemoimmunotherapy who go into remission do so on the first course of chemotherapy and thus do not require a second induction course. The results of maintenance therapy are very early at this time; however, there do seem to be differences emerging between the chemotherapy and the chemoimmunotherapy group and between the two chemotherapy maintenance treatments.

SUMMARY

Three hundred sixty-seven patients have been entered on a comparative study of the value of immunotherapy with MER as an adjuvant induction and two chemotherapy programs in AML. Induction chemotherapy was given with AraC 100 mg/m^2 in a continuous intravenous infusion for 7 days plus daunorubicin 45 mg/m^2 on days 1, 2, and 3 as a direct intravenous injection. In addition, 25% of the patients in induction received immunotherapy with MER. The MER was given in a dose of 1.0 mg, divided into five intradermal sites. Maintenance therapy consisted of monthly 5-day courses of AraC in a dose of 100 mg/m^2 every 12 hr subcutaneously and in the first program patients received in addition TG in a dose of 100 mg/m^2 every 12 hr by mouth. The second maintenance chemotherapy was again monthly 5-day courses of AraC, the same dose as above, and on alternate months the patient received vincristine in a dose of 2 mg/m^2 intravenously on day 1 not to exceed 2 mg plus dexamethasone for 5 days in a dose of 8 mg/m^2 not to exceed 16 mg. The patients were further randomized to receive chemotherapy alone or, in addition to the above chemotherapy programs, the patient received immunotherapy with MER in a dose of 1.0 mg monthly.

The early results of this protocol show that 66% of patients under 60 years of age who were given 7 + 3 plus MER obtained a complete remission compared to 51% of patients receiving induction chemotherapy alone. The age-standardized complete remission rate for chemoimmunotherapy is 53% compared to 45% of patients receiving chemotherapy alone. The results of maintenance therapy have to be considered preliminary at this time, but they do show trends of difference between immunotherapy versus chemotherapy alone and between the two different chemotherapy maintenance arms.

REFERENCES

1. Bodey, G., Coltman, C., Freireich, E. J., Bonnet, J., Gehan, E., Haut, A., Hewlett, J., McCredie, K., Saiki, J., and Wilson, H. (1974): Chemotherapy of acute leukemia. Comparison of cytarabine alone and in combination with vincristine, prednisone and cyclophosphamide. *Arch. Intern. Med.,* 133:260–266.
2. Cuttner, J., Holland, J. F., Bekesi, J. G., Ramachandar, K., and Donovan, P. (1975): Chemoimmunotherapy of acute myelocytic leukemia. *Proc. ASCO,* 16:264.
3. Clarkson, D. B. (1972): Acute myelocytic leukemia in adults. *Cancer,* 30:1572–1582.

4. Crowther, D., Powles, R. L., Bateman, C. J. T., Beard, M. E. J., Gauci, C. L., Wrigley, P. F. M., Malpos, J. S., Hamilton-Fairley, G., and Bodley Scott, R. (1973): Management of adult acute myelogenous leukemia. *Br. Med. J.,* 1:131–137.
5. Gutterman, J. U., Rodriquez, V., Mavligit, G., Burgess, M. A., Gehan, E., Hersh, E. M., McCredie, K. B., Reed, R., Smith, T., Bodey, G. B., and Freireich, E. J. (1974): Chemoimmunotherapy of adult acute leukemia. Prolongation of remission in myeloblastic leukemia with BCG. *Lancet,* 1405–1409.
6. Ellison, R. R. (1973): Acute myelocytic leukemia. In: *Cancer Medicine,* p. 1229 Lea & Febiger, Philadelphia.
7. Yates, J. W., Wallace, H. J., Jr., Ellison, R. R., and Holland, J. F. (1973): Cytosine arabinoside (NSC-63878) and daunorubicin (NSC-83142) therapy in acute non-lymphocytic leukemia. *Cancer Chemother. Rep.,* Part 1, 57:81–48.
8. Gutterman, J. V., Rossen, R. D., Butler, W. T., McCredie, M. B., Bodey, G. P., Freireich, E. J., and Hersh, E. M. (1973): Immunoglobulin on tumor cells and tumor-induced lymphocyte blastogenesis in human acute leukemia. *N. Engl. J. Med.,* 228:169–173.
9. Leventhal, B. G., Halterman, R. H., Rosenberg, E. B., Herberman, R. B. (1972): Immune reactivity of leukemia patients to autologous blast cells. *Cancer Res.,* 32:1820–1825.
10. Powles, R. L., Balchin, L. A., Hamilton-Fairley, G., and Alexander, P. (1971): Recognition of leukemia cells as foreign before and after autoimmunization. *Br. Med. J.,* 1:486–489.
11. Weiss, D. W. (1975): Non-specific stimulation and modulation of the immune response and the status of resistance by the fraction of tubercula bacilli. *Natl. Cancer Inst. Monogr.,* 2,35:157–171.

Question and Answer Session

Dr. Reizenstein: You have a fairly large group of nonevaluable patients. Could you comment on that? And could you please compare the results between the three studies from the Mount Sinai group, your pilot study, your ongoing study, and the earlier study of the same group?

Dr. Cuttner: Regarding the nonevaluable patients, there were no data on thirty-five; ten patients were too early to evaluate, and eighteen patients were ineligible, usually because they had received nonprotocol chemotherapy. Six were lost early, and ten had inadequate records. We should have evaluations on about half of those patients in the next analysis. Comparing the three studies: the chemotherapy arms of the pilot study and the neuraminidase study at Mt. Sinai are identical. In this study, the chemotherapy in maintenance is different. In the study that Dr. Holland reported, MER was not given alone. He reported on neuraminidase cells alone, neuraminidase cells with MER and chemotherapy. My pilot study was MER plus chemotherapy or chemotherapy alone.

Dr. Powles: None of the patients you have described in these studies received neuraminidase cells. Is that right?

Dr. Cuttner: Correct.

Dr. Weiss: Dr. Cuttner, would you discuss the reason for starting MER on Day 1 of induction? When tumor load is still maximal one could argue there would be much less of an effect of an immunostimulatory agent than when tumor is somewhat reduced.

Dr. Cuttner: One of the reasons was that MER has been found in some animal studies to protect against infection. In fact, MER did not prevent patients from becoming infected. The number of infections is equal in both groups.

Dr. Weiss: In the study comparing the efficacy of neuraminidase-treated cells against the controls with or without MER, there was no MER-alone group. It may be that the combination of nonspecific immunomodulation and specific immunological stimulation might in fact be less effective than either one alone. So one would have had to have an MER-alone group in that study in order to be able to make some evaluation of those data comparatively.

Dr. Cuttner: I agree. You can't compare from that point of view, because we didn't have that one group.

Immunotherapy of Cancer: Present Status of
Trials in Man, edited by W. D. Terry and D. Windhorst.
Raven Press, New York © 1978.

Evaluation of *Pseudomonas aeruginosa* Vaccine for Prolongation of Remissions in Adults with Acute Nonlymphoblastic Leukemia Treated with the L-12 Protocol: A Preliminary Report

Timothy S. Gee, Monroe D. Dowling, Isabelle Cunningham,
Herbert S. Oettgen, Donald Armstrong, and
Bayard D. Clarkson

Memorial Sloan-Kettering Cancer Center, New York, New York 10021

The heptavalent lipopolysaccharide *Pseudomonas aeruginosa* vaccine was initially used at Memorial Sloan-Kettering Cancer Center in the L-6 protocol (Fig. 1) from 1970–1974 (1–4) in a randomized controlled prospective study to determine if this form of immunization would prevent a nosocomial

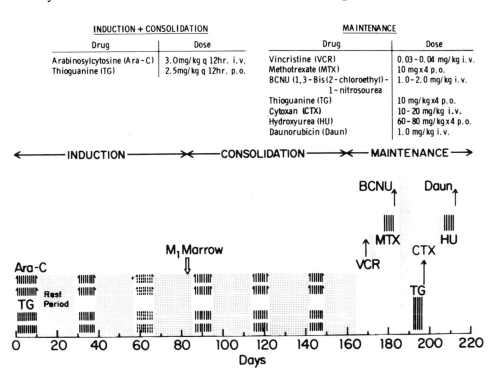

INDUCTION + CONSOLIDATION		MAINTENANCE	
Drug	Dose	Drug	Dose
Arabinosylcytosine (Ara-C)	3.0mg/kg q 12hr. i.v.	Vincristine (VCR)	0.03 - 0.04 mg/kg i.v.
Thioguanine (TG)	2.5mg/kg q 12hr. p.o.	Methotrexate (MTX)	10 mg x 4 p.o.
		BCNU (1,3-Bis(2-chloroethyl)-1-nitrosourea	1.0-2.0 mg/kg i.v.
		Thioguanine (TG)	10 mg/kg x4 p.o.
		Cytoxan (CTX)	10-20 mg/kg i.v.
		Hydroxyurea (HU)	60-80 mg/kg x 4 p.o.
		Daunorubicin (Daun)	1.0 mg/kg i.v.

FIG. 1. L-6 protocol.

415

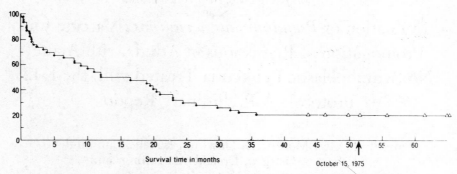

FIG. 2. Survival curve of 46 responders on the L-6 protocol. △, living NED, ●, dead.

infectious complication in patients with acute nonlymphoblastic leukemia. The results of this study (3) revealed a significant number of patients with long-term remissions (>36 months) (Fig. 2). A disproportionately higher number of long-term remissions occurred in patients who had received *P. aeruginosa* vaccine than in the control group. It was because of this finding that *P. aeruginosa* vaccine was incorporated into the L-12 protocol in a prospective randomized trial to determine if this form of nonspecific immunotherapy would prolong remissions.

PATIENTS

Adult patients (>15 years) with acute nonlymphoblastic leukemia and no prior or minimal prior chemotherapy treated on the L-12 protocol were randomized by a computer-generated selection code into a vaccine or control group. Fifty adult patients with previously untreated acute myeloblastic, myelomonocytic, or monoblastic leukemia (AML) have been entered on the L-12 protocol. An additional 10 patients with erythroleukemia and nine pa-

TABLE 1. *L-12 Protocol, previously untreated patients*

	AML	Erythro	PL
Entered	50	10	9
Died during induction	14	0	1
Failure	10	5	0
Died during consolidation (M₁ Marrow)	1	1	2
PR	0	2	0
CR	25	2	6
Relapses	7 (2–10 Mos.)	1 (10 Mos.)	0
Still in CR	18 (1–19 + Mos.)	1 (7 Mos.)	6 (5–17 + Mos.)

AML, acute myeloblastic, myelomonocytic, monoblastic leukemia; Erythro, erythroleukemia; PL, acute promyelocytic leukemia; PR, partial remission.

tients with acute promyelocytic leukemia have been studied, but this discussion is limited only to patients with AML (Table 1). The AML patients consisted of 28 males and 22 females, age range 16 to 71 (median 54 years). In this group of 50 patients, 21 had begun the L-12 protocol *before* the vaccine was included in the study and thus were not randomized. Four of these 21 nonrandomized patients were given *P. aeruginosa* vaccinations after they had attained complete remissions (CR).

The 29 patients who were randomized consisted of 15 males and 14 females with an age range of 16 to 70 years (median 55). Thirteen of the 20 patients were in the vaccine group. Table 2 details some of the initial clinical aspects of the patients randomized to the vaccine and control groups.

TABLE 2. *Clinical information on 29 AML patients randomized for Pseudomonas vaccine study*

| | | | | | | Blasts | | |
| | | | | | | Peripheral blood | | Marrow |
Group	Age	Sex	WBC $\times 10^3/mm^3$	HGB g %	Platelets $\times 10^3/mm^3$	%	Absolute	%
Vaccine								
J. B.	45	M	7.6	10.6	70	43	3.4	37.5
B. N.	16	M	6.1	8.5	12	0	0	20
M. Mc	40	M	21.0	7.9	15	↑	—	37.5
J. K.	48	F	102	9.9	40	74	75.5	2.8
M. M.	43	F	5.2	8.9	37	21	1.1	88.
H. G.	58	M	3.9	9.5	18	3	0.1	21.5
G. D.	44	F	42.6	10.1	40	15	6.4	10
M. B.	61	M	75.	13.5	64	71	53.3	79
J. M.	53	M	11.	7.4	63	60	6.7	35
F. I.	51	M	2.6	8.3	12	2	0.05	23.5
K. S.	57	F	51.9	6.1	70	73	37.8	47
T. S.	68	F	4.0	8.3	27	10	0.4	18.5
J. M.	69	M	19.1	7.4	29	16	3.1	39.5
Control								
R. L.	27	F	16.4	7.7	62	89	14.6	63
R. C.	48	M	14.	13.5	101	14	2.0	14
A. S.	30	F	32.1	10.2	19	87	27.9	75
S. K.	24	F	7.0^a	5.3	87	10	0.7	19
C. L.	18	F	3.	12.8	278	5	0.2	64.5
J. D.	42	F	3.2	7.4	67	48	1.5	74.5
M. S.	61	F	86.	8.7	60	51	43.9	100
G. W.	59	M	2.2	11	49	0	0	6.6
H. D.	67	M	91	8.6	140	29	26.4	18
J. P.	60	M	34.3	11.7	50	0	0	33
S. G.	60	F	36.6	10.8	155	24	8.8	18
P. G.	69	F	0.9	8.6	59	16	0.4	40
G. B.	55	M	9.2	12.9	21	42	3.9	38
G. M.	62	F	1.4	8.5	45	N.D.	N.D.	80
J. Mc	70	M	24.5	12.5	25	24	5.9	10
G. B.	62	M	1.3	9.1	148	30	0.4	90

^{a} Four days after first visit.

↑, Increased blasts; HGB, hemoglobin; N.D., not done; WBC, white blood cell count.

TREATMENT

The chemotherapeutic drugs, dosages, and schedule of the L-12 protocol are graphically represented in Fig. 3.

P. aeruginosa vaccine was administered intramuscularly with a #26 gauge needle beginning on the first day of induction therapy. The dose of vaccine was escalated gradually from 0.25, to 0.50, to 1.0 ml. During the induction therapy the vaccine was given twice weekly and then once weekly through the consolidation phase of the protocol. No prophylactic therapy with antihistamines or antipyretic agents were given for local or systemic reaction to the vaccine.

The severity of local and/or systemic reactions frequently made it difficult to adhere strictly to the vaccination schedule. However the vaccine group received one to 11 (median three) vaccinations during induction and zero to four during the consolidation phase of the L-12 protocol.

RESULTS

Table 3 summarizes the results of the L-12 protocol in adult patients with AML. As demonstrated, there is no apparent difference in remission rate, number of failures, or patients dying during induction between the three groups. In addition to the 14 deaths during induction therapy, seven of the 10 failures have died whereas the remaining three patients who failed the L-12 have continued on other chemotherapeutic regimens or on no therapy.

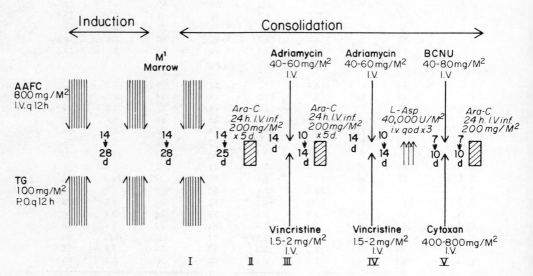

FIG. 3. L-12 protocol for patients with acute nonlymphoblastic leukemia. AAFC, anhydroarabinosylfluorocytosine; TG, 6-thioguanine; Ara-C, arabinosylcytosine; and BCNU, 1,3-bis (2-chloroethyl)-1-nitrosourea.

TABLE 3. Pseudomonas *vaccine, L-12 (AML only)*

	Randomized Vaccine during induction		Not randomized
	PV+	PV−	PV−
Entered	13	16	17
Died during induction	4	4	6
Failure	3	5	3
CR	6	7	8
Not randomized CR given PV during remission	4		
Relapses	1 (7 Mos.)	2 (2–3 Mos.)	4 (3–10 Mos.)
Died in CR			1*
Still in CR	9 (1–19 Mos.)	5 (1–9 Mos.)	3 (1–17 Mos.)
Relapses/CR	1/10		6/15
		p < .18	

PV, *Pseudomonas* vaccine.
a Died in consolidation from infection.

There have been a total of 7/25 relapses from all three groups. The 18 patients still in their initial remissions have remission durations ranging between 1 to 19+ months with a current median of 10+ months.

Of particular interest is the rate of relapses occurring in patients who received the vaccine compared with the control group. There have been 2/7 relapses in the randomized control group and 4/8 relapses in the patients who did not receive the vaccine prior to randomization. Thus a total of 6/15 relapses have occurred in patients who did not receive the *P. aeruginosa* vaccine. In the 10 patients who receive the vaccine (including the four who received the vaccine only after achieving remission) there has been only one patient who has relapsed. The difference is not statistically significant with $p < 0.18$ by Fisher's Exact Test (5).

SIDE EFFECTS OF TREATMENT

With the vaccination dose schedule used, 2/17 (12%) of the patients developed severe local reaction, whereas several more had mild to moderate reaction; all developed fevers of which 15/17 (88%) had a temperature >102°F (38.9°C) within 48 hr after the vaccination. The local reaction generally consisted of a cellulitis type reaction. Because of the severity of some of the local and systemic reactions, the vaccination dose schedule has since been changed to an initial dose of 0.025 ml rather than 0.25 ml i.m. If a severe reaction occurs with the initial 0.025 dose, the next dose is decreased to 0.01 ml. Vaccination in each sequence of the consolidation phase of the

L-12 is withheld until peripheral hematologic recovery from chemotherapy is noted, and given at least 24 hr before the next cycle of scheduled cytotoxic agents. For the present, a desired reaction from the vaccination in patients without fevers or infections is a fever less than 38.5°C, moderate erythema and warmth at the injection site, and/or pain that does not require analgesics.

DISCUSSIONS

The results presented here regarding the use of *P. aeruginosa* vaccine as active immunotherapy in a randomized study in adult patients with AML on the L-12 protocol are relatively premature. However, it does reveal no difference in the remission rate in patients who are vaccinated compared with a control group. Even though the numbers are small and differences not statistically significant, so far there is a lower relapse rate in vaccinated patients. This is consistent with an earlier finding with the L-6 protocol (Fig. 1), when the *P. aeruginosa* vaccine was used as active immunization against a common bacterial infection. The results showed no significant protection for infections by *P. aeruginosa,* but the L-6 protocol produced a CR rate of 56% (49/88 patients) with 12 of the 49 CR (24%) patients considered long-term remissions with remission durations >36 months. The patients with long-term remission have durations of remissions ranging between 38+ to 73+ months. Since all treatment was stopped after 31 to 36 months, these patients have had no therapy for 2 to 37 months. Only one patient has relapsed at 47 months after having been off maintenance therapy for 16 months. The single relapse patient in this subgroup of long-term remission had not received any *P. aeruginosa* vaccine.

In the L-6 study, only 17/88 patients received the *P. aeruginosa* vaccine. There were 13/17 CRs (77%) in the vaccine group compared to 36/71 (51%) in the control group. Seven of the 13 CRs (54%) in the vaccinated group were long-term remissions whereas only 5/36 (14%) were long-term remissions in the control group. The difference is statistically significant with a *p* value < 0.01 by the two-tailed Chi square test (5).

The lower relapse rate in the current study is obviously too early for comparison with the L-6 study but may be an early indicative trend towards a similar result of long-term remissions in the vaccine group.

The intensity of the side effects of vaccination is generally dose related in a single patient, but with significant variability between individual patients. It is unclear whether a local cellulitis or fever is necessary, let alone how severe a reaction or how high a fever should be to be considered an adequate response to the vaccination. For the time being, an adequate vaccination dose is based on occurrence of a moderate local cellulitis or fevers of at least 101°F. Because of the individual or biologic variability of response to the vaccine, the vaccination dose is variable, but generally the vaccination dose for most patients has been 0.25 to 0.5 ml i.m. Serum hemagglutination titres continue to be followed, and at present there continues to be no correlation of the titre to severity of local reactions.

The preliminary results reported justify the continuation of the current study using *P. aeruginosa* vaccine as part of L-12 protocol.

SUMMARY

Fifty adult patients (≥ 15 years) with acute nonlymphoblastic leukemia have been treated on the L-12 protocol. Twenty-nine patients were randomized, 13 to receive *P. aeruginosa* vaccine and 16 to the control group. No difference in remission rate is noted with 6/13 and 7/16 CR in each group, respectively. Twenty-one other patients were not randomized and 12/21 had remissions, also giving a comparable CR rate to the vaccine group. Four of the 12 not-randomized CR patients received the vaccine after attaining their remissions. Thus there are a total of 10 CR patients who received the vaccine and 15 CR patients in the control group.

There have been 6/15 relapses in the control group and 1/10 relapses in the vaccine group. The *p* value is 0.18. Because of the lower relapse rate in the vaccine group, the current study is being continued.

ACKNOWLEDGMENTS

This investigation was supported in part by National Cancer Institute grant nos. CA-08748 and CA-05826.

The authors wish to gratefully acknowledge the assistance of Peggy Dufour in the preparation of this manuscript.

REFERENCES

1. Hanessian, S., Regan, W., Watson, D., Haskell, T. H. (1971): Isolation and characterization of antigenic component of a new heptavalent *Pseudomonas* vaccine. *Nature (New Biol.)*, 229:209–210.
2. Fisher, M. W., Devlin, H. B., and Gnabasik, F. J. (1969): New immunotype schema for *Pseudomonas aeruginosa* based on protective antigens. *J. Bacteriol.*, 98:835–836.
3. Clarkson, B. D., Dowling, M. D., Gee, T. S., Cunningham, I. B., and Burchenal, J. H. (1975): Treatment of acute leukemia in adults. *Cancer,* 36 (2) Suppl.: 775–795.
4. Young, L. S., Meyers, R. D., and Armstrong, D. (1973): *Pseudomonas aeruginosa* vaccine in cancer patients. *Ann. Intern. Med.,* 79 (4):518–527.
5. Armitage, P. (1974): *Statistical Methods in Medical Research.* Wiley & Sons, New York.

Question and Answer Session

Dr. Fahey: Did I understand from one of your figures that there were seven or more patients who had a complete remission lasting for more than four years?

Dr. Gee: Twelve out of forty-nine. And they have been off therapy for three years.

Dr Fahey: Is there any evidence that the vaccine helps protect against pseudomonas?

Dr. Gee: No.

Dr. Hortobagyi: Why was the intramuscular route chosen? Was it on the basis of the infectious disease studies? Also, have you tried alternate routes of administration?

Dr. Gee: The intramuscular route was started by the infectious disease group, and we continued it. We are trying to find out whether it was significant or not. Possibly some of the patients may have received subcutaneous rather than intramuscular, but no other routes have been used.

Immunotherapy of Cancer: Present Status of Trials in Man, edited by W. D. Terry and D. Windhorst. Raven Press, New York © 1978.

Polyriboinosinic:Polyribocytidylic Acid as an Adjunct to Remission Maintenance Therapy in Acute Myelogenous Leukemia

O. Ross McIntyre, *Kanti Rai, **Oliver Glidewell, and †James F. Holland

*Norris Cotton Cancer Center, Dartmouth-Hitchcock Medical Center, Hanover, New Hampshire 03755; *Long Island Jewish-Hillside Medical Center, Division of Hematology, New Hyde Park, New York 11040; **Cancer and Leukemia Group B Operations Office, Scarsdale, New York 10583; and †Department of Neoplastic Disease, Mt. Sinai School of Medicine, New York, New York 10029*

Polyriboinosinic acid:Polyribocytidylic acid (Poly I:Poly C) is a synthetic double stranded RNA that is a highly effective interferon inducer and a potent immunological adjuvant (3,8,11). Following the demonstration that Poly I:C suppressed growth in animal tumor models, several human trials were initiated (1,6,9), most of them on patients with high tumor loads. One preliminary report of a trial in patients with recurrent superficial bladder carcinoma has also appeared (5).

The study reported here grew out of a phase II investigation at the Dartmouth-Hitchcock Medical Center in which Poly I:Poly C was administered to patients with acute myelogenous leukemia following a drug-induced remission (1). In this uncontrolled trial it was demonstrated that the compound could be administered with acceptable toxicity to patients in remission and that significant levels of serum interferon could be demonstrated in the patients following treatment. The results of this nonrandom trial could not be adequately compared with those derived from a historical control group because of differences in the chemotherapeutic programs employed. The duration of remission and survival data for the Poly I:Poly C group, however, suggested a possible benefit from the treatment and provided evidence that, at the very least, the treatment had not been harmful.

METHODS

As a result of the above trial the Cancer and Leukemia Group B (CALGB) designed the study shown in Fig. 1. Patients with acute myelogenous leukemia who achieved a drug-induced remission were randomized to receive one of four chemotherapeutic arms for maintenance. Two of the arms

---

For the Cancer and Leukemia Group B.

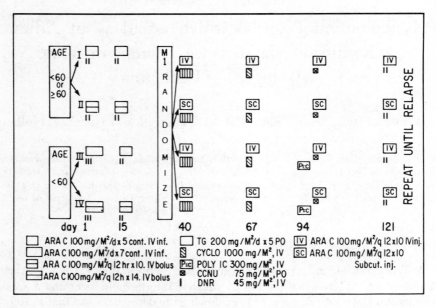

FIG. 1. Study design for protocol #7421.

employed, in addition to the chemotherapy, a single injection of Poly I:Poly C (Poly I:Poly C Lot 10 prepared by Miles Laboratories, Elkhart, Indiana) administered intravenously at a dosage of 300 mg/m² 1 week prior to the third maintenance chemotherapy treatment. A more complete description of the induction and maintenance chemotherapy employed will be published separately. This chapter concerns only the results of the study as they relate to the administration of Poly I:Poly C. Patients who entered remission received the maintenance chemotherapy shown in Fig. 1 at 4-week intervals. Investigators were asked to perform a bone marrow prior to the third course of chemotherapy as well as routine blood counts, history, and physical examination. Patients were randomized by the sealed envelope technique using a Latin square arrangement in order to achieve a balanced distribution. Poly I:Poly C was shipped individually to investigators for each patient who was randomized to receive the agent in order to conserve the limited supply of the drug. The drug was administered over a 10-min period by a slow intravenous infusion. Investigators were cautioned to observe the patient for allergic reactions and to treat these appropriately if they arose. Those patients receiving Poly I:C were given the assigned chemotherapy regimen 1 week later, and the chemotherapy was repeated as indicated for the experimental and control groups at 4 weekly intervals until relapse. Standard CALGB rating criteria and definitions of remission and relapse, as will be reported, were employed in this study (2). Serum specimens were shipped to Dartmouth-Hitchcock Medical Center for measurement of serum interferon by means of a dye uptake assay adapted to a micro technique in this laboratory (7).

RESULTS

The study was activated April 25, 1974, and was closed to patient entry on May 7, 1975. The results represent an analysis of information available at the time flow sheets were submitted in June, 1976. Table 1 displays the outcome of the randomization to Poly I:C or to the control group. Because the induction regimen was more effective than anticipated, a larger than expected number of patients entered the remission phase. The supply of Poly I:Poly C was, therefore, insufficient to treat all patients randomized to this therapy, and 39 evaluable patients actually received the Poly I:C, whereas 67 evaluable patients comprised the control group. Table 2 displays

TABLE 1. *Evaluable patients in experimental and control group*

72 patients were randomized to receive Poly I:C
  14 relapsed prior to its scheduled administration
  18 cases had no Poly I:C available
   1 was disqualified for receiving the drug 7 months late
39 patients are *evaluable* for the Poly I:C
79 patients were randomized to no Poly I:C
  9 relapsed prior to the third maintenance course
  3 were otherwise off prior to the third course (2 died, 1 lost)
67 patients are *evaluable* for the control group

TABLE 2. *Characteristics of evaluable patients*

Characteristic	Control	Poly I:C
% initial marrow > 90% leukemic cells	41	28
Mean age	39	40
% over 60 years	15	24
% males	59	51
% initial hemoglobin < 8.0 g %	33	27
% initial platelets < 50 × 10³	59	54
Median initial WBC × 10³	14.0	19.0
% initial WBC > 50 × 10³	32	21
% circulating blasts > 75%	36	24
% responded to 1 induction course	56	55
% induced with 5 & 2 Inf.[a]	18	33
% induced with 5 & 2 Bol.[b]	15	26
% induced with 7 & 3 Inf.[a]	37	18
% induced with 7 & 3 Bol.[b]	30	23
% i.v. Ara-C in maintenance	49	51
% s.c. Ara-C in maintenance	51	49

AraC, cytosine arabinoside; WBC, white blood cell count.
[a] Ara-C given in 24-hr infusion.
[b] Ara-C given in bolus.

the characteristics and prognostic factors of evaluable patients in the control and Poly I:Poly C groups. Although the control group tended to have a higher bone marrow blast percentage, a higher initial peripheral blast count, and an increased number of patients with white counts in excess of 50, -000/mm, there is no significant difference between the two groups in these characteristics.

Toxicity

All but two patients developed fever (mean $= 39.1 \pm 1.1°C$). Chills, nausea, and occasional vomiting were also noted. One patient developed vasomotor collapse and wheezing, which responded to therapy with epinephrine and antihistamines. No other toxicity was noted.

Interferon Production

Samples of serum obtained 8½ to 25 hr after Poly I:Poly C infusion were received on thirty-three patients for assay of serum interferon. The mean level of serum interferon was 41 IU/ml with a range from 0 to 290 IU. The infusion was stopped on the patient who developed the anaphylactic episode, and no interferon was found in this serum at 20 hr. Four other patients, in whom samples were obtained at 8½, 16, 17, and 20 hr, were found to have undetectable serum interferon. One of these patients did not develop fever or chills, the other three did. Assays conducted on six patients with acute myelogenous leukemia in remission and on patients with a variety of other malignancies failed to show detectable levels of serum interferon in the absence of treatment with interferon inducers, and for this reason, serum specimens for interferon assay were not collected on the control population.

Effect of Poly I:C on Remission Duration

Figure 2 shows the remission duration curves measured from the date of induction treatment for the control and the Poly I:Poly C-treated groups.

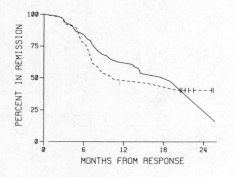

FIG. 2. Duration of remission for patients receiving Poly I:Poly C (------) and control patients (————).

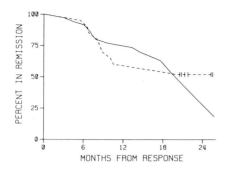

FIG. 3. Duration of remission for patients with normal marrow receiving Poly I:Poly C (------) and control patients (————).

There is no difference in response duration at the time of this analysis. Because of the possibility that the residual tumor load in these patients influences the activity of Poly I:Poly C, an analysis was undertaken of the marrow status in the patients prior to the administration of Poly I:Poly C. Figure 3 displays the response duration curves for the control and the Poly I: Poly C-treated group for those patients with a marrow showing a complete remission (<6% blasts). Figure 4 shows the response duration for the treated and control groups who were noted to have 6 to 20% blast cells in a marrow taken prior to the third maintenance treatment course. Although a significantly shorter response duration was noted for those with the higher leukemic cell residual, there is no evidence at this time that Poly I:Poly C influences the response duration in either the normal or early relapse groups. Figure 5 displays the remission duration for patients who had normal marrow at the time of Poly I:Poly C treatment and who were demonstrated to produce serum interferon. Similar curves are drawn for the group in early relapse in Fig. 6. Marrow information was lacking on an additional five patients. The differences between the control and experimental group shown in these figures is not statistically significant and suggests that the failure to demonstrate an effect secondary to Poly I:C in the earlier figures is not due to the inclusion of patients who failed to produce serum interferon.

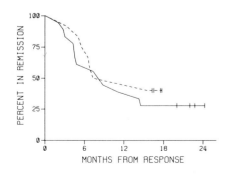

FIG. 4. Duration of response for patients in early relapse who received Poly I:Poly C (------) and control patients (————).

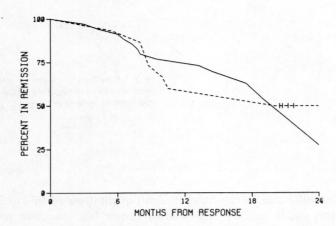

FIG. 5. Duration of remission for patients who had normal marrows (M1) and produced interferon after Poly I:Poly C (------) and control patients (————).

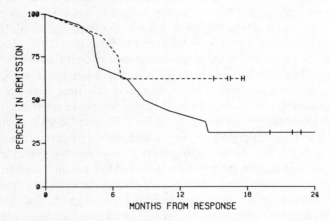

FIG. 6. Duration of response for patients who were in early relapse (M2) and produced interferon after Poly I:Poly C (------) and control patients (————).

DISCUSSION

Patients with acute myelogenous leukemia in remission provide an ideal population for studying the effect of interferon, interferon inducers, and immunological adjuvants. In these patients successful initial chemotherapy causes a minimum of a 1 to 2 log reduction in tumor cell mass as evidenced by a return of the bone marrow to normal and reduction in organ size. Despite continuation of therapy in a variety of maintenance schedules, relapse is rapid. Further reduction in tumor load by adjunctive therapy should be readily discernible in the form of a longer remission.

Although differences in remission duration and survival may yet emerge for the group receiving Poly I:Poly C in this study, at the present time there is no evidence that the administration of Poly I:Poly C in this study has influenced these parameters. In the present study some patients clearly had a lower tumor cell burden following the initial induction phase and were in early relapse at the time Poly I:C was administered. Other patients may have had a lower tumor cell burden during the interval the drug was administered than at the end of the induction. Development of means whereby tumor cell burden could be more adequately measured during remission may assist in the scheduling of this type of therapeutic intervention.

Furthermore, the timing of the adjunctive therapy with respect to the chemotherapy may be of critical importance. Immunological suppression followed by a rebound phenomenon has been demonstrated after chemotherapeutic treatment (4,10). Our phase II studies showed a clear suppression of the *in vitro* correlates of the cellular immune response in patients receiving Poly I:C, which we are attempting to relate to the known adjuvant activity of this agent in studies that are currently under way. It is possible that treatment with Poly I:Poly C and the maintenance chemotherapy arms employed in the present study could produce immunological effects that were independent and additive, or that nullified each other.

Because immunotherapeutic findings derived in certain animal models are not reproducible when applied to other models, it is clear that the information derived from such experimentation should be transposed to man with great caution. A considerable amount of work based upon empirical design is necessary for optimization of immunotherapeutic schedules in man. The demonstration that Poly I:Poly C, Bacillus Calmette-Guerin (BCG) and BCG derivatives may all produce harmful effects in certain animal models, especially those in which the agents are administered prior to tumor cell challenge, makes it imperative to employ adequate concurrent randomized controls in the human trials. The present study indicates that Poly I:Poly C can be administered with reasonable safety in this setting. Considerable additional work is necessary in order to explore the effect of dose level and frequency of administration and to explore possible interactions with concurrent chemotherapy. In view of the activity that this agent has demonstrated in animal tumor models, further human experimentation is indicated despite the lack of effectiveness encountered in this study at this time.

SUMMARY

Poly I:Poly C was administered as a single injection of 300 mg/m^2 i.v. to 39 randomized patients with acute myelogenous leukemia receiving maintenance chemotherapy on CALGB protocol #7421. The duration of remission for the Poly I:Poly C-treated group was compared with that of 67 patients who were randomized to the same chemotherapy maintenance program but who did not receive the agent. The Poly I:Poly C was administered 1 week prior to the third monthly maintenance chemotherapy regimen. At this time 20 of the patients receiving Poly I:Poly C and 35 of the control patients had normal marrows, and the remainder of each group was in early relapse as indicated by the presence of 6 to 20% blasts in the marrow. Twenty-eight of 33 patients tested showed significant amounts of serum interferon following Poly I:Poly C treatment. At this time there is no difference in response duration between the experimental and control groups. In order to investigate the possibility that Poly I: Poly C was more effective in patients with a low tumor cell burden, the duration of remission for that group of patients who received the agent during early relapse was compared to the group who received it at a time the marrow examination was normal. The group in early relapse had a shorter overall duration of response whether or not they received the Poly I:C, and there was no indication that Poly I:C was detrimental in either group. Toxicity was acceptable, and there was no evidence of augmentation of tumor growth.

ACKNOWLEDGMENT

This study was supported by grants CA-04326, CA-11028, CA-16128, and contract NO1-CN-55199.

REFERENCES

1. Cornell, C. J., Jr., Smith, K. A., Cornwell, G. G., III, Burke, G. P., and McIntyre, O. R. (1977): Systemic effects of intravenous polyriboinosinic: polyribocytidylic acid in man. *J. Natl. Cancer Inst.,* 57:1211.
2. Ellison, R. R., Holland, J. F., Weil, M., Jacquillat, C., Boiron, M., Bernard, J., Sawitsky, A., Rosner, F., Gussoff, B., Silver, R. T., Karanas, A., Cuttner, J., Spurr, C. L., Hayes, D. M., Blom, J., Leone, L. A., Haurani, F., Kyle, R., Hutchison, J. L., Forcier, R. J., and Moon, J. H. (1968): Arabinosyl cytosine: A useful agent in the treatment of acute leukemia in adults. *Blood,* 32:507.
3. Field, A. K., Young, C. W., Krakoff, I. H., Tytell, A. A., Lampson, G. P., Nemes, M. M., and Hilleman, M. R. (1971): Induction of interferon in human subjects by poly I:C. *Proc. Soc. Exp. Biol. Med.,* 136:1180.
4. Halterman, R. H., and Leventhal, B. G., (1971): Enhanced immune response to leukemia. *Lancet,* 2:704.
5. Kemeny, N., Yagoda, A., Whitmore, W., Grabstald, H., Young, C., and Krakoff, I. (1976): Randomized prospective therapeutic trial of poly rI:rC in patients with papillomas or superficial carcinomas of the urinary bladder. *Proc. Am. Assoc. Cancer Res.,* 17:171.
6. Levy, H. (1970): Interferon and interferon inducers in the treatment of malignancies. *Arch. Intern. Med.,* 126:78.
7. McManus, N. (1976): Microtiter assay for interferon: Microspectrophotometric quantitation of cytopathic effect. *Appl. Microbiol.,* 31:35.
8. Pidot, A. L. R., and McIntyre, O. R. (1973): Interferon and interferon inducers in cancer chemotherapy. In: *Cancer Medicine,* edited by James F. Holland and Emil Frei III. Lea & Febiger, Philadelphia.
9. Robinson, R. A., DeVita, V. T., Levy, H. B., Baron, S., Hubbard, S. P., and Levine, A. S. (1976): Brief communication: A Phase I-II trial of multiple-dose polyriboinosinic-polyribocytidylic acid in patients with leukemia or solid tumors. *J. Natl. Cancer Inst.,* 57:599.

10. Schwartz, R., Stock, J., and Dameshek, W. (1958): Effect of 6-mercaptopurine on antibody production. *Proc. Soc. Exp. Biol. Med.*, 99:164–167.
11. Turner, W., Chan, S. P., and Chirigos, M. A. (1970): Stimulation of humoral and cellular antibody formation in mice by poly Ir:Cr. *Proc. Exp. Biol. Med.*, 133:334.

Question and Answer Session

Dr. Reizenstein: Did you have about an 18-month median remission duration in your chemotherapy-only arm? This is much better, I think, than most of the people here today have had.

Dr. Smith: These are the results of Protocol 7421, and maybe Dr. Holland would like to comment on it.

Dr. Holland: That's why the starting point for calculation is so critical. This is plotted from the 183rd day of remission, which is the time that the opposite arm plots from, the Poly I:C. So it automatically eliminates some of the early failures and is not to be taken as if it's representative of the total complete remission. It's the comparative arm for the Poly I:C arm.

DISCUSSION: ACUTE MYELOGENOUS LEUKEMIA

Dr. Fahey: We have to consider a series of points in discussing the presentations summarized in Table 1. First, what is the status of BCG immunotherapy in AML?

Dr. Vogler: In our study we demonstrated that a short course of BCG could prolong duration of remission in patients compared to control groups treated on a chemotherapy program which is probably not optimal for maintenance. This may have been of some advantage in pointing out a small effect of BCG, which might have been obscured in some of the other studies by the rather intensive chemotherapy programs that were used. We only gave a little bit of immunotherapy, but we did see an effect.

Dr. Fahey: Dr. Hersh has a more vigorous immunotherapy schedule, and can help answer the question of where and when BCG is really worth giving to patients with AML.

Dr. Hersh: Our data have convinced us that immunotherapy has added something to the survival and perhaps to the remission duration of our patients.

Everybody has to look at these data and decide for themselves what kinds of therapeutic programs to design for their patients. But my concept of multimodality therapy is that we should use as many modalities as seem to be beneficial.

Dr. Hewlett: I don't think the negative results of the Southwest Oncology Group Study can be assumed to be entirely correct. There were a number of problems we ran into, namely, the dose of BCG, which was probably less than optimum, and the number of patients in both arms are relatively small.

TABLE 1.

Investigator	All Immuno Rx in maintenance phase except where otherwise noted Type Immuno Rx	No. of Pts. Contr/Immuno	Median Remission duration (wks) from end induction Contr/Immuno	Median Survival (wks) from end induction Contr/Immuno
Powles	BCG + irrad. allogeneic cells	22/28	27/44	39/73[a]
Reizenstein	BCG + viable allogeneic cells	14/16	22/35	44/89[a]
Peto	BCG + irrad. allogeneic cells	24/47		
Vogler	BCG	33/25	13/25*	
Gutterman	BCG[b]	24[b]/14	52/85	96/145+[a]
Hewlett	BCG	25/20?	55/59	55+/74
Whittaker	BCG i.v.	19/18	27/34	50/69[a]
Holland	1) VCN cells	17/31	26/95*	too early
	2) VCN cells + MER	17/22	26/48	
Cuttner	MER added to induction chemotherapy	?		
Sauter	Viral oncolysate of allogeneic cells	22/22	28/28	52/52
Gee	Pseudomonas vaccine in induction	16/13	too early	
McIntyre	Poly I:C (following 2 maint. courses)	67/39	no difference found	

[a] $p < .05$ or better.
[b] historical controls. All others randomized or alternated.

Another criticism of group studies, which I really don't think applies here, however, is that when a number of the investigators are giving the immunotherapy, in this case, there were 15 institutions involved—there is always a question as to whether it was administered properly and according to the protocol. In this study it was done properly. We contacted each and every investigator to clarify that point, and it was given approximately on schedule and according to the protocol. But the dose was somewhat low and that may make it difficult to interpret this study.

Dr. Fudenberg: Could the panel give their opinions on using the various strains of BCG with comparable numbers of organisms?

Dr. Hersh: I can respond to that. I think that's an important question, and it has been inadequately evaluated in both animal models and in patients. The panel's presentations this morning represent at least three or four different strains of BCG which have profoundly different biologic activities *in vitro* and animal models, at dose ranges well over several logs.

Also, when one administers BCG into the skin, there is very little information on how many organisms one is delivering to the system.

For that reason we see the future of active nonspecific immunotherapy with microbial adjuvants going toward the direction of something that can be standardized. MER, cell-wall skeleton, and P-3 are examples of materials capable of being standardized which we desperately need.

Dr. Fahey: There does not seem to be comparative information, Dr. Fudenberg, to answer your question. But as Dr. Hersh has indicated, uncertainty about how much is administered through the skin was one of the main reasons for Dr. Whittaker to undertake a study where he knew how much he was giving because he put it in intravenously.

Question: Was the same BCG used in the MRC and Powles trials?

Dr. Powles: Yes, it is the same BCG. But the discussion about which BCG is best at this moment in time may be irrelevant. If we address ourselves first to what we are going to measure for our standardizations, we might then see whether it's worthwhile even embarking on comparing different types of BCG.

Dr. Kay: It seems to me the prolongation of survival is the one real effect of BCG, and we wondered whether this was a nonspecific effect on bone marrow cells. There is, however, no real evidence that it's a nonspecific effect. An interesting contrast exists in these patients on immunotherapy between the poor state of their marrow (they tend to have rather hypoplastic marrows) and their overall physical state—they are not in a bad state of health at all. It is my impression that when they get a relapse, they are in a better state than a patient who has AML for the first time. And there are at least two possible reasons for that: One, they have been more closely observed than when a patient first comes along. Alternatively, it is possible the BCG is having an effect. For this reason, it would be very nice to be able to compare the chemotherapy-only relapses with the immunotherapy relapses as regards their state of health. You could measure the incidence of pneumonia, perianal lesions, incidence of septicemia—that sort of thing.

None of the six study groups here is big enough to show a difference, but if all of them put their data together and did a retrospective survey on their chemotherapy relapses and their chemotherapy-immunotherapy relapses, it might be possible to answer the question: Is this a nonspecific stimulation of resistance to bacteria?

Dr. Reizenstein: Powles said he found an increase in the number of colony-forming units in his animal studies, but they didn't resist chemotherapy any better. That would be one effect.

Another effect may be that BCG alters the immunodepression of the patient. There is statistically significantly less immunodepression in patients given immunotherapy than in those who don't get it, and this is probably a BCG effect.

Mrs. Nauts (New York): The Trudeau Institute, under Mackaness' direction, has tested at least 28 or 30 different preparations of BCG, and has analyzed them according to their potency.

Dr. Frei: I would like to propose an explanation for this discordancy of no remission prolongation but prolongation of survival because of duration of survival after relapse. Presumably the patients getting immunochemotherapy are seen more frequently. They get their immunotherapy once a week or every two weeks, and this is done under tight control. It may be that the patients on chemotherapy get their chemotherapy at other institutions for a period of time and come back to the mother institution at two- or three-month intervals.

Is it possible that you are simply picking up the relapses earlier in the immunochemotherapy group, which would shorten their duration of remission relative to the remission of the chemotherapy only, but correspondingly prolong the duration of survival after relapse?

Also, if relapses are picked up earlier, they probably respond to chemotherapy more effectively, that is, for induction of secondary remission.

Dr. Powles: That is a fair comment, but in fact in the study that we did, this didn't apply. The chemotherapy patients were seen at the same institution as the immunotherapy patients. Also, we didn't do routine marrows in that study. We diagnosed the onset of relapse as the appearance of blast cells in the blood or the appearance of bone marrow failure. And we tended in that study to hold back and delay the treatment of relapse.

Dr. Weiss: There has been repeated reference to the variability of living BCG with regard to the number of viable organisms that get in. It must also be emphasized that there is enormous variability as to the infectivity of these organisms once they do get in, relating to the strain of BCG and to the host capacity to handle this material. It's a lost cause to attempt to obtain a standardized BCG preparation in terms of what the numbers of organisms will be after some days or weeks in the tissues of the patients.

In light of the fact that there is very little convincing experimental evidence from animal studies that living BCG is intrinsically superior to non-living materials, I truly wonder why there remains so much focus on a nonstandardizable living entity when the door is open to the use of various factions of nonliving nature where at least standardization is possible.

Dr. Powles: As a physician, I prefer to measure the effect on the patient first, and then dictate the dose of the drug after. What I find happening amongst the people asking "which BCG, where, and when?" is they want to dictate the dose of the drug first and then measure the effect after. I find that the wrong way around.

Dr. Weiss: There are data that at certain dosages you get the opposite of the desired effect, whether on immune function or states of resistance. Thus, by using a living entity in a patient who may or may not be capable of offering strong, moderate, or no defense against the spread of this organism, you create a situation where you have no idea whether you are giving a dosage which is desirable or not desirable.

Dr. Holland: It was these considerations which led us to explore MER.

Dr. Gee: On the point of the prolongation of survival without significant prolongation of remission, there are still other possibilities. Perhaps there are changes where our techniques are not good enough to pick up any stimulation of the normal stem cell.

Dr. Reizenstein: On the question of prolongation of remission versus prolongation of life, Dr. Frei's suggestion here was a valid one and it could probably be answered by the joint study proposed by Dr. Kay looking at the state of the patients when they do relapse.

On the other hand, we are not sure that there is no prolongation of the remission duration. Almost all the studies shown indicate a numerical prolongation but in individual studies it isn't significant.

Dr. Fahey: Let's switch from this discussion of treatment that may have nothing to do with whether the tumor is immunogenic or not to another form of treatment, using modified tumor, which relies on the premise that the tumor is immunogenic. What is the evidence, from giving modified cells, that there is an increased resistance from this maneuver, based on Powles', Reizenstein's, Peto's, and Holland's chapters?

Dr. Smith: I don't think you can evaluate these clinical data because the proper controls weren't done. You should have given a control group normal allogeneic cells in order to be able to discern an effect of the tumor cells.

Dr. Hersh: I believe that's a kind of academic question that is properly asked in a guinea pig and not in a patient.

Dr. Holland: It's very hard to get adequate numbers of normal myeloblasts. The myelocyte is not equivalent to the myeloblast. There are certainly enormous surface differences between the two from antigenic studies. Dr. Bekesi has evaluated normal thymus cells versus leukemic thymus cells in mouse experiments and shows the normal thymus cell does not immunize whereas the leukemic thymus cell does. I don't think that's a necessary control.

Dr. Fahey: Two of the studies used irradiated cells and one used viable cells. There is obviously a different premise there. And the fourth used neuraminidase-treated, but otherwise not altered cells.

Dr. Reizenstein: The reason why we chose viable cells was there were two or three animal studies published where viable cells were more immunogenic than irradiated cells. I think there is no evidence whatsoever that viable cells *in vivo* are any better. In fact, I'm not sure that the cells do anything at all. We might have done just as well with BCG alone. However, using viable cells does save much time and labor, and there has been no evidence at all of tumor takes in the recipients.

Dr. Fahey: You are assessing the Phase I aspect; it's not hazardous to the recipient.

Dr. Reizenstein: Correct.

Dr. Fahey: Do you and Dr. Bekesi concur in that?

Dr. Holland: Well, we don't use plain cells. They are neuraminidase-treated, and those cells have lost their leukemogenicity in susceptible mice.

So I don't think we are putting people at hazard, but we certainly have never seen a tumor grow.

Dr. Fahey: Now, what is the evidence of inducing a specific immune response? Dr. Reizenstein said his data were not complete. Is it complete enough to comment on?

Dr. Reizenstein: We cannot demonstrate any increased lymphocyte activity to autologous blasts after immunization repeatedly with allogeneic blasts.

Dr. Fahey: Is the assay blastogenic or cytogenic?

Dr. Reizenstein: It's a thymidine uptake assay.

Dr. Fahey: That might not be the relevant assay.

Dr. Reizenstein: That is absolutely correct.

Dr. Powles: I can comment on that. We have a cytotoxic assay, and we can show that the patients recognize the allogeneic immunizing cells, and there is excellent cytotoxicity. But I would fully support Dr. Reizenstein that we have never yet detected any evidence of a host reaction against the autologous leukemic cells.

Dr. Mathé: We store leukemic cells in liquid nitrogen and test the patient against autologous cells about five months or six months after they are put in storage. In testing against allogeneic, normal donors, we find the stimulation index is proportionately decreased as the storage time increases.

Thus, what you are trying to measure six months or 12 months later may not be the true assessment of the patient, but the decay of the cell during the storage period.

Also, on a few occasions we were fortunate enough to collect some normal allogeneic cells from the patient who donated the myeloblasts. We treated these with neuraminidase and stored them with the heat denatured neuraminidase and the supernatant. The delayed skin hypersensitivity responses to the allogeneic remission lymphocytes were not the 20 to 30 mm in duration induced by leukemic cells, but were around 2 to 3 mm with comparable numbers of cells.

Dr. Leventhal: Just to add to the confusion, in our experiments, cells stored up to five years in liquid nitrogen do not lose their capacity to stimulate *in vitro*.

Dr. Hersh: We reported the same findings.

Dr. Smith: We also reported the same.

Dr. Fahey: What is the panel's assessment of the evidence that irradiated cells with BCG are better than BCG alone, especially since the better chemotherapy regimens seem to be producing more long-term survivors? Are cells plus BCG better than BCG alone?

Dr. Powles: The information is not available, and there is really very little discussion on this point. A controlled trial to compare them certainly might give an answer, but it would still have to take into account two things: First, are we satisfied with the systems we have for measuring effects in this disease, and second, is that the most important question to ask with the poor availability of patients at the moment?

Dr. Reizenstein: I agree. Actually, the only one who has systematically tried to combine specific and nonspecific immunotherapy is Dr. Holland, and apart from that we just don't have any evidence that I know of that compares BCG plus cells with BCG alone. The questions we have to ask in relation to cells are really three: One, are there cross-reacting antigens, or are there group antigens, or are there individual antigens? If there are not cross-reacting antigens, then obviously there is no sense in using allogeneic cells for immunization. Two, is there really any immune surveillance in the generally accepted sense? That is also a nonproven question. And three, what is the difference between different myeloblasts? We have seen evidence that some are more immunogenic than others, and I think this certainly needs looking into.

So as far as the question of specific immunization concerns, I think we are really very early in the game.

Dr. Sokal: I'd like to raise a completely different kind of question, and that is whether there may be some defects in the schedules of immunotherapy that are being used.

Those reports that are positive show, by and large, an initial beneficial effect which then seems to fade out as immunotherapy is continued. There are at least two possible explanations for this. One is that an initial boost is all that can be expected after which remission duration and survival lines are going to be more or less parallel. The other possibility is that an initial effect is being lost despite continued immunotherapy, and the question must be considered as to whether it is lost because you are losing the immunologic stimulation. I would call your attention to the fact that considered from the standpoint of an immunologist, the schedules that we have been discussing are sort of crazy. All of them give relatively large amounts of antigenic material repeatedly for long periods of time. When as much as 1 g or 10 g of antigenic material is given, the question must be raised as to whether the subject is going to recognize the small amount of specific antigen in this huge mix.

In our experience we have found a definite loss of beneficial effect associated with increasing the intensity of immunologic stimulation with BCG: cell mixtures, but this is probably related to the BCG rather than the cell mixture.

In studies in chronic myeloid leukemia and in malignant lymphoma, we have recorded the duration of the effect on cellular immune responses, and this tends to run on the order of six months, 15 months, sometimes two years, after individual administrations of BCG. So when the immunologic effect that you can measure is a relatively persistent one, what is the logic of stimulation every week or every other week?

Dr. Powles: That's a very valid point. On the other hand, Ceppellini, in raising HLA antibody in normal individuals using normal buffy coat, found that the best way to raise good antibody was to immunize with 10^9 buffy-coat cells weekly. I must admit it doesn't detract from the point you make, which is that a weak antigen may be completely overwhelmed by the presence of strong antigens.

Dr. Edynak: We have had some experience with patients treated with BCG, following these patients sequentially with *in vitro* lymphocyte blastogenesis, four mitogens, and T- and B-cell evaluation. Patients receiving either active specific or active nonspecific therapy, bimonthly for a period of a year, maintained their lymphocyte stimulation indexes on a high normal level. When we cut the twice monthly immunization to once monthly, stimulation indices to the four mitogens fell drastically from 150 to 200 times above unstimulated values to only 75 to 100 times above unstimulated values.

The second thing that has been shown by a number of people is that in the animal systems BCG, depending on the dose, can enhance tumor growth. In C3H mice with breast tumors we found that our vaccine, in conjunction with BCG, can serve both as immunoprophylaxis and immunotherapy. BCG alone will enhance and cause facilitation of death of all animals.

As a third point, in looking at 100 or more patients with different histologic types of cancer, we found that using Tice BCG in a range of about 1 times 10^8 organisms, about 5 to 10 percent of patients are immunodepressed or immunosuppressed, in that their lymphocyte stimulation indices will fall for a period of a week to 10 days or more after receiving such a dose.

Dr. Terry: If you look at all the studies, the effect of adding BCG to chemotherapy varies from slight prolongation (even in Dr. Peto's case, considering only median survival) up to a 100 percent increase in survival if you look at Dr. Reizenstein's numbers.

A reasonable question could be asked by your local medical practitioner: Should patients with AML be receiving BCG as a routine part of the therapy now?

What does the panel think about this, not from the point of view of investigative medicine, but from the point of view of patients who are not being treated in specific clinical trials.

Dr. Reizenstein: We must be sure that it is effective first. Six studies were reported at this panel with either BCG or BCG plus cells, and two were negative.

I agree completely with Dr. Hewlett that we are looking forward to seeing their study with a higher BCG dose. But we still have Dr. Peto's negative study, and before one treats on a nonrandomized or nonscientific basis, we have to have more information.

Dr. Holland: I can't think of a better way to impede progress, than to start treating all AML patients with BCG now.

Dr. Powles: This comes right back to the very matter that should have been vitally addressed on this panel: Is there a statistical observation of an effect or is there not? And if we establish there is not a statistical observation—in other words, the statistical methods fail—then the discussion should be: What methods are we going to use in the future to be able to measure whether there is an effect? If we agree there is an effect, then we can begin to decide where we should address our attentions in future studies.

On that point, I would like to just make one point to Dr. Peto, which I think is an important one. I fully applaud his comment as a mathematician that it would be very nice to have large numbers of patients in each arm. But it is a fact of life that the number of patients that we get is limited and uncontrolled. So instead of saying, "Give us more numbers," I'd say to him, "Give us some hope. Give us an alternative statistical method if this approach doesn't work."

Dr. Fahey: Let's ask you to respond to your query. What do you see up here as a positive observation?

Dr. Powles: If we can accept the mathematics of it, then I think we are compelled to say that there is an effect of immunotherapy, be it BCG and/or cells, on the prolongation of survival after relapse. And that includes Peto's data. That is about as far as we can go at the moment.

Dr. Fahey: I would like to focus attention on Dr. Gee's presentation where he had 12 patients who lived more than four years in their first remission. Part of the goal is to get more patients into that kind of remission.

Dr. Gee: It is still difficult to separate out, obviously, whether it's a pseudomonas vaccine or, perhaps, a combination of our therapy, which has now given us 12 out of 49 responders who have lived from four to seven years now and have been off therapy at least one year. My own feeling, at least from our work on the new protocol, is that the vaccine contributes something of value. This time we are keeping our therapy constant and just adding pseudomonas vaccine, and looking at the relapse rate. This will obviously reflect itself in duration of remission in our group as a whole.

Dr. Fahey: Dr. Cuttner, do you want to comment about parameters of study?

Dr. Cuttner: In a large group study, the number of tests you can use are limited. We have been using skin tests.

The initial impression is that a positive skin test, as a parameter of cellular immunity, indicates a better chance of going into complete remission and survival.

Dr. Gee: There has been much discussion here about how long patients receive BCG and what the schedule is. To add another point, in our initial group of pseudomonas vaccine patients all but one received it during the induction phase and had no maintenance vaccine afterward.

Dr. Holland: The correlations can only come when there are appreciable numbers of patients with long-term survival. As we get to curative disease—and certainly Dr. Gee's long-term, and some of Dr. Hersh's data, and some of our data have these long plateaus of people who are in their first remission —then the correlations with the kinds of responses they have in skin tests or *in vitro* tests are important.

Dr. Peto: Apparent plateaus are a very common artifact—I mean you always think early on in a study that you have a plateau because every actuarial survival curve . . .

Dr. Holland: I'm talking about things after all the patients are gone, Dr. Peto. All the patients are dead. Ours are not apparent plateaus.

Dr. Lipton: It was mentioned that hepatic mixed oxidase function is altered. In our own laboratory we have experienced that this is indeed the case with BCG and with *C. parvum* therapy in certain selected cases.

Is it possible that some of the effect we are seeing is due to what becomes an effective chemotherapy due to a reduction of the metabolic degradation of the chemotherapeutic materials by the concomitant administration of both chemotherapy and immunotherapy?

Dr. Powles: Good point.

Dr. LoBuglio: From someone who is not involved in leukemia trials, the only thing that looks the least bit interesting or exciting in the summary table is the marked and dramatic prolongation of first remission, of two years in length.

Do the chemotherapists here think that the Ad-OAP regimen is so remarkably better than everyone else's treatment that it accounts for that difference, or that the addition of BCG has produced that result?

Immunotherapy of Cancer: Present Status of Trials in Man, edited by W. D. Terry and D. Windhorst. Raven Press, New York © 1978.

Acute Lymphocytic Leukemia and Lymphomas: Status of Chemotherapy

James F. Holland

Department of Neoplastic Diseases, Mount Sinai School of Medicine, New York, New York 10029

It is no accident that acute lymphocytic leukemia is the crucible in which chemotherapy and immunotherapy have both first been launched. Figure 1 shows twenty years of research in acute lymphocytic leukemia of the Cancer and Leukemia Group B, involving two thousand patients. The plateaus, at eight to ten years, give some intimation of cures of this disease. It is easier perhaps to see this plotted in logarithmic fashion. (Fig. 2). The slope, which might be called the death function, changes, showing a progressive decrease. All patients are not getting the same regimen. They are indeed stratified and randomized to several arms within each study and each curve contains worse and better regimens.

A succession of the best regimens of the Cancer and Leukemia Group B from 1963 onward is shown in Fig. 3. One can see plateaus that are now up to 10 years long. There is little likelihood that patients will relapse after several years of plateau (sustained remission in the entire population).

A study done in 1963, (Fig. 4) is a clinical translation of the enormous contribution that Skipper and Schabel and their colleagues have made to cancer medicine: induction, intensive treatment, and other concepts of cell

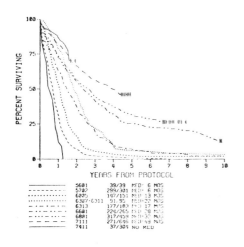

Fig. 1. Childhood acute lymphocytic leukemia— 1956–1976.

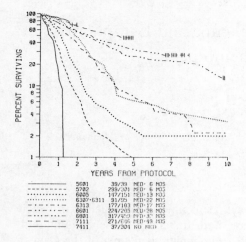

Fig. 2. Childhood acute lymphocytic leukemia—1956–1976.

kinetics relating to the potential for killing cells and for quantifying the number killed. Patients remained untreated after intensive therapy, and we tried to estimate the number of leukemic cells remaining in the marrow, spleen, nodes, liver, and blood. We calculated that 2^{37} cells were present at diagnosis in children. The effect of chemotherapy was to decrease the population "by extrapolated reasoning" to about ⅓ in geometric terms. If we had extended the treatment for 120 days, and if killing had continued at the same rate, it might have led to complete cell killing. We extended the next program to 240 days. Induction was followed by intensive treatment going out for eight months of treatment, sometimes with pulsed reinforcement; then at random some patients were left untreated (Fig. 5).

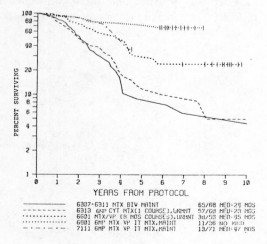

FIG. 3. Best regimen, 1963–1974.

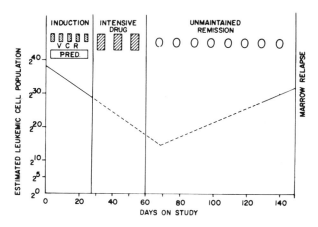

FIG. 4. Model of leukemic cell kinetics.

Patients are plotted in Fig. 6 from the time of last chemotherapy. After eight months or three months of methotrexate courses, these patients were observed without further treatment. Those treated with three courses of treatment had a steep relapse curve. Save one child without relapse at 7 years, none other stayed in remission more than a year-and-a-half. The group of children who received eight months of courses of methotrexate are in unmaintained remission seven and eight years later without treatment; those who received eight months of courses of methotrexate plus vincristine and prednisone reinforcement treatments show the highest proportion of survivors without disease in the seven-to-nine-year period after cessation of treatment.

Therefore, it appears possible to cure acute lymphocytic leukemia with chemotherapy in approximately 20 to 30% using the best arm of this pro-

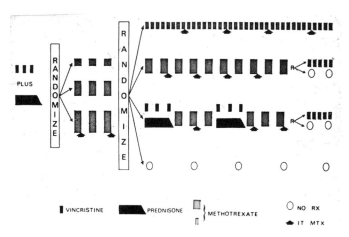

FIG. 5. Study design for protocol.

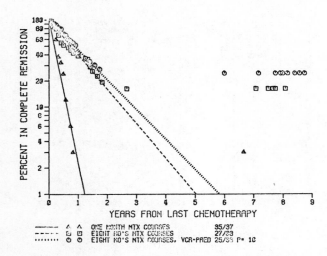

FIG. 6. Acute lymphocytic leukemia, unmaintained remissions.

tocol. We have many times tried to improve upon this by using intensive continued courses of methotrexate and of 6-mercaptopurine. The studies have not gone on for enough years to allow us to say that we have improved on it.

We have embarked on other studies, too, which are continuous maintenance programs instead of intensive treatments. In a continuous maintenance program of 6-mercaptopurine, done many years ago, vincristine and predisone used during the course of the remission, demonstrate reinforcement of the maintenance chemotherapy (Fig. 7).

In 1968 a program was started with five randomizations, 2^5 for 32 arms. Patients up to 21 years received asparaginase or not, vincristine and prednizone with or without daunorubicin, intrathecal methotrexate or not, methotrexate alone or in combination with 6-mercaptopurine, and reinforcement

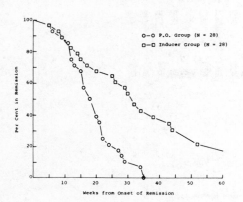

FIG. 7. Duration of remissions maintained by daily oral 6-MP alone or in addition to monthly reinforcement doses of VCR and prednisone.

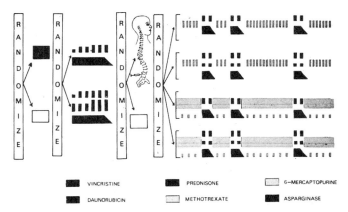

VINCRISTINE   PREDNISONE   6–MERCAPTOPURINE

DAUNORUBICIN   METHOTREXATE   ASPARGINASE

FIG. 8. Study design for protocol.

doses of vincristine and prednisone, or vincristine, prednisone, and dauno-rubicin (Fig. 8). The outcome of this study was that certain of these ran-domizations conveyed specific and particular advantage and others did not. In the best of the arms, 60% of those children in remission, have been in remission for five years and more (Fig. 9). At five years the treatment is discontinued in half the patients at random. We do not know at this point when the proper time to stop the treatment is. We do not think that it is at three years as others have advocated, because relapses are still occurring. The plateau is of considerable importance, suggesting disease eradication. The difference between the two arms is the net effect of giving intrathecal methotrexate.

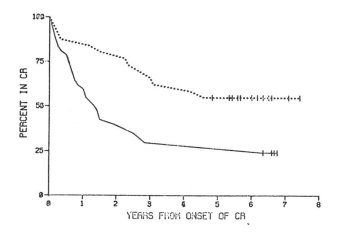

FIG. 9. Acute lymphocytic leukemia, complete remission duration.

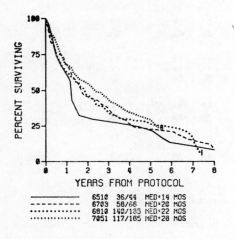

FIG. 10. Lymphosarcoma, 1965–1972.

Survival times in lymphosarcoma, a disease that represents diffuse lymphocytic lymphoma in the new terminology, is shown in Fig. 10. Nodular lymphomas are under-represented in the data of CALGB due to systematic exclusion in years past of giant follicular lymphosarcoma. The same distinct improvement in survival as in ALL is not seen.

In reticulum cell sarcoma or histiocytic lymphoma, as it is called today, (Fig. 11) a much more acute mortality, and then a horizontal, sharp deflection indicates that this is indeed two populations of patients; those who have and those who have not responded to treatment. It could be that there are two diseases.

DeVita and colleagues from the NCI were the first to point out that patients with histiocytic lymphoma aggressively treated—with nitrogen mustard or cyclophosphamide, vincristine, prednisone, and procarbazine—have a long survival off treatment and are apparently cured (Fig. 12).

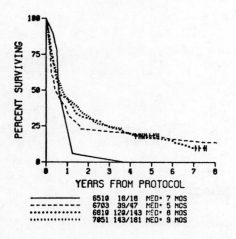

FIG. 11. Reticulum cell sarcoma, 1965–1972.

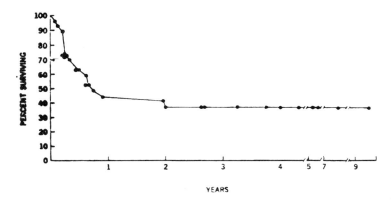

FIG. 12. Life-table analysis of survival of entire group of patients with advanced histiocytic lymphoma. (From DeVita et al., *Lancet*, 1975).

The same phenomenon is apparently reproduced in data of the Cancer and Leukemia Group B (CALGB) for diffuse histiocytic lymphomas. The increasing percentage of patients responding to treatment is reminiscent of the improving survival data for acute lymphocytic leukemia (Fig. 13).

The same phenomenon is recognizable for diffuse lymphocytic poorly differentiated lymphomas, another of Rappaport's unfavorable classifications (Fig. 14).

Data from the NCI show a major prognostic difference between nodular and diffuse lymphomas. The frequency of these types in any series is of utmost importance because of the difference in prognosis.

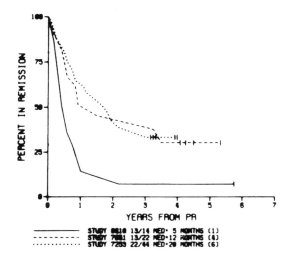

FIG. 13. Complete responders, HD only.

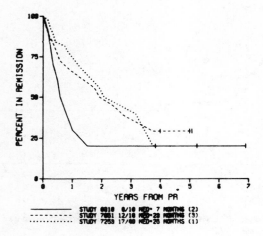

FIG. 14. Complete responders, PLPD only.

Age also exerts a very striking impact. There is not surprisingly a very substantial decrease in the survival of those who are more than 60. For 151 patients who are under 35, however, a surprising decrease in survival was seen (Fig. 15). Histology, nodularity, and age are bases for useful stratification in controlled clinical trials.

New histopathologic classifications appear to be useful. The CALGB is utilizing this approach prospectively and retrospectively. For a sample of one thousand patients who were classified as lymphosarcoma and reticulum sarcoma, we have had a subset of some 700 cases reclassified in accord with

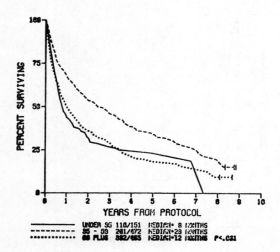

Fig. 15. Survival rates by age in lymphomas, not classified as Hodgkin's disease.

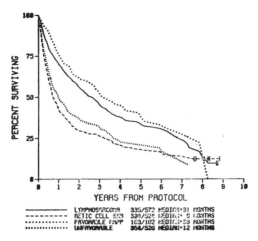

FIG. 16. Survival rates in lymphomas by histological classifications.

the Rappaport scheme. Recognizing that we had excluded some nodular (follicular) lymphomas from clinical trial, we did find that cases reclassified as favorable or unfavorable lymphomas in the Rappaport classification had differences in survival similar to those which had been ascribed to lymphosarcoma and reticulum cell sarcoma (Fig. 16).

Hodgkin's disease, a lymphoma where there is convincing therapeutic progress, is characterized by many histologic subtypes which have prognostic significance. As chemotherapy improves for Stages III and IV disease, there has been an appreciable change in survival (Fig. 17). A substantially im-

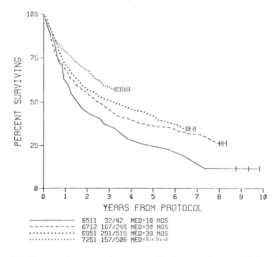

FIG. 17. Change in survival rates in Hodgkin's disease, 1965–1975.

proved therapy has been found ten years after the introduction of mustard, vincristine, prednisone, and procarbazine, the standard MOPP treatment. A combination of CCNU, vinblastine, prednisone, and procarbazine causes at least equivalent remission induction, at least equivalent remission duration and the regimen can be used with substantially less cost in toxicity.

Against this background, I would like to see immunotherapy achieve an augmented or more enduring response.

ACKNOWLEDGMENTS

These studies were supported in part by grants from the National Cancer Institute, CA16118, CA04457, and CA15936.

*Immunotherapy of Cancer: Present Status of
Trials in Man,* edited by W. D. Terry and D. Windhorst.
Raven Press, New York © 1978.

Chemotherapy Followed by Active Immunotherapy in the Treatment of Acute Lymphoid Leukemias For Patients of All Ages: Results of ICIG Acute Lymphoid Leukemia Protocols 1, 9, and 10; Prognostic Factors, and Therapeutic Implications

G. Mathé, L. Schwarzenberg, F. De Vassal, M. Delgado, J. Pena-Angulo,
D. Belpomme, P. Pouillart, D. Machover, J. L. Misset, J. L. Pico,
C. Jasmin, M. Hayat, M. Schneider, A. Cattan, J. L. Amiel,
M. Musset, and C. Rosenfeld

*Institut de Cancérologie et d'Immunogénétique (ICIG), Institut National de la Santé et de
la Recherche Médicale (INSERM), Hôpital Paul-Brousse, and Service d'Hématologie de
l'Institut Gustave-Roussy, Villejuif, France*

In 1963 we started treating acute lymphoid leukemia (ALL) patients of *all ages* with systemic active immunotherapy (SAI) according to the following principles raised by our experimental study (18,29): (a) immunointervention may be as efficient against established neoplasias (which is the definition of immunotherapy) as it may be in their prevention; (b) it can be achieved by the administration of irradiation-sterilized tumor cells or immunity systemic adjuvants, such as BCG, or by the combination of both which is more effective than each one of these means given singly; (c) contrary to chemotherapy, which obeys first order kinetics (40–42) and, therefore, does not kill the last cell (17), SAI is able to eradicate the total neoplastic cell population of a leukemia, provided the number of cells present is $\leqslant 10^5$ (18); and (d) active immunotherapy (AI) is strikingly efficient when applied after cell reduction by chemotherapy (26) or radiotherapy (15).

These observations determine the conditions under which we submit ALL patients to SAI: (a) We first induce an apparently complete remission (CR) and then reduce the number of residual cells by systemic chemotherapy (20,21), intrathecal chemotherapy, and central nervous system (CNS) radiotherapy (30,35) in order that it should be as low as possible (the equivalent of the critical murine number of 10^5). The reason why we chose ALL in 1963 was that, when we started the clinical trials, it was the only leukemia whose cells were sensitive enough to chemotherapy to allow us to surmise that their number could be reduced to this critical number by cytostatics.

(b) We then applied, for SAI, irradiated pooled ALL allogeneic cells i.d., and fresh Pasteur Bacillus Calmette-Guérin (BCG) on scarifications [a method that is effective in SAI of leukemia in mice (16)].

Since 1963 we have conducted nine randomized trials of SAI applied after cell-reducing chemo(radio)therapy[1] (CRC) in the treatment of ALL patients of all ages (20,21).[1]

The results of some of the trials have already been published (22–24). In this chapter, we shall present (a) the follow-up of protocol ICIG 1, which compared the evolution of patients under AI with that of controls left without treatment after CRC, and (b) the results of two unpublished protocols (ICIG 9 and 10) that were set up to answer three questions: (i) Is a long pre-AICRC (25 month) more beneficial than pre-AICRC of moderate length (9 month)? (ii) Is the addition of *Corynebacterium granulosum* to BCG and leukemic cells beneficial to AI? (iii) Are cells cultured in bulk and presenting three markers of the original leukemic cells (37) as efficient as pooled cryopreserved cells? and (c) the comparison of our AI results and those of maintenance chemotherapy (MC) protocols applied in other centers (1,2,10, 13,33,44).

PATIENTS AND METHODS

Our nine ICIG protocols were randomized trials. Patients were of *all ages* (varying from 1 to 80 years).

All patients were treated exclusively by our group. The curves are so-called direct curves (38). The statistical test used is the X_2.

The methods of protocol ICIG 1 have already been published (22,23). Those of protocols ICIG-ALL 9 and 10 are shown in Fig. 1 and the distribution of the patients according to the main parameters of prognosis in Table 1. The percentages of the poor prognoses, the so-called prolymphoblastic, type and of hyperleukocytemic cases are identical for both protocols.

The cytological diagnosis and typing are those of the World Health Organization (WHO) Reference Center for the Histological and Cytological Typing of Neoplastic Diseases of Hematopoietic and Lymphoid Tissues (32). The immunological typing methods have been published previously (5).

RESULTS

1. The 1976 results of the first pilot trial started in 1963, which compared the evolution of 20 patients submitted to AI with that of 10 controls left without treatment after CRC, are maintained today—whereas all the controls relapsed, seven out of the AI group are still in first CR between 10 and 13

---

[1] Some of our patients were not submitted to CNS radiotherapy at the time we compared CNS-irradiated and CNS-nonirradiated patients (20,21).

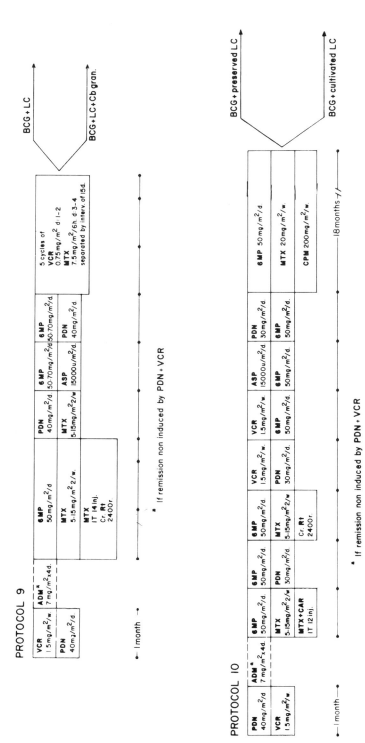

FIG. 1. Protocols ICIG-ALL 9 and 10. The cultured cells belong to the Reh line (37). It presents three markers of the original leukemic cells (chromosome abnormalities, leukemia-associated antigens, and identical electrophoretic mobility). VCR, vincristine; PDN, prednisone; ADM, Adriamycin®; 6MP, 6-mercaptopurine; MTX, methotrexate; ASP, L-asparaginase; CAR, cytosine arabinoside; CPM, cyclophosphamide; LC, leukemic cells; Cb gran, C. granulosum; Cr. Rt, cranial radiotherapy; and CCRRC, complementary cytoreductive radiochemotherapy.

TABLE 1. ICIG-ALL protocols 9 and 10—distribution according to age, sex, cytological types, and initial number of leukemic cells

	Number of patients	Age (Yrs.)	Sex		Cytological types					Leukemic cells in blood		
			M	F	ProLB	MacLB	MicLB	ProLC	Unclas-sified	>10,000/mm³	<10,000/mm³	Unknown
Protocol 9	38	2 to 48	24	14	8 21%	8 21%	4 10%	13 34%	5 13%	15 39%	15	8
Protocol 10	18	1 to 30	10	8	4 22%	6 33%	1 5%	4 22%	3 16%	7 39%	7	4

MacLB, macrolymphoblastic; MicLB, microlymphoblastic; ProLB, prolymphoblastic; ProLC, prolymphocytic.

years after starting AI, and eight are alive in CR (Fig. 2). These patients were randomized, but not stratified according to the parameters of prognosis used today.

2. A comparison of the results of protocols ICIG 9 and 10 (Table 1) answers the three questions raised earlier: (a) Is a long pre-AICRC (25 month) more beneficial than pre-AICRC of moderate length (9 month)? Our results have not produced a positive answer (Figs. 3 and 4), which sug-

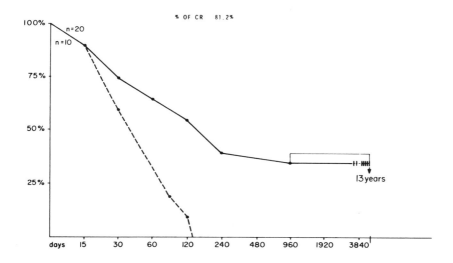

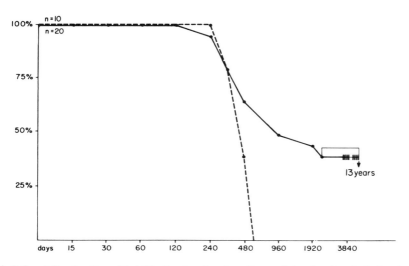

FIG. 2. Cumulative durations of first CR after stopping chemotherapy (*above*) and survival after the beginning of the disease (*below*) of AI and control patients of *all ages* of protocol ICIG-ALL 1, 1963–1976. Note that the time scale is geometrical. •———•, submitted to immunotherapy; •———•, not submitted to immunotherapy; ■, living (*above*) and still in 1st CR (*below*) (5/1/76).

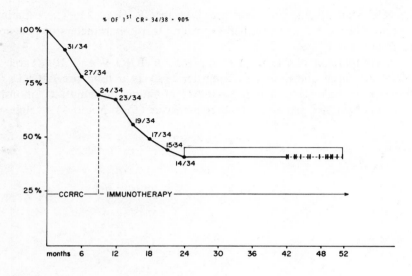

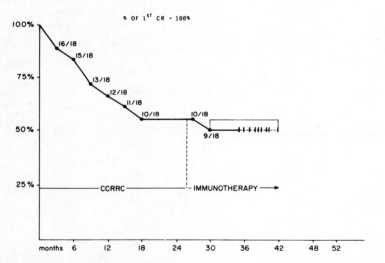

FIG. 3. Cumulative duration of first remission of patients of *all ages* included in protocols ICIG-ALL 9 (*above*, n = 34) and 10 (*below*, n = 18), 1971–1973.

gests that AI is as efficient as MC between the ninth and the 25th months after remission induction. The percentage of patients belonging to the plateau of the remission curves is 41 and 50%, respectively, for protocols 9 and 10, and for the plateaux of survival, 62 to 55% of those who entered remission (respectively, 90 and 100% for protocols 9 and 10). This observation can be likened to that of the EORTC Hemopathy Working Party (8), which found

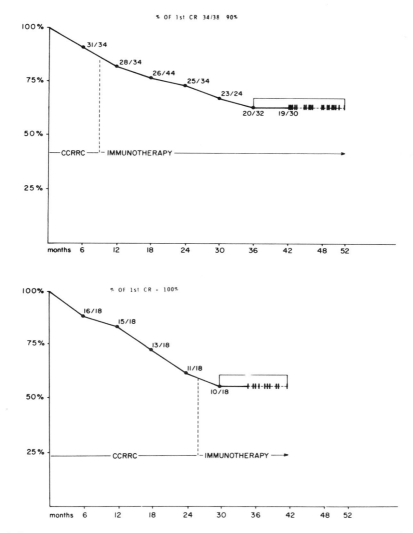

FIG. 4. Cumulative duration of survival of patients of *all ages* included in protocols ICIG-ALL 9 (*above,* n = 34) and 10, (*below*, n = 18).

no significant difference between MC and AI in maintaining remission after the 14th month. (b) Is the addition of *C. granulosum* to BCG and pooled cryopreserved irradiated leukemic cells (PCLC) beneficial for AI? Again, our results have not yielded a positive answer (Fig. 5). (c) Are cells cultured in bulk and presenting three markers of the original leukemic cells as efficient as pooled cryopreserved cells? The answer cannot yet be determined.

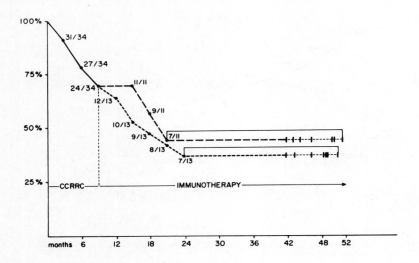

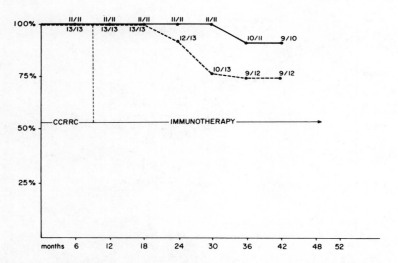

FIG. 5. Cumulative duration of first remission (*above*) and survival (*below*) of ICIG-ALL protocol 9 according to the addition or absence of C. *granulosum* in AI. There is no significant difference. •———•, BCG + LC + Cb gran (n = 11); •‑‑‑‑‑•, BCG + LC (n = 13); LC, leukemic cells; Cb gran, C. *granulosum*.

COMPARISON OF AI AND MC: RESULTS OF TRIALS CONDUCTED BEFORE 1973

The following data considered for comparing AI and MC effects were obtained for AI from the study of 100 patients submitted to this treatment from 1963 to 1971.

TABLE 2. *Side effects of AI in ALL patients*

	Patients	Necessity to stop BCG applications
Temperature $> 39°$ C	9/100	
Chills or sweating	11/100	
Pruritus	78/100	
Localized skin rash	2/100	
Generalized skin rash	1/100	
Ulcers	0/100	
Adenopathy	28/100	
Splenomegaly	18/100	
Hepatic dysfunction	6/100	
Hepatic granulomata	2/8	
Choroiditis	1/100	+

Toxic Cost

The short-term side effects of AI are listed in Table 2 (39). Only one case of choroiditis obliged us to stop treatment. The other manifestations were those of the necessary BCG bacteremia (19). Not one side effect was lethal, a result very different from MC lethal toxicity, which varies between 4 to 28% in MC patients (Table 3) (3,9,11,12,14,25,43,45).

TABLE 3. *Comparative toxic cost of AI and MC in ALL treatment*

G. Mathé et al. (25)[a]	Deaths 0/100 patients[b]	Severe not lethal toxicity 0/100 patients
AI	0/300 patients	
MC		
J. V. Simone (43) (Protocol V)	3/31 patients	
J. V. Simone (43) (Protocol VI)	5/94 patients	
J. V. Simone (43) (Protocol VIa)	2/10 patients	
J. V. Simone (43) (Protocol VII)	4/94 patients	
J. V. Simone (43) (Protocol VIII)	2/92 patients	
	2/17 patients	
R. Aur and J. V. Simone (3)	3/20 patients	6 crippling leuco-encephalopathy/20
Cl. Jacquillat and J. Bernard (10)	6/81 children	
(Protocol 06 LA/66)	6/21 adults	
F. Lampert et al. (11)		
(Early irradiation	4/79 patients	
(Late irradiation)	1/19 patients	
F. Mandelli et al. (13)	2/30 patients	
T. S. Gee et al. (9)	3/74 patients	
A. C. Smyth et al. (45)	2/17 adults	

[a] Cure expectancy of the microlymphoblastic type after AI:85%.

[b] A recent analysis of side effects in 277 ALL patients submitted to AI also reveals no deaths.

No long-term complications of AI, the length of which is 5 years, have been observed, whereas sterility and mutations are feared after long-term chemotherapies (27,28). We regret that we have been unable to find publications on sterility and second neoplasias in ALL patients submitted to long-term MC, although such long-term complications have been described in nephrosis and Hodgkin's disease (28) patients submitted to applications of cytostatics.

Cure Expectancy

Concerning antileukemic effects of AI and MC, it is remarkable that we have obtained second remissions in 94% of patients who relapsed under AI (Table 4) (34), whereas we obtained less than 70% after short-term MC and even less after long MC, a problem that calls for further publications. The cure expectancy in patients who relapsed under AI is noticeable (as illustrated by the comparison of remission and survival curves of protocol 9, whereas it is generally considered low in those who relapsed under MC.

The curve of first remission (32a) and of survival in remission (Fig. 6) for this group of 100 patients of *all ages* whom we started treating with AI in 1963, presents a plateau (no relapses) after 4 years (Table 4) as already indicated in the curves of protocols 1, 9, and 10.

These results are noticeably different from those concerning *only children* published (a) by Lonsdale et al. (13), who maintained less than 15% of their children in remission at 18 months (the authors have not published their curve of survival), (b) by Jacquillat et al. (9), who have observed no plateau on their remission curve before 70 months, the longest follow-up at the time of publication. The comparison with Acute Leukemia Group B (1) and Memphis Group (2,33,44) protocols will need a longer follow-up (36). It is difficult, in any case, to know how the patients submitted to protocols were selected from among the overall populations of ALL patients treated in the different centers. The poor prognosis type that we refer to as "prolymphoblastic" ALL, is often called "undifferentiated" by other centers and not included in ALL trials.

TABLE 4. *Late relapses and second remissions*

	In the 100 patients submitted to AI
Late relapses after 4 years	0
Second remissions after early relapses	94%

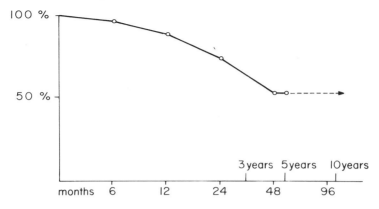

FIG. 6. ALL. Cumulative duration of survival of 100 patients after AI is started. Note that time scale is geometrical.

Prognostic Factors

Particularly striking are the prognosis factor differences in AI and in MC patients.

Age

Figure 7 shows that age, which is a prognostic factor in MC patients, is not so for AI patients. The results in children will be analysed in a separate paper (32b).

Cytological Type

The cytological types that we described in 1971 (31) and that are illustrated in the WHO monograph of the Reference Center for Histological and

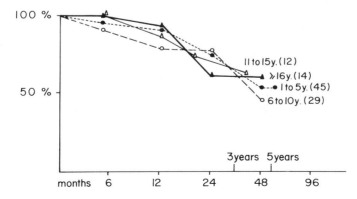

FIG. 7. ALL. Cumulative duration of survival of 100 patients (submitted to AI) according to age. Note that time scale is geometrical.

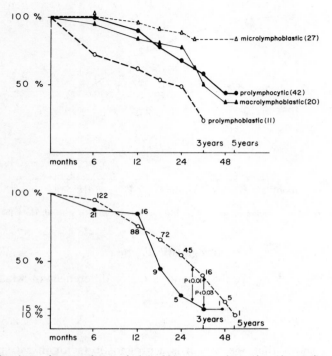

FIG. 8. ALL. Cumulative duration of survival of the 100 patients submitted to AI according to cytological types (*above*). Note that time scale is geometrical. ALL. Cumulative duration of survival of Jean Bernard's patients submitted to MC according to cytological types (*below*). Type I: prolymphoblastic; type II: macrolymphoblastic; type III: microlymphoblastic; type IV: prolymphocytic. (6,11). •———•, Type I (34 cases); •- - - -•, types II, III, and IV (170 cases).

Cytological Typing of Neoplastic Diseases of Hematopoietic and Lymphoid Tissues (32) are of no prognostic value in MC patients, but are a very important factor in AI patients. Figure 8, which compares the prognosis of Jean Bernard's MC patients (6,11) with that of AI patients (both groups having been treated at the same time and in the same city) is very convincing —whereas the curves of survival for the patients are almost identical in the four types in the case of the MC patients, they are different in the case of the AI patients. The curve of the prolymphoblastic type drops to a low level, whereas the curve forms a plateau after 3 years for 85% of the patients submitted to AI, who carry the microlymphoblastic type. The prognosis is intermediate for the other two types, the macrolymphoblastic and the prolymphocytic.

Volume of Neoplasia

The volume of neoplasia was shown in a previous article (32a) to be a prognostic factor. The prognostic value of the combination of cytological types and the volume of the neoplasia will be discussed in another paper (32b).

Immune Markers

The value of the immune markers of the leukemic cells is also different in both groups of patients. Although Brouet and Seligmann (7) do not see any difference in the prognosis of ALL according to the presence of the T markers (Table 5), we find a striking difference in a study concerning more recently treated patients (4). First, it must be stressed that all prolymphoblastic and microlymphoblastic cases are "null" cell ALL, and that half of the macrolymphoblastic and the prolymphocytic cases are T cell ALL whereas half are null. Second, Fig. 9 shows that duration of first remission

TABLE 5. Prognosis according to Seligmann of T and non-T ALL patients submitted to MC

	T	Non-T
Deaths or hematological relapse	9/28	27/69
	NS	

NS, not significant

and survival of our AI null ALL patients is much longer than that of the T patients.

Multiplicity of ALL and Its Incidence on the Constitution of New Protocols

In view of these observations, it appears clear that ALL is not one single disease, and that there are, considering both ALL factors for therapeutic response(s), cytological types and immune markers, two populations of patients—those with high cure expectancy under AI following chemotherapy and those who still have a poor prognosis.

Until both MC and AI are submitted to explorations for these prognostic factors in all trials, no further comparison between their respective values is valid.

However, for AI protocols, practical conclusions can be drawn. It is evidently unethical to submit ALL patients for whom the prognosis is excellent, such as the microlymphoblastic type and the null cell macrolymphoblastic and prolymphocytic types, to the risk of an intensive and long MC. On the other hand, a more intensive preimmunotherapy chemotherapy can be attempted ethically in patients known to have a poor prognosis. This is what we do in our protocols ICIG-ALL 12, the results of which are very encour-

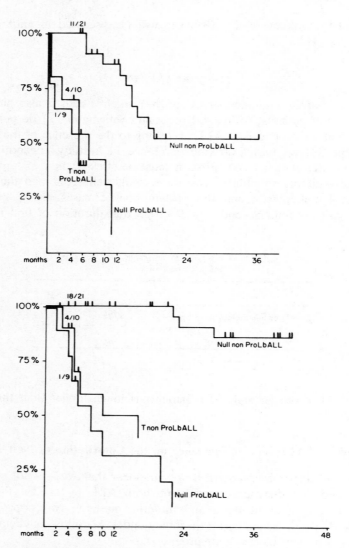

FIG. 9. Cumulative duration of first remission (*above*) and survival (*below*) in the case of our null prolymphoblastic ALL, T nonprolymphoblastic ALL, and null nonprolymphoblastic ALL.

aging (the present plateaux of the first remission and survival curves included, respectively, more than 75 and 85% of the patients).

SUMMARY

Since 1963, we have conducted nine controlled randomized trials on active immunotherapy (AI), applied after cell-reducing CRC in the treatment of acute lymphoid leukemia (ALL) patients of all ages (20,21).

1. The results of the first trial, which compared the evolution of 20 patients of all ages submitted to AI with that of 10 controls left without treatment after chemotherapy, are maintained today—whereas all the controls relapsed, seven out of the AI group are still in first CR between 10 and 13 years after starting AI, and eight are alive in CR.

2. Other trials have been published. In this chapter we consider two protocols that have not yet been published that were set up to answer three questions: (a) Is a long pre-AICRC (25 months) more beneficial than a pre-AICRC of moderate length (9 months)? Our results have not produced a positive answer, suggesting that AI is as efficient as maintenance chemotherapy between the ninth and the 25th months after remission induction. This observation can be likened to that of the EORTC Hemopathy Working Party (8), which found no significant difference between MC and AI in maintaining remission after the 14th month. (b) Is the addition of *C. granulosum* to BCG and PCLC beneficial for AI? Our results have not yielded a positive answer. (c) Are cells cultured in bulk and presenting three markers of the original leukemic cells as efficient as pooled cryopreserved cells? The answer cannot yet be determined.

The percentage of patients belonging to the plateaux of the remission curves are 41 and 50%, respectively, for protocols 9 and 10 and, to the plateaux of survival, 62 and 55% of the patients who entered remission (respectively, 90 and 100%).

3. The results of AI for 100 patients who were submitted to trials started in 1963 and who entered remission, are discussed and compared with those of several MC trials: (a) The AI trials are characterized by the absence of late relapses after the fourth year following immunotherapy, whereas late relapses have been observed after MC with an incidence that is variable from center to center; (b) the rate of second remissions (94%) and that of cure expectancy after a second remission are higher in patients relapsing under AI than under MC; and (c) the lethal toxicity of AI is nil, that of MC varies between 14 to 28%.

4. The prognostic factors seem to be different in AI and in MC patients. Although the cytological subtypes according to Jean Bernard and the surface immune markers according to Seligmann have no value in MC patients, they allow us to distinguish two categories of subjects submitted to AI, respectively, those with high cure expectancy and those with unfavorable evolution. We now apply different protocols according to the prognostic category, and their preliminary results are encouraging.

5. For a valid comparison of MC and AI patients, the author proposes that the smears taken from all patients by groups who conduct trials in ALL be controlled at the WHO Reference Center for Classification of Neoplastic Diseases of Hematopoietic and Lymphoid Tissues (32): (a) because of important differences that this center has observed in cytological diagnosis according to different groups (several groups exclude our poor prognosis

prolymphoblastic type from ALL, calling it undifferentiated), (b) in order to randomize patients into stratified groups, and (c) to adapt the therapeutic risk into prognostic category.

6. The results obtained with protocols 9 and 10 in children, as well as the prognostic value of the combination of cytological types and the volume of the neoplasia, will be discussed in another article (32b).

REFERENCES

1. Acute Leukemia Group B.: *Personal communication.*
2. Aur, R. J. A., Simone, J. V., Hustu, H. O., Verzosa, M. S., and Pinkel, D. (1974): Cessation of therapy during complete remission of childhood acute lymphocytic leukemia. *N. Engl. J. Med.*, 291:1230.
3. Aur, R. J. A., Verzosa, M. S., Hustu, H. O., Simone, J. V., and Barker, L. (1975): Leuco-encephalopathy (LEP) during initial complete remission (CR) in children with acute lymphocytic leukemia (ALL) receiving methotrexate (MTX). *Proc. Am. Assoc. Cancer Res.,* 16:92 (Abstr. 365).
4. Belpomme, D., Mathé, G., and Davies, A. J. S. (1977): Clinical significance and prognostic value of the T-B immunological classifications of human primary acute lymphoid leukaemias. *Lancet, 4*:555.
5. Belpomme, D., Dantchev, D., Du Rusquec, E., Grandjon, D., Huchet, R., Pouillart, P., Schwarzenberg, L., Amiel, J. L., and Mathé, G. (1974): T and B lymphocyte markers on the neoplastic cell of 20 patients with acute and 10 patients with chronic lymphoid leukemia. *Biomedicine, 20*:109.
6. Bernard, J., Weil, M., and Jacquillat, C. (1975): Prognostic factors in human acute leukemias. In: *Workshop on Prognostic Factors in Human Acute Leukemia,* edited by T. M. Fliedner and S. Perry. Pergamon Press, Oxford.
7. Brouet, J.C. Valensi, F., Daniel, M. T., Flandrin, G., Preud'homme, J. L., and Seligmann, M. (1976): Immunological classification of acute lymphoblastic leukaemias: Evaluation of its clinical significance in a hundred patients. *Br. J. Haematol.,* 33:319.
8. Otten, J., (1977): Immunotherapy versus chemotherapy as maintenance treatment of acute lymphoblastic leukemia. (*This volume.*)
9. Gee, T. S., Haghbin, M., Tan, C., Murphy, M. L., Dowling, M. D., and Clarkson, B. D. (1974): Differences in response in adults (15 years) and children with acute lymphoblastic leukemia (ALL) on a single therapeutic regimen. *Proc. Am. Assoc. Cancer Res.,* 15:164 (Abstr. 720).
10. Jacquillat, C., Weil, M., Gemon, M. F., Auclerc, G., Loisel, J. P., Delobel, J., Flandrin, G., Schaison, G., Izrael, V., Bussel, A., Dresch, C., Weisgerber, C., Rain, D., Tanzer, J., Najean, Y., Seligmann, M., Boiron, M., and Bernard, J. (1973): Combination therapy in 130 patients with acute lymphoblastic leukemia (Protocol 06 LA 66-Paris). *Cancer Res.,* 33:3278.
11. Jacquillat, C., Weil, M., Gemon, M. F., Boiron, M., and Bernard, J. (1975): Acute lymphoblastic leukemia in adults. In: *Therapy of Acute Leukemias,* edited by F. Mandelli, S. Amadori, and G. Mariani. Minerva Medica, Rome.
12. Lampert, F., Heinze, G., Wundisch, G. F., Olischlager, A., Klose, K., Usener, M., and Neidhardt, M. (1975): Cranial irradiation and combination chemotherapy of childhood acute lymphoblastic leukemia. In: *Therapy of Acute Leukemias,* edited by F. Mandelli, S. Amadori, and G. Mariani. Minerva Medica, Rome.
13. Lonsdale, D., Gehan, E. A., Fernbach, D. J., Sullivan, M. P., Lane, D. P., and Ragab, A. H. (1975): Interrupted vs continued maintenance therapy in childhood acute leukemia. *Cancer,* 36:341.
14. Mandelli, F., Amadori, S., Anselmo, M. P., Del Principe, D., Deriu, L., Digilio, G., Isacchi, G., and Multari, G. (1975): Total therapy in acute lymphoid leukemias. In: *Therapy of Acute Leukemias,* edited by F. Mandelli, S. Amadori, and G. Mariani. Minerva Medica, Rome.

15. Martin, M., Bourut, C., Halle-Pannenko, O., and Mathé, G. (1975): BCG immunotherapy of Lewis tumor residual disease left by local radiotherapy. *Biomedicine,* 23:337.
16. Martin, M., Bourut, C., Halle-Pannenko, O., and Mathé, G. (1975): Routes other than i.v. injection to mice for BCG administration in L1210 leukemia active immunotherapy. *Biomedicine,* 23:339.
17. Mathé, G. (1967): La dernière cellule. *Presse Med., 75*:2591.
18. Mathé, G. (1968): Immunothérapie active de la leucémie L1210 appliquée après la greffe tumorale. *Rev. Franç. Etudes Clin. Biol.,* 13:881.
19. Mathé, G. (1977): Negative result of "controlled" randomized therapeutic trials and the "dilution phenomenon." *Biomedicine,* 26. (In press.)
20. Mathé, G. (1976): *Active Immunotherapy of Cancer: Its Immunoprophylaxis and Immunorestoration.* Springer-Verlag, Heidelberg.
21. Mathé, G. (1976): *Immunothérapie Active des Cancers: Immunoprévention et Immunorestauration.* Expansion Scientifique Française, Paris.
22. Mathé, G., Amiel, J. L., Schwarzenberg, L., Schneider, M., Cattan, A., Schlumberger, J. R., Hayat, M., and de Vassal, F. (1968): Démonstration de l'efficacité de l'immunothérapie active de la leucémie aigue lymphoblastique humaine. *Rev. Franç. Etudes Clin. Biol.,* 13:454.
23. Mathé, G., Amiel, J. L., Schwarzenberg, L., Schneider, M., Cattan, A., Schlumberger, J. R., Hayat, M., and de Vassal, F. (1969): Active immunotherapy for acute lymphoblastic leukaemia. *Lancet,* 1:697.
24. Mathé, G., Amiel, J. L., Schwarzenberg, L., Schneider, M., Hayat, M., de Vassal, F., Jasmin, C., Rosenfeld, C., and Pouillart, P. (1971): Preliminary results of a new protocol for the active immunotherapy of acute lymphoblastic leukemia: Inhibition of the immunotherapeutic effect by vincristine or adamantadine. *Eur. J. Clin. Biol. Res.,* 16:216.
25. Mathé, G., Amiel, J. L., Schwarzenberg, L., Hayat, M., Pouillart, P., Schneider, M., Cattan, A., Jasmin, C., Belpomme, D., Schlumberger, J. R., de Vassal, F., Musset, M., and Misset, J. L. (1975): Immunothérapie active des leucémies aigues et des lymphosarcomes leucémiques. Bilan de 10 ans. Etude de 200 cas. *Nouv. Presse Med.,* 4:1337.
26. Mathé, G., Halle-Pannenko, O., and Bourut, C. (1974): Immune manipulation by BCG administered before or after cyclophosphamide for chemo-immunotherapy of L1210 leukemia. *Eur. J. Cancer,* 10:661.
27. Mathé, G., and Kenis, Y. (1975): *La Chimiothérapie des Cancers (Leucémies, Hématosarcomes et Tumeurs Solides),* 3rd ed. Expansion Scientifique Française, Paris.
28. Mathé, G., and Oldham, R. K. (editors) (1974): *Complications of Cancer Chemotherapy.* Springer-Verlag, Heidelberg.
29. Mathé, G., Pouillart, P., and Lapeyraque, F. (1969): Active immunotherapy of L1210 leukemia applied after the graft of tumor cells. *Br. J. Cancer,* 23:814.
30. Mathé, G., Pouillart, P., and Schwarzenberg, L. (1975): Meningeal localisation of acute leukemias. *Acta Neuropathol.* (Berl.), 6:235.
31. Mathé, G., Pouillart, P., Sterescu, M., Amiel, J. L., Schwarzenberg, L., Schneider, M., Hayat, M., de Vassal, F., Jasmin, C., and Lafleur, M. (1971): Subdivision of classical varieties of acute leukemias. Correlation with prognosis and cure expectancy. *Eur. J. Clin. Biol. Res.,* 16:554.
32. Mathé, G., and Rappaport, H. (1976): Histological and Cytological Typing of Neoplastic Diseases of Haematopoietic and Lymphoid Tissues. World Health Organization, Geneva.
32a. Mathé, G., de Vassal, F., Delgado, M., Pouillart, P., Belpomme, D., Joseph, R., Schwarzenberg, L., Amiel, J. L., Schneider, M., Cattan, A., Musset, M., Misset, J. L., and Jasmin, C. (1976): 1975 Current results of the first 100 cytologically typed acute lymphoid leukemia submitted to BCG active immunotherapy. *Cancer Immunol. Immunother.,* 1:77.
32b. Mathé, G., De Vassal, F., Schwarzenberg, L., Delgado, M., Weiner, R., Gil, M. A., Pena-Angulo, J., Belpomme, D., Pouillart, P., Machover, D., Misset, J. L., Pico,

J. L., Jasmin, C., Hayat, M., Schneider, M., Cattan, A., Amiel, J. L., Musset, M., and Rosenfeld, C. (1977): Results in children of acute lymphoid leukaemia protocol ICIG-ALL 9 consisting of chemotherapy for only nine months followed by active immunotherapy. *Cancer Immunol. Immunother.*, 2:(*in press*).

33. Mauer, A. M., and Simone, J. V. (1976): The current status of the treatment of childhood acute lymphoblastic leukemia. *Cancer Treatment Rev.*, 3:17.
34. Misset, J. L., Delgado, M., Hauss, G., de Vassal, F., Schwarzenberg, L., Hayat, M., Pouillart, P., and Mathé, G. (1977): Rechutes de leucémie aigue lymphoïde. *Sem. Hop. Paris.* (*in press.*)
35. Pouillart, P., Schwarzenberg, L., Schneider, M., Amiel, J. L., and Mathé, G. (1972): Les méningites lymphoblastiques. Incidence, prévention et traitement. *Nouv. Presse Med.*, 1:387.
36. Powles, R. K. (1976): Pitfalls in analysis of survival in clinical trials. *Biomedicine*, 24:327.
37. Rosenfeld, C., Venuat, A. M., Goutner, A., Guégand, J., Choquet, C., Tron, F., and Pico, J. L. (1975): An exceptional cell line established from a patient with acute lymphoid leukemia. *Proc. Am. Assoc. Cancer Res.*, 16:29 (Abstr. 115).
38. Schwartz, D., Flamant, R., and Lellouch, J. (1970): *L'Essai Thérapeutique Chez l'Homme.* Editions Médicales Flammarion, Paris.
39. Schwarzenberg, L., Simmler, M. C., and Pico, J. L. (1976): Human toxicology of BCG applied in cancer immunotherapy. *Cancer Immunol. Immunother.*, 1:69.
40. Skipper, H. E., Schabel, F. M., and Wilcox, W. S. (1964): Experimental evaluation of potential anticancer agents. XIII. On the criteria and kinetics associated with "curability" of experimental leukemia. *Cancer Chemother. Rep.*, 35:1.
41. Skipper, H. E., Schabel, F. M., and Wilcox, W. S. (1965): XIV. Further study of certain basic concepts underlying chemotherapy of leukemia. *Cancer Chemother. Rep.*, 45:5.
42. Skipper, H. E., Schabel, F. M., and Wilcox, W. S. (1967): Scheduling of arabinocytosine to take advantage of its S-phase specificity against leukaemic cells. *Cancer Chemother. Rep.*, 51:125.
43. Simone, J. V. (1975): Treatment of childhood acute lymphocytic leukemia. In: *Therapy of Acute Leukemias,* edited by F. Mandelli, S. Amadori, and G. Mariani. Minerva Medica, Rome.
44. Simone, J. V., Aur, J., Hustu, H., and Pinkel, D. (1972): "Total" therapy studies of acute lymphocytic leukemia in children. *Cancer,* 30:1488.
45. Smyth, A. C., Wiernik, P. H., and Serpick, A. A. (1975): Therapy of adult acute lymphocytic leukemias (ALL) with thioguanine, oncovin, daraprim and dexamethasone (TODD). *Proc. Am. Assoc. Cancer Res.*, 16:236 (Abstr. 1062).

Question and Answer Session

Dr. Holland: How do you know that the results of Study 9 and Study 10 are in any way related to immunotherapy? How do you know, since you have no control group, that you are not seeing a 35 percent plateau from cytocidal chemotherapy? Why do you say that this result is due to immunotherapy?

Dr. Mathé: I do not say so. I said that with a short chemotherapy and a long chemotherapy we have exactly the same curve, which indirectly indicates that, for this time, immunotherapy does as well as chemotherapy.

Dr. Holland: I could interpret the curves by saying that two thirds of your population is failing on chemotherapy, but one third of the group was cured back in the first three months and eventually becomes the plateau.

Dr. Mathé: This is my second conclusion. We have two kinds of patients

—those who are indifferent to chemotherapy and immunotherapy and those who will give a plateau—no doubt.

Dr. Holland: Can you say with conviction that it is due to BCG and cells or could it be due to the chemotherapy alone? The CALGB has in its own data very good plateaus for chemotherapy alone.

Dr. Mathé: In Protocol 12, when we gave a stronger chemotherapy to the poor prognosis patients, we did better. And this is due to the stronger chemotherapy. Since 1963, when we introduced BCG, we have made no further progress with different forms of immunotherapy for acute lymphatic leukemia. There is no improvement.

Dr. Simone: I have a question for clarification. My understanding is that those 30 patients in the initial study who were randomized received two years of combination chemotherapy before they were randomized. Did they also receive CNS therapy? I ask this question because I am unable to determine this from your papers. Your papers in the *Royal Society of Medicine Proceedings* in April 1975, and in the *Lancet* in 1969 indicated that there was no CNS therapy. In contrast, in the *European Journal of Biological Research* and in the *NCI Monograph* the statement was made that CNS therapy was administered.

Dr. Mathé: In the beginning, all the patients received CNS therapy. However, there was a trial group in which we compared CNS with no CNS therapy. But the patients I presented today all had CNS therapy.

Dr. Simone: In that group of patients who were on therapy for two years and randomized for no further therapy, all relapsed in 130 days. I wish you would give me your view as to why that happened because contemporary studies indicate that with any ten patients who had been on therapy and in remission for that duration of time, it would be extremely unlikely that all ten patients would relapse in 130 days. In my opinion that result is inconsistent with the results of other trials.

Dr. Mathé: The patients who were under immunotherapy relapsed identically. There was a curve of relapses during chemotherapy, which decreased more quickly after stopping chemotherapy.

Dr. Simone: Yes, but that means that with your chemotherapy, all the patients relapsed in four months after two years of complete remission. It does not fit with anybody else's data.

Dr. Mathé: You are speaking of contemporary results. This was the result of chemotherapy at that time.

Dr. Simone: I don't think that is the answer because your results are also inconsistent with those of CALGB which at that time only employed 8 months of chemotherapy.

Immunotherapy of Cancer: Present Status of
Trials in Man, edited by W. D. Terry and D. Windhorst.
Raven Press, New York © 1978.

Immunotherapy Versus Chemotherapy as Maintenance Treatment of Acute Lymphoblastic Leukemia

‡‡‡J. M. Andrien, ‡‡M. P. Beumer-Jockmans, †J. Bury, †J. L. David,
***G. Delalieux, **M. J. Delbeke, ***R. Denolin, **P. De Porre,
†††D. Fiere, *G. Flowerdew, *S. L. George, ‡H. Hainaut,
†J. Hugues, ††Y. Kenis, §§§R. Masure, ***R. Maurus,
§§J. Michel, ***J. Otten, †§M. E. Peetermans,
†M. Reginster-Bous, ††P. A. Stryckmans[1],
*R. Sylvester, *M. Van Glabbeke,
**W. Van Hove, **L. Verbist,
*A. Wennerholm, and §H. Williaert

*E.O.R.T.C. Coordinating and Data Center, Brussels, Belgium; **Akademisch Ziekenhuis,
University of Ghent, Belgium; ***Hôpital St Pierre, Free University of Brussels, Belgium;
†Hôpital de Bavière, University of Liège, Belgium; ††Institut Jules Bordet, Free University
of Brussels, Belgium; †††Hôpital Edouard Herriot, Lyon, France; ‡Clinique de l'Espérance,
Montignée, Belgium; ‡‡Institut Pasteur du Brabant, Brussels, Belgium; ‡‡‡Hôpital Civil,
Verviers, Belgium; §Kindergasthuis Good Engels, Antwerp, Belgium; §§Centre Hospitalier
de Tivoli, La Louvière, Belgium; §§§Clinique de Pédiatrie War Memorial, Brussels, Belgium; †§Algemeen Ziekenhuis Middelheim Antwerp, Belgium

Published data on immunotherapy administered after a prolonged chemotherapy as maintenance treatment of complete remission (CR) in acute
lymphoblastic leukemia (ALL) are still conflicting (1–3).

In Mathé's study (1), patients given immunotherapy were compared to
patients who received no further treatment, and a striking difference in the
number of relapses was noted. The other studies failed to show any effect for
immunotherapy (2,3).

Our study was designed to evaluate the relative effectiveness of immunotherapy and chemotherapy for the maintenance of CR in ALL.

At the time the study was initiated, it was assumed that the possible effect
of immunotherapy was conditioned by the number of leukemic cells still
present when immunotherapy was started. Thus, an eventual failure of immunotherapy could possibly be ascribed to an insufficient consolidation.
Therefore (a) after the induction of CR, a prolonged course of intensive
chemotherapy was given in all patients in order to reduce as much as possible

---

Preliminary results of a randomized trial conducted by the Hemopathies Working
Party of the E.O.R.T.C. (European Organization for Research on Treatment of Cancer).

[1] Secretary of the Hemopathies Working Party.

the leukemic burden before any kind of maintenance treatment was initiated; and (b) two different consolidation regimens were compared for their efficacy in preparing patients to immunotherapy.

Allocation of the patients to either of the two consolidation regimens as well as to either maintenance chemotherapy or immunotherapy was randomly made.

This chapter is a preliminary report of the study that is still in progress and open to new patients.

PATIENTS AND METHODS

Patients under 50 years of age with newly diagnosed ALL are eligible for the trial. Excluded are:

1. patients whose treatment has been initiated elsewhere for more than 2 weeks or has included cytostatic drugs other than 6-mercaptopurine (6MP), corticoids, and/or vincristine (VCR);

2. those with initially localized lymphoma and subsequent leukemic transformation; and

3. those with central nervous system (CNS) infiltration or no CR at completion of induction treatment.

The trial was started in May, 1971. As of October, 1976, 167 patients have been entered into the trial. There have been 140 patients younger than 20 years of age (considered children) and 27 older patients (adults). In view of the low number of evaluable adults, the results refer only to the group of evaluable children. Children and adults were randomized separately.

The patients are contributed by different Belgian and French centers, and all the data are collected and processed at the Data Center of the European Organization for Research on Treatment of Cancer (EORTC).

REMISSION INDUCTION TREATMENT

Induction therapy consists of daily oral prednisolone (40 mg/m^2) and weekly injections of VCR (2 mg/m^2). If after three VCR injections the course of the disease appears unfavorable, weekly daunomycin (60 mg/m^2) is added. All patients receive the induction treatment for at least 4 weeks. If CR is not obtained within 8 weeks, the patient is not entered into the trial. CR is defined as the absence of blasts in the blood, the absence of marrow aplasia, the presence of less than 5% blasts in the bone marrow, and the absence of leukemic infiltration on physical examination.

CONSOLIDATION TREATMENT

As soon as CR is obtained, the patients are randomly allocated to either of two consolidation regimens (Fig. 1). Regimen P, for polychemotherapy,

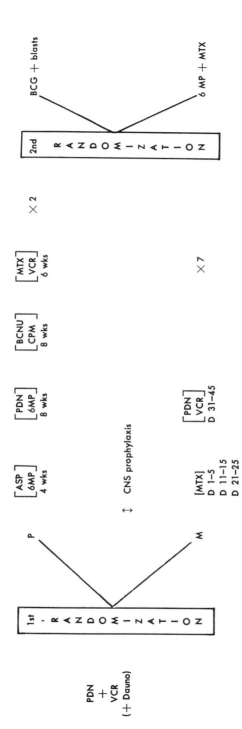

FIG. 1. Schema of the protocol. PDN, Prednisolone; Dauno, Daunomycin; ASP, L-Asparaginase; CPM, Cyclophosphamide.

TABLE 1. *Doses of the drugs and mode of administration during consolidation*

Consolidation P				
L-Asparaginase	150,000 U	/m²	/week	i.v.
6MP	70 mg	/m²	/day	p.o.
Prednisolone	40 mg	/m²	/day	p.o.
Cyclophosphamide	70 mg	/m²	/day	p.o.
VCR	1 mg	/m²	/week	i.v.
MTX	15–20 mg	/m²	2/week	p.o.
BCNU	50–100 mg	/m²	1/month	i.v.
Consolidation M				
MTX	15 mg	/m²	/day	i.v.
VCR	2 mg	/m²	/week	i.v.
Prednisolone	40 mg	/m²	/day	p.o.

consists of four different two-drug combinations given sequentially during 6 months. After the first 6 months, the sequence is repeated so that the whole consolidation extends over 1 year.

Regimen M, for monochemotherapy, consists of methotrexate (MTX) given intravenously daily (15 mg/m²) for 5 days three times a month (15 injections through each month) alternating with prednisolone plus VCR reinductions. The reinductions are given during 2 weeks after each monthly course of MTX. Doses of the drugs are indicated in Table 1.

PROPHYLAXIS OF CNS RELAPSES

Prophylactic therapy of CNS leukemia is given to all patients immediately after CR is obtained. Before July, 1973, the patients received 12 monthly intrathecal injections of MTX (5 mg/m²) and cytosine arabinoside (10 mg/m²) and craniospinal irradiation—1,500 rads to the skull and 1,000 rads to the spine. Later on, the promising results reported by Aur et al. (4) prompted us to adopt their regimen, i.e., 2,400 rads cranial irradiation combined with five intrathecal injections of MTX (12 mg/m²) given over a 16-day period.

MAINTENANCE TREATMENT

The patients who are still in continuous CR after 1 year of consolidation are again randomized, separately for each consolidation arm, to receive either maintenance chemotherapy or immunotherapy.

Maintenance chemotherapy consists of daily 6 MP (90 mg/m²) and weekly oral or i.m. MTX (15 mg/m²).

Patients on immunotherapy receive:

1. two milliliters of fresh fluid Bacillus Calmette-Guérin (BCG) (from the Institut Pasteur, Brussels) by sacrification (20 × 5 cm). The preparation

contains 8×10^7 viable units per ml. It is administered twice a week during 6 months and once a week thereafter.

2. allogeneic nonirradiated leukemic blasts; 4×10^7 blasts are injected intradermally once a week for the first 3 months and then once a month. The blast cells are obtained from the patients before treatment and are cryopreserved at $-196°$ C in the presence of 10% dimethylsulfoxide.

Both types of maintenance treatment were stopped after 4 years, i.e., 5 years from the beginning of consolidation.

COMPLICATIONS OF THERAPY

Of the 167 patients who have been entered into the trial, 13 or 7.8% have died in CR. This number equals the number of patients who died in relapse.

TABLE 2. *Lethal infections in complete remission*

Treatment arm	Number of patients	Number of lethal infections	Etiology
Consolidation P	73	6	Acute interstitial pneumonia (2) Varicella (1) Septicemia (1) Hepatitis (2)
Consolidation M	69	2	Pneumocystis carinii (1) Varicella (1)
Maintenance chemotherapy	34	3	Acute interstitial pneumonia (1) Varicella (2)
Immunotherapy	30	0	

Eleven deaths in CR were caused by infection. The etiology of these infections and their distribution among the different arms of the trial are indicated in Table 2.

It should be stressed that no lethal infection has occurred during immunotherapy.

One patient died of an acute abdominal condition during an asparaginase course, and another died of cirrhosis, which was probably a consequence of MTX.

RESULTS

The median duration of remission calculated from the start of consolidation is 124 weeks for the total number of patients. At 200 weeks, the rate of

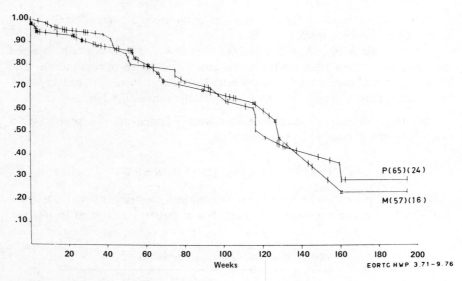

FIG. 2. The probability of remaining in CR as a function of weeks already passed in CR. The first number in parentheses refers to the evaluable patients; the second, to those who relapsed. (See *text*.)

continuous CR is 28%. There is no difference between the two consolidation arms, P and M, either in remission rate (Fig. 2) or in survival (Fig. 3). The calculated survival is 65% at 200 weeks for the whole group.

For comparison of chemotherapy and immunotherapy, the data have been

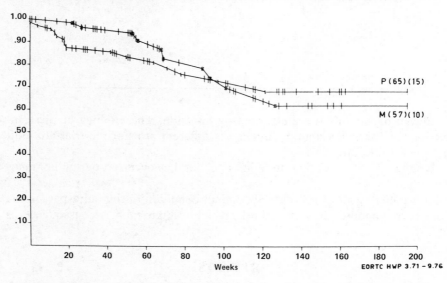

FIG. 3. The probability of surviving as a function of weeks already passed in CR (ages 1 to 21). The first number in parentheses refers to the evaluable patients; the second, to those who died. (See *text*.)

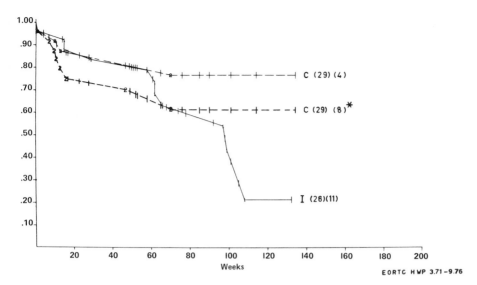

FIG. 4. The probability of remaining in CR as a function of weeks in maintenance therapy (ages 1 to 21). The first number in parentheses refers to the evaluable patients; the second, to those who relapsed. C, chemotherapy; I, immunotherapy; C*, chemotherapy, the patients who died in CR being considered as having relapsed at the time of their death (see *text*). The difference between I and C or C* is not significant.

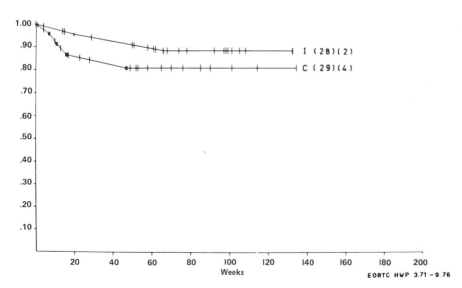

FIG. 5. Probability of surviving as a function of weeks in maintenance therapy (ages 1 to 21). The first number in parentheses refers to the evaluable patients; the second, to those who died. C, chemotherapy; I, immunotherapy.

considered from the end of consolidation. For the patients under maintenance chemotherapy, two modes of evaluation of the CR rate have been used (Fig. 4). The patients who died while in CR have been either assimilated to relapsing patients (*lower C curve*) or considered as leaving the study at the time of death (*upper C curve*).

Up to this time, statistical analysis of the curves shown in Fig. 4 shows no significant difference between chemotherapy and immunotherapy, whatever curve is chosen for the chemotherapy arm.

Survival is similar in both groups; of the patients who completed consolidation, 88% survive in the immunotherapy arm and 81% in the chemotherapy arm (Fig. 5).

DISCUSSION

The purpose of the present trial was twofold. The main question it was designed to answer is how immunotherapy alone compares with a chemotherapy known to be active for the maintenance of CR in ALL (6). A second subsidiary question was whether the kind of consolidation chemotherapy conditions the efficacy of maintenance therapy.

Regimen M was chosen because at the time this study was initiated it was known for having produced some of the best results in remission duration (5). However, the availability of several new efficient cytostatics offered the opportunity to design in parallel another consolidation program based on multiple-drug chemotherapy rather than on monochemotherapy.

At the present time, both consolidation regimens are equally efficacious in CR rate and survival. In this trial at least, multiple-drug chemotherapy is not better than a regimen of monochemotherapy interspersed with reinductions. However, it is not yet possible to conclude whether for those patients who received immunotherapy one of the consolidation treatments is better than the other.

As the main purpose of the trial was to specifically test the value of Mathé's et al. (1) immunotherapy technique compared to chemotherapy, we followed the method of these authors for the type of vaccine used and the mode and schedule of administration.

The maintenance chemotherapy regimen also was chosen because of its known efficacy at the time the trial was designed (6).

As of now, there is no significant difference in remission rate between the two maintenance arms.

This holds true even if the patients who died in CR are not tabulated as relapsing patients (*upper C curve*). It should be stressed that no patient on immunotherapy died while in CR. By contrast, three patients in CR had lethal infections during maintenance chemotherapy.

Complications of immunotherapy were minimal. Some patients experienced fever and local skin inflammation.

The overall toxicity of this immunotherapy thus appears negligible compared to the side effects of chemotherapy.

Survival is the same in the two maintenance arms. This is however a poor criterion for the comparative evaluation of the two modes of treatment because the patients who relapsed while on immunotherapy and who were reinduced in CR further received nonstandardized maintenance chemotherapy.

At the present time, it is not possible to ascertain the influence of immunotherapy and of maintenance chemotherapy on the ultimate survival of this heterogeneous group of patients. The fact that the remission rate remains similar in both maintenance groups, can be interpreted at least two ways:

1. the two types of treatment are equally effective but with a higher toxic cost for chemotherapy or,

2. the aggressiveness of the consolidation regimens is entirely responsible for the long-term remissions observed [see regimen D, study ALGB 6601 (5)], and neither of the two maintenance treatments contributes to the control of disease.

To test the second hypothesis, a control group without maintenance treatment should have been included in the study. At the time the trial was designed, it was not considered ethically acceptable to stop treatment after only 1 year, so a control group was deleted.

With this reservation in mind, this trial is the only randomized controlled clinical study that suggests that immunotherapy and chemotherapy are equally efficient for the maintenance of CR in ALL. As a matter of fact, in two other controlled trials (2,3), immunotherapy with BCG alone failed to prolong remission when compared to the absence of maintenance treatment, and patients who received maintenance chemotherapy had longer remissions than either the control or the BCG-treated patients.

Comparison between those studies (2,3) and the one reported here is difficult however because all studies differ in many respects—duration and type of consolidation therapy, use of or abstention from CNS prophylaxis, origin of the BCG strain and schedule of administration, use of BCG alone (2,3) or combined with blast cells (1), etc.

In the case maintenance immunotherapy and maintenance chemotherapy would remain of equal value in disease control, it is necessary to determine whether these two treatment modalities are equivalent in possible late untoward effects such as impairment of growth, pubertal development, fertility, etc. These questions are currently under study.

SUMMARY

A study was started in May, 1971, to evaluate the efficacy of either chemotherapy or immunotherapy as maintenance treatments of complete remission in ALL.

Through October, 1976, 167 patients in their first complete remission had been randomly allocated to either of two consolidation regimens. One, called P consists of a sequence of four different two-drug combinations. The other called M consists of MTX alternating with VCR-prednisolone reinduction.

After 1 year of this consolidation therapy, the patients are again randomized to receive either maintenance chemotherapy (MTX + 6 MP) or immunotherapy (BCG + blast cells).

No difference in relapse rate or in death rate has been observed between P and M.

For the patients who completed consolidation in CR, no significant difference in survival or in relapse rate has been observed between those receiving maintenance chemotherapy and those receiving immunotherapy. Hitherto, immunotherapy and chemotherapy appeared to be of equal value for the maintenance of CR in ALL.

ACKNOWLEDGMENTS

This work was partially supported by the "Ministère de la Santé Publique et de la Famille, Belgium," by Grant no. 2 R10 CA 11488–06, awarded by the National Cancer Institute, DHEW.

REFERENCES

1. Mathé, G., Amiel, J. L., Schwarzenberg, L., Schneider, M., Cattan, A., Schlumberger, J. R., Hayat, M., and de Vassal, F. (1969): Active immunotherapy for acute lymphoblastic leukemia. Lancet, 1:697.
2. Medical Research Council's Working Party or Leukemia in Childhood (1971): Treatment of acute lymphoblastic leukemia. Comparison of immunotherapy (BCG), intermittent methotrexate, and no therapy after a five month intensive cytotoxic regimen (Concord Trial). Br. Med. J., 4:189.
3. Heyn, R. M., Joo, P., Karon, M., Nesbit, M., Shore, N., Breslow, N., Weiner, J., Reed, A., and Hammond, D. (1975): BCG in the treatment of acute lymphocytic leukemia. Blood, 46:431.
4. Aur, R. J. A., Simone, J., Hustu, H. O., Walters, T., Borella, L., Pratt, C., and Pinkel, D. (1971): Central nervous system therapy and combination chemotherapy of childhood lymphocytic leukemia. Blood, 37:272.
5. Holland, J. F., and Glidewell, O. (1972): Chemotherapy of acute lymphocytic leukemia of childhood. Cancer, 30:1480.
6. Bernard, J., and Boiron, M. (1970): Current status: Treatment of acute leukemia. Semin. Hematol., 7:427.

Question and Answer Session

Dr. Simone: Was the DMSO washed out of the cells prior to administration to the patient?

Dr. Otten: Yes.

Dr. Simone: In the EORTC trial, did all the deaths which occurred during the course of chemotherapy occur during the consolidation phase?

Dr. Otten: No. Six patients died in consolidation regimen P, two in consolidation regimen M, and three during maintenance chemotherapy.

Dr. Terry: Does anyone have a study with similar induction and consolidation, but with a no-maintenance arm? Is there any inkling as to what one could expect without any further therapy?

Dr. Holland: I do not think so, not with polychemotherapy and discontinuation after one year.

Dr. Otten: When our protocol was designed, the question of having a control group that would receive consolidation chemotherapy without any maintenance treatment was heavily discussed. At the time we initiated the study, there were very few studies published in which consolidation chemotherapy was arrested or stopped so soon. Most of the people in the group considered it unethical to treat patients without any maintenance therapy. I agree that one could interpret the present results as reflecting the effectiveness of the consolidation therapy, and it is possible that neither the immunotherapy nor the chemotherapy maintenance is contributing anything.

Immunotherapy of Cancer: Present Status of
Trials in Man, edited by W. D. Terry and D. Windhorst.
Raven Press, New York © 1978.

Intermittent Chemotherapy and BCG in Continuation Therapy of Children with Acute Lymphocytic Leukemia

H. Ekert*, D. G. Jose, K. D. Waters, P. J. Smith, and R. N. Matthews

Department of Clinical Hematology and Oncology and Research Foundation, The Royal Children's Hospital at Parkville, Parkville, Australia

The role of immunotherapy in maintenance of remission in patients with acute lymphocytic leukemia (ALL) is presently unknown. Mathé and colleagues suggested that active immunotherapy [inoculation of nonspecific immunostimulants such as Bacillus Calmette-Guérin (BCG) combined with irradiated leukemic cells] may prolong the duration of remission in patients with ALL who have previously been given intensive chemotherapy for variable periods of time prior to active immunotherapy (1–3). On the other hand, BCG used as the only maintenance agent following induction of remission in ALL did not prolong remission duration when compared with no-treatment control groups (4,5).

In a pilot study, 12 children with ALL in complete remission maintained with continuous chemotherapy for at least 12 months were changed to intermittent chemotherapy and BCG inoculation. In all patients there was improvement in general tests of immunological function and in antibody and blastogenic responses of remission lymphocytes to leukemia cell membrane antigens (7). After 3 years follow-up more of these patients remained in total and bone marrow remission than a matched but not randomly selected group of children maintained on continuous chemotherapy (6). It thus seemed possible that a regimen of continuation therapy combining the cytotoxic effects of chemotherapy with the immunopotentiating effects of BCG could be achieved by the use of intermittent chemotherapy with BCG inoculation during drug-free intervals.

This chapter reports the results of the use of intermittent chemotherapy and BCG inoculation commenced from completion of remission induction and prophylactic therapy to the central nervous system (CNS).

* Present address: Research Laboratory, Oxford Haemophilia Centre, Churchill Hospital, Headington, Oxford OX3 7LJ England.

From Ekert, H., Jose, D. C., Waters, K. D., Smith, P., and Matthews, R. N. (1977): Intermittent chemotherapy and BCG in continuation therapy of children with acute lymphocytic leukemia. *Pediatri. Med. Oncol.* Courtesy of Alan R. Liss, Inc.

PATIENTS AND METHODS

Twenty-eight consecutively admitted children with newly diagnosed ALL were entered into the study. No patient had received any therapy prior to entry to the study. No attempt to differentiate between ALL and lympho-blastic lymphoma with leukemic transformation was made, and all patients whose marrow showed infiltration with lymphoblasts in excess of 40% were accepted into the study. There were 15 boys and 13 girls, and their ages ranged from 1 year and 5 months to 12 years, with a median of 3½ years. The white cell count at diagnosis was greater than $30,000/mm^3$ in mine, between 10 and $30,000/mm^3$ in four, and less than $10,000/mm^3$ in 15. Massive lymphadenopathy was present in seven and splenomegaly in excess of 6 cm in five. Mediastinal enlargement on chest X-ray was present in four, but no patient had leukemic cells in the cerebrospinal fluid at commencement of CNS prophylaxis. Five of the patients with a white cell count greater than $30,000/mm^3$ also had marked lymphadenopathy and splenomegaly, four had mediastinal enlargement, and all had increased numbers of T lymphocytes (E rosettes) in the peripheral blood ($>2,500/mm^3$) [8]. Three also had hot E rosettes, characteristics of thymus lymphocytes or malignant lymphoma cells [9].

REMISSION INDUCTION THERAPY

All patients with a white cell count of less than $30,000/mm^3$ and two patients with a white cell count in excess of $30,000/mm^3$ were induced with six weekly injections of vincristine 2 mg/m^2 and 2 weeks of oral prednisolone 50 mg/m^2. Seven patients, all with a white cell count greater than $30,000/mm^3$, were induced with combination chemotherapy consisting of cytosine arabinoside, cyclophosphamide, and *E. coli* L-asparaginase (May and Baker, United States), because they were considered to be high-risk patients. The cytosine arabinoside and cyclophosphamide were administered intravenously in a dose of 40 mg/m^2 8 hourly for 12 doses (4 days). L-asparaginase was given intravenously in a dose of 30,000 $units/m^2$ from day 4 to 7 [10].

Prophylactic therapy for CNS leukemia (CNS prophylaxis) was given to all patients using cranial irradiation to a dose of 2,400 rads together with four injections of intrathecal methotrexate 12 mg/m^2 at weekly intervals. All patients given combination chemotherapy had remission documented with a bone marrow aspiration prior to CNS prophylaxis, and during it they were given chemotherapy with weekly vincristine 2 mg/m^2 and a 2-week course of prednisolone. A bone marrow aspiration was repeated at the end of CNS prophylaxis.

CONTINUATION THERAPY

This consisted of 3 weeks of chemotherapy followed by a 2-week rest phase in the middle of which BCG was administered. The BCG was derived from a Pasteur strain (Commonwealth Serum Laboratories, Melbourne). This lyophilized preparation had a protein concentration of 75 mg/ampoule, and a viable bacterial count of 6 to 20 $\times$ 10^6/mg semidry weight, i.e., per ampoule contains approximately 0.45–1.2 $\times$ 10^9 organism. Approximately 20 mg of reconstituted vaccine was applied on the skin, and inoculation performed by a heaf gun set to position 1, with four inoculations each consisting of 20 puncture sites. The BCG was allowed to air dry following inoculation. The depth of penetration of the BCG was variable as on some occasions administration of BCG drew blood from the puncture sites, whereas on other occasions no blood was drawn.

Twelve patients in the early phase of the study were given continuation chemotherapy consisting of vincristine 2 mg/m^2 i.v. and methotrexate 120 mg/m^2 i.v. on day 1 and 6-mercaptopurine 65 mg/m^2 orally from day 2 to day 23. BCG was administered on day 30. The development of vincristine peripheral neuropathy in some children and the possibility of inducing leukoencephalopathy in children receiving intravenous methotrexate after cranial irradiation (11) resulted in a change of chemotherapy to oral cyclophosphamide 200 mg/m^2 on day 1, 6-mercaptopurine 65 mg/m^2 day 2 to day 23, and methotrexate 30 mg/m^2 orally on day 2, 9, and 16. All patients who commenced intravenous therapy were changed to this regimen, and 16 patients commenced the oral chemotherapy regimen from the time of remission. All but one patient received the oral regimen for at least 6 months.

Continuation therapy in this manner was continued until relapse in the bone marrow or CNS occurred. Bone marrow aspiration and lumbar puncture were performed only when a clinical or hematological indication arose.

COMPLICATIONS OF THERAPY

These were subdivided into those occurring during the first three courses of chemotherapy and those that occurred subsequently. The complications during the first three courses (15 weeks) could be associated with the toxicity attributed to induction therapy and CNS prophylaxis as well as continuation therapy. It was considered that the bone marrow and immunosuppressive effects of induction therapy would have minimal influence on the toxic reactions observed after 15 weeks. Infections were classified clinically as minor when the illness could be treated at home and subsided within 7 days. Viral infections were diagnosed by the appearance of a typical exanthem or by laboratory confirmation of viral infection. Major infections were defined as those requiring hospital treatment. Chemotherapy was postponed if there was neutropenia (polymorphonuclear neutrophil count $<$1,000/cm^2), thrombocytopenia (platelet count $<$75,000/cm^2), or anemia (hemoglobin $<$9 g/100 ml).

Total remission was defined according to the criteria proposed by the Children's Cancer Study Group (12). In brief the patients were free of symptoms and signs of disease, the blood examination was within normal limits allowing for the effects of chemotherapy, and bone marrow aspiration showed no identifiable leukemic cells and less than 5% blasts. Delayed tuberculin sensitivity was determined by injecting intradermally 0.1 ml purified protein derivative (PPD; Commonwealth Serum Laboratories, Melbourne), 1:1,000, and measuring the diameter of induration at 48 hr.

RESULTS

All children entered into the study achieved complete remission. Twenty-eight children have received from six to 19 courses (median 15) of intermittent chemotherapy and BCG with a median follow-up time of 17 months from diagnosis. Twenty children (71%) remain in continuous total remission and 24 (86%) in continuous bone marrow remission. The incidence of relapse according to the white cell count at diagnosis is shown in Table 1. Relapse occurred most frequently in patients with a white cell count between 10 to 30,000/mm^3. The actuarial complete remission rates are shown in Fig. 1. At 20 months the complete remission rate was 60%.

The response to BCG inoculation was variable. All patients showed local induration and inflammatory response usually after two to three inoculations; it became most marked 3 to 5 days after inoculation and usually faded during the week when the next course of chemotherapy commenced. The intensity of the inflammatory response varied from patient to patient, and in the same patient different intensities of response occurred with different inoculations. Tuberculin sensitivity was determined after at least five inoculations of BCG in 25 patients, and the results are shown in Table 2. Tuberculin sensitivity was not tested prior to relapse in one patient, and two in total remission were not available for testing as they had migrated to another state. The PPD reaction was negative in the three patients who relapsed first in the bone marrow but was positive in four who relapsed first in the CNS. Of 18 patients remaining in total remission only one was tuberculin negative.

TABLE 1. *Incidence of relapse*

White cell count at diagnosis 10^3/mm	No. of patients	Bone marrow release first	CNS relapse first	Bone marrow and CNS relapse
0–10	15	2	1	0
10–30	4	1	2	0
>30	9	0	1	1

All patients who relapsed had had induction therapy with vincristine and prednisolone except for the patient with combined bone marrow and CNS relapse who had been induced with cytosine arabinoside, cyclophosphamide, and L-asparaginase.

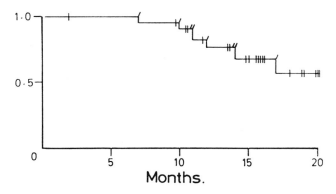

FIG. 1. Actuarial total remission plot. Sloping lines represent a patient who has relapsed.

TABLE 2. *Tuberculin sensitivity*

Response to treatment	PPD positive	PPD negative	Unknown
Total remission	17	1	2
CNS relapse first	4	0	0
Bone marrow relapse first	0	3	0
Simultaneous CNS and bone marrow relapse	0	0	1

$+$ve, an induration in response to PPD $>$ 15 mm diameter; $-$ve, no induration following PPD injection or induration $<$15 mm diameter.

Complications of Therapy

These are shown in Table 3. Neutropenia, minor infections, and postponement of chemotherapy occurred significantly more often during the first three courses of chemotherapy than in all the subsequent courses of intermittent chemotherapy. Viral and major infections were rare during both early and

TABLE 3. *Frequency of complications associated with continuation therapy*

	Incidence during first 3 courses in all patients		Incidence after first 3 courses in all patients		Statistical significance (Chi squared)
	Incidence	Total no. of courses	Incidence	Total no. of courses	
Neutropenia	10	84	10	254	p 0.025
Minor infections	18	84	24	254	p 0.01
Viral infections	1	84	2	254	NS
Postponement of chemotherapy	5	84	4	254	0.05 p 0.01
Major infections	1	84	1	254	NS

NS, not significant

subsequent courses of treatment. Anemia and thrombocytopenia leading to postponement of chemotherapy did not occur. No patients died in remission. The only complications of BCG inoculation were local skin inflammation and irritation. There were no patients with evidence of local or systemic BCG infection.

DISCUSSION

The best results in childhood ALL have been achieved by induction therapy with some form of CNS prophylaxis and either continuous multiple drug continuation chemotherapy or intermittent intensive chemotherapy given to maximum hematological tolerance. Recent studies in ALL reported from St. Jude Children's Research Hospital (study 8) show a 71% complete remission rate with a follow-up of 11 to 37 months in children given multiple drugs continuously (A. M. Mauer, *personal communication*). In earlier studies from the same hospital a total remission rate of approximately 60% was achieved with longer follow-up (13). Infection was a major cause of morbidity in 5 to 10% of patients (14).

The results of intermittent intensive continuation chemotherapy (L2 Protocol) have been reported by Haghbin et al. (15). In this series patients having malignant lymphoma with marrow infiltration were excluded, and the total remission rate was reported to be 83% with a follow-up of 1 to 42 months. Infections occurred most frequently during induction and consolidation but only seldom during maintenance; there being two deaths in 74 patients who achieved remission.

The incidence of total remission in our study is similar to the results reported for continuous multiple-drug continuation therapy (13). The proportion of patients in continuous remission achieved with the L2 protocol is marginally superior to ours (71 versus 83%), but it is difficult to compare these results since patients with malignant lymphoma and marrow infiltration were included in our study but were excluded from the analysis of the L2 protocol, and the induction therapy in the L2 protocol is very different to that used in our study or the St. Jude's Hospital studies.

The total dose of chemotherapy administered in continuation chemotherapy in our patients is approximately three-fifths of the total dose given during a comparable period of continuous chemotherapy. A previous study (16) has shown that in a group of patients who did not receive CNS prophylaxis, the patients given only half-dose continuous multiple-drug continuation therapy had a median duration of remission of only 6 months compared to 15 months in a control group receiving full-dose chemotherapy. However, our protocol is producing results comparable to those achieved by intensive protocols in use in other units. This would indicate that either intermittent administration of chemotherapy produces an enhanced tumoricidal effect making intensive chemotherapy unnecessary or that BCG inoculation is producing a significant antileukemic effect. A controlled study of patients on intermittent continuation chemotherapy randomized to receive BCG or no BCG is underway at present.

It is likely that some late relapses will occur in the patients in our study since the median follow-up is only 17 months. An analysis of actuarial total remission plots for children treated with CNS prophylaxis and multiple-agent continuous chemotherapy (13) or the L2 protocol (15) indicates that the majority of relapses occurred within 16 months. It would therefore seem unlikely that with longer follow-up our results will be significantly inferior than those discussed above.

Mathé et al. (3) have used active immunotherapy as continuation therapy after remission induction, CNS prophylaxis, and consolidation with various drug combinations for 3 to 24 months. They reported a total remission rate in patients under the age of 15 years of approximately 30% with 20 to 64 months follow-up. These results appear to be inferior to those reported in this study, but firm conclusions about the relative merits of these two approaches to immunotherapy require randomized controlled studies.

Intermittent courses of chemotherapy and BCG have resulted in an increase in general immunity and tests of specific immunity to leukemia membrane antigens (6). In this study we have investigated tuberculin sensitivity during the course of treatment. Tuberculin sensitivity among children in our community is very rare. In a study of newly diagnosed children with ALL the tuberculin sensitivity at the time of remission was negative in 20 consecutively tested children (*unpublished observations*). The finding of a positive tuberculin reaction in all but one patient in total remission but a negative tuberculin reaction in the three patients who first relapsed in the bone marrow is of particular interest as it indicates that a failure to show tuberculin hypersensitivity after BCG inoculation is a bad prognostic sign and provides further indirect evidence that immunological responses are related to the outcome of ALL.

The hematological and infectious complications of intermittent chemotherapy and BCG inoculation were minimal and occurred most often in the first 15 weeks after remission induction and CNS prophylaxis. This is probably due to the marrow and immunosuppressive effects of the induction regimen. It is not possible to assess whether the BCG inoculation diminished the incidence of infections since a control group on intermittent chemotherapy only was not studied. The lack of complications with this regimen of therapy allowed the patients 5-week intervals between visits and ensured a good quality of life. The patients were reviewed in the midpoint of the 2-week period off therapy, and BCG was given on this day. If the full blood examination showed no evidence of toxicity then chemotherapy as described was commenced the next week. If hematological toxicity was present on the day BCG vaccination fell due this was still given, but the patient was reviewed with a full blood examination 1 week later, and if the toxicity had resolved then chemotherapy was commenced. As noted in Table 3 postponement of chemotherapy was an infrequent occurrence.

SUMMARY

Continuation therapy using intermittent chemotherapy and BCG inoculation was commenced in 28 children with ALL immediately after remission induction and CNS prophylaxis. At a median follow-up time of 17 months, 71% remain in total remission and 86% in bone marrow remission. Complications of the therapy were minimal. Major infections occurred on two occasions, and there were no deaths in remission. Neutropenia, minor infections, and postponement of chemotherapy occurred most often during the first three courses of treatment. There were no local or systemic BCG infections. Tuberculin sensitivity was tested in 25 patients. It was positive in 17 of 18 in total remission and all four with only CNS relapse. It was negative prior to relapse in three patients who developed bone marrow disease.

ADDENDUM

Since the manuscript was submitted we have had an opportunity to review our experience after 36 months follow-up from the time of remission induction. Our results show that the total remission rate at 36 months is only 40%. A detailed analysis of the reasons for this disappointing total remission rate revealed that children maintained on a course of chemotherapy consisting of vincristine 2 mg/m² day 1 and methotrexate 120 mg/m² day 1 followed by 6-mercaptopurine days 2–23 (Group Y) had a significantly lower remission rate (log rank test $p < .05$) than did those children main-

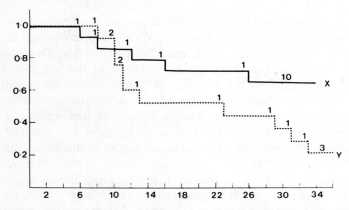

FIG. 2. Complete remission rates in children in Group X and Group Y. Numbers indicate the patients relapsing and the number in remission. Vertical axis, proportion in remission; Horizontal axis, month.

tained on cyclophosphamide 200 mg/m² day 1, 6-mercaptopurine 65 mg/m² days 2–23 and methotrexate 30 mg/m² days 2, 9 and 16 (Group X) (Fig. 2). The presenting features in the 2 groups of patients were not significantly different and in fact there were more patients with WCC in excess of 30,000 in Group X (6 patients) than in Group Y (3 patients). It would seem that the poor response was due to the use of single drug maintenance with consolidation with vincristine and a single dose of methotrexate on day 1 of the therapy cycle in Group Y. It is of interest that the administration of BCG did not improve the remission rate for the patients treated with inadequate chemotherapy.

REFERENCES

1. Mathé, G., Amiel, J. L., Schwarzenberg, L., Schneider, M., Cattan, A., Schlumberger, J. R., Hayat, M., and de Vassal, F. (1969): Active immunotherapy for acute lymphoblastic leukemia. *Lancet,* 1:697.
2. Mathé, G. (1974): Attempts at immunotherapy of 100 acute lymphoid leukaemia patients. In: *Advances in Acute Leukaemia,* edited by F. J. Cleton, D. Crowther, and J. S. Malpas, pp. 143–157. North-Holland Publ., Elsevier, Amsterdam.
3. Mathé, G., Schwarzenberg, L., Amiel, J. L. Pouillart, P., Hayat, M., de Vassal, F. D., Rosenfeld, C., and Jasmin, C. (1975): Immunotherapy of leukemia. *Proc. R. Soc. Med.,* 68:211.
4. Preliminary Report by the Medical Research Council by the Leukaemia Committee and the Working Party on Leukaemia in Childhood. Treatment of acute lymphoblastic leukaemia comprising of immunotherapy (BCG) intermittent methotrexate and no therapy after 5 months intensive cytotoxic regimen (Concord trial). *Br. Med. J.,* 4:189,1971.
5. Heyn, R. M., Joo, P., Karon, M., Nesbit, M., Shore, N., Breslow, N., Weiner, J., Reed, A., and Hammond, D. (1975): BCG in the treatment of acute lymphocytic leukemia. *Blood,* 46:431.
6. Ekert, H., Jose, D. G., Wilson, F. C., Matthews, R. N., and Lay, H. (1975): Intermittent chemotherapy and immunotherapy with BCG in remission maintenance of children with acute lymphocytic leukemia. Effects upon immunological function. *Int. J. Cancer,* 6:102.
7. Ekert, H., and Jose, D. G. (1975): Chemotherapy and BCG in acute lymphocytic leukemia. *Lancet,* 2:713.
8. Jose, D. G., Ekert, H., Colebatch, J. H., Waters, K. D., Wilson, F. C., and O'Keefe, D. (1976): Immune function at diagnosis in relation to response of therapy in acute lymphocytic leukemia. *Blood,* 47:1011.
9. Borella, L., and Sen, K. (1975): E receptors on blasts from untreated acute lymphocytic leukemia (ALL): Comparison of temperature dependence of E rosettes formed by leukemic and lymphoid cells. *J. Immunol.,* 114:187.
10 Lay, H. N., Ekert, H., and Colebatch, J. H. (1975): Combination chemotherapy in children with acute lymphocytic leukemia who failed to respond to standard remission induction therapy. *Cancer,* 36:1220.
11. Price, R. A., and Jamieson, P. A. (1975): CNS in childhood leukemia. II. Subacute leucoencephalopathy. *Cancer,* 35:306.
12. Leikin, S. L., Brubaker, C., Hartman, J. R., Murphy, M. L., Wolff, J. A., and Ferrin, E. (1968): Criteria for chemotherapy in acute leukemia. *Cancer,* 21:349.
13. Simone, J., Aur, J. A., Hustu, H. O., and Pinkel, D. (1972): "Total therapy" studies of acute lymphocytic leukemia in children: Current results and prospects for cure. *Cancer,* 36:1488.
14. Simone, J., Holland, E., and Johnson, W. W. (1972): Fatalities during remission of childhood leukemia. *Blood,* 39:759.

15. Haghbin, M., Tan, C. C., Clarkson, D. G., Miké, V., Buřhenal, J. H., and Murphy, M. L. (1974): Intensive chemotherapy in children with acute lymphoblastic leukemia. ("L2 Protocol"). *Cancer,* 33:1491.
16. Pinkel, D., Hernandez, K., Borella, L., Holton, C., Aur, R. J. A., Samoy, G., and Pratt, L. B. (1971): Drug dosage and remission duration in childhood lymphocytic leukemia. *Cancer,* 27:247.

Immunotherapy of Cancer: Present Status of
Trials in Man, edited by W. D. Terry and D. Windhorst.
Raven Press, New York © 1978.

Acute Lymphoblastic Leukemia: 5-Year Follow-up of the Concord Trial

Humphrey E. M. Kay

Leukemia Trials Office, The Royal Marsden Hospital, London SW3 6JJ England

In the British wing of the Concord trial, patients with acute lymphoblastic leukemia (ALL) received a standard induction and consolidation regime as shown in Fig. 1 (see ref. 1). At the end of this period of 21 weeks (plus delays of up to 8 weeks) they were randomized to receive no further treatment. Glaxo Bacillus Calmette-Guérin (BCG) was given by Heaf gun weekly, or methotrexate twice weekly. In a preliminary report (1) it was shown that the randomized groups were comparable with respect to age, initial white cell count, and other features. There was no significant difference in remission length between the BCG and no-treatment groups, both being inferior to the chemotherapy group. There was some slight evidence that BCG enhanced

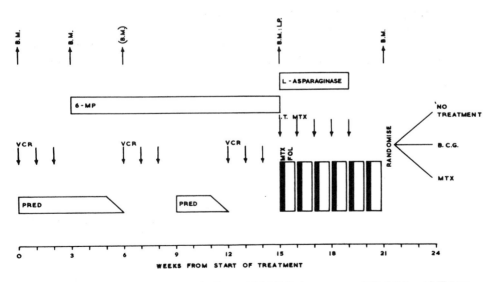

FIG. 1. Initial treatment for ALL cases in the Concord Trial. B.M., bone marrow; FOL, folinic acid; IT, intrathecal; 6 MP, 6-mercaptopurine; MTX, methotrexate; PRED, prednisolone; VCR, vincristine.

On behalf of the Medical Research Council's Working Party or Leukemia in Childhood.

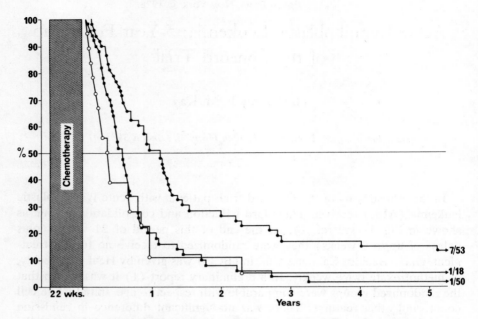

FIG. 2. Remission duration for all randomized patients (entry 1969–1970) still in remission at the end of 22 weeks chemotherapy. O—O, No treatment; ■—■, BCG; MTX, methotrexate, ●—●.

delayed hypersensitivity responses and increased the lymphocyte count in the first 8 weeks of treatment.

Further follow-up has confirmed the initial trends. Figure 2 shows remission duration to 5¼ years with no relapses since then, all patients having

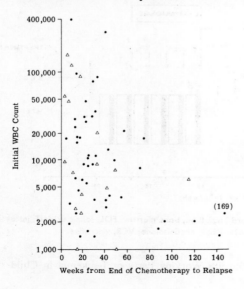

FIG. 3. Relationship of initial leukocyte count to duration of remission in cases having BCG or no treatment. △, No treatment; ●, BCG; WBC, white blood cell count.

reached 6 years since diagnosis. Out of 50 BCG patients one is still in first remission (plus one, the only one, who was switched by a prejudiced trial participant to methotrexate after 7 weeks BCG). This compares with one of 18 controls (plus one of two deviant controls whose initial chemotherapy was unduly prolonged) and with seven of 53 patients on methotrexate. The latter difference is small ($p < 0.05$) but probably real. The results are poor by modern standards since there was inadequate central nervous system (CNS) prophylaxis in the chemotherapy group and inadequate systemic chemotherapy also in the other groups.

BCG was given weekly for 3 years in the few long remitters, but relapses continued to occur, the latest ones being at 111, 137 (local lesion), 163, and 190 weeks from diagnosis. There was also one at 137 weeks in the no-treatment control group. It may be significant that these patients all had rather low initial leukocyte counts (Fig. 3). By chance, the pretrial pilot BCG group has fared rather better with two out of 12 in remission at 7 years.

The survival of these patients has largely depended on treatment received since first relapse, and that was not standardized. A few relapsing BCG and no-treatment patients received CNS prophylaxis, and some of the methotrexate group with meningeal relapse appear to have been successfully treated with long second remissions. At 5 years there were no significant differences —22/53 for chemotherapy, 16/50 for BCG, and 6/18 for no treatment. The survival for all patients in the trial is compared (Fig. 4) with previous and subsequent trials.

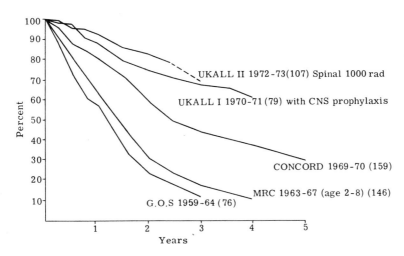

FIG. 4. Comparative survival as of January 1, 1976 in successive Medical Research Council (MRC) trials in ALL involving children ages 1 to 13. UKALL, United Kingdom acute lymphoblastic leukemia; GOS, Great Ormond Street.

REFERENCE

Medical Research Council's Working Party on Leukemia in Childhood (1971): Treatment of acute lymphoblastic leukaemia. Comparison of immunotherapy (BCG), intermittent methotrexate, and no therapy after a five-month intensive cytotoxic regimen (Concord Trial). *Br. Med. J.,* 4:189.

Question and Answer Session

Dr. Powles: It is a bit unfair to totally ignore the survival figures in this study just because they had a hodge-podge of treatment after they relapsed. In a trial of this size, I think it might just be worth looking at survival. The reason I say this is that if the survivals of the BCG group and the methotrexate group are the same, yet the BCG had shorter remissions, then we could draw the conclusion that the immunotherapy group had longer survival after relapse than the nonimmunotherapy group. Similar comments have already been made with regard to AML.

Dr. Kay: We have in fact done those calculations on five-year survivals. The group which was marginally better in the long run was the no further treatment group. Perhaps this was because that group of patients relapsed quickly and received better treatment quickly thereafter and therefore did better. However, the differences are so slight you can say absolutely nothing about it.

Immunotherapy of Cancer: Present Status of Trials in Man, edited by W. D. Terry and D. Windhorst. Raven Press, New York © 1978.

Treatment of Acute Lymphatic Leukemia with Chemotherapy Alone or Chemotherapy Plus Immunotherapy

David G. Poplack, Brigid G. Leventhal,[1] Richard Simon, Thomas Pomeroy, Robert G. Graw, and Edward S. Henderson

Pediatric Oncology Branch and Radiation Branch (TP), National Cancer Institute, Bethesda, Maryland 20014

Stimulated by Mathé's original description suggesting a beneficial effect for immunotherapy in childhood acute lymphocytic leukemia (ALL) (1), we undertook a study designed to compare the effectiveness of chemotherapy plus immunotherapy versus chemotherapy alone as maintenance treatment for this disease. Newly diagnosed patients with ALL were induced into remission with chemotherapy and then randomized to receive either chemotherapy alone or chemotherapy plus immunotherapy with Bacillus Calmette-Guérin (BCG) and allogeneic leukemia cells during a 34-month maintenance treatment period. The results of this study are presented in this chapter.

MATERIALS AND METHODS

Previously untreated children less than 20 years of age with the diagnosis of ALL were eligible for this study. Prior to entrance into the study informed consent for the patient's participation was obtained. All patients were induced with repeated 5-day courses of POMP consisting of prednisone 1000 mg/m^2 i.v. days 1 to 5, vincristine 2 mg/m^2 i.v. day 1 (maximum 2 mg), methotrexate 7.5 mg/m^2 i.v. days 1 to 5, 6-mercaptopurine 125 mg/m^2 i.v. days 1 to 5, and allopurinol 100 mg/m^2 three times a day. Once remission was achieved, patients received "systemic consolidation" with four additional courses of POMP. Following this, all patients underwent central nervous system (CNS) prophylaxis including 2,400 rads to the cranial vault and intrathecal chemotherapy with either methotrexate or cytosine arabinoside given during the radiation and monthly thereafter. After the first 35 patients had been treated on this regimen, it was noted that five patients had devel-

---

[1] Present address The Oncology Center, The Johns Hopkins Hospital, Baltimore, Maryland 21205

oped meningeal disease prior to receiving prophylaxis. Thus, it was felt that systemic consolidation excessively delayed the institution of CNS prophylaxis. The protocol was subsequently adjusted to institute CNS prophylaxis earlier, immediately following attainment of bone marrow remission, and a systemic consolidation regimen was given following prophylaxis consisting of two 5-day courses of cytosine arabinoside (100 mg/m² i.v. or s.c. every 12 hr) plus 6-thioguanine (90 mg/m² p.o. every 12 hr). Following completion of consolidation, all patients began 34 months of maintenance therapy that was divided into six treatment blocks (Fig. 1). Each treatment block consisted of an initial 4-month period (phase 1) during which all patients received identical chemotherapy consisting of vincristine (2 mg/m² maximum 2 mg on days 1, 8, and 15 of the first and third month) together with 15 days of prednisone (100 mg/m² daily p.o.), daily 6-mercaptopurine (75 mg/m² daily p.o.), and weekly methotrexate (15 mg/m² p.o.). In the next 2 months of each maintenance treatment block (phase 2) patients were randomized to receive one of three different maintenance regimens. Group 1 received methotrexate twice a week (20 mg/m² daily p.o.). Group 2 received 5-day courses of methotrexate (15 mg/m² daily p.o.) with 10-day rest intervals. Group 3 received immunotherapy with BCG and allogeneic leukemia cells. Immunotherapy consisted of live allogeneic leukemia cells collected from a single donor at the time of admission and stored in a viable state in dimethyl-sulfoxide (DMSO) in the gas phase of liquid nitrogen (2). After thawing and

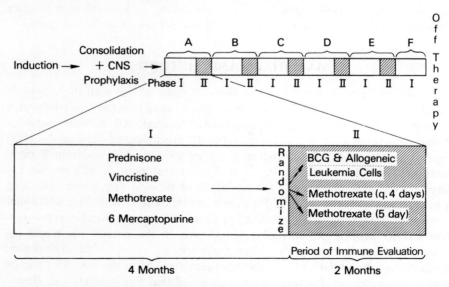

FIG. 1. Scheme of National Cancer Institute Protocol 72–1. Patients were randomized to one of three maintenance treatment groups during phase 2 (shaded boxes). Total duration of maintenance therapy was 34 months.

washing, 4×10^7 cells were injected intradermally on the anterior aspect of the thigh. BCG obtained fresh from the Pasteur Institute and containing 1×10^9 live organisms per ml was applied over the injection sites with a Heaf gun. Immunization was repeated weekly during the first month of each phase 2 maintenance period. Once randomized, all patients received the same phase 2 therapy during subsequent phase 2 periods. Patients in the three maintenance treatment groups repeated phase 1 and 2 five times and then finished their maintenance therapy with a final phase 1 period of chemotherapy for a total of 34 months maintenance treatment.

All patients underwent immune evaluation during each of the phase 2 treatment periods. This included skin testing and measurement of *in vitro* lymphocyte transformation.

RESULTS

Seventy patients entered this protocol. Six failed to achieve remission, one died during induction, one was declared ineligible, and six relapsed before the start of maintenance therapy. Thus, 56 patients were randomized to one of the three different maintenance treatment groups—24 to group 1, 11 to group 2, and 21 to group 3. When it became apparent that the two chemotherapy groups (1 and 2) were similar in efficacy, randomization to group 2 was halted to increase the numbers of patients in groups 1 and 3. Each group was reasonably comparable in terms of prognostic factors. Fifteen of the 35

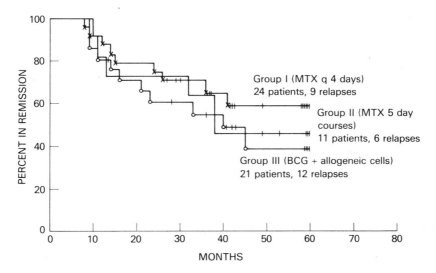

FIG. 2. Percent of patients in continuous extra-CNS remission at 60 months. There is no significant difference in remission duration between the chemotherapy alone (groups 1 and 2) and the chemotherapy plus immunotherapy treatment group (group 3), $p > 25$.

patients in groups 1 and 2 who received chemotherapy alone have had extra-CNS relapses, whereas 12 of the 21 patients in the chemotherapy plus immunotherapy group (group 3) have relapsed outside the CNS. Thus, there is no significant difference ($p > 0.25$) in the relapse rates between those patients who received chemotherapy alone versus those who received chemotherapy plus immunotherapy. Similarily, there is no significant difference in the remission duration between any of the maintenance treatment arms (Fig. 2). At the present time 44% of all patients are in initial complete extra-CNS remission at 60 months. A complete analysis of the results of the CNS therapy on this protocol is in preparation.

In those patients receiving immunotherapy some toxicity was noted. Acute pain with injection of cells was common. Local induration and ulceration occurred at the sites of BCG administration in all patients by the second passage through phase 2 of maintenance. There were two children who developed secondary *Staphylococcus aureus* infections at injection sites. Fever within 48 hr was also common. A generalized papular erythematous rash developed in two patients that did not recur with repeated lower doses of BCG. No patients developed systemic BCG infection.

DISCUSSION

The intent of this study was to compare the effectiveness of maintenance chemotherapy plus immunotherapy with BCG and allogeneic leukemia cells versus chemotherapy alone for the treatment of ALL. The study was designed to expose patients to immunotherapy early, following remission induction, rather than after prolonged periods of chemotherapy. It utilized nonirradiated, live allogeneic cells together with BCG. Immunotherapy was given intermittently in maintenance for periods of 2 months when no chemotherapy was given. It was hoped that this schedule would result in a maximum immunostimulating effect during a period when there were no ongoing suppressive effects of chemotherapy. However, we were not able to see any clinical evidence for either nonspecific or specific immunotherapeutic effects such as diminution in relapse rate or prolongation of remission duration in those patients treated with immunotherapy. Moreover, aside from positive skin test reactions to tuberculin in those patients who received BCG, immune evaluation yielded no evidence for immunostimulation in our patients. On the contrary, we saw progressive immunosuppression over the duration of maintenance therapy in all patient groups (4). Although it could be argued that BCG and allogeneic cells were as effective as chemotherapy during the phase 2 treatment periods, one cannot conclude from our results any advantage for the addition of immunotherapy to chemotherapy. We believe our results, which concur with those of several other recent studies (5–8), fail to confirm those original studies that suggested a beneficial effect for immunotherapy in the maintenance therapy for ALL.

REFERENCES

1. Mathé, G., Amiel, J. C., Schwarzenberg, L., Schneider, M., Cattan, A., Schlumberger, J. R., Hayat, M., and de Vassal, F. (1969): Acute immunotherapy for acute lymphoblastic leukemia. *Lancet,* 1:697–699.
2. Halterman, R. H., Johnson, G. E., and Leventhal, B. G. (1973): Storage method for leukemia blast cell. *NCI Monogr.,* 37:149–151.
3. Poplack, D. G., Simon, R. S., and Leventhal, B. G. *In preparation.*
4. Leventhal, B. G., Poplack, D. G., Johnson, E. G., Simon, R., Bowles, C., and Steinberg, S. (1976): The effect of chemotherapy and immunotherapy on the response to mitogens in acute lymphatic leukemia. In: *Mitogens in Immunobiology,* edited by J. Oppenheim and D. Rosenstreich, pp. 613–623. Academic Press, New York.
5. Preliminary Report to the Medical Research Council by the Leukemia Committee and the Working Party on Leukemia in Childhood (1971): Treatment of acute lymphoblastic leukemia: Comparison of immunotherapy (BCG), intermittent methotrexate, and no therapy after a five-month intensive cytotoxic regimen (Concord trial). *Br. Med. J.,* 4:189–194.
6. Gutterman, J. N., Hersh, E. M., Rodriguez, V., McCredie, K. B., Mavligit, G., Reed, R., Burgess, M. A., Smith, T., Gehan, E., Bodey, G. P., and Freireich, E. J. (1974): Chemoimmunotherapy of adult acute leukemia. *Lancet,* 2:1405–1409.
7. Heyn, R. M., Joo, P., Karon, M., Nesbit, M., Shore, N., Breslow, N., Weiner, J., Reed, A., and Hammond, D. (1975): BCG in the treatment of acute lymphocytic leukemia. *Blood,* 46:431–442.
8. Stryckmans, P. A., and Otten, J. A. (1976): Immunotherapy in acute lymphoblastic leukemia. EORTC Hemopathies Working Party. *Proc. 12th Ann. Mtg. Am. Soc. Clin. Oncol.,* 17:217.

Immunotherapy of Cancer: Present Status of
Trials in Man, edited by W. D. Terry and D. Windhorst.
Raven Press, New York © 1978.

BCG in the Treatment of Acute Lymphocytic Leukemia

R. M. Heyn, P. Joo, M. Karon, M. Nesbit, N. Shore, N. Breslow,
J. Weiner, A. Reed, H. Sather, and D. Hammond[1]

The objectives of a clinical trial undertaken by Children's Cancer Study Group in children with acute lymphocytic leukemia (ALL) were threefold: (a) to evaluate the use of nonspecific immunotherapy with Bacillus Calmette-Guerin (BCG) in prolonging an unmaintained complete remission, (b) to compare the effect of BCG at early and late intervals during remission, and (c) to determine whether the study plan constituted good treatment by evaluating the total duration of control with similar chemotherapy in all treatment groups and the survival in all groups.

PATIENTS AND TREATMENT

The study plan is shown in Fig. 1. No stratification of patients based on initial white cell count or age was made. Children under 16 years of age with previously untreated ALL were induced with 6 weeks of prednisone and weekly vincristine. If the bone marrow was an M_1 rating (less than 5% blasts) or an M_2 rating (6 to 25% blasts) at the end of 6 weeks, an 8-week period of consolidation with intravenous methotrexate was begun. Bone marrow examination was done at the end of the consolidation period. All patients whose marrow was an M_1 rating and who had not developed central nervous system (CNS) leukemia were randomized to one of three primary maintenance regimens. An absolute neutrophil count of $1,500/cm^2$ and absolute lymphocyte count of $500/cm^2$ were requisites for beginning maintenance therapy. The three regimens included regimen 1, no further therapy, regimen 2, BCG, and regimen 3, chemotherapy. The patients in regimen 3 who remained in remission for 8 months were rerandomized into the same three regimens as in primary maintenance. Thus, regimen 4 received no further therapy, regimen 5, BCG, and regimen 6, chemotherapy. If patients on no therapy or BCG in either primary or secondary maintenance developed marrow relapse, they were reinduced and reconsolidated as before and put on maintenance chemotherapy. Patients were off study if they developed an M_3 rating (greater than 25% blasts) while on chemotherapy.

The doses of drugs used in the study are given in Fig. 2. Prednisone, 60

---

[1] Investigators, institutions, and grant support are given in Appendix 1.
For the Children's Cancer Study Group.

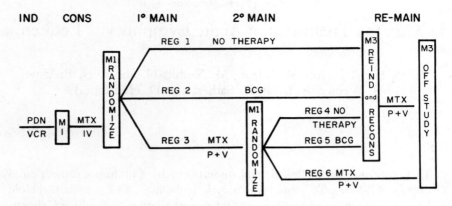

FIG. 1. Schematic plan for the use of immunotherapy with BCG following chemotherapy for induction (IND) and consolidation (CONS). The regimens for primary (1° MAIN) and secondary (2° MAIN) maintenance are designated. IV, intravenous; MI, bone marrow rating, less than 5% blasts; MTX, methotrexate; P + V, prednisone + vincristine; PDN, prednisone; VCR, vincristine.

mg/m² daily, and vincristine, 2 mg/m² weekly were used for induction. Consolidation consisted of four courses of intravenous methotrexate, giving 15 mg/m² daily for 5 days every 2 weeks. Maintenance chemotherapy consisted of methotrexate, 30 mg/m² orally twice a week, and monthly reinducer courses of prednisone for 5 days plus a single dose of vincristine. The doses of prednisone and vincristine were the same as those used during induction.

BCG was obtained from the Research Foundation in Chicago. This strain of BCG was originally obtained from the Pasteur Institute in Paris in 1954. It was grown in pellicle culture and prepared for use as a freeze-dried preparation. Sterile water, 0.7 ml, was added to a single vial to make a reconstituted wet weight of 75 mg/ml. Three drops of the resuspended vaccine were

INDUCTION - 6 weeks

Prednisone	60 mg/m²/d in 3 divided doses
Vincristine	2.0 mg/m²/wk X 6

CONSOLIDATION - 8 weeks

Methotrexate	15 mg/m²/d X 5 q 2W X 4

MAINTENANCE

Methotrexate	30 mg/m² biw orally
Prednisone	60 mg/m² in 3 divided doses X 5 once/month
Vincristine	2.0 mg/m² once/month

FIG. 2. Doses of drugs used for induction, consolidation, and maintenance phases. MTX, methotrexate; Pred, prednisone; Vcr, vincristine.

put on each of two skin sites that were rotated between the upper arms and thighs. A vaccinating disc with 36 prongs was held on a magnet-type holder and applied to the area of skin containing the vaccine. The prongs were imbedded into the skin by pressure applied on the holder. The procedure was repeated at the second skin site. The patients in regimens 2 and 5 were vaccinated twice a week for the first 4 weeks and weekly thereafter until marrow or CNS relapse.

No prophylactic therapy was given to the CNS. When CNS leukemia occurred, the patient was treated with intrathecal methotrexate, 12 mg/m² twice weekly until the spinal fluid was normal. Radiotherapy was used at the discretion of the primary physician. Patients who developed CNS leukemia while on no therapy or BCG were begun on maintenance chemotherapy as described above and continued on study.

STATISTICAL ANALYSIS

In order to insure an adequate number of children would be available for secondary randomization after 8 months of maintenance chemotherapy, the initial randomization placed one-fifth of patients in remission on no therapy, one-fifth on BCG, and three-fifths on chemotherapy. In primary randomization the comparative analysis of remission duration in the three groups was made at 7 months. This was done because patients on chemotherapy in regimen 3 were due to be rerandomized at 8 months. Because the remission duration on no therapy or BCG in primary randomization proved itself to be inferior to drug therapy quite early, randomization was limited as soon as statistically adequate numbers of patients were entered in each of the first two regimens. This change accounts for the difference in the number of children in regimens 1 and 2 compared to regimens 4, 5, and 6. The comparison of remission duration in secondary randomization was made 12 months following the onset of secondary maintenance. Survival curves for all patients on study and for the separate regimens are presented as life table analyses.

RESULTS

Patient entries in the various phases of the study are summarized in Tables 1, 2, and 3. A total of 502 patients was entered on study over a 20-month period. Eighty-six percent achieved an M_1 marrow. Three-hundred and fifty children were randomized to primary maintenance, 31 receiving no further therapy, 34, BCG, and 285, chemotherapy. In secondary maintenance, 153 children were randomized to receive no therapy (52), BCG (44), and chemotherapy (57).

Figure 3 shows the comparative remission durations for the three regimens in primary maintenance. At 7 months, 25% of patients remained in remission on no therapy and 20% continued in remission on BCG. In contrast,

TABLE 1. *Summary of induction phase of 502 patients entered on study*

Status at end of induction	
M_1	432 (86.0%)
M_2	21
M^3	13
Expired during induction	18
Lost to follow-up	8
Toxicity before 42 days	1
Protocol error	9
Total	502
Reasons for not entering consolidation phase	
M_3	13
Expired	18
Lost to follow-up before 42 days	8
Lost to follow-up at 42 days	4 (4 M_1)
Toxicity	2 (1 M_1)
Protocol error, progressive disease	12 (3 M_1)
Total	57
Patients entering consolidation	445

79% of patients on maintenance chemotherapy were still in remission. The difference between the number of patients in remission on regimens 1 and 2 and the number in remission in regimen 3 is statistically significant using the log rank Chi square test ($p < 0.01$). Only one patient in regimens 1 and 2 has not relapsed. This patient received BCG for 3½ years before it was stopped.

Figure 4 compares the remission duration following secondary randomization. Twelve months after randomization, 36% of patients receiving no further therapy and 32% of patients receiving BCG continued in remission. Fifty-six percent of the children who continued on chemotherapy were still

TABLE 2. *Summary of 445 patients entered on consolidation phase*

Status at end of consolidation	
M_1	371
M_2	52
M^3	14
Expired	3
Lost to follow-up	3
Protocol error	2
Total	445
Reasons for not entering primary randomization	
M_2	52
M^3	14
Expired	3
Lost to follow-up	4
CNS leukemia	22
Total	95
Patients randomized to primary maintenance	350

TABLE 3. *Summary of patients randomized and evaluable in primary and secondary maintenance*

Randomized to primary maintenance		350
Regimen 1—no therapy	31 (28)	
Regimen 2—BCG	34 (28)	
Regimen 3—chemotherapy	285 (247)	
CNS leukemia	43	
M₃	35	
M₂ at 8 months	16	
Protocol error	11	
Lost to follow-up	27	
Randomized to regimens 4, 5, 6	153	
Total	285	
Randomized to secondary maintenance		153
Regimen 4—no therapy	52 (49)	
Regimen 5—BCG	44 (41)	
Regimen 6—chemotherapy	57 (48)	

Evaluable patients shown in parentheses.

in remission at the same interval, a difference that is significant ($p < 0.01$). The duration of remission following secondary randomization was longer in regimens 4 and 5 than that following primary randomization to regimens 1 and 2. This is probably accounted for by the selectivity of better-risk patients after 8 months of maintenance therapy. At the present, seven patients

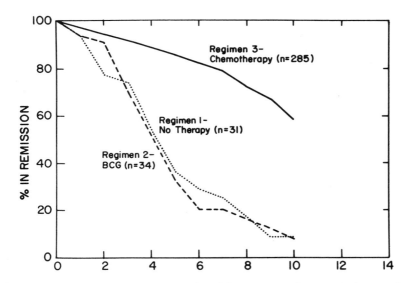

FIG. 3. The duration of remissions in regimens 1, 2, and 3 in primary maintenance is shown as the percentage of patients in remission on each regimen for each month of treatment after randomization. All cases are included in the curves; nonevaluable cases are followed only for periods properly at risk, and evaluable cases are followed until outcome.

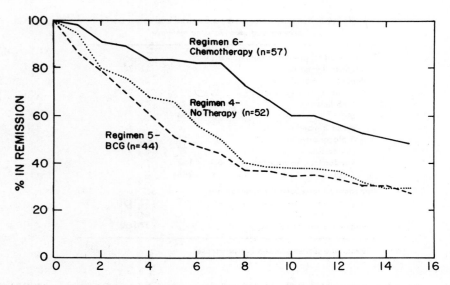

FIG. 4. The duration of remissions in regimens 4, 5, and 6 in secondary maintenance is shown as the percentage of patients in remission on each regimen for successive months after randomization. All cases are included in the curves; nonevaluable cases are followed only for periods properly at risk, and evaluable cases are followed until outcome.

continue in remission on no therapy, eight are in remission on BCG, and 11 continue in remission on chemotherapy.

Follow-up on all patients entered on study is now approaching 5 years. The incidence of reinduction of marrow remission in those patients relapsing while off chemotherapy in regimens 1, 2, 4, and 5 did not show a difference between the patients on no therapy and those on BCG. Patients who relapsed during regimens 1 and 2 had a reinduction rate of 84%. Ninety-six percent of patients relapsing during regimens 4 and 5 achieved a second M_1 marrow. Second remission durations of these four groups of patients receiving the same maintenance chemotherapy were similar, and all were longer than the first remission on primary maintenance.

Median survival of all patients entered on study is between 36 and 37 months. The survival curves for patients on individual regimens suggest an apparent superiority of regimens 4, 5, and 6. However, this must be viewed in light of the selectivity of better-risk patients in these three groups. There is no statistically significant difference in survival between the control and BCG groups from either primary or secondary randomization. If one compares survival in regimens 1 (no therapy) and 2 (BCG) with all patients originally entered on regimen 3 (chemotherapy), there is no significant difference among the three groups, supporting the element of selectivity of better-risk patients in secondary randomization.

TOXICITY

BCG vaccinations were generally well tolerated. Two children were removed from study because of problems with BCG. Both developed exacerbation of the reaction in previous vaccination sites, with each new vaccination causing ulceration and draining. One of the two also developed a secondary rash after multiple vaccinations. The rash was papular, erythematous, and pruritic.

Toxicity to vincristine was easily remedied by lowering drug dose. During consolidation with methotrexate the commonest signs of toxicity were mouth ulcers and respiratory infections. During maintenance chemotherapy, methotrexate toxicity included liver fibrosis, osteoporosis of bones, skin rashes, and respiratory infectious illnesses. Five children expired while in complete remission on maintenance chemotherapy, one with encephalitis, two with pneumocystis carinii pneumonia, one with varicella pneumonia, and one with an unidentified pneumonia. Sixteen children were removed from study with M_1 marrows because of methotrexate liver toxicity. Another three children in remission on chemotherapy were thought to have osteoporosis and were removed from study with M_1 marrows.

DISCUSSION

Although vaccination with BCG as done in this study was successful in immunizing the majority of patients who received it, no effect could be seen on the leukemic process. This is in contrast to Mathé's initial report (2) but similar to the findings of the Concord trial reported by the Medical Research Council in 1971 (3). A subsequent report by Mathé showed that the patients who accounted for the cumulative survival duration plateau following chemotherapy and immunotherapy were those who had morphologic characteristics described as microlymphoblastic and prolymphocytic (4). Other factors that may play a role in the results of the various studies in ALL include the adequacy of dose and delivery of the BCG used and the number of viable organisms present in each of the BCG preparations. A prerequisite to further studies should include the ability to measure these factors more precisely and to measure the adjuvant effect of the immunotherapy used.

SUMMARY

In 1970 Children's Cancer Study Group began a controlled clinical trial to evaluate the use of BCG in children with ALL. A total of 502 children were entered on study. Children in complete remission following induction and a period of consolidation with chemotherapy were randomized into groups receiving no further therapy, BCG, or chemotherapy. Patients on chemotherapy who remained in remission for 8 months were again randomized into the same three groups. BCG failed to prolong remission beyond that of the control group in either the primary or secondary randomization. Patients on chemotherapy had significantly longer remissions in both maintenance periods. The preliminary results of this study were published in 1975 (1).

REFERENCES

1. Heyn, R. M., Joo, P., Karon, M., Nesbit, M., Shore, N., Breslow, N., Weiner, J., Reed, A., and Hammond, D. (1975): BCG in the treatment of acute lymphocytic leukemia. *Blood,* 46:431–442.
2. Mathé, G., Amiel, J. L., Schwarzenberg, L., Schneider, M., Cattan, A., Schlumberger, J. R., Hayat, M., and De Vassal, F. (1969): Active immunotherapy for acute lymphoblastic leukaemia. *Lancet,* 1:697.
3. Preliminary Report to the Medical Research Council by the Leukaemia Committee and the Working Party on Leukaemia in Childhood (1971): Treatment of acute lymphoblastic leukaemia. *Br. Med. J.,* 4:189.
4. Mathé, G., Pouillart, P., Sterescu, M., Amiel, J. L., Schwarzenberg, L., Schneider, M., Hayat, M., De Vassal, F., Jasmin, C., and Lafleur, M. (1971): Subdivision of classical varieties of acute leukemia, correlation with prognosis and cure expectancy. *Eur. J. Clin. Bio. Res.,* 16:554.

APPENDIX I

Investigators	Institution	Grant Support[a]
R. Heyn[b] R. Holland D. Tubergen	Mott Children's Hospital University of Michigan Ann Arbor	CA-02971
P. A. Joo[b]	University of Wisconsin Medical School Madison	CA-05436
R. Chard[b] J. Hartmann	Children's Orthopedic Hospital and Medical Center University of Washington Seattle	CA-10382
S. Leikin[b] N. Movassaghi	Children's Hospital National Medical Center Washington, D.C.	CA-03888
A. Schwartz[b] M. Pierce W. Borges J. Swaney	Children's Memorial Hospital Chicago	CA-07431
M. Karon[b] G. Higgins C. Hyman K. Williams J. Ortega N. Shore S. Siegel J. Lazerson	Children's Hospital of Los Angeles	CA-02649

APPENDIX I (cont.)

W. A. Newton, Jr.[b] I. Ertel S. Kontras J. Wadhwa	Children's Hospital of Columbus Ohio State University Columbus	CA-03750
J. A. Wolff[b] A. Sitarz	Babies Hospital The Children's Medical and Surgical Center New York City	CA-03526
V. Albo[b] P. Gaffney W. Prin S. Orlando	Children's Hospital of Pittsburgh	CA-07439
E. C. Beatty, Jr.[b]	Children's Mercy Hospital Kansas City, Missouri	—
M. Nesbit[b] W. Krivit	University of Minnesota Minneapolis	CA-13539
M. Donaldson[b] A. Evans	Children's Hospital of Philadelphia	CA-11796
W. Hirte[b] J. B. McSheffrey	University of Saskatchewan Saskatoon	—
D. Miller[b] V. Canale	New York Hospital Cornell Medical Center New York City	CA-14557
R. Baehner[b] R. Weetman V. Wagner	James W. Riley Hospital for Children Indiana University Indianapolis	CA-13809
D. Kmetz[b]	Louisville Children's Hospital University of Louisville Louisville	—
M. Sonley[b]	Princess Margaret Hospital Toronto	Ontario Cancer Treatment and Research Fund - Grant 4117
M. E. Lahey[b]	University of Utah Salt Lake City	CA-10198
L. Vitale[b] G. Gill	New Jersey College of Medicine and Dentistry Newark	CA-12637
M. Klemperer[b] G. Segel H. Lee	Strong Memorial Hospital University of Rochester Rochester	CA-11174
J. M. Teasdale[b]	University of British Columbia Vancouver	Vancouver Foundation
L. G. Thatcher[b]	Milwaukee Children's Hospital Marquette University Milwaukee	CA-11075
A. Pyesmany[b]	The Izaak Walton Killam Hospital for Children Halifax	Canadian Cancer Society
J. Finklestein[b] L. Greenberg	Harbor General Hospital Los Angeles	CA-14560

APPENDIX I (cont.)

D. Hammond	Chairman Children's Cancer Study Group University of Southern California Los Angeles	CA-13539
J. Weiner, Dr. P.H. A. Reed, Ph.D. H. Sather, Ph.D.	Statistical Center University of Southern California School of Medicine Los Angeles	CA-13539
N. Breslow, Ph.D.	Department of Biostatistics University of Washington Seattle	CA-10382

[a] All CA grants are U.S. Public Health Service sponsored.
[b] Senior investigator.

Question and Answer Session

Dr. Salmon: It appears that BCG immunotherapy was relatively similar in many of these trials and had similar features even if a different dose, strain or route of administration of BCG was utilized. Perhaps the chemotherapy or the use of intrathecal therapy or nonimmunotherapeutic measures were every bit as important variables as those of immunotherapy. These could account for the different results in apparently negative and apparently positive BCG immunotherapy trials in all.

Immunotherapy of Cancer: Present Status of
Trials in Man, edited by W. D. Terry and D. Windhorst.
Raven Press, New York © 1978.

BCG Immunotherapy Following Chemotherapy-Induced Remissions of Stage III and IV Hodgkin's Disease

*Richard F. Bakemeier, **William Costello, †John Horton,
and ‡Vincent T. DeVita

*University of Rochester, Rochester, New York 14642; **State University of New York at Buffalo, Buffalo, New York 14226; †Albany Medical College, Albany, New York 12208; and ‡National Cancer Institute, Bethesda, Maryland 20014*

Hodgkin's disease is associated with demonstrable defects in cellular immune function. Whereas the role of these defects in the pathogenesis of the disease is unclear, the augmentation of cellular immune function in Hodgkin's disease patients might provide an avenue by which additional therapeutic benefits might be attained. Complete clinical remissions can now be anticipated in over 70% of stage III and IV Hodgkin's disease patients through combination chemotherapy with or without added radiation therapy. In an effort to prolong such remissions, the Eastern Cooperative Oncology Group (ECOG) has conducted a study of stage III and IV Hodgkin's disease in which one-third of patients entering complete remission following intensive chemotherapy were randomly assigned to a maintenance regimen of BCG immunotherapy, no further therapy, or additional chemotherapy. This progress report summarizes the results of the study (EST 2472) to September, 1976.

PATIENTS

All patients had biopsy-proved Hodgkin's disease with slides reviewed by a qualified group of hematopathologists designated by the ECOG. Staging was accomplished by standard procedures, with laparotomy and splenectomy left to the discretion of the investigator. The majority of patients were stage IIIB or IV. Stage IIIA patients were entered from institutions treating such patients with combination chemotherapy rather than radiation therapy. A small number of patients whose Hodgkin's disease had recurred in previously irradiated areas were included. Prior to chemotherapy induction, all cases were stratified according to amount of prior therapy, age, stage, and splenectomy status. Randomization was either to MOPP (nitrogen mustard—

For the Eastern Cooperative Oncology Group.

6 mg/m² i.v., days 1 and 8; vincristine—1.4 mg/m² i.v., days 1 and 8; procarbazine—100 mg/m²/day p.o., days 1–14; prednisone—40 mg/m²/day
p.o., days 1–14 (cycles 1 & 4); repeat every 28 days) chemotherapy or to a
five-drug 1-3-bis-(2-chloroethyl)-1-nitrosourea (BCNU)-containing combination BCVPP (BCNU—100 mg/m² i.v., day 1; cyclophosphamide—600
mg/m² i.v., day 1; vinblastine—5 mg/m² i.v., day 1; procarbazine—100
mg/m²/day p.o., days 1–10; prednisone—60 mg/m²/day p.o., days 1–10;
repeat at 28 days). All patients entering complete remission were further
randomized to a schedule of intradermal Bacillus Calmette-Guérin (BCG)
injections (described below), additional five-drug chemotherapy, or no
further therapy. For purposes of this study, a complete remission was
defined as complete regression of measured lesions and disappearance of all
other objective evidence of lymphoma. A repeat lymphangiogram or laparotomy was not required to document response of abdominal nodes.

TREATMENT

After induction of complete remission, generally with six cycles of the
designated chemotherapy regimen, patients were assigned by previous randomization to no further therapy, BCG injections, or six cycles of five-drug
chemotherapy, the latter following a 3-month rest period (Table 1).

TABLE 1. *EST 2472: Chemoimmunotherapy of stage III & IV Hodgkin's disease*

Induction:	MOPP vs. BCVPP
Maintenance: (of CR)	No treatment
or	BCG: 2×10^6 VU — ID at mos. 1,2,4,6, then q 3 mos.
or	BCVPP $\times$ 6

VU, viable units; ID, intradermal; q, every; CR, complete remission.

BCG injections were given intradermally with a syringe and needle at
1, 2, 4, and 6 months after the final chemotherapy administration and every
3 months thereafter until relapse. Each dose consisted of 0.1 ml, containing
2×10^6 viable units of Tice strain BCG from the Chicago Research Foundation. The ensuing reaction was variable but usually led to a superficial ulceration within 2 weeks with satisfactory healing within 4 months. The intradermal route was chosen in an effort to quantify the BCG dose administered.

STATISTICAL ANALYSIS

Patients were followed with monthly physical examinations and blood
counts. Blood chemistries, appropriate X-rays, and skin tests were repeated
at 3-month intervals. Remission duration and duration of survival were
evaluated. Life table analysis was used to generate the remission duration

and survival curves. Median survivals were read off these curves, interpolating between the points.

RESULTS

To the present, 264 patients on this study are evaluable. Complete remissions were achieved in 92 of 128 on MOPP (72%) and 93 of 135 on BCVPP (69%). Median remission duration after MOPP is 119.1 weeks and after 125.3 weeks (Table 2). One hundred twenty-four patients have entered

TABLE 2. *EST 2472: Remission induction*

	MOPP	BCVPP
Evaluable patients	128	135
CR	92	93
% CR	72	69
Median duration CR	119.1 wks.	125.3 wks.

CR, complete remission.

TABLE 3. *EST 2472: Maintenance therapy*

	CT1	CT2	CT3
Evaluable	43	29	52
Med. duration CR (wks.)	121	120	122

CR, complete remission; CT, coded treatment.

the maintenance phase—43 on coded treatment 1, 29 on treatment 2, and 52 on treatment 3 (Table 3). The median duration of remission in the three groups is 121 weeks, 120 weeks, and 122 weeks, respectively.

Fourteen of the 124 evaluable patients who entered the maintenance phase have died—4 of 43 (9%) on treatment 1, 4 of 29 (14%) on treatment 2, and 6 of 52 (12%) on treatment 3. The median duration of survival has been reached only for the unmaintained group at 181 weeks.

Estimates of percentages of patients surviving for more than 2 years from current survival curves are 97, 84, and 84%, respectively, for the three groups. These are not significantly different.

SIDE EFFECTS

In general, the technique of intradermal injection of 2×10^6 viable units of Tice BCG at intervals of 1 to 3 months was well tolerated. Mild malaise and low grade fever were reported in a minority of patients. Fever to 40°C shortly after injection was reported in some patients. The injection sites usually ulcerated within 2 weeks with satisfactory healing within 4 months. Moderate regional lymph note enlargement occurred in at least half the patients at some time. Several were biopsied, and at least two patients demonstrated Hodgkin's disease in such nodes. One patient developed ulceration of axillary nodes with drainage, which responded to antituberculous therapy. Several patients were placed on antituberculous therapy for suspected systemic BCG infection, but no well-documented occurrences of this complication have been reported.

DISCUSSION

Many patients are still in the study or not completely reported. To date, the three maintenance arms are not significantly different in median durations of remission, and only one arm has reached the median duration of survival. These durations should be viewed as tentative. It appears that neither BCG nor chemotherapy maintenance is prolonging remission durations significantly beyond the unmaintained remission duration. However, only about one-third of each group has relapsed to date.

The frequency of BCG injections has been relatively low (months 1, 2, 4, 6, and every 3 months thereafter) in comparison to more intensive scarification regimens employed in melanoma and in colon and breast carcinoma studies. With sufficient patient accession having been achieved to permit more definitive conclusions eventually, the ECOG has activated a new study (EST 1476) for advanced stages of Hodgkin's disease. BCG will be administered to one-half those patients entering complete remission following either combination chemotherapy or combined chemotherapy–radiation therapy. The tine technique will be employed instead of intradermal injection, in keeping with other ECOG studies and in response to patient preference. A more frequent administration schedule will be employed, specifically weekly for 1 month, biweekly for 2 months, monthly for 6 months, and bimonthly to a total duration of 18 months after complete remission induction. The continuation of these immunotherapeutic approaches to Hodgkin's disease is encouraged by recent reports of Hoerni and co-workers (1) and Thomas and co-workers (2) that have suggested possible beneficial effects of BCG following remission induction in malignant lymphomas, including Hodgkin's disease.

SUMMARY

Stage III and IV Hodgkin's disease patients who achieved a complete remission with one of two combination chemotherapy regimens were randomized either to (a) no further treatment, (b) intradermal injection of Tice strain BCG, or (c) additional combination chemotherapy. One hundred twenty-four patients have entered the maintenance phase. The median duration of remission of patients on the three maintenance arms is each approximately 120 weeks. Only one-third of the patients in each group has relapsed, however, and further observation will be necessary. Only one group has reached the median duration of survival at 181 weeks. A new study with more frequent BCG administration has been started.

REFERENCES

1. Hoerni, B., Chauvergne, J., Hoerni-Simon, G., Durand, M., Brunet, R., and Lagarde, C. (1976): BCG in the immunotherapy of Hodgkin's disease and non-Hodgkin's lymphomas. *Cancer Immunol. Immunother.*, 1:109–112.
2. Thomas, J. W., Plenderleith, I. H., Clements, D. V., and Landi, S. (1975): Observations in immunotherapy of lymphoma and melanoma patients. *Clin. Exp. Immunol.*, 21:82–96.

Immunotherapy of Cancer: Present Status of Trials in Man, edited by W. D. Terry and D. Windhorst. Raven Press, New York © 1978.

Chemoimmunotherapy of Non-Hodgkin's Lymphoma with BCG: A Preliminary Report

Stephen E. Jones, Sydney E. Salmon, *Thomas E. Moon, and **James J. Butler

*Section of Hematology and Oncology, University of Arizona College of Medicine, Tucson, Arizona 85724; *Southwest Oncology Group, Biostatistical Office, Houston, Texas 77030; and **Department of Pathology, University of Texas System Cancer Center, M. D. Anderson Hospital and Tumor Institute, Houston, Texas 77030*

In October, 1974, the Southwest Oncology Group (SWOG) initiated a large scale controlled clinical trial of chemoimmunotherapy in advanced non-Hodgkin's lymphomas (NHL). The protocol (SWOG 7426/7427) compares three remission induction treatment regimens—one consisting of combination chemotherapy plus Bacillus Calmette-Guérin (BCG) with two other regimens consisting of combination chemotherapy alone. Patients achieving complete remission were then rerandomized to unmaintained remission or immunotherapeutic maintenance with monthly BCG scarifications. The study was based in part on the following observations.

1. Some patients with NHL (particularly those with diffuse histologic types) manifest severe immunodeficiency (1).

2. There is evidence of therapeutic effect of BCG in other neoplasms, such as acute leukemia and melanoma (2,3).

3. There is a suggestion of prolonged remission duration in patients with a variety of lymphomas, including Hodgkin's disease (4).

In this trial, major efforts were made to insure quality control by incorporating, for the first time, routine submission of pathologic material for expert histopathologic review (5) and the use of systematic restaging to more accurately define complete remission (6). The documentation of complete remission through restaging was considered an essential decision point before discontinuation of chemotherapy and allocation to either unmaintained remission or BCG maintenance immunotherapy.

It must be emphasized that this clinical trial is still underway, and this preliminary analysis is based on information available in October, 1976 on approximately one-half of the patients entered on the study who are currently evaluable for response.

For the Southwest Oncology Group.

PATIENTS AND METHODS

Only patients with biopsy-proved stage III or IV NHL without prior chemotherapy were eligible for this study. Cases were entered by investigators from 34 SWOG institutions. All lymphomas were classified according to the criteria of Rappaport (7), and original biopsy material from each patient was submitted for additional review by the Lymphoma Pathology Panel and Central Respository (5). Patients were evaluated for extent of disease prior to treatment (8) and staged according to the criteria of the Ann Arbor Conference (9). After obtaining informed written consent, patients were then assigned at random to one of three chemoimmunotherapy or chemotherapy programs intended to induce a complete remission (randomizations were stratified by nodular or diffuse histologic pattern). The details of these three treatments are as follows.

1. COP-Bleomycin (four drugs): *cyclophosphamide* (C), 125 mg/m^2 given orally daily for 14 days starting on day 1; vincristine (Oncovin® [O]), 1.4 mg/m^2 given i.v. on days 1 and 8 (maximum of 2 mg/injection); *prednisone* (P), 100 mg/day given orally on days 1 to 5; and *bleomycin* (Bleo), 4 mg/m^2 given i.v. on days 1 and 8. Courses were repeated every 28 days if the peripheral blood counts were adequate. (Patients with preexisting cardiac disease or mycosis fungoides were assigned to treatment with COP-bleomycin and are listed as "other" in results.)

2. CHOP-Bleomycin (five drugs): *cyclophosphamide,* 750 mg/m^2 given i.v. on day 1; *doxorubicin (hydroxyldaunorubicin* [H]), 50 mg/m^2 given i.v. on day 1; *vincristine,* 1.4 mg/m^2 given i.v. on day 1 (maximum of 2 mg/injection); *prednisone,* 100 mg/day given orally on days 1 to 5; and *bleomycin,* 4 mg/m^2 given i.v. on day 1. Courses were repeated every 21 days if the blood counts were adequate.

3. CHOP-BCG (five drugs): same regimen as in CHOP-Bleomycin therapy except for substitution of high viability Pasteur *BCG* for bleomycin. BCG was given by scarification at a dose of 1 ampoule (6 ± 4 × 10^8 viable units of Pasteur lyophylized BCG) on days 8 and 15 of each 21-day treatment cycle. BCG scarifications were performed on extremities with a standard 5-×-5-cm grid of 10 scratches in each of two perpendicular directions. BCG sites were rotated with each dose so that all major lymphoid drainage pathways from upper and lower extremities were repetitively challenged. Doses of drugs and BCG were modified in accord with standard SWOG guidelines based on toxicity. For example, BCG was reduced to a single-day 15-administrations-per-treatment course if a moderate reaction (i.e., erythema or induration extending more than 1 cm beyond the site with or without mild systemic symptoms) occurred with the previous BCG administration. If the reduced frequency failed to reduce the intensity of reactions, specifically planned reductions in dose of BCG were also recommended. BCG was to be discontinued for signs or symptoms of systemic BCG in-

fection (10). Although not addressed in this chapter, patients underwent immunologic testing including a skin test battery (multiple recall antigens) and studies of circulating lymphocytes and immunoglobulins. These studies were carried out prior to treatment, at the time of restaging, and 6 months thereafter.

The basic design of this study is shown in Table 1. Remission induction therapy for responding patients consisted of eight courses of treatment given at 3 to 4 week intervals, followed by "systematic restaging" if all clinical signs and symptoms of lymphoma had disappeared (6). Patients considered to be free of disease after completing restaging (this was the definition of "complete remission" used in this study) were then assigned at random to receive either no further therapy or BCG by scarification at monthly intervals for 18 months with close follow-up for signs of relapse. Patients who experienced only a "partial response" (at least a 50% regression of all measurable sites of involvement) after the first eight courses of treatment or those who were found to have persistent disease at restaging received another three courses of the same treatment. If a documented complete remission was achieved after 11 courses of induction treatment, patients were then eligible for randomization into the maintenance phase. Patients who failed to achieve at least a partial response after four courses of induction treatment were considered "nonresponders" and taken off study.

A comprehensive, computerized, "updated study analysis" has been performed by the SWOG statistical office every 4 months since the study was begun. Several tests of significance have been employed in these analyses. The Chi square method was employed to compare differences in response rates. Survival and remission duration were calculated by the method of Kaplan and Meier (11), and comparison of survival or remission duration between various groups of patients was made with the modified Wilcoxon

TABLE 1. *SWOG 7426/7427: Treatment plan for patients with advanced non-Hodgkin's lymphoma (October, 1974 to October, 1976)*

CR, complete remission.

test of Gehan (12). The data in this report are based on an analysis performed in October, 1976 on clinical records available through June, 1976. Only patients with a "final evaluation" (those who have completed induction treatment) are considered for the purposes of this report.

RESULTS

As of October, 1976, 514 patients have been entered on this study (as detailed in Table 2), and 262 patients have had final evaluations. The clinical and pathologic characteristics of patients in the three treatment groups are comparable.

The preliminary results according to induction treatment are shown in Table 3. There is no difference in complete remission rates, but the overall remission rate (partial plus complete responses) is significantly higher ($p = 0.03$) for patients receiving CHOP + BCG (92%) compared to those receiving CHOP + bleomycin (78%) or COP + bleomycin (84%). Among patients with final evaluations and completed hematopathology review, there

TABLE 2. SWOG 7426/7427: Chemoimmunotherapy of NHL—patient population, induction phase (10/76)

	Total	CHOP + BCG	CHOP + Bleo	COP + Bleo	Other[a]
Number entered	514	140	149	182	43
Ineligible	21	4	6	6	5
Too early to evaluate	99	33	32	26	8
Not evaluable	6	2	2	2	0
Partially evaluable	43	8	12	16	7
Early death	22	4	5	8	5
Inadequate trial due to toxicity	1	0	0	1	0
Refused further treatment	12	2	5	3	2
Lost to follow-up	6	1	1	4	0
Fully evaluable	345	93	97	132	23

[a] Includes patients with heart disease or mycosis fungoides who received treatment with COP + bleomycin.

TABLE 3. SWOG 7426/7427: Chemoimmunotherapy of NHL—preliminary results, induction phase (10/76)

Treatment	No. with final evaluations	No. with CR (%)	No. with PR (%)	PR + CR (%)
CHOP + BCG	76	44 (58%)	26 (34%)	(92%) ⎤
CHOP + Bleo	86	50 (58%)	17 (20%)	(78%) ⎬[a]
COP + Bleo	100	59 (59%)	25 (25%)	(84%) ⎦
Total	262			

CR, complete remission; PR, partial remission.
[a] $p = 0.03$.

TABLE 4. SWOG 7426/7427: Preliminary response
rates according to histopathology review (10/76)

	Number	No. with CR (%)
Diffuse	104	a⌐ 61 (59%)
Nodular	118	⌐ 83 (70%)

CR, complete remission.
a $p = 0.07$.

is nearly a significant difference ($p = 0.07$) in complete remission rates for those with nodular lymphoma compared to diffuse lymphoma (Table 4). Within each major histologic type of lymphoma, however, there is no significant difference in complete remission rates with respect to the type of induction regimen.

All three induction treatment regimens were generally well tolerated with the major toxicity being leukopenia. The COP + bleomycin regimen was associated with significantly less toxicity ($p < 0.001$) than CHOP + bleomycin or CHOP + BCG. There was no difference in hematologic toxicity between CHOP + bleomycin or CHOP + BCG treatment. The administration of BCG was well tolerated as shown in Table 5. Sixty-three percent of patients experienced no toxicity requiring modification of BCG frequency or dosage. No cases of systemic BCG infection or fatal BCG reactions were encountered.

To date 38 relapses have been observed in patients achieving a complete remission (CHOP + BCG, 7; CHOP + bleomycin, 10; COP + bleomycin, 21), but no significant differences are apparent in the duration of complete remission according to the type of induction treatment. However, patients with nodular lymphomas have had a complete remission duration that is significantly longer than that observed in patients with diffuse histologies ($p = 0.03$).

TABLE 5. SWOG 7426/7427: Chemoimmunotherapy
of NHL—toxicity of BCG by scarification
(101 patients, CHOP + BCG; 10/76)

Toxicity grade	Percentage of patients
None (local inflammatory response ± mild systemic symptoms)	63
Mild (requires BCG dosage modification)	29
Moderate (local BCG abscess formation)	6
Severe (regional node involvement with abscess formation)	2
Life-threatening (systemic BCG infection)	0
Fatal	0

TABLE 6. SWOG 7426/7427: Chemoimmunotherapy of
NHL—preliminary results, maintenance phase (10/76)

	Number	Relapses (%)
No further treatment	64	14 (22%)
BCG once/month	54	12 (22%)

As of October, 1976, 148 patients who achieved complete remission documented by restaging have been registered on the unmaintained versus BCG immunotherapy maintenance program. Of these, 118 are currently evaluable. Twenty-six of the 38 relapses to date have occurred during this phase of the study. These relapses have occurred with similar frequency from groups receiving BCG immunotherapy or in unmaintained remission status (Table 6). There is no difference in duration of complete remission according to the use of monthly BCG immunotherapy or no additional treatment.

Overall survival by initial induction treatment is not different at this time; 63 patients have died (CHOP + BCG, 15; CHOP + bleomycin, 22; COP + bleomycin, 26). When survival was examined by the type of lymphoma according to histopathologic review, none of the patients with nodular lymphoma who received CHOP + BCG has died, and their survival is superior to that observed with CHOP + bleomycin ($p = 0.09$) and COP + bleomycin ($p = 0.15$). For patients with diffuse lymphoma, there is no difference in survival in relation to initial induction treatment, but survival of these patients is significantly less than that associated with nodular lymphoma ($p = 0.02$).

Finally, we compared overall survival of all 345 fully evaluable patients on this study (Table 2) with survival of the fully evaluable patients from the most recently completed SWOG study in which patients received induction chemotherapy with CHOP (without bleomycin or BCG) followed by maintenance chemotherapy for 18 months (13). These two groups of patients are identical in clinical and pathologic characteristics, and the rates of complete remission are also nearly identical. Nonetheless, overall survival in this current program is already superior to that observed in the former study ($p = 0.03$).

DISCUSSION

Nonspecific immune stimulation with BCG has received considerable attention in recent years as a form of cancer therapy. Chemoimmunotherapy with BCG has been evaluated in various types of cancers including melanoma, acute leukemia, breast cancer, and Burkitt's lymphoma (2,3,14,15). In most of these trials survival or duration of remission has been improved by the addition of BCG to chemotherapy, but rates of complete remission have not been increased. These observations may eventually be confirmed in this study of chemoimmunotherapy for patients with NHL, but the results are still too preliminary to be certain. With final evaluations of about one-half of the cases entered on this study, we have demonstrated a significant improvement in overall survival compared to our most recently completed and otherwise comparable trial (13). In addition, we have observed that the overall response rate (partial plus complete) is significantly higher in patients receiving CHOP + BCG compared to treatment with either CHOP + bleomycin or COP + bleomycin, although there is no difference in complete remission rates. There is also a suggestion (not yet significant) that survival of patients with nodular lymphoma might be improved by the addition of BCG to CHOP chemotherapy compared to the regimens without BCG. This is interesting because nodular lymphoma patients appear to be more immunocompetent at the time of presentation (1) and may have better preservation of the T-dependent areas of lymphoid organs. This could be relevant if the BCG immunotherapeutic effect is mediated through T lymphocytes.

After induction of complete remission we have not yet been able to demonstrate any advantage, in terms of prolonging duration of complete remission, to administering BCG at monthly intervals by scarification compared to no further treatment. The majority of relapses observed to date have occurred early (average time from restaging to relapse is 4 months [range 1 to 12 months]), and many of the relapses appear to have occurred in patients whose restaging evaluations were not sufficiently thorough to detect persistent lymphoma (6). Our choice of administering BCG at monthly intervals after restaging, in retrospect, may have been inadequate to enhance immunoreactivity in patients who did not receive the more intensive BCG stimulation during the remission induction phase. It might have been more appropriate to begin maintenance BCG at weekly intervals until strong reactions occurred, followed by reductions in frequency of administration or dosage thereafter.

It must be reiterated that the results of this study are still quite tentative as only half of the patients have been fully analyzed and the length of follow-up, even of these patients, is still short. Much longer periods of observation and analysis of all cases in this ongoing trial are of critical importance.

SUMMARY

A randomized clinical trial of remission induction chemotherapy with either of two combinations including cyclophosphamide, doxorubicin hydrochloride, vincristine, prednisone, and bleomycin versus a similar combination plus BCG by scarification is underway for patients with advanced non-Hodgkin's lymphoma without prior chemotherapy. Patients achieving complete remission as documented at restaging are then randomly assigned to unmaintained remission or monthly maintenance with BCG immunotherapy. Preliminary results of this ongoing trial are based on analysis of 262 evaluable patients from the induction phase and 118 patients followed beyond restaging. Chemoimmunotherapy has been well tolerated. The complete remission rate has not been improved with the addition of BCG, however the total remission rate (complete + partial) is higher ($p = 0.03$). After restaging, early relapses have occurred with similar frequency in unmaintained and BCG-treated groups. Survival of patients with nodular lymphoma who received BCG during remission induction appears better than our concurrent experience with combination chemotherapy alone. Survival of patients with diffuse lymphoma is inferior to that observed in nodular cases and was similar with all three induction regimens. Longer follow-up and further analysis will be required to fully evaluate the effects of BCG on remission duration and survival.

ACKNOWLEDGMENT

The authors' work was supported in part by research grants from the National Institutes of Health—CA-13612 and CA-12014.

REFERENCES

1. Jones, S. E., Griffith, K., Dombrowski, P., and Gaines, J. A. (1977): Immunodeficiency in patients with non-Hodgkin's lymphomas: relation of immune status to histology. *Blood,* 49:335–344.
2. Gutterman, J. U., Mavligit, G., Gottlieb, J. A., Burgess, M. A., McBride, C. E., Einhorn, L., Freireich, E. J., and Hersh, E. M. (1974): Chemoimmunotherapy of disseminated malignant melanoma with dimethyl triazeno imidazole carboxamide and Bacillus Calmette-Guerin. *N. Engl. J. Med.,* 291:592–597.
3. Powles, R. L., Crowther, D., Bateman, C. J. T., Beard, M. E. J., McElwain, T. J., Russell, J., Lister, T. A., Whitehouse, J. M. A., Wrigley, P. E. M., Pike, M., Alexander, P., and Hamilton-Fairley, G. (1974): Immunotherapy for acute myelogenous leukaemia. *Br. J. Cancer,* 28:365–376.
4. Sokal, J. E., Aungst, C. W., and Snyderman, M. (1974): Delay in progression of malignant lymphoma after BCG vaccination. *N. Engl. J. Med.,* 291:1226–1230.
5. Jones, S. E., Butler, J. J., Byrne, G. E., Coltman, C. A., Jr., and Moon, T. E. (1977): Histopathologic review of lymphoma cases from the Southwest Oncology Group. *Cancer (in press.)*
6. Herman, T. S., and Jones, S. E. (1977): Systematic restaging in the management of non-Hodgkin's lymphoma. *Cancer Treat. Rev. (in press.)*
7. Rappaport, H., Winter, W. J., and Hicks, E. B. (1956): Follicular lymphoma: A re-evaluation of its position in the scheme of malignant lymphoma, based on a survey of 253 cases. *Cancer,* 9:792–821.
8. Jones, S. E. (1975): Non-Hodgkin lymphoma. *JAMA,* 238:633–638.
9. Carbone, P. P., Kaplan, H. S., Musshoff, K., Smithers, D. W., and Tubiana, M. (1971): Report of the Committee on Hodgkin's Disease Staging Classification. *Cancer Res.,* 31:1860–1861.
10. Sparks, F. C., Silverstein, M. J., Hunt, J. S., Haskell, C. M., Pilch, Y. H., and Morton, D. L. (1973): Complications of BCG immunotherapy in patients with cancer. *N. Engl. J. Med.,* 289:827–830.
11. Kaplan, E. L., and Meier, P. (1958): Non-parametric estimations from incomplete observations. *J. Am. Stat. Assoc.,* 53:457–481.

12. Gehan, E. A. (1965): A generalized Wilcoxon test for comparing arbitrarily singly-censored samples. *Biometrika,* 52:203–223.
13. McKelvey, E. M., Gottlieb, J. A., Wilson, H. E., Haut, A., Talley, R. W., Stephens, R., Lane, M., Gamble, J. F., Jones, S. E., Grozea, P. N., Gutterman, J., Coltman, C., Jr., and Moon, T. E. (1976): Hydroxyldaunomycin (adriamycin) combination chemotherapy in malignant lymphoma. *Cancer,* 38:1484–1493.
14. Gutterman, J. U., Mavligit, G. M., Burgess, M. A., Cardenas, J. O., Blumenschein, G. R., Gottlieb, J. A., McBride, C. M., McCredie, K. B., Bodey, G. P., Rodriguez, V., Freireich, E. J., and Hersh, E. M. (1976): Immunotherapy of breast cancer, malignant melanoma, and acute leukemia with BCG: Prolongation of disease free interval and survival. *Cancer Immunol. Immunother.,* 1:99–107.
15. Magrath, I. T., and Ziegler, J. L. (1976): Failure of BCG immunostimulation to affect the clinical course of Burkitt's lymphoma. *Br. Med. J.,* 1:615–618.

APPENDIX

Thirty SWOG institutions registered patients on this study. The following tabulates the principal investigators, National Cancer Institute grant support, and the number of patients entered on this study.

	Total number of patients entered SWOG study #7426
Arthur Haut	
University of Arkansas Medical Center, Little Rock, Arkansas	29
Montague Lane—CA-03392	
Baylor College of Medicine, Houston, Texas	25
James Hewlett—CA-04919	
Cleveland Clinic, Cleveland, Ohio	17
Robert Talley—CA-04915	
Henry Ford Hospital, Detroit, Michigan	29
John Costanzi—CA-03096	
University of Texas Medical Branch at Galveston, Galveston, Texas	15
Charles Coltman	
Wilford Hall Medical Center, Lackland Air Force Base, Texas	20
John Bickers—CA-16422	
Louisiana State University School of Medicine, New Orleans, Louisiana	17
Emil Freireich—CA-10376	
M. D. Anderson Hospital, Houston, Texas	12
H. C. Kwaan	
Northwestern University, Chicago, Illinois	4
Richard Bottomley—CA-16957	
Oklahoma Medical Research Foundation, Oklahoma	45
Henry Wilson—CA-04920	
Ohio State University Hospitals, Columbus, Ohio	50
John Bonnet—CA-10187	
Scott & White Clinic, Temple, Texas	22
W. J. Stuckey—CA-03389	
Tulane University School of Medicine, New Orleans, Louisiana	17
Dr. B. W. Ruffner—CA-13643	
University of Virginia School of Medicine, Charlottesville, Virginia	1
John Athens—CA-13238	
University of Utah Medical Center, Salt Lake City, Utah	16
V. K. Vaitkevicius—CA-14028	
Wayne State University School of Medicine, Detroit, Michigan	26
William Tucker	

APPENDIX (cont.)

Borgess Medical Center, Kalamazoo, Michigan   4
Stuart Spigel
Keesler USAF Medical Center, Keesler Air Force Base, Mississippi   3
John Saiki—CA-12213
University of New Mexico School of Medicine, Albuquerque,
   New Mexico   9
Joseph McCracken
Brooke General Hospital, Ft. Sam Houston, Texas   3
Barth Hoogstraten—CA-12644
University of Kansas Medical Center, Kansas City, Kansas   37
Saul Rivkin
Tumor Institute of Swedish Hospital Medical Center, Seattle,
   Washington   8
Stephen Jones—CA-13612
University of Arizona Medical Center, Tucson, Arizona   40
John Falletta
Duke University Medical Center, Durham, North Carolina   1
Francis Morrison—CA-16385
University of Mississippi Medical Center, Jackson, Mississippi   31
Clarence Vaughn
Providence Hospital, Southfield, Michigan   3
Carlos Vallejos
National Cancer Institute–Peru, Lima, Peru   17
Noboru Oishi
University of Hawaii at Manoa, Honolulu, Hawaii   2
Ismail Elsebai
National Cancer Institute, Cairo, Egypt   9
William Fletcher—CA-12279
University of Oregon Health Sciences Center, Portland, Oregon   1

Question and Answer Session

Dr. Macaully: I think that the optimum time to give immunotherapy in ALL may be postinduction or postconsolidation, the idea being to reduce the initial tumor load to the optimum level where immunomanipulation might best have an effect. Do you think an analogous situation might exist with relation to lymphomas?

Dr. Salmon: The Southwest Oncology Group does not yet have an analysis of this information. We think that the optimal timing for immunotherapy is currently unknown. Optimal timing may well vary, depending upon the type of neoplasm. Additionally, as Dr. Jones indicated, a deliberate attempt was made in our protocol to have the BCG drainage sites be in all the major lymphoid areas which might well be involved with the lymphoma itself. If BCG acts through macrophage activation (which is one of the theses), conceivably it might act locally in lymphoma and add to the effects of chemotherapy during induction. Basically we did not know the optimal timing or the efficacy of BCG in non-Hodgkin's lymphomas; therefore, we felt it would be wise to test this independently, both in induction and in maintenance.

Dr. Jones: It also appears that, contrary to our biases, use of BCG in remission induction may have a major advantage that would not be detected if we tested it only during the maintenance phase. The same may be true for MER in acute myelocytic leukemia as Dr. Cuttner reported.

Dr. Gee: On your curves for survival, did you analyze the response to the three induction arms for those patients whose lymphomas had diffuse histology? If so, is there a difference?

Dr. Jones: There is no difference in survival by induction treatment for the diffuse histology; however, I will say that, as in all other studies, the complete remission rate, the duration of remission and survival was significantly greater for patients with nodular lymphoma as compared to diffuse lymphoma. However, the effects that we noted with chemoimmunotherapy for induction in patients with nodular lymphoma were not seen in those patients with diffuse lymphoma.

Dr. Pinsky: Was the survival advantage in the nodular patients who got the BCG for induction only in the responders compared to the non-responders or is it for the whole group?

Dr. Jones: That was for the whole group of patients. However, the differences are very small, and the differences that we have presented here today must be viewed as tentative. On the other hand, these are differences that now have been apparent through two sophisticated statistical analyses done by the Southwest Group's office, and I anticipate that these trends would probably hold up.

Dr. Pinsky: During the discussion period perhaps those investigators who waited until remission to add the immunotherapy might comment on why they did that. Why has it become so ingrained that for the lymphocytic malignancies one should wait until remission has already been obtained to introduce the immunotherapy?

Dr. Sokal: We have two studies in which we have added BCG to the induction chemotherapy. These are quite different schedules of chemotherapy. One of them is a small study, but it is completed and is now in press, and there was a statistically significant advantage for the BCG patients. The second study is not yet ready for evaluation, but the trend seems to be in the same direction.

DISCUSSION: ACUTE LYMPHATIC LEUKEMIA AND LYMPHOMAS

Dr. Simone: Dr. Mathé, you state that there is a 50 percent cure expectancy with active immunotherapy in your studies, and you showed us a curve that purportedly demonstrates that. However, it should be pointed out that the curve starts from the point that active immunotherapy starts, which, of course, segregates out a considerable number of patients before that. Perhaps you could tell us why you present the data that way.

In your chapter you said that it was difficult to interpret the data from St. Jude's Hospital, that you were unable to find detailed analysis of initial features. The prognostic features in our patients were analyzed in great detail in the Ulm Symposium.

Finally, I wish you would address yourself to the question of why you think the later trials reported here have been unable to reproduce your results.

Dr. Mathé: For Protocols 9, 10, and 12, the data concern all the patients who entered remission, which were 90 percent in Protocol 9, 100 percent in Protocol 10, and 100 percent in Protocol 12. I think that these data can be compared with your data.

Dr. Holland: Dr. Mathé, could I follow the line of inquiry I started before. I am not against immunotherapy.

But I would like you to persuade me that the results that you describe are not due to good chemotherapy. And without a control for comparison, where you don't give immunotherapy, I do not see how you can ascribe the effect to immunotherapy, rather than to the combination. And, since you changed chemotherapy and immunotherapy simultaneously, it becomes impossible to talk about the impact of one or the other.

Dr. Mathé: No, if we compare Protocols 9 and 10 it is because there is no difference in the two branches of immunotherapy in those protocols that we can compare.

Dr. Holland: But one was with preserved cells and one with fresh cells.

Dr. Mathé: Yes, but there are no differences with *C. parvum* or without *C. parvum* and no differences in cryopreserved cells.

Dr. Holland: Right, which makes me wonder whether or not it is due to the chemotherapy. If we describe 20 and 30 percent long-term survivors— and that is what you are describing, we could get about the same results from chemotherapy used at the same time. Now with newer chemotherapy we get better results, about 60 percent long-term survival. Therefore, I do not see how you cannot wonder whether or not your chemotherapy hasn't made the same progress as our chemotherapy?

How do you know your immunotherapy is ever a factor? Don't you think it would be good to have a controlled trial?

Dr. Mathé: I think the MRC did it.

Dr. Holland: And saw nothing.

Dr. Mathé: No, they saw the same result of immunotherapy and chemotherapy.

Dr. Otten: The EORTC did not see any difference between chemotherapy and immunotherapy during the maintenance phase, but I agree also that, because of the progress in the consolidation treatments we and other groups give, it is at the present very difficult, without a control group receiving no maintenance treatment to decide whether immunotherapy really does something. I think that that controlled trial really remains to be done.

Dr. Salmon: One of the statisticians has a question to which he would like Dr. Mathé to respond:

Except for Mathé's 1969 study with twenty treated and ten rapidly dead controls, all the controlled studies of ALL immunotherapy are negative. In conversation, some seem to doubt the results of the study and therefore raise questions about the nature of patient allocation in the initial trial. Was this truly a randomized trial based on random allocation of patients or was it decided who would be a control or who would be an immunotherapy patient? How many unpublished dropouts were there?

Dr. Mathé: These were patients during 1963 who were in remission and who were randomized between ten for controls and twenty for immunotherapy: a third for BCG, a third for cells, and a third for BCG and cells. These cases were randomized; there was no stratification at that time, as we do now.

Dr. Gehan: How was it there were only ten patients in one group and twenty in the other?

Dr. Mathé: Because we thought we could do something. At that time, very few people survived.

Dr. Peto: One thing that is puzzling to me about that original trial is the point that was raised earlier: why did the controls do so badly? They did much worse than controls should have done at that time. The difference is partly because the treated patients did somewhat better than average but the major difference in that trial is because the controls did much worse than they should have.

Dr. Mathé: The relapse was exactly the same.

Dr. Peto: No, it was much worse than anybody else was getting at the time. It is very odd that ten patients stopping chemotherapy should all relapse so rapidly. This is not the experience that other people had at that time.

There are two reasons you can get a difference between two treatments: Either the treatment works or you put a lot of patients who are going to do badly anyway, into the control group.

Dr. Mathé: We have no difference in the medians of the control and of the immunotherapy groups. Both groups relapsed identically. We only had the break of the curve and a plateau.

Dr. Peto: But all the world has to indicate that immunotherapy works in ALL is ten control patients who did much worse than they should have in 1969. Don't you sort of feel that it is very shaky evidence on which to base such a great structure?

Dr. Mathé: Well, the structure—I did not make it myself.

Dr. Holland: The chemotherapy administered to those thirty patients was not identical. I recall from prior conversations with Dr. Mathé that there was a period of chemotherapy—about ten patients—on a modification of ALGB 6313 protocol. That chemotherapy, done in 1963, is different; we don't have any long-term survivors. Certainly not seven out of twenty from the chemotherapy that was done in 1963. So it isn't just a question of the poor controls. They are indeed poor. But Mathé has made an extraordinary observation. Seven patients treated in 1963 are still alive and they are still well, and they haven't had chemotherapy since.

I would love to see a justification that it is not the chemotherapy that is working now, because I'm not very impressed with Studies 9 and 10. Those are lower, it seems to me, than our long-term plateaus. They are in the 35 percent range.

Dr. Mathé: We have a 60 percent plateau for survival.

Dr. Holland: But not in the first remission. The first remission is what counts, not survival, because you are treating them with other things after relapse.

Dr. Heyn: Dr. Mathé, you have included in your studies patients of all ages, but in your analysis you have never made any stratification in terms of either age or initial white count.

The Children's Cancer Group A data suggest that the white count at presentation is probably the single most significant prognostic factor. It would be very nice to see your study analyzed by this criterion.

Children with ALL can be divided into different risk groups. For example, children who are between 3 and 7 years of age and have white counts of less than 10,000 at the time of diagnosis have a survival of 90 to 92 percent at 3.5 years.

Children beyond the age of seven with low white counts have about a 70 percent survival at about 3.5 years. And then you have, as you pointed out, a poor survival group that will go down to the 50 percent survival at this same time follow-up. I think that we must stratify our patients for known prognostic factors in order to compare them.

Dr. Mathé: As we have indicated, number of lymphoblasts is a prognostic factor in our patients.

Dr. Salmon: Certainly when dealing with small numbers of patients a detailed prognostic analysis of the matchings of your groups would be of value. This comment applies to some of the immunotherapy trials for other tumor types too.

I would like the panel to review the various BCG treatment programs for ALL that have been presented here.

Dr. Leventhal and Dr. Otten, as far as I can see, you used the same type of Pasteur BCG as used by Dr. Mathé although the schedules may have varied a bit.

Dr. Leventhal: Our BCG schedule differed a great deal. We felt that there would be a plateau out at the point at which we had completed chemotherapy. We were hoping that immunotherapy would provide a new method of attack on the disease, and we reasoned that the people who badly needed the new attack were those who relapsed early, not those who were still in remission at the end of three years of chemotherapy. And we therefore elected to intersperse the immunotherapy with the chemotherapy.

The other part of our study about which I was unhappy related to using cells from a single donor. I believe that Dr. Mathé's approach of pooling allogeneic cells makes a great deal of sense. We had to use a single donor because of considerations of our Human Experimentation Committee, which asked if it didn't work and the patients relapsed, how were we going to transfuse them?

Dr. Mathé, have you had any difficulty supporting patients with platelet transfusions or blood transfusions after they relapse? Has immunization with a pool of cells interfered with later supportive care of the patients?

Dr. Mathé: Not so far as I know.

Dr. Otten: We had no problems as far as I know.

Dr. Sokal: Our patients are immunized with BCG and cultured leukocytes and do show early and moderately severe reactions to transfusions. We haven't had any great difficulty. They do show a sensitivity to buffy coat.

Dr. Powles: Similar to the importance of remission achieved in AML, in ALL it is absolutely vital we keep our patients in remission at any cost. When a patient relapses with ALL, that is a failed patient. If he has got HLA antibodies going around in relapse this is much less important than the failure of primary therapy.

I feel there is a very strong case for controlled immunotherapy trials in ALL. And this hasn't to do with the plateau that Professor Mathé discussed, but rather with the long-term outcome of these patients who have been on intensive chemotherapy. What is going to happen to these patients in 10 to 20 years? If we conduct controlled immunotherapy trials, we may also have an additional and highly important bonus of information concerning the long-term morbidity of chemotherapy.

Dr. Mathé: I would like to correct you. We have 92 percent secondary remissions in patients who are in immunotherapy, while in patients we have seen in relapse under maintenance chemotherapy given in other services, the rate is much lower, in the range of 60 percent. And the chances of a patient who enters secondary remission getting to the plateau of survival is still 50 percent.

Dr. Powles: How many of your reinduced ALLs have become cures?

Dr. Mathé: I don't say cures, but plateaus—50 percent.

Dr. Frei: Dr. Leventhal, your experimental design was really interesting and quite different from the others, because you had a block of chemotherapy, a block of immunotherapy, in one group, and sequential blocks of chemotherapy in the other.

First, I would like to hear your response to a criticism of that chemotherapy approach, because I think from principles of first order kinetics that it would be the wrong thing to interrupt chemotherapy for blocks of two

months during the first year, and that that would adversely affect chemotherapeutic response in a very serious way.

On the other hand, in contrasting your sequential chemotherapy arm to
that with chemotherapy plus immunotherapy, the fact that they were comparable would suggest to me that immunotherapy might have been effective
in that setting, because it was at least as good as methotrexate.

Dr. Leventhal: Well, my study has been criticized from that point of view
before, and I accept that criticism. The problem that I was concerned about
at the time was the opposite one: that immunotherapy might be ineffective
with the chemotherapy coming so soon after it. We certainly had evidence in
terms of the reaction to the BCG and the development of tuberculin positivity that the patients were immunocompetent. They did become tuberculin
positive at the end of the first two-month block and remained so throughout
the period of immunotherapy. I can't speak to the kinetic theories nearly as
well as you.

Dr. Frei: But am I correct in saying you were able to replace chemotherapy in a critical period early in a period during remission with immunotherapy and not lose?

Dr. Leventhal: Yes.

Dr. Frei: It seems to me that that is a plus for immunotherapy. Did your
early relapses occur during immunotherapy?

Dr. Leventhal: All our patients did not fall off during the time they were
receiving immunotherapy.

Sir Michael Woodruff: Are there any hard grounds or even soft reasons
for speculating that the extreme frequency of administration of immunotherapy which we heard about in so many studies today is likely to be optimal? Is there any evidence to think that giving it less often would be less
dismal, if I might put it that way, than some of the things that have actually
happened?

Dr. Salmon: How often do you give your BCG, Dr. Mathé?

Dr. Mathé: Once a week.

Dr. Otten: We give BCG twice a week for six months and once a week
thereafter for four years.

Dr. Ekert: We give 4×10^8 organisms once every five weeks.

Dr. Kay: We gave BCG weekly.

Dr. Leventhal: We gave BCG once a week for four weeks, one month out
of six.

Dr. Heyn: The question was raised as to why the Children's Cancer Study
Group did what we did, and I think that both the Concorde trial and ours
were trying to show whether Dr. Mathé's original study was valid on a larger
scale. Certainly I think we all based our initial concepts on Dr. Mathé's
mouse work. We waited until we had children in remission and gave them
some consolidation chemotherapy in addition based on the mouse work that
Dr. Mathé reported. In that work, the animals did not respond to immuno-

therapy unless the leukemic burden was reduced to 10^4 or 10^5 cell population. The object was to have the lowest leukemic cell population at the time immunotherapy started. This is why we designed our study as we did. We felt if children who were in complete remission and who had, presumably, the least cell numbers left after another eight months of continuous treatment, these children might respond more favorably. We gave our BCG twice a week for two months and then every week.

Dr. Pinsky: I don't think Dr. Mathé's mouse data represent a true chemoimmunotherapy trial. If you plan to give chemotherapy on a continuous basis, and immunotherapy on a continuous basis, the test of whether it is necessary to wait for the tumor cell number to go down has not been carried out. For most tumor types we have not determined whether the effects of immunotherapy might be reversed by continued intermittent chemotherapy interspersed with the immunotherapy.

Dr. Salmon: The study that Dr. Jones presented addresses that question and I think some data will eventually come out for that tumor and also for certain other tumors.

Dr. Hobbs: I think BCG is very good in generating reactions against BCG, and we find a total dissociation between PPD reactivity and other immune function tests, such as the mixed lymphocyte reaction. We have immunized well-informed subjects, mainly doctors and spouses, with irradiated tumor cells and we have got eleven responses out of eleven volunteers. We have immunized 180 tumor-bearing patients with irradiated tumor cells. We have got a total of nine responses in that 180, and those happened to be nine of the twelve who had a positive mixed lymphocyte reaction (MLR). All the rest didn't have an MLR.

Now, I think the MLR is a very good test of capacity to respond to foreign cells, and I think if you give BCG until you are blue in the face, if you haven't got an MLR, BCG won't give it back to you. Have others done the MLR and determined if their so-called nonspecific immunotherapy can resurrect it?

Dr. Salmon: MLR reactivity is one of the potential correlates of *in vivo* hypersensitivity. However, from data available to date there are no direct, clearly translatable *in vitro* tests which predict *in vivo* results of immunotherapy of cancer.

Dr. Weiss: I know this is not supposed to be a forum for mouse doctors, but I must nonetheless express my amazement at finding immunology rediscovered at this meeting, not only in this session but throughout. And by that I mean there seems to be a near total divorce in the design of clinical trials, from an abundant amount of experimental information in many different species of animals.

With regard to the specific question that came up here, the overwhelming majority of studies with BCG, MER, and a variety of other factors indicate that the hazards of overscheduling are much greater than the hazards of underscheduling. And in comparing identical experimental circumstances of hundreds of animals treated once or twice with those treated repeatedly or comparing animals in which the repetition of treatment is close, the overwhelming tendency is the less the treatment in terms of frequency and the further apart it is, generally the more efficacious it is, the better the result.

Now, I know one cannot jump from mouse, guinea pig, rabbit, rat, ape, or ass to the human being; nonetheless, I just wonder why we have to rediscover all of immunology when we turn to the clinic and not consider anything that has come among the primitive creatures or below man?

Dr. Terry: At the risk of jumping in the other direction, I think that a lot of this discussion is premature in the sense it is all predicated on the assumption that there is an effect of BCG in ALL. I must again go back to the questions that Dr. Holland was asking before.

You can interpret Dr. Otten's study in one of two ways: Either BCG is as good as maintenance chemotherapy and could be used in place of maintenance chemotherapy to achieve an effect, or both BCG and maintenance chemotherapy are as good as doing nothing at all. We can't choose between these possibilities because we don't have the appropriate control group at this time.

Given that situation, and given the absence of controlled studies by Dr. Mathé, I think we have to start from the point where all we can say is that we don't know. Therefore we don't have to worry about whether we are giving the BCG the right way or the wrong way. Until somebody sets up a critical test to determine whether or not the administration of BCG at some stage in ALL is indeed efficacious, we really can't answer any of these questions about frequency or dosage.

Dr. Kay: There was one point about ALL that we left in the air and that was the necessary length of chemotherapy. Although three years is often thought to be a necessary length, there is no evidence that two years is not just as good. In fact, I think we have evidence that it is just the same. Therefore, if the immunotherapists are going to start at 25 months, they must have a notreatment control group there to show that there is any difference, because I believe 25 months is just about enough chemotherapy to achieve long-term maintenance-free survival.

Dr. Eckert: I have several comments.

1. The Concorde and the Children's Cancer Group studies did not use CNS prophylaxis and therefore possible foci of leukemic cells which might predispose to early relapse were not eradicated. It is possible that these patients represent a group in which favorable effects of a form of adjuvant therapy could not be demonstrated.

2. Chemotherapy of 9 and 25 months duration followed by immunotherapy produced similar duration of remission. This suggests that immunotherapy can maintain a certain proportion of patients free of relapse as there

is no evidence from other studies that a similar proportion of patients can be maintained in remission without further treatment after only 9 months of chemotherapy.

3. There were no deaths in remission in patients maintained with immunotherapy while death in remission regularly occurs in a proportion of patients undergoing intensive chemotherapy.

Dr. Morton: I wanted to come back to something that Dr. Mathé said about the difference in responses between the anergic and the allergic patients to BCG, because I think there is something very important here in terms of dosage that we should not forget. BCG is a living organism. If it is placed into the body, it will proliferate there until the patient's immunity gets to a certain point capable of shutting off its proliferation.

Now, that point is going to vary from patient to patient. This shut-off period time is likely to occur sooner with an allergic patient than with an anergic patient. I think the dose of BCG actually changes in the body. This is quite different from the dead materials like MER or *C. parvum,* where you put a certain dose in there, and whether it's the right dose or the wrong dose, it's there.

As Dr. Weiss has said, in experimental animal systems it's very clear that there is a dose-response curve that goes up, and then falls down. As one gets beyond a certain point, inhibition results. A patient who develops systemic BCG-osis becomes completely anergic. They may be immunologically competent, but if they get an overwhelming dose of BCG organisms, then this in itself is immunosuppressive.

I think, as Dr. Weiss has said, if one is uncertain, it is probably better to err on the low side of dosage, but with frequent administration. Let the body do the immunomodulation by how much it lets the BCG proliferate, rather than go beyond this point where a progressive systemic BCG infection results.

Dr. Leventhal: Dr. Jones, could you interpret your study as showing that adriamycin and bleomycin have some sort of antagonistic effect on one another, accounting for the disparity between the two arms?

Dr. Jones: We have a prior large experience with CHOP without the bleomycin, and the results of that study are virtually identical to the results we are seeing with CHOP plus bleomycin. That is, I do not think the bleomycin adds or detracts from the results of the basic CHOP regimen alone. This is pretty low-dose bleomycin. What we are seeing is a significant difference in the results with BCG added to the basic CHOP regimen.

Dr. Leventhal: But wasn't your COP plus bleomycin better than your CHOP plus bleo? I may be getting my data confused, but your lowest arm was CHOP plus bleo.

Dr. Jones: In the COP-bleomycin arm, there was a slight imbalance in favor of patients with nodular lymphoma. We have a higher response rate in the COP-bleomycin arm, and I think that accounts for it.

At the current time, the patients with diffuse lymphoma have exhibited significantly shorter remission duration when they received treatment with COP-bleomycin compared to either one of the adriamycin-containing induction arms. However, there is no difference with respect to the addition of bleomycin or BCG to CHOP-treatment arms. In terms of remission duration in patients with diffuse lymphomas, however, these arms were significantly better than the remission duration seen with COP-bleomycin. So, although the initial response rate appears to be higher in diffuse lymphomas with COP-bleomycin, there is a more rapid relapse rate when treatment is stopped or BCG is administered than with adriamycin-containing combinations.

Dr. Green (Memphis, Tennessee): Dr. Jones, you implied that BCG during the remission induction was helpful because it improved the number of partial responders to your therapy. What evidence do you have that attaining a partial response in diffuse lymphomas is of any value? Can you salvage those patients, or do they go on and relapse rapidly and die?

Dr. Jones: I did not imply it was helpful. I indicated that the overall response rate, partial plus complete, was higher in patients receiving CHOP plus BCG. I am sure you are aware of the data from the National Cancer Institute concerning histiocytic lymphoma that suggest that partial response is not of any benefit. In our trial, patients have stayed on continued treatment if they have not achieved documented complete remission. We do not know yet what effect additional partial remission rate might have on overall survival or remission duration. That remains to be seen. I am not suggesting that is helpful at the moment. The only thing I can say is that in a randomized, well-controlled clinical trial, the overall response rate when patients receive BCG was significantly higher than when they did not receive BCG. And this was largely made up of additional responses of the partial-response type. It was not seen in a complete remission rate. How this will be translated in the long term remains to be seen.

Immunotherapy of Cancer: Present Status of
Trials in Man, edited by W. D. Terry and D. Windhorst.
Raven Press, New York © 1978.

Clinical Trials of Immune RNA in the Immunotherapy of Cancer

*Yosef H. Pilch, **Kenneth P. Ramming, and †Jean deKernion

*Department of Surgery, University of California Medical Center, San Diego, San Diego, California 92103; **Department of Surgery/Oncology, University of California, Los Angeles, School of Medicine, Center for the Health Sciences; and †Department of Surgery/ Urology, University of California, Los Angeles, School of Medicine, Center for the Health Sciences, Los Angeles, California 90024

Since 1967, our laboratory has been studying the mediation of anti-tumor immune responses by RNA preparations extracted from the lymphoid organs of animals previously immunized with tumor cells. Such immunoreactive RNA extracts of lymphoid tissues have been termed "Immune RNA" (I-RNA) and have been shown to mediate tumor-specific immune responses *in vitro* and *in vivo* in a variety of animal tumor systems (1–30,32–36). Of particular interest has been the activity of I-RNA in transferring anti-tumor immune responses across species lines, i.e., with xenogeneic sources of I-RNA (2,3,5,8,11–13,15,16,18,19,21–30,32,33,35).

Recently, the successful immunotherapy of transplantable spontaneously metastasizing mammary adenocarcinoma 13762 in female Fischer 344/N rats with xenogeneic or syngeneic I-RNA was demonstrated in our laboratory. In this model, when growing primary tumor transplants are surgically excised 18 days after transplantation, local recurrence does not occur. However, all animals go on to die of metastases to lung and other organs if no additional treatment is given. An experiment was performed in which immunotherapy with I-RNA was utilized as an adjuvant to surgical excision of the primary tumor transplant. With no treatment at all, all animals died within 70 days. With excision of the primary tumor transplant alone, all animals died of metastases within 96 days. Xenogeneic I-RNA was extracted from the lymph nodes and spleens of Hartley guinea pigs 2 weeks following immunization with mammary adenocarcinoma tissue. This I-RNA was administered at a dose of 1.0 mg in 1 ml of buffer containing 10 mg/ml of a potent inhibitor of ribonuclease—sodium dextran sulfate (molecular weight 500,000). Twenty-five one-hundredths of a milliliter of this mixture was administered into each of the four footpads of a group of rats, every other day for 10 doses (i.e., 20 days), beginning 10 days prior to surgical excision of the primary tumor transplant. Of the animals so treated, 80% survived and remained free of disease for 180 days. When xenogeneic I-RNA was administered at a dose of 1 mg every other day for 10 doses beginning at the day of surgical excision of the primary tumor, 67% of animals so treated survived and remained free of disease for 180 days. Syngeneic I-RNA was extracted from the spleens of Fischer rats bearing growing transplants of the mammary adenocarcinoma. When this syngeneic I-RNA was administered, at the same dosage schedule, pre- and postoperatively to another group of rats, 50% of the animals so treated survived and remained free of disease for 180 days. These studies suggested that immunotherapy with I-RNA might be clinically efficacious.

We also were able to demonstrate that xenogeneic I-RNA extracted from the lymphoid organs of sheep or guinea pigs immunized with human tumor cells mediates cytotoxic immune responses that are specifically directed against tumor-associated antigens of human tumor cells (16). Peripheral blood lymphocytes both from healthy donors and from cancer patients became markedly more cytotoxic for human tumor target cells following incubation with I-RNA extracted from the lymphoid organs of guinea pigs or sheep that had been immunized with cells of the same tumor type. Tumors studied included gastric carcinoma, malignant melanoma, and carcinoma of the breast. Lymphocytes incubated with RNA from animals immunized with complete Freund's adjuvant only evidenced no increased cytotoxic activity. RNA extracted from the lymphoid organs of the animals immunized with normal skin fibroblasts, when incubated with normal allogeneic lymphocytes, also mediated cytotoxic immune reactions against tumor target cells. These immune responses presumably were directed against normal histocompatibility antigens. However, when lymphocytes that were autologous with respect to the immunizing tumor and/or the tumor target cells were incubated with RNA from animals immunized with autologous normal fibroblasts, no increase in cytotoxicity against autologous tumor target cells was observed. Only I-RNA extracted from animals specifically immunized with tumor cells mediated cytotoxic antitumor immune responses when incubated with autologous lymphocytes. It was concluded that a recognition of self occurred during the course of those reactions, and, therefore, no immune reactions against self cell surface antigens were initiated by xenogeneic I-RNA. Only I-RNAs directed against foreign (not self) antigens were able to initiate cytotoxic antitumor immune reactions following incubation with human lymphocytes.

Recently, in our laboratory, new experiments were designed and carried out that included normal fibroblast cell lines as target cells (13). These important controls, because of technical reasons, could not be included in our previous reports, which had been performed exclusively with established tumor cell lines as target cells. Additional evidence that xenogeneic I-RNA can mediate immune responses specifically against human tumor-associated antigens was obtained from new studies of two autologous melanoma systems *in vitro*. In these systems malignant melanoma target cell cultures, matching normal fibroblastic target cells, lymphocyte effector cells, and melanoma and normal skin tissue used to immunize RNA donor animals were derived from the same autochthonous hosts. These experiments demonstrated that, although xenogeneic antitumor I-RNA mediated immune reactions against normal cell surface antigens on incubation with allogeneic lymphocytes, only immune reactions against tumor-associated antigens were detected when anti-tumor I-RNA was incubated with autologous lymphocytes. When incubated with autologous lymphocytes, I-RNA extracted from the lymphoid organs of donor animals immunized with melanoma tissue mediated immune reactions against autologous melanoma target cells *in vitro*. I-RNA from animals immunized with normal skin tissue from the autochthonous host did not increase the cytotoxicity of autologous lymphocytes for autologous melanoma cells. Using autologous fibroblasts as target cells, no increase in cytotoxicity was detected when autologous lymphocytes were incubated with RNA from animals immunized with either melanoma tissue or normal skin tissue from the autochthonous host. By contrast, when allogeneic lymphocytes were used as effector cells, RNA extracted from animals immunized with either melanoma tissue or normal skin mediated cytotoxic immune reactions against both melanoma target cells and normal fibroblast target cells derived from the same patient.

The successful transfer of cell-mediated immune responses to human tumor-associated antigens *in vitro* by xenogeneic I-RNA provided a logical basis for preliminary trials of immunotherapy of human cancer with I-RNA. This form of immunotherapy offered several specific theoretical advantages. First, large quantities of I-RNA could be produced without dependence on human donors. Secondly, since histologically similar human tumors appear to share tumor-associated antigens, many patients with the same tumor type could be treated with I-RNA from an animal immunized with a single patient's tumor.

Because the evidence from accumulated laboratory studies in animal models suggested that I-RNA could induce clinically relevant anti-tumor immune responses and because of the many potential advantages of this form of immunotherapy in the human situation, a clinical study was designed to examine the feasibility of I-RNA immunotherapy of human neoplasms. The aim of this initial study was to assess toxicity and to establish dose-response relationships associated with I-RNA immunotherapy. It also was intended to document possible changes in host immunity secondary to I-RNA therapy. It, therefore, appeared appropriate to include only patients with gross disease, especially patients for whom no effective therapy was available or in whom standard therapy for metastases had failed. It is known that such patients have little chance of responding to immunotherapy of any type, and therefore clinical response, although sought, was not expected as a primary goal. Similarly, controls were not included since clinical response was not the major determinant of the study. Later in the clinical trial, some patients who were rendered free of gross disease by surgery but who had a significant probability of developing local recurrence and/or distant metastases (minimum residual disease) were included. In these patients, disease-free interval was determined as well as changes in immunologic parameters. These patients were included only after a significant number of patients with metastatic disease were treated and found to develop no signs of toxicity.

MATERIALS AND METHODS

The xenogeneic I-RNA was extracted from lymphoid tissues of sheep immunized with a human tumor in the following manner (22). A thick suspension of viable tumor cells prepared in 3 ml of medium was emulsified in an equal volume of complete Freund's adjuvant and injected intradermally into all four extremities of a sheep at weekly intervals for 3 consecutive weeks. Ten days after the last injection the animals were sacrificed and the spleens and mesenteric lymph nodes excised and immediately frozen in dry ice for RNA extraction.

The frozen lymphoid tissues homogenized in 10 ml/g of an extraction medium, consisting of equal parts of buffer (0.1 M Tris buffer pH 5.0 containing 0.5% sodium dodecyl sulfate (SDS), 0.5% (1.5) naphthalenedisulfonic acid, and 2 μg/ml polyvinyl and sulfuric acid potassium salt and buffer-saturated phenol. Homogenization was carried out at 0°C for three 1-min periods. The homogenate was then heated for 6 min in a 65°C water bath and cooled rapidly in an ice water slush. The homogenate was centrifuged at 2,000 × g for 20 min at 4°C and the aqueous phases combined and reextracted three to five times in one-half volume of buffer-saturated phenol. The combined aqueous phases were then extracted five times with an equal volume of cold ether to remove phenol, and nitrogen was then bubbled through the solution to remove the ether. The solution was made 0.1 M with respect to NaCl, and 2½ volumes of cold ethanol was added and the RNA precipitated overnight at −20°C. The RNA was then reprecipitated twice from solutions made 2 M with respect to potassium acetate, treated with pronase (to remove contaminating protein), and again reprecipitated from 2 M potassium acetate. The RNA was then dialyzed against sterile distilled water, sterilized by passage through 0.22-μm millipore filters and lyophylized. The RNA was resuspended in normal saline prior to injection.

The RNA preparations were assayed for RNA, DNA, and protein concentration. The pronase treatment and reprecipitation method reduced the protein concentration to very low levels. However, traces of sheep protein remained, possibly complexed to the RNA. Sterility of each preparation of RNA was determined by routine bacterial and fungal cultures. In no instance was any RNA preparation found to be contaminated. The integrity of the RNA was determined by sucrose density gradient analysis and by disc gel electrophoresis. Preparations found to be degraded were discarded, although this was a rare occurrence. The I-RNA was stored at −75°C, although lyophylized preparations stored at room temperature for 30 days were found to have undergone no degradation.

Immediately before administration, the I-RNA was resuspended in sterile saline and injected intradermally in multiple wheels of 0.1 ml near lymph node-bearing areas (groins or axillae). When possible, each patient received I-RNA prepared against autologous tumor tissue. If this was not feasible, I-RNA prepared against allogeneic tumor tissue of the same histologic type was used. Doses of I-RNA ranged from 2 to 60 mg/week in single or divided doses but were usually 4 or 8 mg/week. As noted above, a purpose of this study was to determine dose-response relationships. As far as could be determined, there was no significant difference in response of patients to small or large doses. However, since measurable objective responses were rare, as would be expected in patients with such far advanced disease, assessment of proper dosage was difficult. However, quantitative measurements in our laboratory of lymphocyte cytotoxicity *in vitro* mediated by I-RNA suggested a relationship between the concentration of I-RNA and the magnitude of the response. It was found that incubation of effector cells with I-RNA concentrations of 500 μg/ml or greater produced maximal cytotoxicity, whereas reducing the concentration to 250 μg/ml usually caused a decrease in cytotoxicity. Further reduction in the concentration usually resulted in further diminution of cytotoxicity (14,18,30,35). Wang et al. have also reported a dose-response curve based on *in vitro* cytotoxicity (37). Further clinical experience is necessary before an *in vivo* dose-response relationship can be detected.

Immune responses of treated patients were monitored by response to dinitrochlorobenzene (DNCB) and common antigens and by changes in lymphocyte-mediated cytotoxicity to tumor target cells. Patients were sensitized and subsequently challenged with DNCB according to the method of Eilber and Morton (6). They were retested at 8 to 12 week intervals throughout their treatment with DNCB and common antigens. Lymphocyte cytotoxicity to tumor target cells was determined by a microcytotoxicity test that has been previously reported (16,17,30). Peripheral blood samples were obtained serially prior to and during the course of therapy. Lymphocytes were isolated on Ficoll-isopaque gradients and were frozen in the vapor phase of liquid nitrogen at 1°C/min. Viability of the frozen lymphocytes varied from 60 to 80%. Details of this method have previously been reported (16, 30). The target cells for the microcytotoxicity assay were allogeneic tumor cells of the same histologic type as the tumor of the patient under study.

RESULTS

Immunotherapy of Advanced Disease

Malignant Melanoma

Patients in the advanced disease category had either unresectable local or regional recurrence, or visceral metastases, or both. In all instances, histologic diagnosis of malignant melanoma had been made at some time in the patient's course. In many instances, the metastatic lesion(s) was proved by biopsy. Over half the patients had failed one or more chemotherapeutic regimens. I-RNA immunotherapy consisted of weekly intradermal injections of 4 to 8 mg of I-RNA. In several cases where a patient's autologous tumor tissue was available, the I-RNA was extracted from lymph nodes and spleens of sheep immunized with the patient's own tumor. In other instances, the I-RNA administered was from sheep immunized with melanoma tissue from another patient. Patients were treated for a minimum of 2 months, and therapy was continued thereafter until progression occurred. A total of 15 patients with advanced melanoma received I-RNA. Progression occurred within 2 months in six of the patients. One patient has shown no progression of his disease over a 7-month treatment interval and is alive. One patient had temporary stabilization of multiple pulmonary metastases for a 3-month period, as indicated by serial chest X-ray. His disease then slowly progressed, and he died 10 months after the initiation of I-RNA therapy. One patient had slow progression of pulmonary metastases. He died with brain metastases 12 months after initiation of therapy. One patient had stabilization of his metastases for a period of 5 months and died of brain metastases at 6 months. Of all 15 patients, 10 are dead at the time of this writing, four are alive with obviously progressive disease despite I-RNA therapy, and one patient is alive with no progression of his disease after 7 months of therapy. There were no 1-year survivors.

It is of interest that despite the advanced stage of disease in these patients when first seen, all reacted to DNCB skin tests prior to therapy. Two of the patients actually showed increasing reactivity to DNCB despite progression of their disease. Seven patients showed no change in cutaneous reactivity to DNCB when serially tested. The patient who had the most advanced disease with lung, brain, and intraabdominal metastases was the only patient to become anergic to DNCB and showed no cutaneous reactivity when tested shortly before death.

All patients' lymphocytes were sampled prior to treatment and serially during therapy and tested for cytotoxic activity against melanoma target cells. In all but one of these patients, the target cell was derived from the same allogeneic human melanoma cell line. A significant increase in lymphocyte cytotoxicity, compared to pretreatment levels, was noted in five of the patients while they were receiving I-RNA therapy, despite progressive tumor growth. In three of these patients, lymphocytes were tested against the skin of the melanoma target cell donor as well as the melanoma target cells themselves. In each instance, a high level of cytotoxicity was noted against the melanoma target cells, and only minimal cytotoxic activity was noted against the skin fibroblasts.

Colon Carcinoma

Two patients with far advanced adenocarcinoma of the colon were treated. The I-RNA was obtained from lymphoid organs of sheep immunized with human colon cancer. One patient had pulmonary metastases, and the other patient had intraabdominal recurrence. The first patient was treated for 2 months. During this time, his carcinoembryonic antigen (CEA) level increased from 16 to 150, and he had obvious clinical progression of disease. He was initially anergic to DNCB but had a slight reaction when retested 8 weeks after the onset of therapy. He is alive and receiving chemotherapy at this time.

A second patient who underwent resection of an intraabdominal recurrence of colon carcinoma was clinically stable for 6 months while receiving I-RNA. Her CEA remained approximately 2.0 during this period. However, she then required surgery for another intraabdominal recurrence that clearly was progressing while she was receiving treatment. She reacted strongly to DNCB both prior to and while receiving I-RNA therapy. She is currently alive and receiving chemotherapy.

Hypernephroma

Twenty patients with metastatic hypernephroma (renal cell carcinoma) have been treated with I-RNA. This I-RNA was obtained from sheep immunized with allogeneic human hypernephroma tissue. Weekly intradermal doses of 4 to 8 mg of I-RNA were given. Twelve patients had pulmonary metastases only, whereas five had extrapulmonary metastases as well (to bone, brain, or liver). One patient had a large mass of metastatic hypernephroma in superior mediastinal lymph nodes, proved by biopsy. Eight of the 20 patients presented with metastases at the time of original diagnosis and underwent palliative nephrectomy prior to receiving I-RNA treatment. The survival of these patients, plotted by the life table method is depicted in Fig. 1. In this group, three patients have been under treatment for less than 6 months. The longest follow-up has been a patient who is alive and well after 35 months, with biopsy-proved mediastinal lymph node involvement. Eight patients have died. Therefore, the median survival has not yet been reached.

Survival appears to correlate not only with extent of disease, but also with location of metastases. Those patients with metastases confined to the lungs had a better prognosis than those with metastatic involvement elsewhere. Four of five patients with extrapulmonary involvement died with a mean survival of 8.5 months.

Eleven patients with metastatic hypernephroma had serial measurements of lymphocyte-mediated cytotoxicity against allogeneic hypernephroma target cells. In six of these patients, cytotoxicity did not increase at any time during therapy, which ranged from 5 to 19 months. Three of these patients are alive, two at 17 and one at 19 months, and three died at 6, 11, and 12 months. Five patients evidenced significant increases in lymphocyte cytotoxicity while receiving I-RNA therapy. Three of these patients then had a decrease in cytotoxicity that correlated with progression of disease, and these

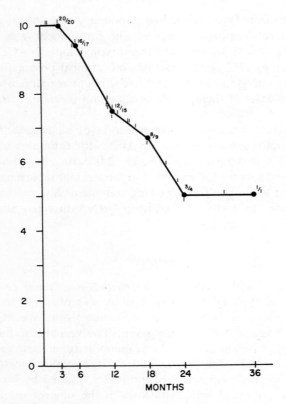

FIG. 1. Survival of patients with metastatic hypernephroma treated with I-RNA.

patients died at 12, 18, and 24 months. Two patients with stable metastatic disease are alive at 13 and 35 months. In both of these patients, the cytotoxic indices have remained high.

It is of interest that 10 of the patients with advanced metastatic disease did not respond to initial testing with DNCB. There appeared to be little correlation between this cutaneous anergy and tumor burden, since patients with very small amounts of tumor as well as patients with extensive metastatic disease were included in this group. However, regardless of initial response, an increase in sensitivity to DNCB was correlated with stabilization of growth or unusually slow progression of metastases observed in six of the 20 patients. The converse was not true, since some patients who appeared to have temporary stabilization of growth of metastases did not have an increase in DNCB skin test reactivity.

Miscellaneous Tumors

Seven other patients have received I-RNA for advanced malignancies. They include one patient with gastric carcinoma, three with sarcomas, one with metastatic lung cancer, and one patient with breast carcinoma. These patients were treated during the very early phase of our pilot study, and it is not possible to draw any conclusions from review of their clinical courses.

One of these patients, however, merits a comment. This 9-year-old girl presented with an irresectable alveolar soft part sarcoma of the pelvic soft tissues and pulmonary metastases. She received I-RNA from a sheep immunized with her own tumor. Her pulmonary metastases did not progress at all while on therapy, and a few decreased slightly in size. After 8 months and after this favorable clinical response, the patient was placed on chemotherapy and has had further regression. She is currently alive 15 months after diagnosis. Her lymphocytes exhibited a moderate increase in cytotoxicity against allogeneic sarcoma target cells. Her DNCB reactivity also increased significantly during treatment.

Adjuvant Immunotherapy

Patients in this category were at high risk for recurrence following potentially curative surgical resection of all clinically detectable tumor. Immunotherapy was initiated within 10 weeks of operation. All patients received 4 mg of I-RNA weekly. Whenever possible, each patient received I-RNA from a sheep that had been immunized with his own autologous tumor cells. Alternatively, each patient received I-RNA from a sheep immunized with allogeneic tumor cells of the same histologic type. If progression of disease was noted, I-RNA therapy was discontinued and alternative therapy instituted. If no recurrence developed, treatment continued for 2 years and was then stopped.

Malignant Melanoma

Ten patients with malignant melanoma at high risk for recurrence were included in this pilot study. Another patient had had multiple recurrences of tumor in the left axilla and chest wall. These had been locally excised six times within 4 years, the longest interval between recurrences being 8 months. An eighth patient was treated following excision of a mass of recurrent melanoma from the right groin less than 1 year after a groin dissection for lymph node metastases. Four patients were treated who did not have lymph node involvement. Two of these patients had not undergone node dissection, and two had been subjected to node dissection without evidence of nodal involvement. Of these four patients, one had a lower extremity melanoma with invasion to Clarke's level III and three had melanomas of the trunk with invasion to Clarke's level IV or V.

The survival free of disease (recurrence rate) of these 10 patients, plotted by the life table method, is presented in Fig. 2. The median follow-up is 17 months, and the mean follow-up is 18 months. Two patients have been

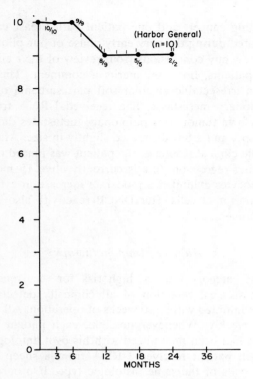

FIG. 2. Survival free of disease of patients with stage II malignant melanoma receiving adjuvant immunotherapy with I-RNA.

treated for 24 months, and their therapy has been discontinued. Only one patient has developed a recurrence. The patient from whose groin a mass of recurrent melanoma had been excised prior to entry into the study developed another recurrence in the same groin after 7 months of I-RNA immunotherapy. She was treated with radiation therapy and chemotherapy and had a complete response. She remains alive and in complete remission over 1 year later.

In one of the melanoma patients receiving I-RNA immunotherapy, a 28-year-old white male with innumerable deeply pigmented nevi, a marked vitiliganous change developed in most of the nevi after 1 year of I-RNA treatment. Photographs of two of these nevi are presented in Fig. 3A and B. Vitiliganous change in pigmented nevi has occasionally been observed by other investigators in melanoma patients undergoing other forms of immunotherapy.

All patients tested exhibited cutaneous responses to initial challenge doses of DNCB prior to beginning therapy, and in all patients the level of reactivity to subsequent DNCB challenges increased during therapy. Four of the seven

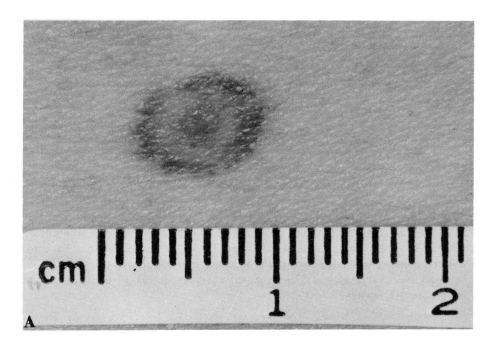

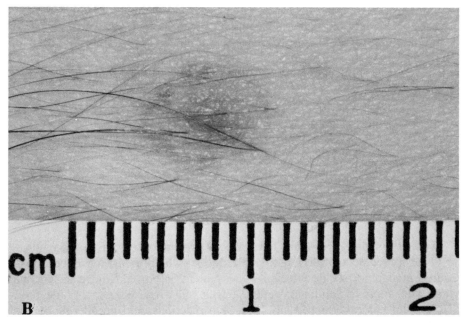

FIG. 3A & B. Cutaneous nevi on the trunk of a melanoma patient showing vitiliganous change after 1 year of immunotherapy with I-RNA.

patients tested had significant increase in lymphocyte cytotoxicity during treatment, and three patients had no increase whatsoever.

Colorectal Cancer

A prospectively randomized trial of adjuvant immunotherapy with I-RNA in patients with Dukes' B$_2$ or Dukes' C colorectal cancer was begun in September of 1975. In this study patients are randomized postoperatively into either treatment or no-treatment groups. Treated patients receive 4 mg of I-RNA weekly for 2 years, unless recurrence or metastases develop. To this date, 10 patients have been entered into this study—six in the treatment group and four in the control group. The six patients receiving I-RNA have been followed for 2, 4, 7, 10, 12, and 16 months, without evidence of recurrence. Three of these patients are receiving I-RNA from sheep immunized with autologous tumor tissue. CEA levels in all of these patients have remained below 2.0. Of the four patients in the control group, one patient developed liver metastases at 5 months and the others remain free of disease at from 2 to 10 months.

Hypernephroma

Patients in this category underwent radical nephrectomy and regional lymphadenectomy for hypernephroma and had findings at surgery that indicated a high probability of recurrence, i.e., microscopically positive resection margins, invasion of the inferior vena cava, metastases to regional lymph nodes, or resection of metastatic tumor deposits. Eight patients have been followed for 7, 9, 12, 14, 16, 20, 26, and 36 months, with a mean follow-up of 17.5 months. All are alive without evidence of recurrence. Three patients developed modest rises in lymphocyte-mediated cytotoxic responses to renal carcinoma cells *in vitro*. Skin test data were unpredictable. Two of the patients who are clinically free of recurrence have never demonstrated a response to DNCB, and the remainder has shown progressive increases in cutaneous sensitivity on sequential DNCB testing.

DISCUSSION

Toxicity of the I-RNA has been absent or minimal. Total doses of up to 600 mg (over 36 months) and single doses as high as 60 mg have not resulted in significant side effects. A few patients reported mild transient malaise and anorexia, and one patient developed a transient low-grade fever. No patient has experienced any local skin reactions, and no allergic or anaphylactoid reactions have occurred.

In reviewing our clinical results in advanced disease, it must be remembered that clinical remissions were not expected at this stage of our work, and any clinical responses reported must be considered anecdotal. In these initial phase I trials, the objectives were (a) to establish the safety (or toxicity) of sheep I-RNA, (b) to evaluate dosage schedules and routes of administration, and (c) to monitor any possible effects of I-RNA treatment on immunologic parameters, both tumor specific and nonspecific. The optimum dosage, route, and frequency of administration of I-RNA are not known. Certainly, we have not as yet approached a toxic dose of I-RNA.

In our previous animal experiments (2,3,24,28,29), it appeared desirable to administer I-RNA in a medium containing a strong ribonuclease inhibitor (e.g., SDS). However, since we have not as yet received approval from the Food and Drug Administration to administer SDS experimentally in man, we have not incorporated a ribonuclease inhibitor into our I-RNA preparations. Perhaps by so doing we might significantly increase the efficacy of I-RNA therapy.

Although treatment of lymphocytes *in vitro* with I-RNA has been shown to induce such lymphocytes to effect anti-tumor immune responses *in vivo* and *in vitro* (13,14,16–18,30,33,35), we have not, as yet, treated any patients by the intravenous infusion of autologous lymphocytes preincubated *in vitro* with I-RNA. This reluctance has been due to the fear of inducing untoward allergic reactions related to small amounts of sheep protein that contaminate the RNA and might be expected to remain with the lymphocytes even after several washes. However, this method of utilizing I-RNA therapeutically may offer promise of greater efficacy.

The influence of the therapy in patients with extensive disease was difficult to assess. Complete regression did not occur in any patient treated. Several patients, however, had temporary stabilization of growth of metastases documented to be progressively growing prior to the initiation of I-RNA therapy. Three patients with malignant melanoma and one patient with alveolar soft part sarcoma appeared to have temporary arrest of growth of metastatic lesions. Stabilization of growth of pulmonary metastases was noted in several hypernephroma patients. However, the peculiar natural history of hypernephroma makes interpretation of such temporary changes in growth patterns difficult. Erratic growth of pulmonary nodules with periods of growth arrest is known to occur in patients receiving no therapy, and occasional spontaneous regressions have also been reported (38).

Failure of I-RNA therapy to influence extensive disease is not surprising. Immunotherapy in any form appears to be effective only in the presence of a minimal tumor burden. However, survival of some hypernephroma patients did appear to be increased by I-RNA treatment.

Survival of patients with metastatic hypernephroma has not been shown to be influenced by currently available methods of therapy. Johnson et al. (10) reported approximately 25% 1-year survival in 93 patients with metastatic hypernephroma. The 2-year survival was 13%. Rafla (31) reported a higher 2-year survival—28%. However, Mostofi (20), in a review of 1,700 cases of patients with metastatic renal carcinoma, reported only two survivors after 2 years in patients who had metastases at the time of diagnosis, regardless of therapy. When compared to these published statistics, the patients with metastatic hypernephroma treated with I-RNA seemed to have had an increase in survival from the time of onset of metastases. However, only by prospectively randomized studies can any true alteration of survival or growth of metastases be attributed directly to I-RNA immunotherapy.

Patients with a minimum residual disease and patients with a high probability of recurrence following curative surgery are more suitable candidates for immunotherapy. Twenty-four patients in this category (10 melanoma, six colon carcinoma, eight hypernephroma) have received adjuvant immunotherapy with I-RNA and have been observed for 2 to 25 months. Only one of these patients has developed evidence of recurrence during this period. Our preliminary results in the adjuvant immunotherapy of malignant melanoma with I-RNA suggest a decreased recurrence rate of the same order of magnitude as that reported by other investigators who have treated similar groups of melanoma patients with BCG or BCG plus allogeneic melanoma cells (7,9). Although our initial results are encouraging, the number of patients is small, and longer follow-up is necessary. Furthermore, factors such as patient selection, histology, and thoroughness of surgical excision influence the probability of recurrence. The definitive interpretation of the efficacy of I-RNA immunotherapy in this category of patients, therefore, awaits the results of randomized clinical trials. One such randomized trial of adjuvant immunotherapy with I-RNA in patients with Dukes' B_2 and Dukes' C colorectal cancer is already in progress.

Evidence for stimulation of host immunity by I-RNA was assessed through skin test responses to DNCB and assessment of lymphocyte-mediated cytotoxicity to tumor target cells in vitro. In most patients, DNCB response correlated with progression of disease. Initial skin test responses in hypernephroma patients, however, often did not correlate with tumor burden. Furthermore, the subsequent clinical course in many cases was not reflected by changes in DNCB response. In all patient groups, increases in skin test responses were frequently noted after the institution of I-RNA therapy.

Similarly, changes in lymphocyte-mediated cytotoxicity values are difficult to interpret. Increases in cytotoxic indices in some patients were clearly attributable to the I-RNA therapy, but in others no significant changes were noted. There was no good correlation between changes in lymphocyte-mediated cytotoxic activity and clinical course.

Administration of I-RNA, intradermally, undoubtedly results in degradation of a significant portion of the nucleic acid by endogenous ribonucleases. We have attempted to compensate for this eventuality by employing doses of I-RNA far in excess of those required for the mediation of antitumor immune responses in vitro. At the present time no effective ribonuclease inhibitors are available for human use. Further investigation of such agents and their incorporation into clinical trials may be necessary before maximum effect of intracutaneous administration of I-RNA can be assessed. Incubation and re-infusion of autologous lymphocytes with the xenogeneic RNA, as described above, is an alternative method for minimizing the influence of endogenous ribonucleases. This approach merits further investigation.

The mechanism of action of I-RNA remains unclear. Identification of the active fraction and the mechanism by which it transfers immunologic information may be necessary before rapid advances in the field are possible. Furthermore, the specific aspect of host immunity that is influenced by I-RNA must be elucidated. The appropriate *in vitro* assays can then be identified that will detect effects of the therapy relevant to *in vivo* effects.

Finally, it is clear that sheep I-RNA, when prepared as described above and administered intradermally in the doses and schedules described, is completely free of significant local or systemic toxicity and is very well tolerated. Much more work is required to evaluate the possible efficacy of I-RNA as an immunotherapeutic modality.

ACKNOWLEDGMENTS

This work was supported in part by grants CA-21664, CA-12582, and CA-16042 and by contract no. 4-444996–32691 from the National Institutes of Health, U.S. Public Health Service.

REFERENCES

1. Deckers, P. J., and Pilch, Y. H. (1972): Mediation of immunity to tumor-specific transplantation antigens by RNA: Inhibition of isograft growth in rats. *Cancer Res.*, 32:839–846.
2. Deckers, P. J., and Pilch, Y. H. (1971): RNA-mediated transfer of tumor immunity—A new model for the immunotherapy of cancer. *Cancer*, 28:1219–1228.
3. Deckers, P. J., and Pilch, Y. H. (1971): Transfer of immunity to tumor isografts by the systemic administration of xenogeneic "Immune" RNA. *Nature (New Biol.)*, 231:181–183.
4. Deckers, P. J., Ramming, K. P., and Pilch, Y. H. (1973): The transfer of tumor immunity with syngeneic RNA. *Ann. NY Acad. Sci.*, 207:442–453.
5. deKernion, J. B., Ramming, K. P., Skinner, D. G., and Pilch, Y. H. (1977): The clinical experience in the therapy of renal carcinoma with Immune RNA. In: *Immune RNA in Neoplasia*, edited by M. A. Fink. Academic Press, New York. (*In press.*)
6. Eilber, F. R., and Morton, D. L. (1970): Impaired immunologic reactivity and recurrence following cancer surgery. *Cancer*, 25:362–367.
7. Eilber, F. R., Morton, D. L., Holmes, E. C., Sparks, F. C., and Ramming, K. P. (1976): Adjuvant immunotherapy with BCG in treatment of regional lymph node metastases from malignant melanoma. *N. Engl. J. Med.*, 294:237–240.
8. Fritze, D., Kern, D. H., Chow, N., and Pilch, Y. H. (1977): Production of cyto-toxic antibody to a benz (a) pyrene-induced sarcoma in mice receiving xenogeneic anti-tumor Immune RNA. *Cancer Immunol. Immunother.* (*In press.*)
9. Gutterman, J. U., Mavligit, G. M., Kennedy, A., McBride, C. M., Burgess, M. A., and Hersh, E. M. (1976): Immunotherapy for malignant melanoma. In: *Neoplasms of the Skin and Malignant Melanoma*, pp. 497–531. Year Book Medical Publ., New York.

10. Johnson, D. E., Kaesler, K. E., and Samuels, M. (1975): Is nephrectomy justified in patients with metastatic renal carcinoma? *J. Urol.*, 114:27–32.
11. Kern, D. H., Chow, N., and Pilch, Y. H. (1976): Kinetics of synthesis and immunologically active fraction of anti-tumor Immune RNA. *Cell. Immunol.*, 24: 58–68.
12. Kern, D. H., deKernion, J. B., and Pilch, Y. H. (1976): Intracellular localization of anti-tumor "Immune" RNA. *Cell. Immunol.*, 22:11–18.
13. Kern, D. H., Drogemuller, C. R., Chow, N., Holleman, D. D., and Pilch, Y. H. (1977): Specificity of anti-tumor immune reactions mediated by xenogeneic Immune RNA. *J. Natl. Cancer Inst.* (*In press.*)
14. Kern, D. H., Drogemuller, C. R., and Pilch, Y. H. (1974): Immune cytolysis of rat tumor cells mediated by syngeneic "Immune" RNA. *J. Natl. Cancer Inst.*, 52: 299–302.
15. Kern, D. H., Drogemuller, C. R., and Pilch, Y. H. (1976): The mediation of immune responses to tumor antigens in vitro by Immune RNA. *Ann. NY Acad. Sci.*, 276:278–302.
16. Kern, D. H., Fritze, D., Drogemuller, C. R., and Pilch, Y. H. (1976): Mediation of cytotoxic immune responses to human tumor associated antigens by xenogeneic Immune RNA. *J. Natl. Cancer Inst.*, 57:97–103.
17. Kern, D. H., Fritze, D., Schick, P. M., Chow, N., and Pilch, Y. H. (1976): Cytotoxic immune responses against human tumor associated antigens mediated by allogeneic Immune RNA. *J. Natl. Cancer Inst.*, 57:105–109.
18. Kern, D. H., and Pilch, Y. H. (1974): Immune cytolysis of murine tumor cells mediated by xenogeneic "Immune" RNA. *Int. J. Cancer*, 13:679–688.
19. Kern, D. H., and Pilch, Y. H. (1977): Mediation of anti-tumor immune responses with I-RNA. In: *Immune RNA in Neoplasia*, edited by M. A. Fink. Academic Press, New York. (*In press.*)
20. Mostofi, F. R. (1967): Pathology and spread of renal cell carcinoma. In: *Renal Neoplasia*, edited by J. S. King, pp. 41–85. Little Brown, Boston.
21. Pilch, Y. H., and deKernion, J. B. (1974): Immunotherapy of cancer with "Immune" RNA: Current status. *Semin. Oncol.*, 1:387–395.
22. Pilch, Y. H., deKernion, J. B., Skinner, D. G., Ramming, K. P., Schick, P. M., Fritze, D., Brower, P., and Kern, D. H. (1976): Immunotherapy of cancer with "Immune" RNA: A preliminary report. *Am. J. Surg.*, 132:631–637.
23. Pilch, Y. H., Fritze, D., and Kern, D. H. (1976): Mediation of immune responses to human tumor antigens with "Immune" RNA. In: *Clinical Tumor Immunology*, edited by J. Wybran and M. Staquet, pp. 169–190. Pergamon Press, Oxford.
24. Pilch, Y. H., Fritze, D., deKernion, J. B., Ramming, K. P., and Kern, D. H. (1976): Immunotherapy of cancer with Immune RNA in animal models and cancer patients. *Ann. NY Acad. Sci.*, 277:592–608.
25. Pilch, Y. H., Fritze, D., Waldman, S. R., and Kern, D. H. (1975): Transfer of anti-tumor immunity by "Immune" RNA. *Curr. Top. Microbiol. Immunol.*, 72: 157–190.
26. Pilch, Y. H., Fritze, D., Ramming, K. P., deKernion, J. B., and Kern, D. H. (1977): The mediation of immune responses by I-RNA to animal and human tumor antigens. In: *Immune RNA in Neoplasia*, edited by M. A. Fink. Academic Press, New York. (*In press.*)
27. Pilch, Y. H., and Ramming, K. P. (1970): Transfer of tumor immunity with ribonucleic acid. *Cancer*, 26:630–637.
28. Pilch, Y. H., Ramming, K. P., and Deckers, P. J. (1973): Induction of anti-cancer immunity with RNA. *Ann. NY Acad. Sci.*, 207:409–429.
29. Pilch, Y. H., Ramming, K. P., and Deckers, P. J. (1973): Studies in mediation of tumor immunity with "Immune" RNA. In: *Methods in Cancer Research*, Vol. 9, edited by H. Busch, pp. 195–254. Academic Press, New York.
30. Pilch, Y. H., Veltman, L. L., and Kern, D. H. (1974): Immune cytolysis of human tumor cells mediated by xenogeneic "Immune" RNA: Implications for immunotherapy. *Surgery*, 76:23–34.
31. Ralfa, S. (1970): Renal cell carcinoma: Natural history and results of treatment. *Cancer*, 25:26–40.

32. Ramming, K. P., and Pilch, Y. H. (1970): Mediation of immunity to tumor isografts in mice by heterologous ribonucleic acid. *Science,* 168:492–493.
33. Ramming, K. P., and Pilch, Y. H. (1971): Transfer of tumor-specific immunity with RNA: Inhibition of growth of murine tumor isografts. *J. Natl. Cancer Inst.,* 45:735–750.
34. Ramming, K. P., and Pilch, Y. H. (1970): Transfer of tumor specific immunity with RNA: Demonstration by immune cytolysis of tumor cells *in vitro. J. Natl. Cancer Inst.,* 45:543–553.
35. Veltman, L. L., Kern, D. H., and Pilch, Y. H. (1974): Immune cytolysis of human tumor cells mediated by xenogeneic "Immune" RNA. *Cell. Immunol.,* 13:367–377.
36. Waldman, S. R., and Pilch, Y. H. (1975): Specific MIF release by rat lymphocytes following incubation with syngeneic anti-tumor "Immune" RNA. *Cell. Immunol.,* 18:246–250.
37. Wang, B. S., Deckers, P. J., and Mannick, J. A.: *Personal communication.*
38. Werf-Meffing, B. van der, and Van Gilse, H. A. (1971): Hormonal treatment of metastases of renal carcinoma. *Br. J. Cancer,* 25:423–427.

Question and Answer Session

Dr. Morales: Dr. Pilch, have your patients received any other therapy besides nephrectomy, such as hormones?

Dr. Pilch: A number of those patients did not even have nephrectomy. No patient received any treatment other than immune RNA while receiving the substance. Some of the patients still had the primary tumor in place in addition to their metastatic disease at the time of presentation.

The philosophy with those patients was to begin immunotherapy with RNA and see if stabilization occurred. We usually waited two to three months to allow for stabilization. If, and only if, stabilization took place, was a nephrectomy performed, and then immune RNA continued. Since the mortality of nephrectomy in the presence of metastatic disease is 2 to 7 percent, we felt that nephrectomy was not justified without stabilization. A number of the patients had failed Provera prior to presenting to our study.

Dr. Sinkovics: I would like to know whether or not these patients produced any sheep-type antibody?

Dr. Pilch: We sent about 150 sera to Dr. Fisher and Dr. Adler at St. Jude's. With their techniques, they were not able to demonstrate any evidence of sheep globulin.

Dr. Spitler: Dr. Pilch, since we are spending so much time at this meeting discussing study design, in the colorectal study, I calculate that in order to detect a 20 percent effect of your immune RNA, and be fairly certain of detecting this, you would have to have at least 100 patients in each arm. And since your accrual was 11 patients in the last year, I'm wondering how long you are planning to continue the study?

Dr. Pilch: Well, our statisticians calculated 60 in each arm, and it is on this basis that we began the study. The first year's accrual is not representative of what the accrual will be, because there is always some tooling-up time. But our statisticians tell us that 60 in each arm will do it, and we hope to reach this number in three years.

Dr. Rosenberg: Were there objective responses in the metastatic hypernephroma group?

Dr. Pilch: Yes. Of the nine that we call stabilization, there were four objective partial regressions. Time doesn't permit me to show the X-rays. There were not complete regressions. But in four patients there was a measurable, obvious contraction of lesions.

Dr. Hobbs: Have you shown that patients' lymphocytes in the test tube can be transformed with your immune RNA?

Dr. Pilch: Many times.

DISCUSSION: NEW APPROACHES TO IMMUNOTHERAPY

Dr. Rapp: In developing a discussion for a session called "New Approaches to Anything," it would seem appropriate to say something about previous or current approaches. I suppose what we have been hearing about in this volume is a pretty fair representation of what's going on now. Based on what I've heard I really am not discouraged—I suppose there is cause for discouragement in what we have heard, but I must say I'm still at least as enthusiastic as I was about the use of immunotherapy in cancer as before the presentations.

I'd like to throw some ideas at you that have been suggested from the experimental laboratory. I want to present these ideas because this is the other side of the coin of "new approaches." There are several ideas from basic immunology that need to be tested, but I think they should be tested in a way that facilitates evaluation of results. I know some of the things I'd like to see done may be extremely difficult or impossible to do because of clinical limitations, but I think we ought to shoot for the best we can.

Let me start by telling you that when John Ziegler came back from Africa, where he studied Burkitt's lymphoma, he told us that it was fairly easy to get patients to participate in some of the immunotherapy studies because traditionally doctors in that area for centuries have rubbed herbs and other medicinals into malignant lesions. They know that if you are going to use immunopotentiation for cancer, you should administer the potentiator intralesionally.

I was impressed by Dr. Whittaker's presentation. I think he has taken a step in the right direction by giving the BCG intravenously. But there is one more step that needs to be taken, and this was almost alluded to by Dr. Pinsky; you ought to think about using immunotherapy before chemotherapy.

Also, you should think about the use of BCG cell walls—not the cell-wall skeletons, but the undegraded cell wall. This would solve many problems in the preparation, storage and standardization of BCG vaccine. It would also eliminate the chance of BCG infection. Experimentally, cell walls in an oil and water emulsion are just as active as living BCG without being infectious. Moreover, cell walls of mycobacteria other than BCG, e.g., smegmatis, are active when used in the Ribi-type vaccine, i.e., incorporated into oil droplets emulsified in water.

Almost all the ideas I have about how to apply immunotherapy to cancer really lead back to Edmund Klein and to William B. Coley. I think if you go back and see what Dr. Klein has done in the past and what he is doing now, you will have the basis for direction. I think we are all familiar with Dr. Klein's work, there are others who have looked at this kind of approach, and I'd like to mention the work of Professor Pillat from Vienna, who died last year.

We became interested in his work recently because Dr. Bast, Dr. Borsos, Dr. Ohanian, and others have pretty good evidence that when you inject certain chemotherapeutic agents directly into tumors, you not only get rid of the injected tumor but the recipient also develops tumor-specific immunity. So it would appear that this approach might actually be chemoimmuno-therapy. In looking around for additional examples of chemoimmunotherapy, we found the work of Dr. Pillat. He treated lid carcinomas in many patients by injecting a chemotherapeutic agency (E-39) directly into the tumor. He claimed success with this treatment in about 100 cases (A. Pillat, *Wiener Med. Wochenschr.* 110:975, 1960).

I would like to mention a clinical cancer which happens to occur in a cow. This is a metastasizing squamous cell carcinoma that occurs naturally and at high frequency in several breeds of cattle, notably Herefords. It is agnogenic but sunlight has been postulated as an etiologic factor. It can start on the cornea, the corneoscleral junction, the lacrimal lake, the nictitating membrane or the eyelid. It is almost always metastatic to lymph nodes and sometimes to lung. If left untreated, it invariably leads to the death of the animal.

Current therapies for this disease are unsatisfactory. In a recent study of the efficacy of immunotherapy for bovine ocular squamous cell carcinoma, 24 animals were treated by intralesional injection of BCG cell wall vaccine. Seventeen of them either had complete regression of their disease (some for more than one year so far) or are still alive with no apparent progression of disease since they were treated. Among 18 control animals all either have progressive disease or have been killed because of the pain accompanying advanced disease. Nine of the control animals were untreated and nine received vaccine with the BCG cell walls in the aqueous rather than the oil phase. Although experiments are not yet completed to determine whether metastases were present at the time of treatment, the success achieved in the treatment of relatively large primaries suggests that metastases have been affected. Autopsy of 12 animals killed because of advanced disease showed that 10 had lymph node metastases and one a lung metastasis.

These results suggest that a major cooperative study should be carried out on the treatment of those human squamous cell carcinomas for which current therapies may not be satisfactory. Several clinicians have told me that among the malignancies that might be candidates for intralesional immunotherapy are those that occur in the mouth, the lower part of the esophagus, the anus, or the penis. It has been suggested that bronchogenic squamous cell carcinoma occurring at the carina might be treated successfully by intralesional immunotherapy.

Dr. Weiss: I should like to discuss briefly a comment referring to the possibility of *in vitro* sensitization of effector cells. I refer to the work of Dr. Eli Kedar and his group. An intensive effort has been made by him in our laboratories in the past two years on *in vitro* sensitization (or "education") and the results to date point encouragingly to a new approach to immunotherapy. Dr. Kedar has been concentrating on tumor systems in which it is difficult or impossible to demonstrate immunization against tumor *in vitro* or sensitization of effector cells *in vitro*.

Now, it turns out that the addition of as little as 1 microgram per milliliter of MER, or less, to the cell education mixture *in vitro* makes for very effective sensitization, in two phases—a highly specific sensitization towards the educating tumor cells in the mixture, and a nonspecific sensitization phase in which effector cells, even in the absence of any neoplastic cells, become highly cytotoxic to a variety of tumor cells *in vitro*. We then tested these effector cells in both Winn-type assays and in passive or adoptive immunotherapy experiments; these *in vitro* educated effector cells were seen to be highly effective in both.

We have now reached the point of doing this with human peripheral blood lymphocytes against a variety of autochthonous malignant cells in culture, and are observing that even where there is no *in vitro* sensitization in the absence of an immunostimulator, the presence of such very small amounts of MER makes for an effective specific and nonspecific sensitization process. It has also been shown that prolonged preservation of peripheral blood effector cells does not affect adversely their ability to be educated *in vitro* or to exhibit effector action. These observations have direct clinical implications for therapy with autochthonous cells obtained from patients, preferably in remission, sensitized *in vitro*, cryopreserved, and reintroduced early in relapse or otherwise as indicated.

I mention this also because it bears on an ongoing dialogue between Dr. Rapp and myself: whether it is really a generality that nonspecific immunostimulators have to be introduced directly into a tumor lesion in order to be effective. I cannot accept this as a *general* rule and Kedar's *in vitro* studies indicate that nonspecific immunostimulators can work *directly* on the level of effector cell sensitization, specifically and nonspecifically.

Perhaps our current emphasis on *in vitro* development of cytotoxic effector cells is also indicative of something else. When people do not know what they are talking about in several different fields, they go and study the interface between them. So, we are here focusing on the interface between specific and nonspecific sensitization, still knowing very little about the molecular mechanisms of either, and coming up with a rather interesting phenomenon.

Dr. Hersh: Dr. Rapp has emphasized the local, or what I prefer to call the regional, effect repeatedly over the years, and I think there is great merit in it.

Some of our own data in melanoma support this. You will recall our failure to affect IV-B disease arising from head and neck primaries. In contrast, we have observed an apparent improved response in regional lymph node areas in Stage IV-B melanoma. There have been a couple of reports now showing that intravenous immunotherapy with *C. parvum* has in itself caused objective regression of tumor. This has been mainly in the liver and lung and these are the areas where *C. parvum* localizes when administered intravenously. In our own very recent study with *C. parvum* in melanoma, we have seen a dramatic improvement in survival.

I really do not think there is only one pathway to the clearing in the woods, and I'd like to think that there will eventually develop a multimodality approach to immunotherapy in which we will be able to characterize the individual immunological problems and will be able to tailor our immunotherapy to those. I think that the regional approach and the suggestion that immunotherapy come before conventional therapy is an important one.

Dr. Rapp: My working hypothesis, for which there is good evidence, is that no matter what method you use, unless you end up with a specific immune response detrimental to the tumor, no immunotherapeutic modality is going to work. To consider the use of BCG or MER as nonspecific immunotherapy only is inadequate. It involves elements of nonspecificity, but the final result is systemic tumor-specific immunity.

Dr. Weiss: In this light I would consider agents like BCG and MER as nonspecific aids to the development of specific immunity.

Dr. Rapp: I agree. And if you can do it by *in vitro* sensitization or by any other means I think you are going to be successful.

Dr. Nauts: I am very glad that Dr. Hersh brought up the fact that there are some other things besides BCG that can be used, such as endotoxins. There have been many positive findings with mixed bacterial vaccines known as Coley's toxins. They were given without chemotherapy because chemotherapy was not in existence in those days. There were five-year survivals in at least 240 of 590 inoperable cases. The importance of injections into the tumor was also quite apparent, and so, Dr. Rapp, I think your point is well taken. A few early experiments on dogs showed that you could produce complete regression with injections remote from the tumor. But it took a great deal longer to achieve a therapeutic effect and you might lose control of the tumor during that period. In recent years we have learned that certain bacteria can increase immunogenicity of substances but to do so they must be very close to the target tissue.

Dr. Rosenberg: The clinical problems we are attacking are complex, but we must maintain a scientific attitude towards the work we perform in patients. With that in mind, I would like to pose some questions.

First, Dr. Pilch, you presented to us data relating to an uncontrolled trial of patients with Stage II melanoma that consisted of 10 patients. I wonder if you think there is any conclusion that could be drawn from those data and, if so, what do you think scientifically is the strongest conclusion that one might make?

Dr. Pilch: Those 10 patients with minimum residual melanoma were part of a Phase I experiment to determine whether administration to humans of immune RNA made in sheep produced any toxicity. We found that xenogeneic immune RNA made in sheep injected intradermally in the dosages that we used (up to 40 mg) was completely safe, even when given over very extended periods. Prospectively randomized Phase II trials are now needed to see if there is a useful immunotherapeutic effect against cancer by immune RNA.

In the hypernephroma series, the data are perhaps more useful because this was a gross disease where lesions could be measured. Survival is hard data. But without a control population it is very difficult to draw any conclusions, and randomized studies will be necessary.

Dr. Rosenberg: Dr. Rapp, I don't know what you want us to take away from the fact that in animals that have a local tumor, one can inject material and make the tumor go away. What do you think one can conclude from that work as it relates to the clinical problems that we face in patients with malignant disease? For example, do you have evidence that any disease other than local disease has been affected?

Dr. Rapp: We have prevented the development of metastases.

Dr. Rosenberg: But do you have any evidence that established metastatic disease was affected at all by the therapy?

Dr. Rapp: There is indirect evidence and direct evidence is now being sought. But metastasis is not the only justification for trying immunotherapy. If you have a situation which is difficult to handle surgically, you ought to consider immunotherapy.

Question: To continue Dr. Rosenberg's comments on the intratumoral chemotherapy in one hundred patients with squamous cell carcinoma of the eyelid, there are data showing that such patients can be treated very effectively with radiation alone.

Dr. Morton: I think many of us agree that if you have a choice, it's better to put the BCG into the lesion. There is a very long clinical history in malignant melanoma indicating that intralesional injection can cause regression of cutaneous lesions. However, the problem has been that the patients with gross disease in visceral organs do not respond. Now, I don't think this invalidates the concept that you proposed, Dr. Rapp. The problem is that in dealing with human cancer, one has to have a suitable treatment control. If I were to design your study in cattle, I think it would be necessary to compare cattle treated with radiation therapy, and a group of cattle treated with radical surgery, including a regional lymph node dissection, because that's comparable to what we have to deal with clinically. I think there is really no objection to carrying these concepts into the clinic, but it has to be done, I think, in a carefully controlled trial.

Dr. Rapp: Yes, I agree. But immunotherapy should be tested in primary disease, not recurrent disease. Under ideal conditions, immunotherapy should be used when there are no metastases. On the basis of present knowledge, immunotherapy should not be used in advanced cancer, even if you reduce the tumor burden. Before I could even think about how to treat advanced cancer immunologically I would need to see experimental justification and to have the confidence that might be obtained from human trials of intralesional BCG for early squamous cell carcinoma.

Dr. Mickshe: I would like to make a comment on new approaches to immunotherapy in the treatment of squamous cell carcinoma, especially in the lung. Since 1969 a group under the direction of Professor Wraba has been treating patients with inoperable lung cancer by administering high doses of vitamin A orally. Our initial purpose was to potentiate chemotherapy, radiotherapy, or active specific immunotherapy (injection of extracts of lung cancer tissue). By following up patients it turns out this is a form of immunotherapy, and this is now well documented in animal studies.

By giving vitamin A alone to lung cancer patients with very depressed immune responses, we found a restoration of the responses. Patients given vitamin A pretreatment had more objective remission and longer survival.

Based on these results, vitamin A is being used together with active specific immunization, in the form of solubilized tumor antigen, in a randomized prospective trial for inoperable squamous cell carcinoma of the lung. This form of treatment is being compared to polychemotherapy and to symptomatic therapy. In summary, after having treated more than 140 patients by administration of large doses of vitamin A, it can be stated that this form of treatment has a local effect on the tumor itself; approximately 20 percent objective remissions were obtained. In addition, there was potent immunostimulation. Therapy studies in other localizations of squamous cell carcinomas are now being performed with vitamin A alone or with other treatment modalities.

Dr. Woodruff: May I comment on your remarks about the use of immunotherapy in metastatic disease, Dr. Rapp? I couldn't agree more that in gross metastatic disease you are not going to get anywhere with immunotherapy. But to the surgeon, and we will hear more about this, the critical problem in cancer is the invisible, small metastasis that is beyond the reach of surgery. It's a cinch to remove a little tumor below the eye or somewhere. It may leave a bit of a scar. But what is totally beyond surgery is to deal with the scattered cells, and it seems to me that in solid tumors of the kind surgeons deal with, this is the test of immunotherapy. Either it can do that or it's of no use.

Dr. Rapp: In guinea pigs with a primary tumor and a few cells in the draining lymph node, injection of BCG into the primary tumor not only eliminates the injected tumor but the microscopic metastases as well. If it weren't for that, I wouldn't be interested in BCG at all. Our job now is to determine whether in the cow disease, BCG treatment affects metastases. I think we have indirect evidence that it does, because the anecdotal experience is that local surgery doesn't work regularly with tumors of the size that are easily cured by BCG.

Immunotherapy of Cancer: Present Status of Trials in Man, edited by W. D. Terry and D. Windhorst. Raven Press, New York © 1978.

Therapy of Colorectal Carcinoma

Philip S. Schein and Daniel F. Hoth

Division of Medical Oncology, Vincent T. Lombardi Cancer Research Center, Georgetown University School of Medicine, Washington, D.C. 20007

Colorectal carcinoma is a major health problem in the United States. It ranks second to skin cancer in overall incidence, with approximately 100,000 new cases diagnosed each year or 15% of all cancer. Almost 50,000 deaths per year are directly attributable to this disease or 13% of all cancer mortality—second only to lung cancer in this category (1). Although it has been one of the most extensively investigated malignancies with regard to therapy, relatively little progress has been made, as reflected in the rather static survival statistics over the past three decades. For this reason, a major emphasis in clinical research has been directed toward surgical adjuvant therapy, an approach first evaluated in the late 1950s.

The design and analysis of any clinical trial of adjuvant therapy is significantly improved by the identification of patients at high risk for relapse. Accumulated experience in the treatment of colorectal cancer has resulted in an appreciation of some of the major prognostic variables that serve to identify these patients.

A heavy emphasis has been given to the Dukes' classification, which correlates the degree of penetration of the colonic wall and involvement of lymph nodes with ultimate survival prospects (2). This classification system has undergone a series of adaptations, and at the present time the Astler–Coller modification is widely accepted (3). Patients with tumor that has invaded through the muscularis and serosa or that has spread to lymph nodes have a relatively poor survival after surgical resection with curative intent. These data represent an approximation of survival statistics from several large series (4–8). In particular, they demonstrate the importance of distinguishing between lymph node-positive cases that do or do not have transmural invasion of the bowel wall, C_1 versus C_2. Although experience differs from center to center, the population of patients who present with stage B_2 and C disease represents a substantial proportion of all cases of colorectal cancer—in the range of 40 to 70%.

Both the number and location of involved nodes have been correlated with prognosis. Copeland has demonstrated a progressive decrease in survival with increasing number of involved nodes; 5-year survival for patients with one or two involved nodes was 30%, whereas patients with five or more positive nodes had a 5-year survival of only 10% (6). Dukes analyzed his C cases according to location of involved nodes; those patients with involvement of only the paracolic nodes demonstrated a 41% 5-year survival, whereas if the involvement extended along the lymphovascular pedicle to the highest point of ligature, survival was reduced to 14% (2).

It is important to recognize that the reported incidence of nodal involvement may be a function of the method and diligence of the pathologic search. Nodes may be identified either by gross dissection or, more satisfactorily, by a technique referred to as "clearing." In this method, the entire specimen is treated with agents that render the tissue translucent. Thus the quality of pathologic review is an important variable when one attempts to analyze the validity of results from treatment programs.

Histologic grading has also been shown to correlate with survival. Using Broder's system, Sanfelippo and Beahrs reviewed 391 cases at the Mayo Clinic and reported survival of 56% for grades I and II, versus 32% for the more undifferentiated grades III and IV at 5 years (9). Dukes, utilizing his own grading system, reported 5-year survivals of 77% for low-grade tumors compared to 61% for average-grade and 29% for high-grade malignancies (2).

Although histologic grade and other pathologic features, such as venous invasion, serve as indices of prognosis, it is unlikely that they function as independent variables but rather co-relate to the two major and apparently independent variables of the Dukes staging system—depth of penetration of bowel wall and involvement of regional nodes.

Of particular interest are the early data of Holyoke and co-workers that suggest the preoperative serum carcinoembryonic antigen (CEA) concentration may have significant prognostic value. In a preliminary report, patients with Dukes' C lesions were divided retrospectively into two groups according to their preoperative CEA level. Among 10 patients with levels below 2.5 ng, only two relapsed, whereas among 11 patients with values greater than 2.5 ng, there were seven relapses (10,11). These data suggest that preoperative CEA may provide significant prognostic information that is additive to the Dukes' staging system. If these data are confirmed in further reports, it will be important to know the results of analyses of this type in any study purporting to demonstrate improved treatment results.

The first controlled clinical trials of adjuvant therapy in colorectal cancer involved the use of alkylating agents thio-tepa and nitrogen mustard. In 1957 the Veterans Administration Surgical Adjuvant Group (VASAG) randomized resected patients to receive either thio-tepa (given both intraoperatively and postoperatively) or placebo. The overall results favored the placebo-treated group, which had a 57% 5-year survival compared to 50% for the chemotherapy group (11). An independent study with similar results was reported by the university hospitals (12).

Following the demonstration that the fluorinated pyrimidines 5-fluorouracil

(5-FU) and the deoxyriboside 5-fluorodeoxyuridine (5-FUdR) were capable of producing objective regressions in advanced disease, attention was directed toward the use of these drugs in the surgical adjuvant setting.

In patients with advanced disease, it is generally accepted that an objective response of 20% can be achieved with the use of 5-fluorouracil (13). It should be emphasized that despite our 19 years of experience with 5-fluorouracil in the treatment of colorectal cancer, controversy persists about the optimal method of administration. A wide range of dose schedules and routes of drug delivery has been recommended. We have now achieved some clarification from the results of recently completed controlled clinical trials.

The original dose schedule for 5-fluorouracil, 5-day intravenous high-dose loading courses followed by alternate day therapy, frequently produced serious and life-threatening toxicity (14). We have since learned that such adverse reactions are not a prerequisite for maximum response, although a mild-moderate degree of leukopenia is required to ensure that a biologically active dose has been administered (15).

There have been strong proponents for the use of oral 5-fluorouracil, particularly for patients with hepatic metastases; response rates of 50 to 70% have been reported in uncontrolled trials (16,17). The original rationale for this approach was the direct delivery of the drug to the liver via the portal venous system.

Three controlled trials that compared oral versus intravenous 5-fluorouracil for metastatic colorectal cancer have been completed. All have demonstrated the superiority of the intravenous route of administration (18–20). Pharmacologic studies have demonstrated erratic blood levels of biologically active drug after oral administration (21).

The Central Oncology Group has compared four basic schedules of 5-fluorouracil administration in patients with advanced measurable adenocarcinoma of the colon in a randomized controlled trial (20). The standard for comparison was the so-called intravenous loading course of 12 mg/kg daily for five consecutive days followed by alternate day treatment with 6 mg/kg until toxicity. These patients were subsequently placed on weekly maintenance therapy with 15 mg/kg. This regimen produced a 38% objective response rate that was significantly higher than the 10 to 15% response obtained with the popular weekly intravenous treatment, a low-dose (500 mg) intravenous loading course, or the oral route. This study has been questioned because the response rate for their high-dose loading course—38%—is significantly higher than the usual remission rate achieved with this single agent. In spite of this, survival was not prolonged for patients receiving the more toxic intravenous loading regimen.

In view of these data, it is fortunate that the major controlled trials of fluorinated pyrimidines when used as surgical adjuvant chemotherapy have employed what is now considered the optimal method of administration—intravenous loading courses.

The Veterans Administration Group has conducted three controlled trials of adjuvant chemotherapy using fluorinated pyrimidines (22–24). As the results of these studies are identical, only the most recent trial is reviewed here.

In this study patients with colorectal cancer who were considered to have a poor prognosis based upon a histologic review of the resected specimen were randomized to receive either 5-FU or no further treatment. 5-FU was administered at an intravenous dose of 12 mg/kg for four successive days. The first course was given 2 weeks following operation, and repeated courses were administered at 6- to 8-week intervals until the 19th postoperative month. Between 1969 and 1973, 522 patients who had undergone a "curative" resection were entered into the trial. The 5-year survival of treated cases is 49% compared to 44% for controls, not a statistically significant difference. In addition, 163 patients with proved residual disease after surgery were also randomized; the survival at 2 years was 31% in the treated group compared to 25% in controls, again a small but not statistically significant difference (24,25).

It has been demonstrated that optimal response rates for 5-FU in colorectal cancer require that a moderate degree of myelosuppressive toxicity be produced (15). One of the criticisms of the Veterans Administration prolonged intermittent therapy study was that relative few patients developed leukopenia during the 19 months of treatment.

However, a more intensive trial of 5-FU adjuvant chemotherapy has been conducted by the Central Oncology Group (26). Patients undergoing curative or palliative resection were randomized to receive either 5-FU or no further treatment until relapse. 5-FU was administered intravenously using a dose schedule of 12 mg/kg daily for four days followed by 6 mg/kg on alternate days for 5 additional days. Following a 7 to 14 day rest, weekly maintenance chemotherapy of 12 mg/kg was continued for 1 year. In contrast to the VA study, 60% of patients developed some degree of leukopenia. As of March of this year (1976), 372 patients had been entered on this study, of which 81% were acceptable for analysis, including 92 patients with Dukes' B and 97 patients with Dukes' C colorectal cancer who had undergone surgical resection with curative intent.

The disease-free interval for the Dukes' curative resection cases approached statistical significance ($p = 0.06$) with a median of 24 months for the chemotherapy group versus 16 months for control. However, this has not been translated into an increased survival for the treated group ($p = 0.18$). The prognostic importance of drug-induced leukopenia was analyzed. The disease-free interval was significantly longer ($p = 0.004$) for patients in whom the white blood cell count was reduced below 4,000 with chemotherapy, but once again there was no impact on survival.

In spite of a few isolated, uncontrolled series that have suggested benefit with postoperative 5-FU, the consistent conclusions reached by the prospective randomized trials cited above make it painfully clear that all future use of 5-FU as single agent adjuvant therapy in colorectal cancer is similarly doomed to failure and that new approaches are required.

Wherever significant advances have been made in the chemotherapy of cancer, it has largely come about through the development and effective use of drug combinations. Of the many anticancer agents that have been adequately evaluated for activity in colorectal cancer, none has proven superior to 5-fluorouracil (27,28). The chloroethyl nitrosoureas 1-3-bis-(2-chloroethyl)-1-nitrosourea (BCNU), 1-(2-chloroethyl)-3-cyclohexyl-1-nitrosourea (CCNU), and methyl CCNU have all demonstrated a response rate of 10 to 15% in patients with advanced disease (29). Attention has largely shifted to methyl CCNU, which in one controlled trial demonstrated activity equivalent to 5-fluorouracil (30).

There have been many attempts to develop effective drug combinations using the limited number of agents available. Combinations of 5-fluorouracil and BCNU or mitomycin-C reached response rates that were no better than those demonstrated with 5-fluorouracil as a single agent (31). Nevertheless, despite these initial disappointing trials investigations continued, and in 1974 Falkson and co-workers reported a 43% response with the combination of 5-fluorouracil, BCNU, vincristine, and dimethyl triazeno imidazole carboxamide (DTIC) (32). Subsequently, Moertel and co-workers reported the results of a controlled clinical trial in which the combination of 5-fluorouracil, methyl CCNU, and vincristine was compared to 5-fluorouracil as a single agent (33). The combination produced a 43.5% response rate, which was statistically superior to the 19.5% for the single agent. The activity of the regimen, with or without vincristine, has been confirmed in the studies of the Southwest Oncology Group (34) and by Falkson and co-workers (35). Similarly at the Vincent Lombardi Cancer Center we have reported a 40% partial response with weekly 5-fluorouracil administered in the same regimen (36).

Despite the increased percent of response there appears to have been no significant impact on the survival. This observation separates colorectal cancer from most other malignancies in which response usually translates into increased survival, and dramatizes the need for continued clinical investigation in the management of advanced large bowel cancer. However there is some expectation that the 5-fluorouracil—methyl CCNU regimen may be more successful in the surgical adjuvant setting in patients with microscopic residual tumor.

The other leads that have aroused new interest in surgical adjuvant therapy are the early results of immunotherapy and immunochemotherapy with Bacillus. Calmette-Guerin (BCG) and oral 5-FU for Dukes' C colorectal cancer (see chapter by Mavligit et al., this volume). The use of a retrospective control, the failure to provide a detailed analysis of the pathologic features, and the use of oral 5-FU has raised serious questions regarding the validity of these data (37).

The Mayo Clinic has used the methanol extracted residue of BCG, or

MER, in 33 patients with advanced measurable colorectal cancer and observed three instances in which patients achieved a 50% or greater regression of disease with associated improvements in symptoms.

These new approaches are now being objectively tested by the Gastrointestinal Tumor Study Group. Patients with Dukes' B_2 and C colon cancer who have undergone surgical resection are being randomized to chemotherapy with 5-FU + methyl CCNU, immunotherapy with MER, chemoimmunotherapy, or a no-treatment control. A positive result in any of the treatment arms should be quite convincing because of the optimal design of the study.

Rectal cancer requires separate consideration because of the potential role of radiation therapy. The rational for radiation therapy is based on (a) its radiosensitivity and (b) its unique pattern of local recurrence without distant metastases in a substantial proportion of patients.

In contrast to previously held concepts, there is little question that rectal cancer is sensitive to radiation. Effective symptomatic palliation and objective regression in locally unresectable and recurrent disease can be effected in 80% of patients (38,39). However less than 10% of such cases achieve long-term benefit. As with chemotherapy, there is reason to believe that radiation therapy might be maximally effective in a patient with minimal residual disease.

Gunderson has provided us with a valuable analysis of sites of relapse found at reoperation following curative resection for rectal cancer (40). In a series of 75 patients undergoing a second operation, 52 were found to have recurrent tumor. Distant metastasis as a sole expression of relapse was uncommon and was demonstrated in only 8% of cases. However local failure and regional lymph node metastasis occurred frequently; they were the only site of failure in 50% of cases and were a component of relapse in 92%. This pattern of failure was predictable based on anatomic factors, specifically (a) the direct extension of the tumor to contiguous tissues and organs and (b) lymphatic drainage patterns; that is, the upper rectum drains to lymph nodes that follow the superior hemorrhoidal and inferior mesenteric arteries. The latter vessel inserts into the aorta at about the level of the second lumbar vertebrae. The lower rectum drains inferiorly to the internal iliac nodes. The major importance of this study is the demonstration that a high percentage of relapses following surgery in rectal cancer occurs in an anatomic distribution that is readily encompassed within a pre- or postoperative radiation port.

The largest single experience with preoperative radiation as a surgical adjuvant for rectal cancer has been reported by Memorial Hospital. Between 1939 and 1951, 727 of a total of 1,276 cases seen were treated preoperatively at dose levels of 1,500 to 2,000 rads. In a nonrandomized comparison 37% of the Dukes' C cases who received radiation therapy were alive at 5 years compared to 27% for a nonirradiated Dukes' C group (41). A subsequent randomized study performed at the same institution utilizing 2,500 rads failed to demonstrate any survival benefit with radiation (42). In addition, in both studies radiation therapy did not alter the relative incidence of Dukes' C (lymph node-positive) cases, a claim that is now being made in several other studies (43–45).

In 1964 VASAG initiated a randomized trial of preoperative radiation therapy using 2,000 rads to a pelvic port. A total of 700 patients was entered into this study. Among 453 patients in whom a curative resection was possible, the group treated with radiation had a 5-year survival of 49% versus 39% for the control group, which was not statistically significant ($0.05 < p < 0.1$) (43,44).

The data were also analyzed for the type of operation performed. For 414 patients who had an abdominoperineal resection, both curative and palliative, the 5-year survival was 41% with radiation, statistically better than the 28% for controls ($p < 0.02$). However, if these data are analyzed only for patients who had curative abdominoperineal resection (i.e., no gross evidence of residual disease), the difference is no longer statistically significant, nor is it significant if the Dukes' C cases are specifically analyzed as a subgroup. In addition, there was no observed difference in survival when resection other than the abdominoperineal approach was employed for lesions above the peritoneal reflection. The VA study did find a reduction in involved nodes in patients who had received preoperative radiation therapy. These data have also been confirmed by both Kligerman and the University of Oregon using higher doses of radiation (45,46).

It is quite clear that, despite the extensive past trials of surgical adjuvant therapy for colorectal cancer, we are still at an early stage of development. Nevertheless, there is reason for cautious optimism for the future.

Unfortunately however, there are physicians who are using regimens such as 5-FU and methyl-CCNU or BCG as routine surgical adjuvant therapy for colorectal cancer even though there are no clear data to support these approaches.

In view of the extensive negative past experience with adjuvant therapy for this disease, it is essential that the efficacy of these newer and potentially toxic regimens be subjected to rigorous controlled trials before they are accepted as normal postoperative practice.

REFERENCES

1. Seidman, H., Silverberg, E., and Holleb, A. I. (1976): Cancer statistics, 1976. A comparison of white and black populations. *Cancer,* 26(1):2–29.
2. Dukes, C. E., and Bussey, H. J. R. (1958): The spread of rectal cancer and its effect on prognosis. *Br. J. Cancer,* 12:309.
3. Astler, V. B., and Coller, F. A. (1954): The prognostic significance of direct extension of carcinoma of the colon and rectum. *Ann. Surg.,* 139:846.
4. Turnbull, R. A. (1975): The no touch isolation technique of resection. *JAMA,* 231:1181.
5. Thomas, W. H., Larson, R. A., Wright, H. K., and Cleveland, J. C. (1969): Analysis of 830 patients with rectal adeno-carcinoma. *Surg. Gynecol. Obstet.,* 129:10.

6. Copeland, E. M., Miller, L. D., and Jones, R. S. (1968): Prognostic factors in carcinoma of the colon and rectum. *Am. J. Surg.,* 116:875.
7. Stearns, M. W., and Schottenfeld, D. (1971): Techniques for the surgical management of colon cancer. *Cancer,* 28:165.
8. Gilbersten, V. A. (1967): Improving the prognosis for patients with intestinal cancer. *Surg. Gynecol. Obstet.,* 124:1253.
9. Sanfelippo, P. M., and Beahrs, O. H. (1972): Factors in the prognosis of adenocarcinoma of the colon and rectum. *Arch. Surg.,* 104:401.
10. Herrera, M., Chu, T. M., and Holyoke, E. D. (1976): Carcinoembryonic antigen (CEA) as a prognostic and monitoring test in clinically complete resection of colorectal carcinoma. *Ann. Surg.,* 183:5–8.
11. Veterans Administration Surgical Adjuvant Cancer Chemotherapy Group (1965): Adjuvant use of HN2 (NSC-762) and thio-tepa (NSC-6396): Progress report. *Cancer Chemother. Rep.,* 44:27–30.
12. Dixon, W. J., Longmire, W. P., Jr., and Holden, W. D. (1971): Use of triethylenethiophosphoramide as an adjuvant to the surgical treatment of gastric and colorectal carcinoma: Ten-year follow up. *Ann. Surg.,* 173:26.
13. Carter, S. K. (1976): Large bowel cancer: The current status of treatment. *J. Natl. Cancer Inst.,* 56:3–10.
14. Ansfield, F. J., and Curreri, A. R. (1959): Further clinical studies with 5-fluorouracil. *J. Natl. Cancer Inst.,* 22:497–507.
15. Moertel, C. G., Reitemeier, R. J., and Hahn, R. G. (1969): Therapy with the fluorinated pyrimidines. In: *Advanced Gastrointestinal Cancer,* edited by C. G. Moertel and R. J. Reitemeier, pp. 86–107. Harper (Hoeber), New York.
16. Khung, C. L., Hall, T. C., Piro, A. J., and Sederick, M. M. (1966): A clinical trial of oral 5-fluorouracil. *Clin. Pharmacol. Ther.,* 7:527–533.
17. Lahiri, S. R., Boileau, G., and Hall, T. C. (1971): Treatment of metastatic colorectal carcinoma with 5-fluorouracil by mouth. *Cancer,* 28:902–906.
18. Hahn, R. G., Moertel, C. G., Schutt, A. J., and Bruckner, H. W. (1975): A double blind comparison of intensive course 5-FU by oral vs intravenous route in the treatment of colorectal carcinoma. *Cancer,* 35:1031–1035.
19. Bateman, J., Irwin, L., Pugh, R., Cassidy, F., and Weiner, J. (1975): Comparison of intravenous and oral administration of 5-fluorouracil for colorectal carcinoma. *Proc. Am. Soc. Clin. Oncol.,* 16:242.
20. Ansfield, F. (1975): A randomized phase III study of four dosage regimens of 5-FU: A preliminary report. *Proc. Am. Soc. Clin. Oncol.,* 16:224.
21. Cohen, J. L., Irwin, L. E., Marshall, G. J., Darvey, H., and Bateman, J. R. (1974): Clinical pharmacology of oral and intravenous 5-fluorouracil (NSC-19893). *Cancer Chemother. Rep.,* 58:723.
22. Dwight, R. W., Humphrey, E. W., Higgins, G. A., and Keehn, R. J. (1973): FUDR as an adjuvant to surgery in cancer of the large bowel. *J. Surg. Oncol.,* 5:243.
23. Higgins, G. A., Dwight, R. W., Smith, J. V., and Keehn, R. J. (1971): Fluorouracil as an adjuvant to surgery in carcinoma of the colon. *Arch. Surg.,* 102:339.
24. Higgins, G. A., Humphrey, E., Juler, G. L., LeVeen, H. H., McCaughan, J., and Keehn, R. J. (1976): Adjuvant chemotherapy in the surgical treatment of large bowel cancer. *Cancer,* 38:1461.
25. Higgins, G. A. (1976): Chemotherapy adjuvant to surgery. *Clin. Gastroenterol.,* 5:795.
26. Grage, T., Cornell, G., Strawitz, J., Jonas, K., Frelick, R., and Metter, G. (1975): Adjuvant therapy with 5-FU after surgical resection of colorectal cancer. *Proc. Am. Soc. Clin. Oncol.,* 16:258.
27. Moertel, C. G. (1976): Chemotherapy of gastrointestinal cancer. *Clin. Gastroenterol.,* 5:777.
28. Carter, S. K., and Friedman, M. (1974): Integration of chemotherapy into combined modality therapy of solid tumors. II. Large bowels carcinoma. *Cancer Treat. Rev.,* 1:114–128.
29. Moertel, C. G., Schutt, A. J., Reitemeier, R., and Hahn, R. G. (1976): Therapy for gastrointestinal cancer with the nitrosoureas alone and in drug combination. *Cancer Treat. Rep.,* 60:729.

30. Moertel, C. G. (1975): Clinical management of advanced gastrointestinal cancer. *Cancer,* 36:675–682.
31. Moertel, C. G., Reitemeier, R. J., and Hahn, R. G. (1970): Combination chemotherapy in advanced gastrointestinal cancer. *Cancer Res.,* 30:1425–1428.
32. Falkson, G., Van Eden, E. G., and Falkson, H. C. (1974): Fluorouracil, imadazole carboximide dimethyltriazeno, vincristine and bis-chloroethylnitrosourea in colon cancer. *Cancer,* 33:1207–1209.
33. Moertel, C. G., Schutt, A. J., Hahn, R. G., and Reitemeier, R. J. (1975): Therapy of advanced colorectal cancer with a combination of 5-fluorouracil, methyl-1, 3-cis (2-chloroethyl)-1-nitrosourea and vincristine. *J. Natl. Cancer Inst.,* 54:69.
34. Baker, L. H., Talley, R. W., Matter, R., Lehane, D. E., Ruffner, B. W., Jones, S. E., Morrison, F. S., Stepheus, R. L., Gehan, E. A., and Vaitkevicius, V. K. (1976): Phase III comparison of the treatment of advanced gastrointestinal cancer with bolus weekly 5-FU vs methyl CCNU plus bolus weekly 5-FU. *Cancer,* 38:1.
35. Falkson, G., and Falkson, H. C. (1976): Fluorouracil, methyl-CCNU and vincristine in cancer of the colon. *Cancer,* 38:1468.
36. Kisner, D., Schein, P., Smith, L., Cohen, P., Smythe, T., and Duvall, C. (1977): 5-fluorouracil, methyl-CCNU and vincristine (FMV) for colorectal carcinoma: Confirmation of increased response rate using weekly 5-FU. *Cancer Treat. Rep.* (*In press.*)
37. Wood, C. B., Gillis, C. R., and Blumgart, C. H. (1976): Use of historic controls in cancer studies. *Lancet,* 2:251.
38. Kligerman, M. R. (1976): Radiation therapy for rectal carcinoma. *Semin. Oncol.,* 3:407.
39. Gunderson, L. L. (1976): Radiation therapy: Results and future possibilities. *Clin. Gastroenterol.,* 5:743.
40. Gunderson, L. L., and Sosin, H. (1974): Areas of failure found at reoperation (second or symptomatic look) following "curative surgery" for adenocarcinoma of the rectum. *Cancer,* 34:1278.
41. Quan, S. H. (1966): Preoperative radiation for carcinoma of the rectum. *NY State J. Med.,* 66:2243.
42. Stearns, M. W., Deddish, M. R., Quan, S. H., and Learning, R. H. (1975): Preoperative roentgen therapy for cancer of the rectum and rectosigmoid. *Surg. Gynecol. Obstet.,* 138:584.
43. Higgins, G. A., Conn, H. J., Jordan, P. H., Humphrey, E. W., Roswit, B., and Keehn, W. S. (1975): Preoperative radiotherapy for colorectal cancer. *Ann. Surg.,* 181:624–631.
44. Roswit, B., Higgins, G. A., and Keehn, R. J. (1975): Preoperative irradiation for carcinoma of the rectum and rectosigmoid color: Report of a National Veterans Administration randomized study. *Cancer,* 35:1597.
45. Kligerman, M. M. (1975): Preoperative radiation therapy in rectal cancer. *Cancer,* 36:691–695.
46. Stevens, K. R., and Allen, C. V. (1977): Preoperative radiotherapy for adenocarcinoma of the rectosigmoid. (*Submitted for publication.*)

*Immurotherapy of Cancer: Present Status of
Trials in Man,* edited by W. D. Terry and D. Windhorst.
Raven Press, New York © 1978.

A Controlled Evaluation of Combined Immunotherapy (MER-BCG) and Chemotherapy for Advanced Colorectal Cancer

C. G. Moertel, M. J. O'Connell, R. E. Ritts, Jr., A. J. Schutt,
R. J. Reitemeier, R. G. Hahn, S. K. Frytak, and J. Rubin

Mayo Clinic, Rochester, Minnesota 55901

Although it seems unlikely that immunotherapy alone will find a significant role in the management of advanced and metastatic malignant disease, there is realistic hope that immune stimulation can contribute to the effectiveness or safety of systemic chemotherapy. It is speculated that this contribution can be made either by the addition of an immunotherapeutic effect or by counteracting a deleterious immunosuppressive effect of chemotherapy. Such considerations, as well as a scattering of optimistic early reports, have formed the background for the current interest in combined immunotherapy–chemotherapy trials as well as for the study reported here.

For our study we elected to employ the methanol extraction residue of Bacillus Calmette-Guerin (MER-BCG) as a nonspecific immunostimulant. Weiss and associates (2) have reported that this nonviable preparation is a potent immunostimulant in animal models. There has also been suggestive evidence that MER added to chemotherapy produces a ·prolongation in survival of patients with acute myelogenous leukemia. For concomitant chemotherapy, we chose three drug combinations that have evidence of anti-tumor activity in advanced colorectal cancer—5-fluorouracil (5-FU) plus methyl cyclohexyl nitrosourea (methyl CCNU), 5-FU plus methyl CCNU plus vincristine, and 5-FU plus cis-diamminedichloroplatinum (CACP).

PATIENTS

All patients selected for study had histologic confirmation of unresectable recurrent or metastatic adenocarcinoma with the primary lesion established as colonic or rectal in origin. All had a measurable area of malignant disease that could be used as an objective indicator of response to therapy. Lesions that could not be directly measured with a ruler or caliper were not included in this category, i.e., extrarectal or pelvic masses, malignant ascites, etc. Malignant hepatomegaly was accepted if the liver measured at least 5 cm below the xyphoid or costal margins on quiet respiration. A lesion noted on liver scan was acceptable if there was a clearly defined perfusion defect measuring at least 5 cm in greatest diameter.

All patients were ambulatory and were maintaining a reasonable state of nutrition prior to treatment. Patients were excluded if they were totally disabled [Eastern Cooperative Oncology Group (ECOG) score 4], if they had significant leukopenia (white blood cell count less than 4,100/mm³) or thrombocytopenia (platelets less than 130,000/mm³), and they were also excluded if there was any evidence of renal insufficiency (creatinine greater than 1.5 mg). No patient was included who had had any previous immunotherapy or any previous chemotherapy with 5-FU, a nitrosourea, vincristine, or CACP. Therapy was deferred for a minimum of 30 days after any abdominal surgery involving resection or anastomosis, for 15 days after abdominal exploration and biopsy only, and for 30 days after any previous chemotherapy or radiation therapy.

TREATMENT

Prior to therapy patients were stratified according to performance status (ECOG score) and according to the distribution of their metastatic malignant disease, e.g., pulmonary, hepatic, abdominal, etc. They were then randomized to one of the following chemotherapy regimens—5-FU plus CACP, 5-FU plus methyl CCNU, or 5-FU plus methyl CCNU plus vincristine. Within each chemotherapy regimen patients were also randomized to receive either concomitant immunotherapy with MER-BCG or no immunotherapy.

Combined CACP and 5-FU: CACP was administered on day 1 in a single intravenous dose of 20 mg/m². 5-FU was administered by rapid i.v. push at a dose of 400 mg/m² daily for 5 days from day 1 through day 5. The same course of combined CACP and 5-FU was repeated on days 36 through 40. Dosages for the second course were reduced if excessive toxicity was experienced with the first course.

Combined 5-FU and methyl CCNU: Methyl CCNU was administered on day 1 in a single oral dose of 175 mg/m². 5-FU was administered by rapid i.v. push at a dosage of 350 mg/m² daily for 5 days from day 1 through day 5. 5-FU, 400 mg/m², was also administered on days 36 through 40. The dosage for this second course of 5-FU alone was reduced if excessive 5-FU toxicity was experienced with the first course.

5-FU + methyl CCNU + vincristine: Methyl CCNU was administered on day 1 in a single oral dose of 175 mg/m². 5-FU was administered by i.v. push at a dosage of 350 mg/m² daily for 5 days from day 1 through day 5. 5-FU, 400 mg/m², was also administered on days 36 through 40. Dosage for the second course was reduced if excessive 5-FU toxicity was experienced with the first course. Vincristine was administered at a dosage of 1 mg/m² on day 1 and on day 36.

MER-BCG: For the first 99 patient entries, those patients assigned to MER received this treatment on days 1, 7, 21, 36, and once every 5 weeks thereafter. When a preliminary analysis of these patient experiences showed increased hematologic toxicity for the MER-BCG-treated patients and no apparent therapeutic advantage, the MER-BCG schedule was changed so that immunotherapy was initiated 3 weeks after initiation of chemotherapy. For these remaining 82 patients, those assigned to MER-BCG received treatment on days 21, 36, and once every 5 weeks thereafter.

On each day of treatment a total dosage of 2 mg of MER-BCG was administered. MER-BCG was given by intradermal injections on the back or flanks, each individual injection containing 0.4 mg.

Before treatment all patients had a complete medical examination, including measurement of indicator lesions. The following laboratory studies were also planned within 72 hr prior to initiation of treatment—routine urinalysis; hemoglobin; leukocyte count; platelet count; differential count; serum creatinine, bilirubin, alkaline phosphatase, glutamic-oxalacetic transaminase, calcium, chest X-ray; skin test with purified protein derivative, mumps, dermatophytin, *Candida,* and SK-SD; dinitrochlorobenzene (DNCB) sensitization; circulating T and B cells; lymphocyte blastogenesis with three dilutions of phytohemagglutinin (PHA), Concanavalin A (Con A), and pokeweed mitogens; and immunoglobulins IgA, IgM, and IgG.

Following therapy patients had white blood counts obtained twice weekly and platelets once weekly. Patients were reevaluated at 5 weeks and at 10 weeks with a general medical assessment, measurement of indicator lesions, and repetition of all pretreatment laboratory studies. If at 10 weeks the patient had shown progression of malignant disease, treatment was discontinued. If he had remained objectively stable without clinical deterioration or if he had shown objective regression, treatment with 5-FU and CACP was continued at 5-week intervals, and cycles of combined 5-FU and methyl CCNU or combined 5-FU, methyl CCNU, and vincristine were repeated every 10 weeks. MER-BCG injections were repeated every 5 weeks for those patients randomized to immunotherapy. Occasionally because of excessive cutaneous reactions it was necessary to reduce dosage of MER or to increase the interval between injections.

STATISTICAL ANALYSIS

All patients randomized on study were initiated on therapy, and all patients initiated on therapy are considered in our analysis of results. Specifically, patients were not considered unevaluable in case of early death or inability to continue therapy. All such patients were considered as having shown progressive disease. All patients initiated on study are also included in our survival analysis. Patients were not excluded if they were suspected, or even known, to have died from causes unrelated to malignant disease. The following criteria were employed in declaring objective regression.

1. There must have been a reduction by at least 50% of the product of the longest perpendicular diameters of the most clearly measurable mass lesion chosen prior to therapy as the primary indicator lesion.

2. If the liver was the primary indicator lesion, there must have been a reduction of the sum of measurements below each costal margin at the midclavicular lines and xyphoid process by at least 30%. If a liver scan was employed in the absence of measurable hepatomegaly, there must have been a 50% reduction in the product of the longest perpendicular diameters of the most clearly defined perfusion defect.

3. There could be no increase in any other areas of malignant disease, and no new areas of malignant disease could appear.

4. There could be no significant deterioration in weight or performance status.

5. This result must be observed at least 2 months after the onset of therapy.

A patient was declared to have shown objective progression if there was an increase in any measurable lesion by greater than 25% of the product of longest perpendicular diameters of any area of malignant disease, if new areas of malignant disease appeared, or if there was significant deterioration in weight (greater than 5%) or decrease in performance status (one level by ECOG score).

RESULTS

The overall distribution of patient characteristics are summarized specifically with regard to the immunotherapy comparison in Table 1. Some prognostic factors were different between the two groups; very well-differentiated tumors were found in a larger proportion of the MER-BCG-treated group and poor performance scores and prior chemotherapy were found in a larger proportion of the group who did not receive MER-BCG. Our prior experiences indicated that each of these factors would weigh in favor of MER-BCG-treated group both in terms of objective response and patient survival. The pretreatment immunologic status of the two patient groups are presented in Table 2; there was a greater proportion of recall skin tests

TABLE 1. *Distribution of pretreatment patient characteristics*

	No MER-BCG	MER-BCG
Characteristic		
Male/female	46/46	44/45
Age: mean	61	59
Grade 1	0	5
2 & 3	87	82
4	4	2
Performance score[a]		
0 & 1	54	60
2 & 3	38	29
Prior radiation	10	11
Prior chemotherapy	28	18
Chemotherapy assignment		
5-FU + CACP	28	28
5-FU + MeCCNU	33	29
5-FU + MeCCNU + VCR	31	32

MeCCNU, methyl CCNU; VCR, vincristine.
[a] ECOG score: 0, fully active, to 4, totally disabled.

TABLE 2. *Pretreatment immunologic determinants*

Assay	No MER-BCG		MER-BCG		Normal range
Recall skin tests					
% tests positive	42	(373 tests)	38	(393 tests)	—
% patients anergic	7	(85)	18	(90)	—
Lymphocytes (mean/mm³)					
Total	1450	(86)	1456	(87)	1820 ± 550
T cells	1261	(61)	1229	(75)	1271 ± 520
B cells	271	(70)	292	(72)	217 ± 43
Lymphocyte blastogenesis (mean cpm × 10³)					
PHA	37	(67)	35	(77)	81 ± 27
Con A	35	(67)	35	(77)	55 ± 23
PWM	28	(67)	28	(77)	32 ± 16
Immunoglobulins (mean ng/ml)					
IgA	2.49	(73)	2.62	(76)	0.3 — 3.0
IgM	1.43	(73)	1.54	(76)	0.2 — 1.4
IgG	11.49	(73)	10.89	(76)	6.4 — 14.3

Number of patients studied in parentheses. Cpm, counts per minute; PWM, pokeweed mitogens.

positive among total skin tests performed in the MER-BCG group, but this group also had a greater proportion of anergic patients. In all other respects, the groups were closely comparable.

Objective response rates are shown in Tables 3 and 4 according to completeness of response, whether or not the patient received immunotherapy, and whether the immunotherapy was administered simultaneously with the onset of chemotherapy or was delayed for 3 weeks after the onset of immunotherapy. It is of interest that our response rates for the regimens incorporating 5-FU plus methyl CCNU are less than we and others have previously observed. This will be the subject of a future publication. It would seem reasonable, however, to conclude that MER-BCG treatment, regardless of when it was initiated, did not have a significant influence on either frequency or completeness of objective response.

TABLE 3. *Objective response according to regimen*

Regimen	Patients	Complete response	Partial response
5-FU + CACP	28	1	6
5-FU + CACP + MER-BCG	28	2	5
5-FU + methyl CCNU	33	3	4
5-FU + methyl CCNU + MER-BCG	29	0	3
5-FU + methyl CCNU + vincristine	31	4	2
5-FU + methyl CCNU + vincristine + MER-BCG	32	2	7

TABLE 4. Objective response rate with and without immunotherapy

		Objective response rate			
		No MER-BCG		MER-BCG	
Early MER	Complete response	4/48	(8%)	3/51	(6%)
	All responses	13/48	(27%)	10/51	(20%)
Delayed MER	Complete response	2/44	(5%)	3/38	(8%)
	All responses	8/44	(18%)	8/38	(21%)
All patients	Complete response	6/92	(7%)	6/89	(7%)
	All responses	21/92	(23%)	18/89	(20%)

Figure 1 displays the duration of objective response as measured from the onset of therapy. It incorporates all patients in both part 1 of our study (early immunotherapy) and part 2 (delayed immunotherapy). Again no advantage can be demonstrated for the patients treated with MER-BCG.

In Fig. 2 we have shown the relationship between immunotherapy and

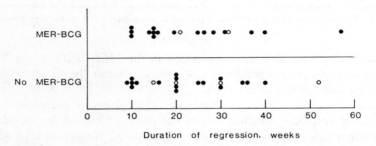

FIG. 1. MER-BCG therapy and duration of objective response. ●, Regression terminated; ○, regression continues.

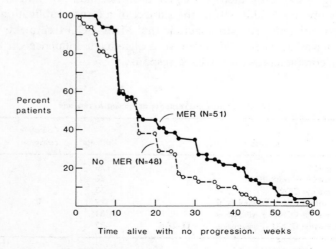

FIG. 2. MER-BCG therapy and time to progression (early MER-BCG).

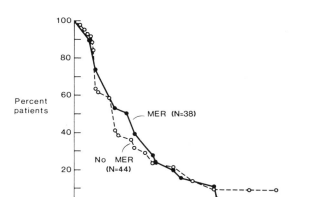

FIG. 3. MER-BCG therapy and time to progression (delayed MER-BCG). (Actuarial presentation. Method of Paul Meier. Twelve patients have not shown progression.)

time to progression in Part 1 of our study (early immunotherapy). The median time to progression is 15 weeks for each group. There is some advantage for the MER-treated group in terms of time to progression, but this is not at a statistically significant level. In part 2 (delayed immunotherapy) the interval to progression seemed totally uninfluenced by immunotherapy (Fig. 3).

Comparative survival times for part 1 of this study are shown in Fig. 4. Survivorships with and without immunotherapy are essentially identical. Data for survival in part 2 are still too incomplete to justify any conclusions, but a preliminary analysis shows no difference.

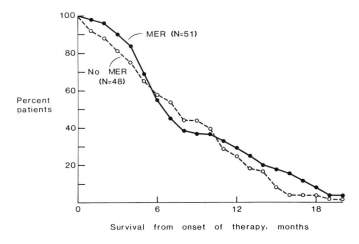

FIG. 4. MER-BCG therapy and patient survival (early MER-BCG).

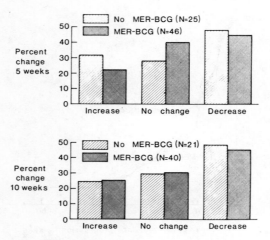

FIG. 5. MER-BCG therapy and change in number of positive recall skin tests (early MER-BCG).

Figures 5 through 10 display changes in recall skin tests, lymphocyte counts, and lymphocyte blastogenesis assays at 5 and 10 weeks after the onset of therapy. These studies, as well as DNCB reactions and immunoglobulins, failed to indicate any demonstrable effect of MER-BCG therapy.

Side Effects of Treatment (toxicity)

The incidence of mucocutaneous and gastrointestinal toxicity to chemotherapy did not seem to be in any way influenced by concomitant immunotherapy.

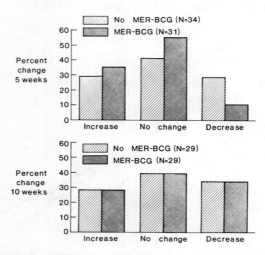

FIG. 6. MER-BCG therapy and change in number of positive recall skin tests (delayed MER-BCG).

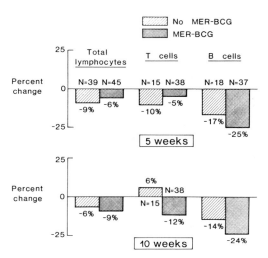

FIG. 7. MER-BCG therapy and change in mean lymphocyte counts (early MER-BCG).

The overall hematologic toxic reactions to chemotherapy are shown in Table 5 with regard to our immunotherapy comparison. It was surprising that immunotherapy initiated simultaneously with chemotherapy was associated with a significantly greater incidence of severe leukopenia as well as a moderate increase in the overall incidence of thrombocytopenia. This was observed in spite of the fact that the patients not treated with MER-BCG had a greater frequency of previous chemotherapy as well as a greater

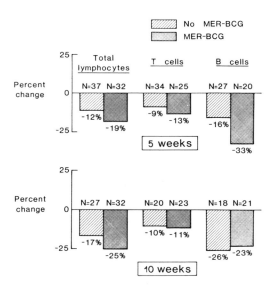

FIG. 8. MER-BCG therapy and change in mean lymphocyte counts (delayed MER-BCG).

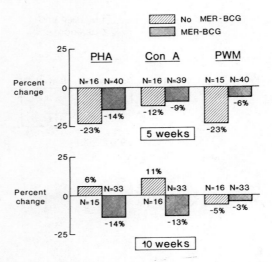

FIG. 9. MER-BCG therapy and change in lymphocyte blastogenesis counts (early MER-BCG). PWM, pokeweed mitogen.

frequency of significant impairment of performance status. When immunotherapy was deferred for 3 weeks after the onset of chemotherapy, there
was, if anything, a slightly greater frequency and severity of hematologic
toxicity in the patients not receiving immunotherapy.

Although occasional mild and transient febrile episodes occurred, the only

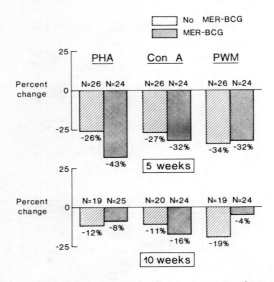

FIG. 10. MER-BCG therapy and change in lymphocyte blastogenesis counts (delayed MER-BCG). PWM
pokeweed mitogen.

TABLE 5. Toxic reactions with and without immunotherapy

	No MER-BCG		MER-BCG	
Early MER				
Leukopenia				
None	12/43		14/51	
< 4,000 > 1,500	27/43	(63%)	25/51	(49%)
1,500 or <	4/43	(7%) p < 0.05	12/51	(24%)
Thrombocytopenia				
None	24/43		18/48	
< 150,000 > 50,000	12/43	(28%)	21/48	(44%)
50,000 or <	7/43	(16%)	9/48	(19%)
Delayed MER				
Leukopenia				
None	10/38		11/35	
< 4,000 > 1,500	21/38	(55%)	20/35	(57%)
1,500 or <	7/38	(18%)	4/35	(11%)
Thrombocytopenia				
None	9/40		16/43	
< 150,000 > 50,000	18/40	(45%)	18/43	(42%)
50,000 or <	13/40	(32%)	9/43	(21%)

significant toxic reaction we observed to immunotherapy was cutaneous in nature. The intensity of MER-BCG cutaneous reactions at this relatively high dosage level was in most cases moderately severe to severe. We have described these in greater detail with an earlier publication (1). Although this toxicity is not life threatening in nature, it is nevertheless most distressing to patients and could only be considered tolerable if there were an associated great gain in therapeutic effect.

DISCUSSION

In this controlled evaluation of immunotherapy with MER-BCG given concomitantly with systemic chemotherapy for colorectal cancer, we were unable to demonstrate any therapeutic advantage for the immunotherapy-treated patients. Certainly such therapy cannot be recommended for further investigation in this patient population. It must be emphasized, however, that all of these patients had very far advanced malignant disease, and quite probably this does not represent the most ideal setting for demonstrating an immunotherapeutic effect. It is also quite possible that immunosuppression resulting from concomitant chemotherapy could have totally abrogated any possible therapeutic gain that immunotherapy may have produced if used alone.

SUMMARY

One hundred eighty one patients with advanced colorectal cancer and measurable disease were treated with combinations of 5-FU plus CACP,

5-FU plus methyl CCNU, and 5-FU plus methyl CCNU plus vincristine. Within each chemotherapy regimen patients were randomized to receive either immunotherapy with MER-BCG or no immunotherapy. In the first half of the study, immunotherapy was initiated simultaneously with chemotherapy; in the last half, it was initiated after a delay of 3 weeks.

Early immunotherapy was associated with significantly more frequent severe leukopenia. Delayed immunotherapy added only its cutaneous lesions to the toxicity of chemotherapy.

Objective responses were observed in 18 of 89 (20%) patients with added immunotherapy, compared to 21 of 92 (23%) patients with no added immunotherapy. Immunotherapy did not produce any significant advantage in completeness of response, duration of response, interval to progression, or patient survival. Under the conditions of this study and by the immunologic assays employed, MER-BCG did not show any evidence of an immunostimulatory effect.

ACKNOWLEDGMENT

The work reported here was supported by grant no. NO 1–CM–02066, Division of Cancer Treatment, National Cancer Institute.

REFERENCES

1. Moertel, C. G., Ritts, R. E., Schutt, A. J., and Hahn, R. G. (1975): Clinical studies of methanol extraction residue fraction of Bacillus Calmette-Guerin as an immunostimulant in patients with advanced cancer. *Cancer Res., 35:*3075–3083.
2. Weiss, D. W. (1972): Nonspecific stimulation and modulation of the immune response and of states of resistance by the methanol-extraction residue fraction of tubercle bacilli. *Natl. Cancer Inst. Monogr., 35:*157–171.

Question and Answer Session

Dr. Weiss: The dosage of MER employed in the study was 2 mg at each time of administration, and the first 90-odd patients were given this in the beginning at weekly intervals and then once every four weeks. This, together with the observation that there was no change in the immunological activity of these patients, which is in contrast to the observations of several groups dealing with MER, suggest the possibility that there may have been overdosage here.

There is increasing evidence in our hands—and I understand from several other groups—that when one exceeds the optimum dose, whatever that is, and that, of course, has to be determined empirically—one obtains a zero or even negative effect in terms of immunological capacity. So, whether it is the advanced stage of the disease or the intensive chemotherapy or, as I have a tendency to think, the 2 mg dose (most other groups use 1 or less and only once a month), it may well be that the negative therapeutic results are directly related to the lack of effect on immunological reactivity. In other words, in light of the no effect on immunological capacity, it would have been rather amazing to find an effect therapeutically.

Dr. Moertel: I think Dr. Weiss's points are very well taken, and certainly we know little regarding dosage of this or any other immunostimulant used in the human setting.

We are currently evaluating MER at two dosage levels, at 0.5 and 2, as well as a placebo control in the controlled trial. The results of the study are still preliminary, but we have not found any meaningful difference between the 0.5 mg dosage and the 2 mg dosage.

Dr. Morton: In this regard, Dr. Moertel, didn't you report that MER did influence immunological reactivity?

Dr. Moertel: Yes, that's interesting. We originally made the assumption that when skin tests turn on and when PHA gets better and when lymphocyte counts go up, this is the effect of the immunostimulant. At that time, however, we were also wise enough to put in a little codicil saying, "We are not really sure this is so."

We did this controlled study to see what really happens to people who are randomized to no treatment versus patients who are randomized to immunotherapy. We were rather surprised to note that the placebo-treated patients will have skin tests that turn on, have PHAs that get better, and have lymphocyte counts that improve, in spite of the fact that they have an advanced and progressive disease. So I do not feel the original evidence we presented is at all convincing of an immunotherapeutic effect.

Dr. Morton: I certainly would echo this. We have data in lung cancer and in melanoma patients where the control group had identical increase in reactivity to that of the patients treated with presumed immunostimulant. I think our results had something to do with repeated skin testing inducing sensitization.

Question: If you compared the responders in the chemotherapy studies only versus the responders in the chemoimmunotherapy groups, was there any difference in survival?

Dr. Moertel: Among those who responded, was there a difference? I must say I have not analyzed the data that way, but my impression is that there was no difference.

Mrs. Nauts: Might it be well to try immunotherapy for a short time prior to chemotherapy, to try to raise the immune status of the patient? I don't know whether you're aware of the beneficial effects reported in one of your Mayo Clinic patients by Black. An acute streptococcus infection developed in an inoperable patient. They had given him a colostomy and sent him home to die, and pretty soon he came back again and said, "I wish you would close the colostomy." They opened him up again and found that it had completely regressed—you know the case.

Dr. Moertel: The patient also had in this interval 4,000 rads of radiation therapy, which wasn't mentioned very prominently in the report.

Dr. Fudenberg: Since these patients were surgically "unresectable," might it not be wise to remove as much of the tumor as possible, even though you can't get it all, so that there would be less tumor cells for the presumably immunologically induced reaction to work against? Might not that aid in getting some beneficial results, and could you perhaps, if you are contemplating a new trial, include that as one of the limbs?

Dr. Moertel: Well, I'm not sure that I could convince my surgical colleagues to start whittling on diffuse peritoneal metastases, pulmonary metastases, and hepatic metastases, which are the main presentations of these patients. I certainly would agree in theory, but from practical considerations I don't really feel that the majority of patients would be at all amenable to such a surgical approach, nor could I urge it, really. Maybe Dr. Morton would want to comment on that.

Dr. Morton: There is only so much you can do with debulking. Even I would stop at some of those patients you described.

Immunotherapy of Cancer: Present Status of
Trials in Man, edited by W. D. Terry and D. Windhorst.
Raven Press, New York © 1978.

Fluorouracil Versus Fluorouracil + BCG in Colorectal Adenocarcinoma

Paul F. Engstrom, Anthony R. Paul, Robert B. Catalano,
Michael J. Mastrangelo, and Richard H. Creech

*Department of Medicine, American Oncologic Hospital, Fox Chase Cancer Center
Philadelphia, Pennsylvania 19111*

In 1974, we initiated a comparative, randomized trial to determine if the addition of Bacillus Calmette-guerin (BCG) to 5-fluorouracil (5-FU) (NSC-19893) chemotherapy of advanced colorectal carcinoma would (a) improve the response rate over 5-FU alone or (b) prolong the response duration and/or patient survival over 5-FU alone. A program of weekly fluorouracil was selected based on data from the Eastern Oncology Cooperative Group (6) and the Western Cooperative Cancer Chemotherapy Group (7). Intermittent intradermal immunization with BCG was selected based on prior studies by Donaldson (3) who found a beneficial response with BCG combined with methotrexate in head and neck tumors. A feasibility study in our own clinics utilizing intradermal BCG + weekly 5-FU showed good patient tolerance with acceptable antitumor effect (4).

PATIENTS

Between April 11, 1974 and December 22, 1975 all patients referred to the American Oncologic Hospital's department of medicine with advanced or recurrent adenocarcinoma of the colon or rectum were considered for this study if they met the following criteria.

1. No prior chemotherapy or immunotherapy.
2. Life expectancy in excess of 4 months and an ambulatory performance status.
3. Measurable tumor parameters, especially in the lung or subcutaneous tissue. Hepatomegaly, due to metastatic tumor as demonstrated by liver biopsy or liver scans consistent with metastatic disease, was accepted if the liver edge was greater than 5 cm below the costal margin.
4. No concomitant serious underlying illness, dehydration, sepsis, severe electrolyte imbalance, or concomitant steroid therapy.
5. Total dose of any prior radiotherapy not in excess of 3,000 rads to the pelvis and no measurable tumor in a previous radiation portal.

TABLE 1. *Patient characteristics of treatment groups*

Characteristics	5-FU group	5-FU + BCG group
Total patients	24	23
Male/female	11/13	10/13
Age range in years	41 → 82	35 → 81
Mean age in years	62	63
Site of measurable recurrence[a]		
Nodes/skin	6	4
Lung	7	6
Liver	16	13
Abd/perineal	6	8
Pretreatment PPD skin test reaction		
Positive	1	6
Negative	13	14
Unknown	10	3
Diagnosis to systemic therapy interval		
Range in months	1 → 72	1 → 72
Mean	23	12
Median	22	5

[a] Some patients in each treatment group had more than one measurable site of recurrence.

6. A normal blood count, platelet count; blood urea nitrogen and liver function studies less than twice the upper limit of normal.

7. Informed patient consent.

Patients were stratified by sex and by predominant site of measurable tumor (i.e., metastases in skin and/or lymph node sites, lung metastases, liver metastases, or local perineal/abdominal metastases) and were randomized to receive 5-FU or 5-FU + BCG therapy. Information on skin test reactivity to major antigens [purified protein derivative (PPD) mumps, *Candida*] was requested but not required prior to randomization.

Table 1 summarizes the characteristics of the 47 patients who comprise this study. The groups are comparable except that the mean interval from diagnosis and/or resection to systemic therapy was longer in the 5-FU-alone group (mean 23 months) compared to the 5-FU + BCG group (mean 12 months).

TREATMENT

The induction course of chemotherapy consisted of 5-FU 600 mg/m² i.v. every week for eight doses. The dosage of 5-FU was calculated to the nearest 50 mg and did not exceed 1,000 mg per injection for the first four courses. If there was no alteration in the white blood count (WBC) below the pretreatment level or below 4,000 mm³, 5-FU was escalated to 700 mg/m² on a weekly basis. One-half the dosage of 5-FU was given if the WBC was

<3,000/mm² or the platelet count was <90,000/mm². Maintenance chemotherapy was instituted after completion of the initial 8 weeks of therapy and if the evaluation showed no evidence of progressive disease. This therapy consisted of the maximum induction dosage given every 2 weeks until disease progression.

The immunotherapy program utilized BCG Glaxo strain, which was supplied as a freeze-dried compound by Eli Lilly & Co., for this study (Bureau of Biologic Investigational New Drug permit #775). Prior to each immunization one ampule of this commercial preparation was reconstituted with 1 ml sterile water for injection that contained no preservative; this solution was allowed to equilibrate for 1 min. One-tenth of a milliliter of the final solution equals one immunizing dose of BCG containing not less than 800,000 and not more than 2,600,000 colony-forming units of BCG. Each patient randomized to the immunotherapy schedule received five 0.1 ml intradermal injections (five immunizing doses) in the shoulder area every 2 weeks for four courses. Maintenance immunotherapy consisted of five immunizing doses of BCG every month until disease progression. In patients who experienced severe local or systemic reactions to BCG, the next scheduled immunotherapy course was reduced to two immunizing doses.

Supportive therapy consisting of antibiotics for urinary tract infection or respiratory tract infections, acetominophen + codeine for fever and/or pain, and flurazepam for sleep was given as needed. No patient received isoniazide or streptomycin. No concomitant radiotherapy was given to patients in this study.

At the time of disease progression, the 5-FU and the BCG were discontinued. Eligible patients were randomized to phase 2 protocol studies using methyl 1-(2-chloroethyl)-3-cyclohexyl-1-nitrosourea (methyl CCNU) (NSU-95441) or Imperial Cancer Research Foundation (of Britain) Compound 159 (ICRF-159) (NSC-129943).

RESULTS

Patients were considered evaluable for toxicity and for response if they completed a minimum of 60 days treatment on this protocol. Response categories were complete remission (CR), partial remission (PR), and no response (NR). CR indicates regression of all measurable lesions resulting in no evidence of disease. PR is defined as a greater than 50% decrease in the sum of the products of the perpendicular diameters of all measurable disease for at least 1 month. A decrease of at least 30% in the sum of three hepatic border measurements perpendicular to the costal margin qualified a patient with malignant hepatomegaly for a PR. The NR category includes patients who had clinical stabilization of their disease (< 50% decrease in measurable parameters and no worsening in their performance status). This group of stable patients was evaluated for duration of stable disease response and

TABLE 2. *Antitumor response after 2 months induction therapy*

		5-FU		5-FU + BCG	
		N	%	N	%
Responders	CR	0	21[a]	1	34[b,c]
	PR	5		7	
Nonresponders	Stable	9	37	13	57
	Progr.	10	42	2	9
	Total	24		23	

[a] 95% confidence range 8.6 to 39.6.
[b] 95% confidence range 17.8 to 59.1.
[c] $p = 0.458$ (Fisher exact test).

for survival in an attempt to define more subtle effects of BCG on systemic disease. NR also includes patients who at 2 months had documented progression of disease ($> 25\%$ increase in the sum of the products of the perpendicular diameters of any one measurable lesion).

Only one patient in this study achieved a CR (a 2-cm pulmonary nodule disappeared for 106 days on 5-FU + BCG). As summarized in Table 2, the percent antitumor response (CR + PR) at the end of induction therapy did not differ significantly ($p = 0.458$) between the treatment groups. The response duration (Fig. 1) was longer in patients receiving chemoimmunotherapy (mean 179 days versus 76 days for 5-FU, $p = 0.028$). However, the

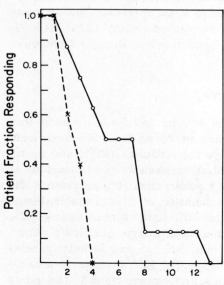

FIG. 1. Duration of response of patients with large bowel carcinoma in CR or PR. ✕, 5-FU; ○, 5-FU + BCG.

COLORECTAL ADENOCARCINOMA

TABLE 3. *Response and survival duration in days*

		5-FU		5-FU + BCG	
Response duration					
CR + PR	Mean	76		179[a]	
	Median	73		140	
	Range	50 → 108		51 → 365	
Stable	Mean	114		88	
	Median	90		82	
	Range	20 → 400		14 → 187	
Survival duration					
CR + PR	Mean	356		325	
	Median	322		370	
	Range	110 → 622		190 → 505	
Stable	Mean	277		271	
	Median	217		213	
	Range	110 → 495		77 → 500	
Progr.	Mean	228		341	
	Median	175		90	
	Range	125 → 763		90 → 592	
Fraction surviving					
		6 Mos.	12 Mos.	6 Mos.	12 Mos.
CR + PR		4/5	2/5	8/8	4/8
Stable		8/9	2/9	10/13	4/13
Progr.		6/10	2/10	1/2	1/2

[a] Using the two-tailed T-test, the probability that the means are equal is $p = 0.028$ assuming unequal variances.

mean survival duration (Table 3) was essentially the same for both treatment groups. As expected, patients who experienced antitumor response had the longer mean survival (12 months for CR + PR; 9.8 months for stable disease; 9.6 months for progressive disease).

All 14 patients who had negative PPD skin tests prior to therapy converted to positive after 2 months of immunotherapy.

SIDE EFFECTS

No patient refused or had therapy discontinued because of adverse side effects from 5-FU. As summarized in Table 4, the induction course of treatment was well tolerated. We observed more gastrointestinal side effects in the 5-FU + BCG-treated patients. Only one patient experienced transient life-threatening leukopenia, which was managed by 5-FU dose alteration. Eight patients described transient incoordination that we attributed to 5-FU-induced cerebellar ataxia. On the average, the patients in the 5-FU-alone group received 90% and those in the 5-FU + BCG group 95% of their calculated drug dosage.

All patients who received BCG immunization experienced mild to moderate local and systemic toxicity (Table 5). Most patients noted low grade

TABLE 4. Toxicity observed during the induction chemotherapy or chemoimmunotherapy course

Toxicity	5-FU		5-FU + BCG	
Nadir WBC $\times 10^3$				
3.0–3.4	11/24	(46%)	12/23	(61%)
2.0–2.9	0	(0)	5/23	(22%)
1.0–1.9	0	(0)	0/23	(0)
0–0.9	1/24	(4)	0/23	(0)
Nadir platelet count $\times 10^3$				
90–130	6/24	(25%)	11/23	(48%)
50–89	6/24	(25%)	6/23	(27%)
25–49	0		0	
0–24	0		0	
Hematocrit %				
28–32	4/24	(16%)	6/23	(23%)
24–27	3/24	(12%)	0	(0)
<24	0		1/23	(4%)
Gastrointestinal toxicity				
Nausea	9/24	(37%)	3/23	(17%)
Nausea & emesis	0		1/23	(4%)
Diarrhea	0		4/23	(17%)
Anorexia	0		8/23	(35%)
Neural toxicity				
Cerebellar ataxia	3/24	(12.5%)	5/23	(17%)

TABLE 5. BCG toxicity

Local:	Erythema	2/23
	Erythema + induration	5/23
	Erythema + ulceration	8/23
	Erythema + ulcer + drainage	8/23
Systemic:	None observed	12/23
	Fever > 99.6°–102° F	6/23
	Flu-like syndrome	2/23
	Fever > 103° F–chills	3/23

fever to 99.6° F with malaise on the night of the BCG immunization. Local skin irritation or pustule formation was usual and in four patients necessitated decreasing the maintenance immunization to two immunizing doses per course. Nine patients received 4 or more months (one patient 12 months) of BCG immunization without hazard. We did not diagnose systemic tuberculosis or disseminated granulomas in any of the patients in this study.

DISCUSSION

The accepted response rate for the 5-FU treatment of colorectal carcinoma is 20%, although there are reported series with response rates as low as 8 and as high as 85% (10). In two separate cooperative group trials utilizing weekly injections of 5-FU 15 mg/kg, Horton et al. (6) observed a 20% response rate and Jacobs et al. (7) a 16% response rate. In this trial, we achieved response rates consistent with the larger cooperative group trials; the chemoimmunotherapy regression rate is not significantly different from 5-FU chemotherapy alone.

The duration of maintained remission has been poorly defined and frequently undocumented in chemotherapy trials of large bowel cancer. Moertel and Reitmeier (9) report that the 31 patients treated with repeated courses of intraveneous 5-FU had a response duration ranging between 2 and 25.5 months (mean 7.3 months). Our mean response duration was 2.7 months for chemotherapy alone whereas our 5-FU + BCG response duration was 6.4 months.

We could not demonstrate an improved survival duration as the result of the concomitant use of immunotherapy with 5-FU. Our mean survival duration was approximately 12 months for both treatment arms; this is considerably poorer than the Mayo Clinic experience (9), which was a 17-month survival duration for 5-FU responders versus a 7-month survival for nonresponders and untreated patients with advanced disease. A comparison of patients from each of our treatment arms matched for pretreatment disease interval suggests that the inequalities of our patient groups for this characteristic did not affect our survival data. This study again confirms the fact that achievement of disease stabilization is not a clinically useful goal for cancer treatment.

Chemoimmunotherapy as administered in this trial was well tolerated and of low toxicity, but it was also of minimum clinical benefit. Several factors could account for these findings. Hersh et al. (5) have emphasized that the efficacy of BCG vaccine depends on strain, quantities of viable organisms, dose, route, and scheduling of administration. These investigators favor the fresh liquid pellicle-grown Pasteur strain BCG vaccine given as 6×10^8 organisms by scarification weekly. Bluming et al. (2) compared 0.1 ml of Glaxo intradermal BCG with dermal scarification using a 0.5 ml suspension of Pasteur Institute BCG and observed that the nonspecific potentiating effect on cellular immunity and the malignant melanoma postoperative remission duration was significantly better in the patients receiving scarification therapy. They attributed the difference in response to the lower dose of organisms in the Glaxo preparation. We selected the Glaxo strain (Lilly) based on our experience in the successful treatment of malignant melanoma by intralesional administration (8). Patients randomized to 5-FU + immunotherapy receive 0.5 ml BCG injected as equal volumes (0.1 ml) in five separate intradermal sites. Thus, each patient received not less than 4×10^6 and not more than 13×10^6 colony-forming units every 2 weeks. With this dosage local pustule formation, systemic fever, and PPD skin test conversion were routinely observed. In an attempt to sensitize lymphocytes draining from the abdominal cavity via the thoracic duct, the skin over the shoulder was the preferred immunization site in the study. Our schedule of administering immunotherapy with chemotherapy injections could have resulted in antagonistic effects on the tumor and on the immune system.

No patient in this study experienced persistent or widely disseminated BCG infection, activation of old dormant acid-fast infections, or hypersensitivity reactions (1).

In conclusion, there was no significant difference between the two groups in percent antitumor response or in median survival duration. However, the median response duration in the 5-FU + BCG treated patients was significantly longer than in the 5-FU treated patients. Investigators contemplating chemoimmunotherapy studies in large bowel carcinoma should consider more effective cytoreductive therapy than 5-FU coupled with more advantageous scheduling of the immunostimulants.

SUMMARY

Adult patients with measurable recurrent or primary advanced (stage IV) adenocarcinoma of the colon and rectum were prospectively randomized to receive 5-FU alone or 5-FU + BCG, Glaxo strain. Treatment groups were matched for age, sex, and measurable disease (i.e., lung, liver, local, lymph node). All 47 patients received 5-FU 600 mg/m^2 i.v. weekly for eight weeks and then every 2 weeks if patients had no evidence of progression. In addition to the 5-FU 0.1 ml reconstituted BCG was given to half the patients in five injection sites intradermally every 2 weeks for four weeks and then every month as maintenance therapy.

The objective response rates (CR + PR) did not differ significantly: five of 24 5-FU versus eight of 23 for 5-FU + BCG ($p = 0.458$). There was an increase in response duration for the 5-FU + BCG group (mean, 179 days versus mean, 76 days for 5-FU alone) ($p = 0.028$). However, no evident benefit in patient survival was noted in the BCG-treated group (mean survival from start of treatment was 12 months in both arms). No adverse or severe toxicity was observed in this treatment trial.

We conclude that 5-FU + BCG as administered in this study is safe, well-tolerated therapy. It does not appear to offer any therapeutic or survival advantages over 5-FU alone in the treatment of advanced, large bowel carcinoma.

ACKNOWLEDGMENT

This study was supported in part by grant no. CA-06551 from the U.S. Public Health Service.

REFERENCES

1. Aungst, C. W., Sokal, J. E., and Jager, B. V. (1975): Complications of BCG vaccination in neoplastic disease. *Ann. Intern. Med.,* 82:666–669.
2. Bluming, A. Z., Vogel, C. L., Ziegler, J. L., Mody, N., and Kamaya, G. (1972): Immunological effects of BCG in malignant melanoma: Two modes of administration compared. *Ann. Intern. Med.,* 76:405–411.
3. Donaldson, R. C. (1972): Methotrexate plus bacillus Calmette-Guerin (BCG) and Isoniazid in the treatment of cancer of the head and neck. *Am. J. Surg.,* 124:527–534.
4. Engstrom, P. F., Catalano, R. B., Creech, R. H. and Mastrangelo, M. J. (1975): Chemoimmunotherapy of colo-rectal carcinoma with 5-FU + BCG. *Cancer Res.,* 16:234 (Abstr. #1052 Proc. Am. Soc. Clin. Oncol.)
5. Hersh, E. M., Gutterman, J. U., Mavligit, O. M., Reed, R. C., and Richman, S. P. (1976): Topics in oncology: BCG vaccine and its derivatives: Potential, practical considerations, and precautions in human cancer immunotherapy. *JAMA,* 235:646–650.
6. Horton, J., Olson, K. B., Sullivan, J., Reilly, C., and Shnider, B. (1970): 5-Fluorouracil in cancer: An improved regimen. *Ann. Intern. Med.,* 73:897–900.
7. Jacobs, E. M., Reeves, W. S., Jr., Wood, D. A., Pugh, R., Braunwald, J., and Bateman, J. R. (1971): Treatment of cancer with weekly intravenous 5-Fluorouracil: Study by the Western Cooperative Cancer Chemotherapy Group. *Cancer,* 27:1302–1305.
8. Mastrangelo, M. J., Bellet, R. E., Berkelhammer, J., and Clark, W. H. (1975): Regression of pulmonary metastatic disease associated with intralesional BCG therapy of intracutaneous melanoma metastases. *Cancer,* 36:1305–1308.
9. Moertel, C. G. and Reitemeier R. J. (1969): *Advanced Gastrointestinal Cancer: Clinical Management and Chemotherapy.* Harper & Row, New York.
10. Schein, P. S., Kisner, D., and MacDonald, J. S. (1975): Chemotherapy of large intestinal carcinoma. *Cancer,* 36:2418–2420.

Question and Answer Session

Dr. Mavligit: I have several comments. First of all, you show that disease-free interval, or the period from resection to the beginning of therapy at the time of development of metastatic disease, was significantly shorter in the BCG group. I looked into this, and I can say that if someone has a Duke's B lesion at the time of resection and another person has a Duke's C, when they subsequently develop metastatic disease the post-relapse survival is significantly shorter in the patient who was originally Duke's C than in the Duke's B patient.

Your data suggest that you have patients with more advanced disease in the BCG group, and that should obviously indicate that the results which you achieved are indeed positive in that this worst prognostic group did as well if not better than the group receiving 5-FU alone.

Comment number 2 concerns the use of Glaxo BCG. I know Dr. Baldwin can comment on that more in an expert way, but there is evidence to suggest that the Glaxo is inferior to other BCGs.

Finally, in your data, pretreatment CEA appears to correlate inversely with the response rate. In our series, if the pretreatment CEA in metastatic disease is less than 30, then the response rate is highest. If it is over 100, the response rate is below 5 percent. So I wonder if there was any difference in the pretreatment CEA between the two groups that could explain the small difference in therapeutic effect?

Dr. Engstrom: I think what you're saying is possibly true. We had a worse group of patients in the 5-FU/BCG group.

Glaxo BCG, as I indicated, was utilized because it's been of use in the past and the fact that in reported cases of solid tumors that have responded to chemoimmunotherapy or an immunotherapy program it was Glaxo BCG that had been used.

We did do serial CEAs in all of our patients. Sera were collected but have not been run as yet.

Dr. Hersh: Am I correct in understanding that you gave the BCG on the same day as the chemotherapy?

Dr. Engstrom: That's correct.

Dr. Hersh: It seems to me from the point of view of chemical immuno-suppression that probably wasn't an ideal timing of administration.

Dr. Engstrom: It was done out of convenience to the patient and to the clinic. However, as you can see, the reaction to the BCG lasts for weeks in these patients and may last months, so I think we are getting a continuous stimulation regardless of when the intradermal injection is made.

Dr Hersh: But it is true that if you give an antigen or an immunostimulant and at the same time apply a chemotherapeutic agent, you are likely at least to modify the response to that agent.

Dr. Gehan: I would like to make a brief statistical comment. With 25 patients in each group, it would have been possible to pick up only something of the order of 40 percent difference between groups. While this study is not statistically significant, that does not necessarily mean that it's not biologically important.

The 9 percent progression rate in the 5-FU/BCG group is quite a bit less than the 42 percent rate in the 5-FU alone group and, taken together with the fact that patients may have had more advanced disease in the BCG group, suggests the possibility that this study should be continued, at least for further evaluation of the BCG group.

Dr. Morton: I think that is a very worthwhile comment. Particularly when dealing with advanced disease, it is a mistake to attempt to draw conclusions on such small numbers followed for such short periods of time. For example, Dr. Moertel mentioned that his apparent response rate in advanced colon cancer with the same combination of chemotherapy (5-FU and methyl CCNU) has dropped from 43 percent to about 27 percent. This illustrates a major problem of trials utilizing small numbers of patients.

Immunotherapy of Cancer: Present Status of
Trials in Man, edited by W. D. Terry and D. Windhorst.
Raven Press, New York © 1978.

Systemic Adjuvant Immunotherapy and Chemoimmunotherapy in Patients with Colorectal Cancer (Dukes' C Class): Prolongation of Disease-Free Interval and Survival

Giora M. Mavligit, Jordan U. Gutterman, Mary Anne Malahy,
Michael A. Burgess, Charles M. McBride, André Jubert,[1]
and Evan M. Hersh

Departments of Developmental Therapeutics, National Large Bowel Cancer Project and Surgery, University of Texas System Cancer Center, M. D. Anderson Hospital and Tumor Institute, Houston, Texas 77030

Since the results from surgical treatment of colorectal cancer seem to have reached a plateau (9), the administration of surgical adjuvant therapy appears to be the rational approach for achieving further improvement in the prognosis of these patients (1). The need for systemic adjuvant therapy is particularly urgent in patients with Dukes' C lesions, i.e., those in whom the primary tumor has involved the regional mesenteric lymph nodes. The natural history of this group of patients, with an approximately 70 to 75% chance for surgical failure and recurrent tumor, strongly indicates that foci of micrometastasis were present already in adjacent structures or in distant organs at the time of surgery. Systemic adjuvant therapy should therefore be directed against those foci of micrometastasis with the hope of increasing the surgical cure rate or prolonging the tumor-free interval and/or the overall survival.

MATERIALS AND METHODS

From April, 1973 to April, 1976, a total of 112 patients with carcinoma of the large bowel—Dukes' C classification—were entered onto a clinical trial of adjuvant therapy consisting of immunotherapy with Bacillus Calmette-guerin (BCG) by scarification or a combination of immunochemotherapy with BCG plus oral 5-fluorouracil (5-FU). Treatment evaluation, in terms of disease-free interval and overall survival, was compared with the same clinical parameters in a consecutive series of comparable (by the major prognostic criteria) surgical control patients with Dukes' C lesions operated on at M.D. Anderson Hospital in 1963–1973. Control patients who died in the immediate postoperative period (60 days) and a few who died of causes

---

[1] Present address: St. Mary's Hospital, Grand Rapids, Michigan.

other than cancer (when this could definitely be established) were excluded. Control patients not operated at the M.D. Anderson Hospital were also left out since—in general, patients are not referred to M.D. Anderson unless a relapse has occurred. In other words, we could not consider the outside patients a homogenous and representative group in the absence of those who, apparently cured by surgery, were never sent to M.D. Anderson Hospital. On the other hand, in order to answer the question, Is surgery at M.D. Anderson equal to surgery elsewhere in postoperative disease-free interval and survival? we compared these parameters, considering only those patients who had a tumor relapse after surgery and excluding those who remained free of disease. We found virtually no difference in either the disease-free interval or the survival between M.D. Anderson patients and those operated on elsewhere. This has allowed us to include the patients who did receive adjuvant therapy regardless of their place of surgery. Further details of the randomization to treatment arms, the treatment regimen, dosages and schedule, criteria for exclusion from this study, and the statistical methods for data analysis have been discussed at length in our previous publications on this study (6,7).

RESULTS

Forty-eight patients received BCG alone and 64 patients received the combination of BCG + 5-FU. Twelve and 16 patients, respectively, have relapsed (Fig. 1). The disease-free interval for both adjuvant treatment groups is estimated to be significantly prolonged compared to the surgical controls ($p = 0.02$). No advantage of one adjuvant treatment over the other was noted ($p = 0.76$).

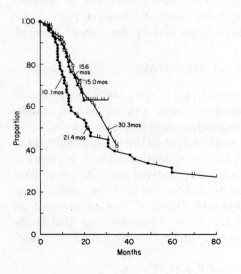

FIG. 1. Dukes' C lesions in colorectal cancer. Disease-free interval from surgery to relapse for group receiving BCG alone (O) and that receiving BCG + 5-FU (▲). Forty-eight out of the total seventy-three controls (●) have relapsed. See text for further details.

The median disease-free interval for patients receiving BCG alone can be estimated at 30.3 months compared to 21.4 months in the controls. For patients receiving BCG + 5-FU this parameter has not yet been reached.

The overall survival curves for the two treatment groups are shown in Fig. 2. The overall survival for each treatment group appears to be significantly prolonged when compared to controls ($p = 0.018$, $p = 0.007$), whereas no difference has been noted as yet between the two treatments ($p = 0.88$). Five patients from each treatment group have died. The median survival times have not been reached yet, but the 75 percentile could be estimated for patients receiving BCG alone at 32.3 months as compared to 16.6 months among the surgical controls.

Since both treatments seem to be equally beneficial at this time, we lumped together the two groups of patients into one group of 112 patients for further analysis and comparison to Dukes' B patients.

The disease-free interval (Fig. 3) of those 112 Dukes' C patients receiving adjuvant therapy, although significantly prolonged when compared to surgical Dukes' C control patients ($p = 0.004$), still falls short of the disease-free interval of surgically treated patients with Dukes' B lesions $(p = 0.01)$. Nevertheless, the overall survival (Fig. 4) of those 112 Dukes' C patients receiving adjuvant therapy was not only significantly prolonged when compared to surgical Dukes' C control patients ($p = 0.001$), but the survival curve almost overlaps that of surgically treated Dukes' B patients $(p = 0.35)$.

To further confirm that the natural history of patients with Dukes' C lesions did not change over time (by the quality of surgery and other unknown factors) and to examine their comparability to the patients receiving adjuvant therapy, we have divided the group of Dukes' C surgical controls

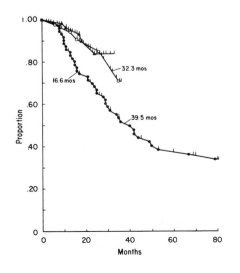

FIG. 2. Dukes' C lesions in colorectal cancer. Survival curves for BCG-alone group (O) and BCG + 5-FU (▲). Deaths were 5/48 and 5/64, respectively. For controls (●) deaths were 41/73. See text for further details.

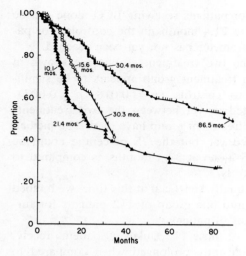

FIG. 3. The disease-free interval from surgery to relapse for Dukes' C patients receiving both types of adjuvant therapy (O) compared with that for Dukes' C controls (▲) and surgically treated patients with Dukes' B lesions (●). Relapsed patients were 28/112, 48/73, and 56/143, respectfully, for the three groups. See text for further details.

into two groups, namely those who were operated on between 1963–1967 and those who were operated on between 1968–1972. The disease-free interval and overall survival curves for both groups of patients were almost identical (Figs. 5 and 6) with $p = 0.42$, $p = 0.31$, respectively. Furthermore, the nodal status of surgical Dukes' C controls was not different from that of the patients treated with adjuvant therapy (Table 1). The mean number of lymph nodes examined in the surgical specimen was similar, and the mean number of nodes involved with tumor was slightly increased among the patients receiving adjuvant therapy. This should, if anything, confer on them a slightly poorer prognosis compared to the surgical controls.

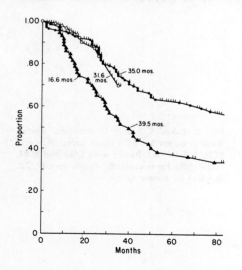

FIG. 4. Overall survival of surgically treated Dukes' B patients (●) compared to Dukes' C patients receiving adjuvant therapy (O) and Dukes' C controls (▲). Deaths were 49/143, 10/112, and 41/73, respectively, for the three groups. See text for further details.

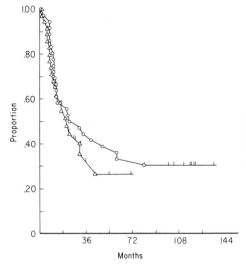

FIG. 5. The disease-free interval from surgery to relapse of 1963–1967 Dukes' C patients (O) compared with that of 1968–1972 Dukes' C patients (△). The number of relapses per group total was 25/36 and 23/37, respectively, for the two groups. See text for further details.

The pattern of relapse among patients receiving adjuvant therapy is shown in Table 2. Among 78 patients with primary carcinoma of the rectosigmoid portion of the large bowel, there were 22 relapses of which 15 occurred locally. In contrast, there were six relapses among 34 patients with primary carcinoma arising proximal to the rectosigmoid of which only one occurred locally ($p < 0.05$). The occurrence of distal metastasis was equally distributed between the primary sites mentioned above.

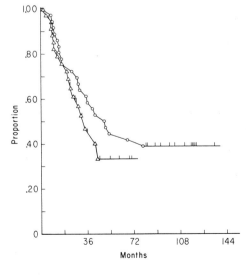

FIG. 6. Survival from surgery to death of 1963–1967 Dukes' C patients (O) compared to survival of 1968–1972 Dukes' C patients (△). The number of deaths per group total for each group was 22/36 and 19/37, respectively. See text for further details.

TABLE 1. *Comparison of nodal status in patients with Dukes' C lesions*

Nodal status	Historical (Surgical) Controls		Adjuvant Rx
	1963–1967	1968–1972	1973–1976
No. of patients	36	37	112
No. of nodes examined (mean)	14.9	15.2	13.8
No. of nodes with tumor (mean)	3.6	3.4	4.3

TABLE 2. *Failure on adjuvant therapy according to site of primary tumor*

Primary site	No. of pts. entered	No. with recurrence			
		Local	Distal	Both	All
Rectosigmoid	78	8[a]	7	7[a]	22
Proximal to rectosigmoid	34	1[a]	5	0	6

[a] $p < 0.05$ for local recurrence.

DISCUSSION

Systemic adjuvant therapy following surgical resection of colorectal carcinoma of the Dukes' C classification appears to confer a significant degree of protection manifested by the prolongation of both the disease-free interval and the overall survival of these patients. Although the concept of systemic adjuvant therapy is not new, its utilization in this group of patients is particularly attractive based on the unfavorable natural history.

The results of this study do not provide—as yet—clear-cut evidence that 5-FU is indeed of any benefit when added to BCG. It is possible, however, that a protective effect of 5-FU was either relatively weak and therefore covered by the more effective protection conferred by BCG or perhaps somewhat delayed so that a longer follow-up may be necessary to fully evaluate its role as an adjuvant therapy. It is noteworthy that although some studies have shown a notable benefit from 5-FU (5,8), others suggested only a marginal, if any, effect at all (3,4). It is also possible that the effect of 5-FU in this study was minimal because of its oral administration as opposed to the more predictable effect resulting from the intravenous route (2). Be that as it may, the protective effect of BCG is suggested in this study, and this agent might be considered the starting point of combinations of adjuvants to be used in this disease in future studies.

In fact, the pattern of tumor recurrence in patients receiving adjuvant therapy, with predominance of local recurrence in patients with primary lesions arising from the rectosigmoid portion of the large bowel, has already led us to include in our next protocol selective postoperative radiotherapy in addition to a sequential regimen consisting of 5-FU (given intravenously) and BCG + pulses of *Corynebacterium parvum*. It is anticipated that with these additional therapeutic modalities we will be able not only to shift the prognosis of Dukes' C patients toward something similar to that of Dukes' B patients, as demonstrated by this study, but perhaps even surpass it.

The controversy regarding the validity of historical controls exposes both ethical and scientific problems. Identical criteria defining Dukes' C lesions were used both in our control and in the study patients. Furthermore, the most important prognostic factor, i.e., the nodal status, was identical in both groups, if not slightly in favor of the controls. Finally, the routine use of serial carcinoembryonic antigen determination in the study patients, but not in the controls, has definitely expedited the early diagnosis of recurrent tumor among the former compared to the latter. This factor lends further support to our results showing longer disease-free interval in patients receiving adjuvant therapy.

SUMMARY

The poor postsurgical prognosis in patients with colorectal cancer of Dukes' C classification has prompted a clinical trial of adjuvant immunotherapy versus chemoimmunotherapy intended to prolong either the disease-free interval or the overall survival, or both. One hundred and twelve patients have been entered on this study. Forty-eight patients received BCG alone and 64 patients received the combination of 5-FU and BCG. The disease-free interval and the overall survival were compared with similar parameters in a group of historical controls with similar prognostic characteristics who were operated on in our institution prior to the initiation of the current study. There has been no difference as yet between BCG alone and the combination of 5-FU + BCG in terms of both the disease-free interval and the survival. Both treatments, however, were significantly better than the controls. Adjuvant therapy, especially with BCG, is advocated for patients with colorectal carcinoma, Dukes' C class, following potentially curative surgery.

ACKNOWLEDGMENTS

This work was supported by U.S. Public Health Service grant no. 1 R26 CA-15458-01 and in part by Hoffman-LaRoche grant no. 169196. Giora M. Mavligit and Jordan U. Gutterman are the recipients of career development awards CA1 KO 4 CA-00130-01 and CA-71007-01, respectively, from the National Institutes of Health. The contribution of patients from Ferguson Hospital, Grand Rapids, Michigan, is acknowledged.

REFERENCES

1. Burchenal, J. H. (1976): Adjuvant therapy—Theory, practice, and potential. *Cancer,* 37:46–57.

2. Hahn, R. G., Moertel, C. G., Schutt, A. J., and Bruckner, H. W. (1975): A double-blind comparison of intensive course 5-fluorouracil by oral vs. intravenous route in the treatment of colorectal carcinoma. *Cancer,* 35:1031–1035.
3. Higgins, G. A., Dwight, R. W., Smith, J. V., and Keehn, R. J. (1971): Fluorouracil as an adjuvant to surgery in carcinoma of the colon. *Arch. Surg.,* 102:339–343.
4. Lawrence, W., Jr., Terz, J. J., Horsley, S., III, Donaldson, M., Lovett, W. L., Brown, P. W., Ruffner, B. W., and Regelson, W., (1975): Chemotherapy as an adjuvant to surgery for colorectal cancer. *Ann. Surg.,* 181:616–623.
5. Li, M. C., and Ross, S. T. (1976): Chemoprophylaxis for patients with colorectal cancer. *JAMA,* 235:2825–2828.
6. Mavligit, G. M., Gutterman, J. U., Burgess, M. A., Khankhanian, N., Seibert, G. B., Speer, J. F., Jubert, A. V., Martin, R. C., McBride, C. M., Copeland, E. M., Gehan, E. A., and Hersh, E. M. (1976): Prolongation of postoperative disease-free interval and survival in human colorectal cancer by BCG or BCG plus 5-fluorouracil. *Lancet,* 1:871–876.
7. Mavligit, G. M., Gutterman, J. U., Burgess, M. A., Khankhanian, N., Siebert, G. B., Speer, J. F., Reed, R. C., Jubert, A. V., Martin, R. C., McBride, C. M., Copeland, E. M., Gehan, E. A., and Hersh, E. M. (1975): Adjuvant immunotherapy and chemoimmunotherapy in colorectal cancer of the Dukes' C classification. *Cancer,* 36:2421–2427.
8. Rousselot, L. M., Cole, D. R., Grossi, C. E., Conte, A. J., Gonzalez, E. M., and Pasternack, B. S. (1972): Adjuvant chemotherapy with 5-fluorouracil in surgery for colorectal cancer. *Dis. Colon Rectum,* 15:169–174.
9. Silverberg, E., and Holleb, A. I. (1975): Major trends in cancer: 25 year survey. *CA,* 25:2–7.

GENERAL DISCUSSION: GASTROINTESTINAL CANCER

Question: You have reported 36 patients in a five-year period, 37 patients in the next five-year period, for a total of 73 patients in the 10-year period between 1963 and 1972, and yet you report 121 patients in a four-year period following that. This suggests that there might be some selection differences among the various groups, and I was just wondering, since this is so important in using historical controls, whether you have examined that question?

Dr. Mavligit: Yes, we have. All 73 patients who served as the controls are a homogeneous group who had their surgery at M. D. Anderson Hospital. I've used this group because when I originally compared patients operated on elsewhere with those operated on at M. D. Anderson, there was a marked difference in favor of M. D. Anderson patients. This is because only those who relapsed were referred to M. D. Anderson Hospital. Referral patients are not a homogeneous group representative of Duke's C lesions. Therefore, I decided to use only M. D. Anderson patients as the historical control group.

The 127 patients in the treatment group are both M. D. Anderson patients and referrals from other places. Therefore, you can see the difference in terms of the number of patients and number of years.

Question: I think the referral pattern of patients going to a center like M. D. Anderson is going to depend upon what you have to offer those patients. In one situation you might have referrals with very ominous disease and hence a bad prognosis. In another situation there might be other considerations, such as young female patients who are known to have a better prognosis in colorectal cancer.

Dr. Wanebo: Could you elaborate on the effectiveness of oral 5-FU? I notice that you have no difference between that and your BCG-alone group, and one wonders whether oral 5-FU is really contributing anything.

Also, I really didn't get straight how many of the patients in your treated group were only from M. D. Anderson.

Third, in using a historic control, although there may be some validity for it, there are also some serious questions. It's not just stage of disease that determines prognosis. For example, a person can have a perforated colon cancer with a Duke's C lesion, which has a far worse prognosis than a Duke's C with two or three positive nodes.

I think there are many variables to be considered. Another example might be the level of the highest positive node. If you have a series of patients with higher positive nodes, that would make it a worse prognosis group. I'm wondering if all of those factors were considered in stratifying these two groups.

Dr. Mavligit: Regarding the oral 5-FU, as I have pointed out, there is no difference between the BCG/5-FU and BCG alone. It is clear that BCG is highly effective, and the question is, what is the role of oral 5-FU? It could be that the effect from BCG has overwhelmed the marginal effect caused by 5-FU. It could also be that oral administration is less effective. We decided, therefore, to go the intravenous route, which may be more predictable in terms of level in the blood. It could be, also, that oral 5-FU will have its effect later on in the game. Further follow-up is required to fully assess the role of oral 5-FU under the circumstances.

Regarding M. D. Anderson's surgery versus surgery elsewhere, I looked into this, and I found no difference if I compared comparable groups. I took the patients who relapsed at M. D. Anderson and compared their prognosis to that of patients who relapsed after surgery elsewhere, and the curves for postsurgery disease-free interval and the survival after relapse are exactly the same. Thus, I could conclude, at least to my satisfaction, that surgery at M. D. Anderson is not different from surgery at other institutions.

Regarding the comment on level of positive nodes, I agree. This information was not routinely available in pathology reports until 1973, and I could not include it in my analysis. I agree that the level of the nodes may be very important in terms of prognosis.

Dr. Morton: Since this is such an important point about the comparability of these two series, perhaps we could have each one of the panel members comment on this problem.

Dr. Schein: I'm sure you are familiar with a letter to the editors of *Lancet* following the publication of one of your initial reports. As you know, these investigators in Glasgow analyzed the patients in their large tumor registry dealing with colorectal cancer, using your inclusion and exclusion factors to analyze their results.

They found a relatively low survival for all their Duke's C cases, but a much higher survival for the patients who they feel fit your inclusion criteria. And the point they made was that they could achieve the same type of statistics for survival that you've achieved if they used the same patient selection but did not treat with BCG. I wonder if you could perhaps comment on that.

In addition, the other point that has been made is that there are Duke's Cs and there are Duke's Cs, and you have to separate them out. Certainly a patient who has transmural involvement (the so-called Duke's C-2) has a survival in all series in which this has been evaluated, which is quite a bit different from the patient with only lymph node involvement, where the disease remains within the muscularis (the so-called Duke's C-1). I think this and the location of the nodes, and perhaps preoperative CEA levels are all important variables that need to be considered.

Dr. Mavligit: My definition of Duke's C is when the tumor has pentrated through into the pericolic sac and lymph nodes are involved. In any case where other structures are involved, such as the ovaries, uterus, posterior wall of the vagina, this is no longer in Duke's C and was not included, either in the study group or in the controls. That is what I would call Duke's D-1, that is, locally advanced disease and these patients have prognoses as poor, or almost as poor, as patients who have widely metastatic disease.

I'm not sure from the description of the Glasgow data whether they indeed included the patients according to my definition of Duke's C. In other words, I have repeatedly found investigators who consider patients to have a Duke's C lesion even if the bladder is involved and part of it was removed, only because lymph nodes were involved. I think this is an important point to make, because it makes a considerable difference in the subsequent progression of these patients. I don't think they gave enough details about their inclusion criteria.

Dr. Schein: I think their concern was that you didn't give enough details, and that they couldn't adequately analyze it. Certainly the strict criteria you just described for selecting cases are not included, at least in your most recent publications. I think it's important to analyze this, and I think many people would include in the Duke's C category a patient who could have an "en bloc" resection, even though there was extension to adjacent small intestine or the bladder. It probably would segregate out cases and one wonders whether or not that has been adequately controlled for in your trial.

Dr. Mavligit: I looked at every single pathology and operative report for the 121 patients and they conformed to the definition I just gave. This also was the definition used for the controls. So from that point of view the study patients and the controls were the same.

Dr. Engstrom: The only question I have is whether the number of lymph nodes was stratified in any way in your series?

Dr. Mavligit: Yes. We stratified them as less than five positive nodes and greater than five and in each of the subcategories the results are just about the same.

Dr. Engstrom: So that patients with five or more lymph nodes have the same recurrence rate and same survival rate as patients with four or fewer lymph nodes?

Dr. Mavligit: No, the prognosis is worse among patients with greater than five positive nodes. What I was trying to say is that the fraction of patients with more than five and less than five nodes is the same in the current study as compared to the historical control.

Dr. Moertel: There is a phenomenon that has developed in colorectal cancer that I have a bit of difficulty coming to terms with. All controlled studies are negative when they are randomized and prospective in design, and all of the controlled studies that are historically controlled are uniformly positive. I suspect that there is clearly a message here for those who wish to have positive studies.

I have been confused as to how you conclude that the results of surgery at M. D. Anderson are no different from the results of surgery elsewhere in the Southwest.

How have you reached that conclusion? How do you know that the surgery was performed in the same way? How do you know the pathology review was performed in the same way, and that the quality of pathology examination was the same?

Dr. Mavligit: The majority of the hundreds of patients who were referred to M. D. Anderson for treatment of colorectal cancer already had metastatic disease at the time that they were referred. I took those who had potentially curative surgery at the place where they came from and measured their disease-free interval and survival and compared that to the same intervals for patients who were originally seen at M. D. Anderson and who had their curative procedure at M. D. Anderson Hospital. If I take only the relapses, those patients who have not been cured, and measured their disease-free interval, plus the post-relapse survival, and compare between M. D. Anderson and the rest, there is no difference. The curves exactly overlap each other.

Based on this, I can say that surgery seems to be the same and it is the biology of the tumor rather than the surgical hand that determines the fate of the patient. I would like to hear a surgeon say that that is not the case.

Dr. Nystrom: Was the postoperative CEA used in any way to screen eligibility for your most recently treated BCG population?

Dr. Mavligit: Since CEA was not done on the historical controls, we did not exclude a single patient, even if he had an elevated level of CEA after surgery and at the initiation of immunotherapy.

Another factor that should be mentioned is that we have excluded all postoperative deaths from the controls; that is, patients who died within 60 days after surgery, because if they had died in our current study we would never have seen them. So from that point of view there was comparability too.

Dr. Baker: You conclude that your current BCG and BCG-FU groups survived longer than the historical controls. In order to convince me, you would have to assure me that the current groups, the BCG and BCG-FU groups, were not treated after their recurrences with new or additional modalities, like hyperalimentation, like resection of solitary pulmonary nodules, like additional chemotherapy to prolong their survival. Can you reassure us that the historical control and your current groups were identical in these respects?

Dr. Mavligit: Of those patients who relapsed on this study, none had had any hyperalimentation; none had resection of solitary pulmonary nodules; and as for some magic chemotherapy, I wish we had it.

Dr. Holland: Don't you think this audience is giving you some sort of message in doubting your 70-odd historical controls? Wouldn't you think it would be advisable in your next study to randomize between BCG (something that you say is indeed beneficial and superior to the current available surgical treatment) and the new program? Could you tell me the ethics of not doing that? I think your studies must cost millions of dollars, and the results are of enormous importance for hundreds of thousands of people. Yet you haven't persuaded significant numbers of physicians here. Dr. Moertel is one, and I'm another.

Dr. Hersh: I think that the point that Dr. Holland has raised is extremely important, and I think that the critical question in going on to the next study is not only the question of what further improvements we can add to the current treatment regimen, but how best can we make an estimate of either possible improvement or possible detriment. Certainly every time we go on to a new study that possibility is real.

It's my understanding from my discussions with our biomathematical colleagues that the most efficient way to make such an estimate is not to do a randomized study between the past treatment program and the new idea, but to do a consecutive series and compare it to the recently completed historical control. I would like to hear some biomathematical discussion on this, because I think there are two points of view on this. My objective is to make the best and fastest estimate of what we are doing so that, what is most important, we can avoid doing harm.

Dr. Salmon: In the historical background which Dr. Schein gave it's not clear to me that the comment that there is no difference between adjuvant treatment versus no treatment after surgery is actually, in fact, correct. In each of the large-scale studies that he showed, there was a *p*-value of about 0.1, with the treated patients in groups of 200 doing somewhat better than the controls in each and every instance with radiotherapy, chemotherapy, or whatever. A *p*-value of 0.1 means there is a nine-out-of-ten chance that there is some difference between those groups, which, although it's not the magical 0.05, suggests that there might be some difference. This could mean that there are subgroups which are doing extremely well, but which have not been identified or segregated out.

I would also comment that if Dr. Mavligit's treatment is in fact any good as an adjuvant to surgery, at some point there should be a break in the curve. If the patients continue to relapse and die, then the strategy of adjuvant therapy has not succeeded. Therapy given after surgery is designed to try to eradicate the residual tumor stem cells if at all possible, and the differences will become dramatic if the curve flattens out. The study will stand on its own if that ever happens.

Dr. Morton: The problems that Dr. Hersh brought up are very important and are central to this entire volume. It is obvious at this point that immunotherapy, if it has any activity at all, is going to have limited activity as a single agent. This being the case, the problem becomes a biomathematical one of designing critical trials to determine how to detect a difference that is small —10 percent, 20 percent, maybe 30 percent at the most. I would like to call on some of the biostatisticians here to discuss this problem. Dr. Gehan, may I ask you to speak first?

Dr. Gehan: First of all, although Dr. Mavligit and I are at the same institution and we have conferred from time to time, I haven't participated in this particular analysis.

It seems to me the most important thing to observe in a study of this type is consistency of treatment effect across subgroups of patients divided into prognostic categories.

What I think would be definitely worth doing before claiming a definite advantage for the BCG or the 5-FU/BCG would be to continue the study of prognostic factors to see if consistent advantages over the control group are present in all circumstances.

I think that in the future study that Dr. Holland has made the major point about, it would be reasonable to randomize a certain fraction of patients to the past treatment and another fraction to the proposed treatment. I wouldn't think that it should be a 50–50 randomization. It could be a one out of three or one out of four going to the previous treatment.

The decision not to randomize would be of less importance than it was in the previous study. In the new study you're going to have the same selection criteria; the same types of patients are going to be coming into the study. So whether this one is randomized or not, it wouldn't be the major issue. I think we'd have a much better handle on the prognostic factors. But I still would have questions about the previous study.

Dr. Holland: Dr. Gehan, what about the different house staff, and the different antibiotics, and the different blood bank materials, and the different anesthesias, and different transportation systems, and even different surgeons? Are they all completely negligible?

Dr. Gehan: My physicians tell me yes. They take care of patients in both groups.

Dr. Byar: It's apparently very hard to avoid getting emotional on this subject. It reminds me of theological arguments in the Middle Ages. Naturally, like all those theologians in the Middle Ages, I have my own beliefs.

I have tried to be as restrained as possible here and not jump up every time I saw something I didn't like, because if I did, I would have been constantly on my feet. However, I cannot help but emphasize that the same observation Dr. Moertel made about studies in colorectal cancer might apply as well in the leukemias, in melanoma, and lung cancer. I don't know about breast cancer yet, because we haven't discussed it. If you look through Abstract Nos. 3, 9, 14, 31, 49, and 52, you have a list of very convincing, positive studies. The only thing is that they're all based on historical control groups.

I would not be one to say, despite my faith in the randomized trial as the most efficacious method for assessing a new therapy, that all randomized trials are well done. There are a great many problems in running them. They also can be misinterpreted. There is an additional complication caused by what appears to me to be some tendency for the people who don't like to do randomized trials to have what appear to be the brightest ideas.

Since they're interested in making rapid progress, you can never really pin them down. By the time they're reporting the results of their last historical control study, they've already changed the regimen; and it's like trying to hit a moving target.

Now, I would agree completely in the case at hand that the data are unconvincing, because I know personally the hazards of doing studies with historical controls. I do them myself. For example, when you want to look at something where a trial hasn't been done yet, the most reasonable thing to do is to look at your past experience.

I know the importance of prognostic factors; I also know how incomplete and inadequate most historically collected data are for assessing these factors. I know that, even if we had perfect data on all those prognostic factors, it's only the ones that you know about; and often the prognostic factor which is going to be discovered in three months from now may have a larger effect than any treatment effects you've seen.

The great advantage of a well-conducted randomized trial is that it controls as well for those factors that you cannot identify or don't know about as it does for those that you do.

So, although I think there is a role for nonrandomized studies, I think they are being misused and they're regarded too much as being on a par with well-conducted randomized studies. If you have the same disease and the same kind of patients treated and the same treatment and put a randomized study next to a historical control study, there's not any question about which one to believe. I think in situations like this you must do the randomized controlled study to convince everyone and yourself—if you're really intellectually honest—before modifying the therapy and continuing in that fashion.

Dr. Gehan: (These comments are included here as "extended" discussion.)

Since this volume was planned to summarize the "present status of trials in man," it is to be expected that the studies reported would be in varying stages of completion. The remarks that follow are not meant to be critical of studies that are still in progress, especially when the report given was a preliminary one.

From a biostatistical viewpoint, issues were raised in this volume which bear on the question of randomized vs nonrandomized studies, small vs large studies, and multi vs single institution studies. There was considerable variation in the way statistical methodology was handled in the chapters. In some chapters, there was a careful statement of the methods used and it is rare that a biostatistician attending a medical conference hears such phrases as "logistic regression analysis," "Kaplan-Meier method of estimating survivorship function," "generalized Wilcoxon test for comparing two groups," etc. In contrast, some authors delivered papers which gave as much emphasis to significance levels (p-values) as to response rates, length of response, or survival. Statistical tests were considered "significant" if the p value achieved was less than .05 and "not significant" otherwise. Some attention to statistical methodology is of importance, especially since there appears to be general agreement that immunotherapy is expected to have only a small-to-moderate effect on the prognosis of patients. In such a situation, efficient analytical methods would be relatively more important than in studies in which large effects on prognosis were expected. However, it is also true that there can be an over-emphasis on the results of statistical tests. The p values were quoted by some authors as if they conferred scientific validity on the results of the study. The p values represent a measure of the strength of the evidence against the hypothesis of no difference between treatment groups and that is all. The most informative studies presented were those which yielded precise estimates of response rate, length of response, or survival and a statement about the effectiveness of immunotherapy in the particular disease category.

Both the randomized and nonrandomized studies presented in this volume can be criticized, obviously some studies more severely than others. In general, the randomized studies, except those conducted by cooperative clinical groups, had small numbers of patients in each of the treatment groups, sometimes as small as 10 or so. Those reporting the results with small numbers of patients emphasized the significance levels of comparisons between groups, while it should be evident that one is unlikely to find statistically significant results with small numbers of patients. The following table, abstracted from (1), gives the number of patients needed in experimental

TABLE 1. *Number of patients needed in an experimental and control group for a given probability of obtaining a significant result (one-sided test) Significance level = 5%, Power = 80%*

Smaller Proportion of success	Larger minus smaller proportion						
	.10	.20	.30	.40	.50	.60	.70
.20	230	63	36	23	15	10	8
.40	310	76	37	23	13	—	—

and control groups for a given probability of obtaining a significant result (one-sided test).

Note that the number of patients required becomes smaller the larger the difference between groups that is to be detected and the number also depends upon the significance level and power of the test. This table would be pertinent if one were doing a randomized study comparing patients treated with chemotherapy plus immunotherapy vs those treated with chemotherapy alone to determine whether immunotherapy led to a *better* response rate. The number of patients would be larger for a corresponding two-sided test of whether immunotherapy added to or subtracted from the benefits of chemotherapy. Note from the table that when there are only 23 patients in each group, it might reasonably be expected to detect only a 40% difference in response rate between groups. To detect differences of 20% or less requires at least 63 patients in each group (depending upon the response rate for the control treatment). It has often been stated that "statistical significance is not equivalent to biological significance." It should be equally recognized that "not statistically significant in a small number of patients is not equivalent to lack of biological importance." When reporting a study with a small number of patients, authors should state what differences in effectiveness the given numbers of patients had a reasonable chance of detecting. Alternatively, authors could report negative results with small numbers of patients in each treatment group as follows: "This study has demonstrated that there is no X% difference in the order of effectiveness between treatment groups." For example, if there were 15 patients in each group, then X = 50%. Small studies might reasonably be expected to provide leads for confirmation in larger studies, but not statistically significant results.

In the nonrandomized studies, the numbers of patients tended to be much larger than for the randomized studies; however sometimes insufficient attention was paid to adjustment for prognostic factors. On the positive side, a large number of patients enables one to *estimate* the effectiveness of a given treatment with more precision and this should not be overlooked. For example, the standard error of the estimate of response rate and the width of a 95% confidence interval for the response rate on an experimental treatment are reduced by approximately 29% when all patients are put on the experimental treatment in comparison with a randomized study when one-half of the patients are put on experimental treatment and one-half on control. When comparing results with a historical control series, a nonrandomizer is obliged to demonstrate no differences in important prognostic characteristics between groups. Multivariate methods, such as logistic regression analysis or Cox's regression analysis (2), could be utilized to test for treatment differences adjusting for multiple prognostic factors between groups. Nonrandomizers should recognize that their results will be treated with skepticism so that they should analyze their data from many different viewpoints; if all viewpoints demonstrate a treatment effect, then it is more likely to be a real one.

Concerning single vs multi-institutional studies, the single institute studies tended to be much smaller, especially when the studies were randomized. It was also true, however, that the single institute studies could be designed to give more aggressive chemotherapy and immunotherapy than multi-institute studies. While a precise statistical study was not done on this point, I believe that the dosages of both immunotherapy and chemotherapy tended to be higher in single institute studies. In studies of chemotherapeutic agents, it is generally accepted that phase II studies of new agents can be done better at one or a small number of institutions rather than by all the institutions in a cooperative group. It is probably true that the study of immunotherapy for many diseases is in a phase II state, i.e., it is important to determine whether the immunotherapy has any effectiveness or not. On general grounds, such studies could probably be done more precisely by single institutions with confirmatory phase III studies done better in the large cooperative groups.

What are the implications of these remarks for future studies of immunotherapy? The first principle in planning clinical studies is: "The best clinical trials are those that have the best treatments in them." Future studies should concentrate on adding immunotherapy to the best available treatments, and chemotherapy was the form utilized most often in studies reported at the conference. To some extent, the studies of immunotherapy should also be regarded as exploratory, since the appropriate type, schedule, dosage, and route of administration are not yet known. Information can be learned about the effectiveness of immunotherapy, both from randomized studies in which a group receiving chemotherapy plus immunotherapy is compared to a group receiving chemotherapy alone or nonrandomized studies in which a series of patients receive chemotherapy plus immunotherapy with comparison made to a historical control series. For both the randomized and nonrandomized studies, there should be a sufficiently large number of patients receiving immunotherapy to make reasonably precise *estimates* of the effectiveness of immunotherapy; obviously, it will be easier to achieve these large numbers if all patients are put in one group rather than divided among more than one. The validity of the nonrandomized study will depend upon whether prognostic factors have been adjusted for in the planning and analysis of the study. For the randomized studies, the test should almost certainly be a one-sided one, namely, designed to answer the question is chemotherapy plus immunotherapy significantly *better* than chemotherapy alone? Randomization could be designed on a 1:1 basis or, when a previous control series was available, a higher proportion of patients might receive chemotherapy plus immunotherapy.

The ethical question is of great importance in planning any cooperative study. If preliminary data suggest that immunotherapy is going to be greatly beneficial, then it is not appropriate to plan a randomized study. One should not plan a randomized study unless one would be willing to be a patient in the study.

The evidence that immunotherapy is beneficial to patients is going to come primarily from well conducted studies that are carefully analyzed and the effects are consistently observed by others. The primary question one should ask is not whether the study was randomized or not, but whether the study was well done and whether the results are worth confirming. For studies that appear to have negative results, the question should be asked whether the study was sensitive enough to detect a reasonable effect of immunotherapy.

REFERENCES

1. Gehan, E. A. and Schneiderman, M. (1973): Experimental design in clinical trials. In *Cancer Medicine,* edited J. Holland and E. Frei, pp. 499–519. Lea & Febiger, Philadelphia.
2. Cox, D. R. (1972): Regression models and life tables. *J. Royal Stat. Soc.* (B), 34:187–220.

*Immunotherapy of Cancer: Present Status of
Trials in Man,* edited by W. D. Terry and D. Windhorst.
Raven Press, New York © 1978.

International Registry of Tumor Immunotherapy: The Contributions of an Information Service to a New Specialty

Dorothy Windhorst

Division of Medical Research, Hoffmann–La Roche, Inc., Nutley, New Jersey 07110

The International Registry of Tumor Immunotherapy is simple in both concept and operation. It is a sharply defined information system which provides a service in the form of a regular publication of concise information about active projects in the field. It should be noted, however, that there are several unique features about this effort (Table 1).

The most important of the special qualities of the Registry is its relevance. Each of the four issues of the Compendium of Immunotherapy Protocols that appeared between 1973 and 1976 reflected clinical trials that were actually in progress at the time the volume was published. Staff work between editions of the Compendium was largely devoted to updating all of the information and determined efforts were made to put the information before the Registry's constituency (its contributing investigators) with minimal delay. In addition, the Compendium listings give the full address and phone number of all investigators. Thus the Registry, through the Compendium, has provided a current, annotated listing of work actually being done in a specific field and has facilitated direct communications between those investigators. Clinical experiments in cancer require careful advance planning and several years of patient accumulation and treatment before evaluations can be made. Thus the Registry, by providing information that is useful to investigators planning new trials, promotes the development of optimum experimental approaches to work that is performed in human subjects. In this sense, the Registry serves not only a scientific but also an ethical function.

TABLE 1. *Unique features of the registry*

---

1. A major effort is devoted to keeping information up-to-date.
2. The Registry interacts closely with its clientele:
   Most protocols come directly from investigators
   Compendium entries and revisions are verified with investigators
   Physicians on the general mailing list must regularly reaffirm their interest
3. Limited use is made of machine technology to facilitate the primary logistical goal of regular dissemination of *current* information.

EARLY HISTORY

In 1972, the basic science of immunology had been undergoing a tremendous expansion in technology, particularly with regard to *in vitro* assays for cell-mediated immunity. At the same time, a parallel conceptual development regarding the use of the immune response for therapy of cancer had led to the initiation of a number of clinical trials.

Also at that time, new funds were made available for the application of modern immunologic methods to the field of cancer research, including immunotherapy. In order to distribute these funds wisely, it was necessary to know exactly what was already being done and planned in the area of clinical trials.

A small group of investigators from the National Cancer Institute and various university-affiliated cancer research centers met in November of 1972 to discuss the state of knowledge in the field of immunotherapy. Participants in this meeting recognized the need to know about clinical trials in progress, and recommended that a centralized information resource to obtain and disseminate such information be explored. The participants in this initial conference, all of whom offered advice to the Registry coordinator over the succeeding months and years, were: Drs. Evan Hersh (Houston); Myron Karon (Los Angeles); A. B. Miller (Toronto); Carl Pinsky (New York); H. F. Seigler (Durham); Richard Simmons (Minneapolis); J. W. Thomas (Vancouver, B.C.); from the NCI, Drs. Mary Fink; Ronald Herberman; Brigid Leventhal; Herbert Rapp; Steven Rosenberg; John Schneider; William Terry; Dorothy Windhorst; and John Ziegler.

ORIGINAL GOALS

Although the members of the original planning group had various opinions about both the desirability and the proper role that an information resource might play, a number of goals were agreed upon. Specifically, the group agreed that the major need was for information on protocols (that is, the scientific/medical questions being asked) rather than any data on individual patients, with the added requirement that the information be focused on work that was actually ongoing rather than information already at the publication stage. Also, the worldwide activity in immunotherapy required that the Registry be international in scope. It was felt the Registry might eventually provide a useful forum for publishing negative results and a mechanism for rapid dissemination of unexpected toxicity in ongoing trials. It was agreed that not only should complex phase II and III trials be studied, but that anecdotal and phase I trials should be included for the sake of the primary goal of complete information exchange. The International Cancer Research Data Bank in the office of the Director of The National Cancer Institute, recognized the usefulness of this approach, and provided funding for the Registry from the beginning.

EARLY EFFORTS

In 1973, with the aid of a small support contract, the Registry coordinator developed protocol abstract forms and prepared a newsletter. These were sent to a mailing list derived from a number of different sources in an effort to locate all individuals conducting trials in immunotherapy of human cancer. In addition, a number of announcements appeared in several relevant journals, and by June of 1973, almost 50 protocols by some 35 different investigators had been submitted.

During 1973 and early 1974, major efforts were directed towards expanding the population of clinical investigators with whom the Registry was interacting. This included a direct postcard mailing to all 2,500 clinicians registered with the cancer clinical cooperative groups. In addition, the Registry coordinator personally visited several major European Cancer centers in 1974 to encourage their cooperation with the Registry. The listing of clinical trials (1) prepared at Villejuif by Dr. T. Flamant was particularly useful during this time. These activities resulted in registration of significantly increased numbers of protocols, and a second Compendium was published in the summer of 1974.

ESTABLISHMENT OF A MACHINE DATA BASE

As the mailing list for the Registry Letter and the Compendium investigators expanded, it was entered into a simple, machine-based data bank providing mechanisms for cross-filing and updating. The mailing list is kept current and requires active expression of interest by the recipients. This can be regarded as a measure of the usefulness of the Registry function.

Although the volume of protocols has never been sufficient to require a machine capability, in one sense, the desire to be able to update the information about protocols and to print completely updated compendia of the protocols at frequent intervals made automation desirable. During 1974 and 1975, therefore, the major effort of the Registry coordinator and the support contractor was to develop a system for standardizing summaries of clinical protocols for printing in the Compendium. The first edition of the Compendium to provide protocol abstracts drawn from the machine file was in October of 1975.

TABLE 2. *Investigators and protocols*

| | (By Compendium Editions) | | | |
	#1 1973	#2 1974	#3 1975	#4 1976
Protocols, Total	50	129	262	347
Principal Investigators, Total	35	76	160	236
Countries Other Than U.S.	6	10	15	17
Protocols	9	33	52	90
Principal Investigators	9	23	38	63

TABLE 3. *Tumors studied under protocol*

| | (By Compendium Editions) | | | |
	#1 1973	#2 1974	#3 1975	#4 1976
Melanoma	18	46	68	82
Lung Cancer	9	29	35	54
Leukemias	9	17	32	47
Multiple Cancers (all tumors)	2	2	35	44
Breast Cancer	6	14	20	28
GI	6	7	21	28
GU (and Gynecologic)	6	11	15	23
Head and Neck	5	8	11	17
Sarcomas	4	12	13	11
Lymphomas		4	4	5
Hodgkin's Disease	1	1	3	4
Myelomas			2	1
Miscellaneous		7		
Neuroblastoma	1	3	1	3
Cutaneous	2	3	2	2
Brain			2	2
Bone		2	1	1

TABLE 4. *Immunotherapeutic agents in protocols*

| | (By Editions of the Compendium) | | | |
	#1 1973	#2 1974	#3 1975	#4 1976
Antigens (allogeneic, autologous, tumor . . .)		3	5	8
BCG	43	99	148	198
BCG, CWS			1	4
C. parvum		5	51	69
Cells, allogeneic	5	10	25	30
Cells, autochthonous	9	8	12	12
Cells, other	2	5	8	14
Extracts, tumor and thymic		1	5	6
Freund's complete adjuvant			1	2
Levamisole		4	12	27
Lymphocytes	3	1	2	6
MER		1	28	36
Plasma, human			1	1
Poly A: Poly U			1	1
Poly I: C		1	1	3
Sera, anti-T cell			1	1
Transfer factor	2	2	11	16
Vaccines, tumor			3	8
Vaccines, bacterial		1	2	4
Vaccines, viral		2	3	4
Vitamin A			1	3
Miscellaneous[a]		1	9	18

[a] Baker's antifole, antiserum (high titered), bone marrow, coenzyme Q-10, cryoimmunotherapy, dextromisole, diribiotine, DNCB, IPM, leukapheresis, neoplastic tissue, PPD, RNA, tilorone, viscum album

It is clear that many details and other subtleties of individual projects were lost in the formating and abstracting process. However, the primary goals of promptness and frequency of input of new information are best served by this approach, and the Registry can thus maintain its currency. Precise use of any Registry information by an investigator requires that he contact the original source of the information, using the addresses and phone numbers provided in the Compendium.

For the year 1975 to 1976, a determined effort was made to clarify the details of both information and systems design that had been neglected for the sake of other goals in the past. Thus, Compendium #4, published in August, 1976, was the culmination of several different major thrusts in a specialized information systems. Tables 2 to 5 review the evolution of the Registry in numerical terms.

TABLE 5. *International participation*

NON-U.S. ADDRESSES	
Canada	90
France	52
England	49
Belgium	40
Switzerland	21
Japan	16
Austria	14
Australia	9
Israel	8
Argentina	7
South Africa	6
Sweden	5
Greece	4
Scotland	4
Denmark	4
West Germany	4
Italy	3
Brazil	3
Peru	2
The Netherlands	2
Bulgaria	2
Czechoslovakia	2
Taiwan	2
Poland	1
Uruguay	1
Columbia	1
U.S.S.R.	1
Yugoslavia	1
Norway	1
Uganda	1
Mexico	1
Hungary	1
Ireland	1
TOTAL	**359**

[a] Mailing List Addresses as of October 10, 1976 = 2,340

IMPACT ON THE FIELD

No formal attempt has been made to evaluate the impact of this specialized service on the field of immunotherapy, although numerous anecdotal episodes indicate that there has been substantial use of the Registry's publication, the Compendium, by investigators planning new studies and by others attempting to evaluate this new discipline.

Several considerations should be borne in mind when evaluating the Registry:

1) The nature of the benefit provided is one of efficiency of communication at a policy/planning level of medical research.
2) The impact has occurred in several directions, especially the following:
   a. Information for government funding agencies.
   b. Information for investigators to use in designing future studies.
   c. An international and comprehensive exchange of information about research at a stage several years before publication of results could be expected.
3) The development of the Registry was initiated at the time of the most rapid expansion of activity in the field, thus its services came at a time when a maximum efficiency of contribution could be expected.
4) In an indirect way, the Registry has acted as an educational medium as well as an information exchange service. The interaction of registry personnel with investigators inevitably resulted in improved understanding of protocol design and the problems of the conduct of clinical trials. (2)

One indication of the impact of the Registry lies in the response of investigators asked to submit protocols and of other clinicians asked whether they wished to remain on the Registry mailing list. In both instances, an active effort is required by the respondant. The average percentage response to such requests from the Registry has been well above 80%. This aspect of the Registry, that of its immediate interest to the people it serves, is probably the most critical, and has guided the planning and execution of the service from the beginning.

One of the most important problems faced by scientists in this era of expanding technical and scientific information is one of keeping abreast of new developments. The Registry offers an example of how investigators can be helped in this task.

REFERENCES

1. Armitage, P., Flamant, R., and Gehan, E. A. (1974): The methodology of controlled therapeutic trials in cancer. In: *Controlled Therapeutic Trials in Cancer* UICC Technical Report Series, Volume 14, International Union Against Cancer, Geneva, Switzerland.
2. Windhorst, D. (1976): The international registry of tumor immunotherapy. *Med. Clin. N. Amer.*, 60(3):641–648.

*Immunotherapy of Cancer: Present Status of
Trials in Man,* edited by W. D. Terry and D. Windhorst.
Raven Press, New York © 1978.

Natural History of Breast Cancer: A Brief Overview

Bernard Fisher, James T. Hanlon, James Linta, and Edwin R. Fisher

*University of Pittsburgh, School of Medicine, Pittsburgh, Pennsylvania 15261; and
Department of Pathology, Shadyside Hospital, Pittsburgh, Pennsylvania 15232*

In the not too distant past, a consideration of the natural history of breast cancer evoked a rather simplistic recital. The classic paper of Bloom and associates in 1962 (5) has supplied information about the fate of patients with breast cancer who, for one reason or another, were untreated. A review of 250 untreated cases on record at Middlesex Hospital in London between 1805 and 1933 indicated that the mean duration of life from onset of symptoms was 3 years; 18% survived 5 years, 3.6% survived 10 years, and 0.8% survived 15 years. The longest survival was 18 years, 3 months, and three other patients survived longer than 13 years. Similar survival rates have been reported by Phillips in 1959 (34) and by Daland in 1927 (10). Whether the natural history of breast cancers occurring at the present time has changed, as determined by the fate of untreated patients, is conjectural and of little pertinence.

At one time, a knowledge of the natural history of untreated cases provided a background against which the worth of treatment could be judged. Such information today is not relevant. What is of significance is that there be universal awareness that the term "breast cancer" is an eponym employed to designate a biologically heterogeneous group of cancers of the breast residing in a biologically heterogeneous group of women. As a consequence of the multiple host–tumor permutations, consideration of the natural history of breast cancer as a single phenomenon is an anachronism. The varied individual natural histories determine the results of treatment that, in turn, influence the subsequent natural history of the disease.

Bloom demonstrated an awareness of this variation of the tumor when he noted that histologic grade of malignancy was correlated with prognosis in 86 untreated cases. The 5- and 10-year survival rate for patients harboring tumors of low-grade malignancy (grade I) was 22 and 9%, respectively, whereas the survival for highly malignant (grade III) tumors was 0% at 5 years.

What are some of the more pertinent variables in the equation that influence the fate of a patient with breast cancer and that influence the design and interpretation of the results of therapeutic strategies? The following seem most important to these reviewers and are presented to indicate that with the accumulation of more biologic information, the more complex becomes the breast cancer problem and the more complex is likely to be the therapeutic approach necessary for its resolution.

BREAST CANCER IS A SYSTEMIC DISEASE

The time-honored concept on which the surgical treatment of cancer has been based is that a growing tumor remains localized for a finite period of time, then, at some point during its growth, disseminates to regional lymph nodes. After a further interval associated with increase in tumor size, systemic dissemination ensues. Adequate operation performed prior to dissemination was thought to ensure cure. Since it was deemed that there was a certain "orderliness" about tumor spread and that clinically recognizable cancer was in many instances a loco-regional disease, it was considered more curable if the surgeon would only be more expansive in his interpretation of what constituted the "region." These anatomic considerations concerning breast cancer spread have persisted for almost a century.

More recently, there has arisen reason to believe that breast cancer is frequently a systemic disease at the time of its diagnosis and may be a systemic disease from its inception. When it is appreciated that a 1 cm tumor, which is usually the minimal size capable of physical diagnosis and which is looked on as an early tumor, has already progressed through 30 of the 40 doublings lethal to a patient, it is not surprising that it is a systemic disease. That a cancer may have only 6 to 10 more doubling times before death strongly implies that the designation "early" may actually signify only an early clinical period of the late stages of the disease.

Data recently reported by us (17) regarding the percent of treatment failures and survival 10 years following radical mastectomy for what were considered to be clinically "curable" breast cancers strikingly emphasize the systemic nature of that cancer at time of surgery. The finding that three of four patients with positive axillary nodal involvement and that almost 9 of 10 with four or more such nodes containing tumor at surgery become treatment failures lends confirmation to such a contention. That one of four patients *without* lymph node involvement develops metastases is also supportive. Because some patients never develop metastases is no indication that the operation has eliminated every cancer cell, that the disease was completely loco-regional in extent, and that dissemination had not taken place. The residual cell burden following tumor removal may have been sufficiently minimal for its eradication by host factors that play a significant role in the success or failure of the operative procedure. It is impossible to estimate the number of micrometastases that may have been so aborted by removal of a primary tumor. Such a concept is at present still too discordant for general acceptance by surgeons and others who care for cancer patients.

Correlating the information concerning the fate of patients having breast cancer with what is known about growth rates and other features regarding the kinetics of cells from such tumors and employing certain assumptions, calculations have been made (40) of the residual tumor cell burden that might be expected in a host following primary tumor removal, i.e., the number of viable cancer cells that are beyond the reach of surgery. It has been estimated that postoperative patients with negative nodes have a lesser residual body burden of tumor than those with one to three positive nodes, who, in turn, have a lesser tumor burden than those with four or more positive nodes. Whether this is true or whether patients who ultimately develop a treatment failure, regardless of nodal status, in fact have the *same* residual tumor burden is not known. Thus, the question of utmost importance with respect to residual tumor burden remaining to be answered is, Do breast cancer patients who have negative nodes and subsequently develop treatment failures (25% of patients) have a residual tumor burden equivalent to that of those with positive nodes who ultimately develop treatment failures, or, is there a quantitative difference in the tumor burden of the negative node patients? Similarly, Is the residual burden of those with one to three positive nodes similar to that in the four or more positive node patients who fail? In other words, do the proportion of patients with negative nodes who develop treatment failures differ in their tumor burden following operation from those with one to three or four plus positive nodes who ultimately fail, or do they have the same tumor burden? Is there simply a smaller proportion of those patients who fail in the negative node group? This is of fundamental importance in planning systemic therapy strategies. For if the former is true (i.e., that there is less tumor burden in negative node patients who fail), less intensive systemic therapy may be required to eliminate treatment failures in this group. On the other hand, if the second hypothesis is true (i.e., that tumor burden is the same in patients who become treatment failures regardless of their nodal status), then no less systemic therapy should be employed in negative node patients than would be employed in positive node patients.

In summary, tumor cell dissemination probably takes place close, if not immediately subsequent, to tumor inception. Failure of all patients to develop metastases is no argument against this. Host–tumor factors determine the incidence and magnitude of metastases. For improved end results, systemic therapy is mandatory.

BREAST CANCER IS A MULTICENTRIC DISEASE

Many, if not all, breast cancers may be multicentric in origin (9). Although several investigators (20,21,32) have addressed themselves to this, it is difficult to be certain how many multicentric, independent cancers might have been present since no clear distinction about actual site or pathologic type of lesion encountered was provided. In an examination of 904 cases (19) in a National Surgical Adjuvant Breast Project (NSABP) study, in order to circumvent the difficulty, if not impossibility, of distinguishing a focus of carcinoma in the quadrant of the primary as an integral part of the primary versus a true *de novo* lesion, data were collected only from quadrants in which the primary was not encountered, except in those instances in which it was beneath the nipple or in the tail of the breast. Either invasive or noninvasive cancers regarded as independent cancers were found in 13.4% of the 904 patients. The probability of detecting such lesions increased with the number of quadrants available for examination rather than with the study of any particular quadrant. The incidence of invasive and noninvasive multicentric cancers was 4.1 and 9.3%. The types of noninvasive cancers encountered were intraductal (66.7%), lobular carcinoma *in situ* (22.6%), and a combination of both (10.7%), All of the invasive forms were of the infiltrating duct not otherwise specified (NOS) type.

Similarly evidence has appeared to indicate that the incidence of cancer in the contralateral breast may be *much* greater than previously supposed (46,47). The disturbing fact is that, despite the significant incidence of multifocal lesions in both breasts of a woman with a primary breast cancer, only extremely rarely is there evidence of two or more clinically overt primary cancers in the same breast. Similarly, the presence of synchronous bilateral tumors are uncommon, and the incidence of a second asynchronous primary tumor in the involved breast fails to approach the incidence of occult lesions detected by random biopsy or autopsy (41). For example, it has been noted that the incidence of clinically latent intraductal carcinomas in breasts of women over the age of 70 who died from causes other than mammary carcinoma is 19 times greater than the reported incidence of clinical breast cancer (25). Such findings are highly suggestive that all cancers do not progress to overt lesions or may even undergo regression. That such a possibility is not remote is shown by the fact that neuroblastomas of the adrenal in children, thyroid carcinomas, and carcinomas of the prostate are found more frequently in random pathologic material than they are found clinically in comparable populations (8). It is of utmost urgency that the natural history of multicentric cancers, their clinical significance, and their influence on treatment, if any, be ascertained. At present, it is difficult for those resorting to orthodox principles of cancer management to accept the possibility that "a cancer may not be a cancer of clinical significance." From a biologic viewpoint, there is need for information relating the kinetics of the growth of such tumor foci to those of the primary tumor. Does the presence or absence of a primary tumor affect their growth? Are their kinetics similar to those of distant metastatic foci? Will they become more susceptible to destruction by antitumor agents following removal of the primary?

In summary, multicentricity is a reality. Its clinical and biologic significance is one of the most important aspects of breast cancer that must be evaluated.

BREAST CANCER IS A PATHOLOGICALLY HETEROGENEOUS DISEASE

Aside from its role in establishing the diagnosis of a lesion, the histopathologic study of tumors may provide (a) discriminants that could be of prognostic significance and (b) biologic information concerning the genesis and progression of mammary cancer. For an in-depth analysis of the pathology of invasive breast cancer the reader is referred to a recently published syllabus (18) that presents pathologic findings from 1,000 cases of breast cancer entered into NSABP Protocol #4. The following identifies those pathological and clinical characteristics found associated with lymph node metastases and treatment failure rates (Tables 1 and 2).

A variety of breast cancers with different histopathologic characteristics are recognized, and prognosis has been reputed to vary according to the tumor type. Infiltrating duct carcinomas in which no special type of histologic structure is recognized are designated not otherwise specified or NOS and are by far the most common duct tumors, accounting for about 50% of breast cancers. They frequently metastasize to axillary lymph nodes, and their prognosis is the poorest of the various tumor types. Another 28% of tumors are infiltrating duct NOS with another tumor type in combination.

There are several other types of invasive carcinomas that arise from large ducts, each having its own distinct histopathologic picture. The *medullary carcinoma,* comprising 5 to 7% of all mammary carcinomas, is a circumscribed lesion that attains large dimensions and demonstrates low-grade, infiltrative properties. The 5-year survival rate following removal of such a tumor is considered better than average. A tumor in which tubule formation is evident (1%) is known as *tubular carcinoma.* This tumor has a high nuclear grade with some existing polarity of its cells, and its prognosis, al-

TABLE 1. *Consistent associations with nodal status*

≥ 4 Nodes positive for metastases
Clinically positive axilla
≥ 4.1 Cm tumor size
Nuclear grade 1 (most anaplastic)
Histologic grade 3 (most malignant)
Lymphatic invasion
Blood vessel invasion
Perineural space invasion
Nipple involvement
Cancer in vicinity of dominant mass
Stromal elastosis
Absent nodal sinus histiocytosis
Capsular extension of nodal metastasis

TABLE 2. *Associations with treatment failure rate*

Age < 50 years
Clinically positive axillary nodes
Pathologically positive axillary nodes
Location tumor in subareolar area
Tumor size 6.1 + cm > 5.1–6.0 > 4.1–5.0 > 3.1–4.0 > 2.1–3.0 > 1.1–2.0 > 0–1.0
Noncircumscribed tumor (macro and microscopic)
Histologic type—NOS; NOS + lobular > NOS + tubular; medullary; lobular invasive; NOS + mucinous > NOS + papillary; NOS + lobular + tubular > mucinous; tubular
Nuclear grade—1 > 2 > 3
Histologic grade—3 > 2 > 1
Tumor necrosis
Lymphatic invasion
Blood vessel invasion
Cell reaction to tumor
Mucin—absent/slight > moderate > marked
Intraductal component of cancer—comedo > solid or papillary > adenocystic or combinations
Microscopic involvement of skin overlying tumor
Nipple involvement
Capsular extension of nodal metastases
Intralymphatic extension in quadrants remote from primary tumor

---

though regarded as better than infiltrating duct cancers, is less favorable than that of the medullary carcinoma, despite the fact that the cells of the medullary carcinoma tumor are more poorly differentiated than are those of the tubular carcinoma. Another tumor type, the *mucinous or colloid carcinoma,* comprises about 3% of all mammary carcinomas. This ductal carcinoma is characterized on microscopy by its nests and strands of epithelial cells floating in a mucinous matrix. It is usually slow-growing and can reach bulky proportions. When the tumor is predominantly mucinous, the prognosis tends to be good. This probably reflects a higher degree of tumor differentiation. This association is in keeping with findings about nuclear and histologic grades and histologic type considered to indicate the degree of tumor differentiation.

One type of tumor that has been attracting considerable attention in recent years is the *lobular carcinoma* that arises from the small end-ducts of the breast. The noninvasive variety, the so-called lobular carcinoma *in situ,* is characterized by clusters of anaplastic small cells of high nuclear grade that lie within lobules. This lesion, extending beyond the boundary of the lobule or terminal duct from which it arises, is known as *invasive lobular carcinoma* and may be indistinguishable from the conventional infiltrating duct carcinoma. At that point its prognosis is poor. The true incidence of lobular carcinomas is uncertain, but it is about 5%.

Although a number of reports show that a lymphoid cellular reaction within a tumor may indicate a host immune response and thus a more favorable prognosis, our findings disclose the converse. The associations between cell reaction and other parameters showing a high degree of malignancy indicate that such a finding is related to the degree of malignancy rather than some immune response to tumor *per se*. Tumor necrosis does achieve importance as a prognostic factor. It and patient age are the *only* characteristics related to treatment failure in patients with Stage I cancer. Microscopic involvement of the skin over a tumor as well as intralymphatic extension, another manifestation of inflammatory cancer, are associated with low survival rates.

A variety of characteristics have been found statistically related to nodal status (Table 1). Tumor size, degree of nuclear anaplasia, and histologic grade relate to nodal involvement, as does the finding of intralymphatic, perineural space, blood vessel, and nipple invasion. Sinus histiocytosis was found absent more frequently in nodes of positive node than negative node patients. Although this might support reports that marked sinus histiocytosis is a favorable prognostic indicator, the converse (i.e., that patients without nodal metastases reveal marked sinus histiocytosis) was not observed. Moreover, the absence of sinus histiocytosis was not a significant parameter associated with treatment failure. Because of this and other considerations expressed elsewhere we are skeptical that sinus histiocytosis is a significant indicator of a favorable host immunologic response to tumor.

In summary, findings indicate that the propensity of most breast cancers for regional and/or systemic metastases is related to quantitative and qualitative histopathologic features that reflect their growth characteristics. Awareness of these discriminants is essential for proper stratification of patients in future clinical studies of breast cancer, and they must be taken into account when assessing studies of breast cancer relating to survival or treatment failure.

BREAST CANCER PRODUCES HETEROGENEOUS TUMOR AND HOST IMMUNE RESPONSES

There is increasing evidence that immune mechanisms play an important role in the natural history of breast cancer. Aside from those morphologic characteristics commented on elsewhere in this review, which are reputed to relate to an immunologic response of the host, a large number of investigations have attempted to measure cell-mediated immune competence of breast cancer patients by a variety of techniques. These have included delayed hypersensitivity reactions to common antigens (29,31,38,43,45), blastogenic transformation of lymphocytes in response to mitogens such as phytohemagglutinin (PHA) (7,13,31,38,49,50), counts of rosette-forming cells (T lymphocytes) (31), migration inhibition assays of regional lymph node and peripheral blood lymphocytes (3,12,37,45), *in vitro* cytotoxicity tests (1,11), indirect measures of macrophage activity (2), thymidine uptake in regional lymph nodes (14), and counts of peripheral blood lymphocytes (33). Although some have tried to correlate depression of these parameters with gradually progressive disease (33), significant depression has only been noted in patients with recurrent or advanced disease (31,50). Cell-mediated immunity seems to remain intact until the disease is advanced.

A number of circulating antigens, both tumor specific and tumor nonspecific, have been studied in an attempt to gauge prognosis and response to therapy. It has been considered that the presence of circulating antigen in postmastectomy patients represents subclinical disease (42,44). If so, such a finding could be used to help select patients who would benefit from adjuvant therapy. The nonspecific antigen studied most extensively in patients with breast cancer has been carcinoembryonic antigen (CEA) (26,42,44). A majority (70 to 80%) of patients with metastatic breast cancer and approximately 30% with localized breast cancer have elevated CEA levels, and the incidence of positive CEA levels increases with advancing stage of disease. In addition, it has been shown that in patients with metastatic disease undergoing chemo- and/or hormonal therapy the trend of serial CEA values in general correlates with the response to treatment. This raises the question whether those patients who have clinical Stage I and II disease and elevated CEA levels might not be patients in whom the tumor has spread beyond the confines of the breast and regional lymph nodes and in whom, therefore, adjuvant therapy would be more likely to be beneficial. Unfortunately, neither CEA nor any other single test presently known demonstrates an abnormality in all patients with disease spread. This emphasizes the heterogeneous behavior of invasive breast cancer (4), and, for this reason, performance of a battery of tests in these patients has been advocated.

Tissue antigens have been identified in breast cancer extracts, in extracts of fibrocystic and fibroadenomatous breasts, and in normal breast tissue (1,22). Some appear to be specific to cancerous tissues, whereas others occur in both cancerous breasts and in those with benign breast disease. Still others are found in both cancerous and normal breasts. In general, tests utilizing cytotoxicity testing and skin testing have implied a fairly extensive crossreactivity between benign and malignant hyperplastic disease of the breast, and the place of tissue antigens in the evaluation of patients with breast cancer is yet to be elucidated.

Humoral factors in the serum and tissue of breast cancer patients have also been studied. Immunoglobulin levels in extracts of cancerous breasts have been compared with levels in extracts from normal breasts and from breasts with benign disease (35,36,39). In general, IgG and IgA levels are significantly decreased in malignant breast tissue when compared with benign and normal tissue. On the other hand, IgM levels, which are detected in only approximately one-third of carcinomas, when present, are significantly elevated compared with benign and normal tissue. It is not known whether this is associated with a good prognosis or with other manifestations of host resistance. In general, the total immunoglobulin and IgG content in malignant tumors correlates with plasma cell infiltration. Unfortunately, the serum immunoglobulin levels may not reflect local antibody production in the tissue. Some reports indicate that serum immunoglobulin levels are normal in breast cancer patients, whereas others have shown elevated serum levels. Even in those studies in which the immunoglobulin levels were abnormal in breast cancer patients, these abnormal levels did not appear to correlate with prognosis (39).

Antibodies to breast cancer antigen and to normal breast antigen have been identified in approximately 50% of patients with breast cancer, and in approximately one-fourth to one-third of patients with benign breast disease (6,23,24). There has been no correlation between tumor type and the presence of serum antibody, although one study indicates that severe sinus histiocytosis in the regional lymph nodes is approximately four times more common in breast cancer patients who have detectable serum antibody (23). The failure to detect serum antibody to breast cancer antigen in approximately half of breast cancer patients could be due to either the lack of antigen(s) in the tumors of these patients similar to those in the test reagents or the absorption of enough antibody by residual body tumor to render it undetectable by present methods. A report from a small series (23,24) lends credence to the latter interpretation, in that 11 of 13 patients with positive lymph nodes and *negative* antibody recurred within 1 year, whereas only three of 18 with positive lymph nodes and *positive* antibody developed recurrence within 2 years. More follow-up and larger series are necessary to test this theory adequately. In any event, the finding of antibody in only half the breast cancer population and in one-fourth to one-third of patients with benign breast disease raises questions about the true value of a positive serum antibody in early diagnosis. It must be emphasized that the central problem is the lack of a specific standard test reagent.

Nontumor-specific autoantibodies, such as antinuclear antibody (ANA), smooth muscle antibody (SMA), antibody against glomerular elements (GA), and mitochondrial antibody (MA), have been studied in patients with breast cancer with conflicting results. One group (48) found a higher incidence of ANA and SMA in breast cancer patients and has equated their early presence with a poor prognosis, whereas another group (30) failed to substantiate these results.

In summary, breast cancers have been found to result in a multitude of host immunologic responses. Their true significance for the natural history of the disease and for therapeutic planning may at present be said categorically to be obscure.

BREAST CANCER IS HETEROGENEOUS AT THE MOLECULAR LEVEL

Although the natural history of breast cancers relates to their varied pathologic discriminants and their capabilities to incite a diversity of immune responses, recent information regarding receptor sites in the cytoplasm of cells of such tumors provides further evidence of their heterogeneity (28). The demonstration that a proportion of breast cancers have or do not have cells containing a cytoplasmic protein that binds estrogen (ER) with high affinity and specificity is in itself significant. The finding of a relationship between the presence or absence of such a receptor and the response of the tumor to endocrine therapies makes such an observation more important. The demonstration of other receptor sites, such as progesterone and prolactin, in cells of some breast cancers is of equal significance. How the presence or absence of receptor sites influences the natural history of breast cancer aside from its response to endocrine therapy remains to be fully ascertained. At an international workshop in 1974 (27), there was suggestive, but not necessarily conclusive, evidence that (a) tumors from postmenopausal patients contain higher ER values than from premenopausal patients, (b) there is no correlation between the histologic type of tumor and the presence of ER, although there is a suggestion that morphologically undifferentiated tumors (grade III) less often contain ER, (c) there is a negative correlation between size of a primary tumor and the presence of ER, (d) there is no correlation between the clinical stage of a patient and tumor ER, (e) there is no correlation between positive or negative axillary nodes and the presence of ER in the primary tumor, (f) there is no correlation between tumor location and ER, (g) there is no correlation between disease-free interval and ER, and (h) there is no correlation between the absolute ER value and the duration of remission.

In summary, the finding of receptor sites in some breast cancers and not others is apt to be only one example of the heterogeneity of such tumors at the molecular level. The future may well demonstrate a multitude of differences on the cell membrane and within the cell itself. It would be naive to anticipate that such dissimilarities are not responsible for variations in tumor growth, host reaction, and response to therapy.

OTHER FACTORS FOR CONSIDERATION

Age or Menopausal Status

NSABP studies over the years have consistently indicated a close correlation between the age of patients and menopausal status. A division of age into those 49 or younger and 50 or older will delineate pre- and postmenopausal patients within a few percent. Consequently, for practical purposes the two may be used interchangeably.

The recent findings that systemic chemotherapy may be more effective in pre- than in postmenopausal patients (15) reevokes the question whether the disease is different in pre- and postmenopausal patients.

Data are conflicting in that regard. Our present NSABP protocol indicates that in radical mastectomy patients having an average follow-up of 3 years, those who are premenopausal with negative nodes have a 17% treatment failure, whereas in those with one to three positive axillary nodes and those with four or more positive nodes, treatment failure is 31 and 64%, respectively. In postmenopausal patients those subgroups display a failure of 8, 23, and 56%, respectively. A report of a previous NSABP study (17) indicated that 5 years following operation, premenopausal patients did less well than those who were postmenopausal, but by 10 years the treatment failures were quite similar.

Location

The long-established principle that the location of a breast cancer influences prognosis was reassessed utilizing NSABP data (16), and it was observed that location *per se* failed to influence a patient's prognosis. Only in patients with four positive nodes having subareolar or diffuse tumors was survival found to be worse. As a result of these findings reported in 1969, it was concluded that there was no reason to anticipate that the utilization of a specific approach for the therapy of breast cancer based on tumor location would be more rewarding than any other. That opinion remains unchanged.

CONCLUSIONS

From the foregoing, it becomes apparent that to talk about breast cancer as if it were a single entity is no longer justifiable. This is particularly relevant when one considers the results of treatment. This reviewer has spent almost a professional lifetime emphasizing the need for proper controls when evaluating treatments and has pointed out the pitfalls of comparing results from divergent series of cases. In that regard, the increasing popularity of different investigators to participate in different arms of a common protocol is not acceptable.

Such considerations indicate the absolute need for accrual of sufficient numbers of patients in clinical trials that are properly stratified in as many discriminants as possible if one wishes to obtain credible information regarding the effect of therapy on various subsets of patients. For, as emphasized with the use of adjuvant chemotherapy, it is unlikely that all patients will be best served by a universal therapy.

Lastly, a few comments concerning the use of immunotherapy. There must be a firm biologic basis for all therapeutic modalities in order to legitimize their use. Just as the surgeon is vaguely aware of what he has accomplished by an examination of the specimen removed, the radiation therapist by the isodose curves he has employed, and the chemotherapist by the bone marrow depression and other toxicity invoked, so would it be wished that the immunotherapist have some equally "poor" gauge of his efforts. For, as repeatedly pointed out, the greatest fear is that what is judged as a therapeutic failure may in reality have never been a therapeutic contest.

REFERENCES

1. Avis, F., Avis, I., Newsome, J. F., and Haughton, G. (1976): Antigenic cross-reactivity between adenocarcinoma of the breast and fibrocystic disease of the breast. *J. Natl. Cancer Inst.* 56:17–25.
2. Baum, M., Sumner, D., Edwards, M. H., and Smythe, P. (1973): Macrophage phagocytic activity in patients with breast cancer. *Br. J. Surg.* 60:899–900 (Abstr.)
3. Black, M. M., Leis, H. P., Jr., Shore, B., and Zachra, R. E. (1974): Cellular hypersensitivity to breast cancer. Assessment by a leukocyte migration procedure. *Cancer*, 33:952–958.
4. Black, M. M., Zachra, R. E., Shore, B., and Leis, H. P., Jr. (1976): Biological considerations of tumor-specific and virus-associated antigens of human breast cancers. *Cancer Res.* 36:769–774.
5. Bloom, H. J. G., Richardson, W. W., and Harries, E. J. (1962): Natural history of untreated breast cancer (1805–1933). Comparison of untreated and treated cases according to histological grade of malignancy. *Br. Med. J.* 2:213–221.
6. Boehm, O. R., Boehm, B. J., and Humphrey, L. J. (1974): The natural history of the antibody response to breast antigens. *Clin. Exp. Immunol.*, 16:31–40.
7. Bolton, P. M., Whitehead, R. H., Newcombe, R. G., James, S. L., and Hughes, L. E. (1975): The relationship between prognosis and lymphocyte response to PHA in breast cancer. *Br. J. Cancer*, 31:262–263 (Abstr.)
8. Burnet, F. M. (1967): Immunological aspects of malignant disease. *Lancet*, 1:1171–1174.
9. Cheatle, G. L., and Cutler, M. (1931): *Tumors of the Breast: Their Pathology, Symptoms, Diagnosis, and Treatment.* Lippincott, Philadelphia.
10. Daland, E. M. (1927): Untreated cancer of the breast. *Surg. Gynecol. Obstet.*, 44:264–268.
11. Deodhar, S. D., Crile, G., Jr., and Esselstyn, C. B., Jr. (1972): Study of the tumor cell-lymphocyte interaction in patients with breast cancer. *Cancer*, 29:1321–1325.
12. Ellis, R. J., Wernick, G., Zabriskie, J. B., and Goldman, L. I. (1975): Immunologic competence of regional lymph nodes in patients with breast cancer. *Cancer*, 35:655–659.
13. Fisher, B., Saffer, E. A., and Fisher, E. R. (1972): Studies concerning the regional lymph node in cancer. III. Response of the regional lymph node cells from breast and colon cancer patients to PHA stimulation. *Cancer*, 30:1202–1215.
14. Fisher, B., Saffer, E. A., and Fisher, E. R. (1974): Studies concerning the regional lymph node in cancer. VII. Thymidine uptake by cells from nodes of breast cancer patients relative to axillary location and histopathologic discriminants. *Cancer*, 33:271–279.
15. Fisher, B., Carbone, P. P., Economou, S. G., Frelick, R., Glass, A., Lerner, H., Redmond, C., Zelen, M., Katrych, D. L., Wolmark, N., Band, P., and Fisher, E. R. (1975): L-Phenylalanine mustard (L-PAM) in the management of primary breast cancer: A report of early findings. *N. Engl. J. Med.* 292:117–122.
16. Fisher, B., Slack, N. H., Ausman, R. K., and Bross, I. D. J. (1969): Location of breast cancer and prognosis. *Surg. Gynecol. Obstet.*, 129:705–716.
17. Fisher, B., Slack, N., Katrych, D., and Wolmark, N. (1975): Ten year follow-up of breast cancer patients in a cooperative clinical trial evaluating surgical adjuvant chemotherapy. *Surg. Gynecol. Obstet.*, 140:528–534.
18. Fisher, E. R., Gregorio, R. M., and Fisher, B., with the assistance of Redmond, C., Vellios, F., Sommers, S. C., and cooperating investigators. (1975): The pathology of invasive breast cancer. A syllabus derived from findings of the National Surgical Adjuvant Breast Project (Protocol No. 4). *Cancer*, 36:1–85.
19. Fisher, E. R., Gregorio, R., Redmond, C., Vellios, F., Sommers, S. C., and Fisher, B. (1975): Pathologic findings from the National Surgical Adjuvant Breast

Project (Protocol No. 4). I. Observations concerning the multicentricity of mammary cancer. *Cancer,* 35:247–254.

20. Foote, F. W., and Stewart, F. W. (1945): Comparative studies of cancerous versus non-cancerous breasts. *Ann. Surg.,* 121:5–53.
21. Gallager, H. S., and Martin, J. E. (1969): The study of mammary carcinoma by mammography and whole organ sectioning. *Cancer,* 23:855–878.
22. Hollinshead, A. C., Jaffurs, W. T., Alpert, L. K., Harris, J. E., and Herberman, R. B. (1974): Isolation and identification of soluble skin-reactive membrane antigens of malignant and normal human breast cells. *Cancer Res.,* 34:2961–2968.
23. Humphrey, L. J., Estes, N. C., Morse, P. A., Jr., Jewell, W. R., Boudet, R. A., Hudson, M. J. K., Tsolakidis, P. G., and Mantz, F. A. (1974): Serum antibody in patients with breast disease: Correlation with histopathology. *Ann. Surg.,* 180:124–129.
24. Humphrey, L. J., Estes, N. C., Morse, P. A., Jr., Jewell, W. R., Boudet, R. A., and Hudson, M. J. K. (1974): Serum antibody in patients with mammary disease. *Cancer,* 34:1516–1520.
25. Kramer, W. M., and Rush, B. F. (1973): Mammary duct proliferation in the elderly—A histopathologic study. *Cancer,* 31:130–137.
26. Marcus, D. M. (1975): Immunologic aspects of cancer of the breast. *Am. J. Clin. Pathol.,* 64:786–791.
27. McGuire, W. L. (1975): Current status of estrogen receptors in human breast cancer. *Cancer,* 36:638–644.
28. McGuire, W. L., Carbone, P. P., Sears, M. E., and Escher, G. C. (1975): Estrogen receptors in human breast cancer—An overview. In: *Estrogen Receptor in Human Breast Cancer,* edited by W. L. McGuire, P. P. Carbone, and E. P. Vollmer, pp. 1–7. Raven Press, New York.
29. Mitchell, R. J. (1972): The delayed hypersensitivity response in primary breast carcinoma as an index of host resistance. *Br. J. Surg.* 59:505–508.
30. Mittra, I., Perrin, J., and Kumaoka, S. (1976): Thyroid and other autoantibodies in British and Japanese Women: An epidemiological study of breast cancer. *Br. Med. J.,* 1:257–259.
31. Nemoto, T., Han, T., Minowada, J., Angkur, V., Chamberlain, A., and Dao, T. L. (1974): Cell-mediated immune status of breast cancer patients: Evaluation by skin tests, lymphocyte stimulation, and counts of rosette-forming cells. *J. Natl. Cancer Inst.,* 53:641–645.
32. Nicholson, G. W. (1921): Carcinoma of the breast. *Br. J. Surg.,* 8:527–528.
33. Papastas, A. E., and Kark, A. E. (1974): Peripheral lymphocyte counts in breast carcinoma. An index of immune competence. *Cancer,* 34:2014–2017.
34. Phillips, A. J. (1959): A comparison of treated and untreated cases of cancer of the breast. *Br. J. Cancer,* 13:20–25.
35. Roberts, M. M., Bass, E. M., Wallace, I. W. J., and Stevenson, A. (1973): Local immunoglobulin production in breast cancer. *Br. J. Cancer,* 27:269–275.
36. Roberts, M. M., Bass, E. M., and Wallace, I. W. J. (1972): Antibody production in breast cancer. *Br. J. Surg.,* 59:904 (Abstr.)
37. Roberts, M. M., and Bass, E. M. (1975): The Immune reaction to human breast cancer tissue. *Br. J. Surg.,* 62:660–661 (Abstr.)
38. Roberts, M. M., and Jones-Williams, W. (1974): The delayed hypersensitivity reaction in breast cancer. *Br. J. Surg.,* 61:549–552.
39. Roberts, M. M., Bathgate, E. M., and Stevenson, A. (1975): Serum immunoglobulin levels in patients with breast cancer. *Cancer,* 36:221–224.
40. Skipper, H. E. (1974): *Combination Therapy, Booklet 13,* p. 1. Southern Research Institute, Birmingham, Alabama.
41. Slack, N. H., Bross, J. D. J., Nemoto, T., and Fisher, B. (1973): Experience with bilateral primary carcinoma of the breast in a cooperative study. *Surg. Gynecol. Obstet.,* 136:433–440.
42. Steward, A. M., Nixon, D., Zamcheck, N., and Aisenberg, A. (1974): Carcino-embryonic antigen in breast cancer patients: Serum levels and disease progress. *Cancer,* 33:1246–1252.
43. Stewart, T. H. M., and Orizaga, M. (1971): The presence of delayed hyper-

sensitivity reactions in patients toward cellular extracts of their malignant tumors. 3. The frequency, duration, and cross-reactivity of this phenomenon in patients with breast cancer, and its correlation with survival. *Cancer,* 28:1472–1478.

44. Tormey, D. C., Waalkes, T. P., Ahmann, D., Gehrke, C. W., Zumwatt, R. W., Snyder, J., and Hansen, H. (1975): Biological markers in breast carcinoma. I. Incidence of abnormalities of CEA, HCG, three polyamines, and three minor nucleosides. *Cancer,* 35:1095–1100.

45. Turnbull, A. R., and Jones, B. M. (1975): Clinical correlates of cell-mediated reactivity to autologous tumor antigens in breast cancer. *Br. J. Surg.,* 62:660 (Abstr.)

46. Urban, J. A. (1967): Bilaterality of cancer of the breast. Biopsy of the opposite breast. *Cancer,* 20:1867–1870.

47. Urban, J. A. (1969): Biopsy of the 'normal' breast in treating breast cancer. *Surg. Clin. North Am.,* 49:291–301.

48. Wasserman, J., Glas, U., and Blomgren, H. (1975): Autoantibodies in patients with carcinoma of the breast. Correlation with prognosis. *Clin. Exp. Immunol.,* 19:417–422.

49. Whitehead, R. H., Bolton, P. M., Newcombe, R. G., James, S. L., and Hughes, L. E. (1975): Lymphocyte response to PHA in breast cancer: Correlation of predicted prognosis to response to different PHA concentrations. *Clin. Oncol.,* 1:191–200.

50. Whittaker, M. G., and Clark, C. G. (1971): Depressed lymphocyte function in carcinoma of the breast. *Br. J. Surg.,* 58:717–720.

Immunotherapy of Cancer: Present Status of Trials in Man, edited by W. D. Terry and D. Windhorst. Raven Press, New York © 1977.

Levamisole Action in Breast Cancer Stage III

Alejandro F. Rojas, Julio N. Feierstein, Horacio M. Glait, and Américo J. Olivari

Centro Oncológico de Medicina Nuclear, Facultad de Medicina (UNBA) y Comisión Nacional de Energía Atómica, Instituto de Oncología "Angel H. Roffo," Buenos Aires, Argentina

A variety of microbial products have traditionally been used as immuno-modulators. Recent studies have shown that low-molecular-weight compounds including thiazole derivates (11) and polynucleotides (2) may have an effect on the immune system as well.

Levamisole [L (-) 2, 3, 5, 6 tetrahydro-6-phenylimidazo (2, 1b) thiazole hydrochloride] is an agent that has had wide clinical use as antihelminthic with few untoward side effects (15). In animal studies, Renoux et al. demonstrated that levamisole increased resistance to infections and stimulated cell-mediated immune reactions (12).

Based on these findings, a clinical trial of levamisole was begun in 1972 in patients with inoperable breast cancer [stage III (UICC) classification] (13). We reported that levamisole increased the reactivity to 2, 4 dinitrochloroben-zene (DNCB), the disease-free interval, and survival after radiation therapy.

MATERIALS AND METHODS

At this institution, breast cancer stage III (UICC classification) is treated primarily by radiation therapy. The radiation treatment was delivered by a cobalt source, 4,000 R (rads) to the chest wall in internal and external tangential fields, 4,000 R to the supraclavicular area, and 3,000 R to the posterior axillary field. This treatment was given over a mean of 2 months. The diagnosis was confirmed histologically in all cases. After completion of radiation therapy, patients were assigned alternately to either the control group or the levamisole-treated group. The control group (23 patients) received no further treatment until there was evidence of recurrent disease. The treated group (20 patients) took levamisole (provided by R. Garrido, Cyanamid Argentina) 150 mg orally daily on 3 consecutive days, every other week, until there was evidence of progressing disease.

Follow-up of patients consisted of a monthly physical examination, bimonthly liver function tests, complete blood count, and differential and platelet count. Skeletal survey, bone scan, and chest X-ray were repeated every 3 to 5 months or earlier if warranted by the patients' symptoms.

TABLE 1. Age, menopausal status, and parity of patients prior to radiotherapy

	Control (23)	Levamisole (20)
Average age	58.3 (39–80)	60.0 (34–82)
Average age at menopause	49.1 (41–57)	49.5 (42–56)
Number of premenopausal patients	3	2
Average number of children	2.2	1.8

The distribution of the patients in each group according to age, menopausal status, and parity is shown in Table 1; both groups were comparable. The distribution in each group according to tumor-node-metastases (TNM) classification is shown in Table 2.

To confirm the validity of this first trial, a retrospective study of 70 stage III breast cancer patients, irradiated between 1971 and 1974, was carried out. This historical control group was compared to 33 breast cancer stage III patients treated with levamisole. Table 3 shows the distribution of the pa-

TABLE 2. Distribution of patients according to TNB classification (UICC)

TNM classification	Control		Levamisole	
$T_3 N_1 M_0$	34.8%	(8)	30.0%	(6)
$T_3 N_2 M_0$	26.1%	(6)	35.0%	(7)
$T_3 N_3 M_0$	13.0%	(3)	10.0%	(2)
$T_4 N_1 M_0$	4.3%	(1)	5.0%	(1)
$T_4 N_2 M_0$	17.4%	(4)	5.0%	(1)
$T_4 N_3 M_0$	4.3%	(1)	15.0%	(3)
Total No. of patients	23		20	

TNM, tumor node metastasis; UICC, Union International Contra el Cancer.

TABLE 3. Age and menopausal status of patients in retrospective study prior to radiotherapy

	Historical control (70)	Levamisole (33)
Average age	59.1 (23–88)	55.8 (33–82)
Average age at menopause	49.3 (40–59)	49.2 (42–56)
Number of premenopausal patients	22	12

Irradiated between 1971 and 1974.

TABLE 4. *Distribution of patients according to TNM classification (UICC) in historical control and 33 levamisole-treated patients*

TNM classification	Historical control	Levamisole
$T_3 N_1 M_0$	21.4% (15)	30.3% (10)
$T_3 N_2 M_0$	32.9% (23)	36.4% (12)
$T_3 N_3 M_0$	5.7% (4)	9.1% (3)
$T_4 N_1 M_0$	22.9% (16)	12.1% (4)
$T_4 N_2 M_0$	10.0% (7)	3.0% (1)
$T_4 N_3 M_0$	7.1% (5)	9.1% (3)
Total No. of patients	70	33

TNM, tumor node metastasis; UICC, Union International Contra el Cancer.

tients according to age and menopausal status. Table 4 shows the distribution in each group according to the TNM classification.

The patients (except the historical controls) were sensitized after completion of radiotherapy using 2 mg of DNCB dissolved in 0.1 ml of acetone applied on the right arm within the confines of a plastic ring. The acetone was allowed to evaporate, and the site was covered with a dressing for 4 days. Fourteen days later, challenge doses of 25 and 100 μg were applied to the right forearm and covered with dry dressings for 48 hr. Reactions were read at 48 hr and classified as:

Negative		0	No response
		1	Erythema
Positive	Weak positive	2	Erythema + induration
	Strong positive	3	Erythema + induration + vesicle
		4	Erythema + induration + bulla

An intradermal skin test was performed on the left forearm with 0.1 ml of *Candida albicans* antigen (1/1,000) (Laboratories Rivero). Reaction was read at 48 hr and graded as negative (< 5 mm induration), 1+ (5 to 9 mm), 2+ (10 to 19 mm) 3+ (20 mm or more), or 4+ (25 mm or more with central necrosis).

Curves of disease-free interval and survival were calculated with the actuarial method and were analyzed with the generalized Wilcoxon test (8).

RESULTS

Recurrence

Figure 1 shows the disease-free interval for the randomized study. The median interval was 8.9 months for the control group and 22.5 months for the treated group ($p < 0.01$ generalized Wilcoxon test). At 42 months 0% of the control patients and 23.9% of the levamisole-treated patients were free

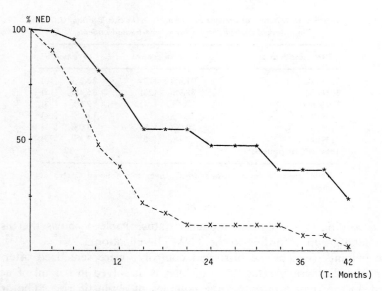

FIG. 1. Disease-free interval for levamisole (20) and control (23) group. *—*, Levamisole; x----x, control; NED.

of disease. Twenty-five percent of the patients were free of disease at 14 months in the control group and at 40.5 months in the treated group.

The sites and frequency of metastasis in both groups are summarized in Table 5. We found a higher frequency of lung metastasis in the treated group (61.9%) than in the control group (21.7%) ($p < 0.05$, X^2 with Yates correction).

After 30 months we have noted an increase in the frequency of local progression but with no statistical significance up till now.

Figure 2 shows the disease-free interval for the historical control group and 33 levamisole-treated patients. For the first group the median disease-free interval was 7.5 months, and at 15 months only 25% were disease free.

TABLE 5. *Comparison of sites of metastasis in randomized group*

Site of metastasis	Control		Levamisole	
Local recurrence	26.1%	(6/23)	30.8%	(4/13)
Skin	17.4%	(4/23)	7.7%	(1/13)
Nodes	21.7%	(5/23)	15.4%	(2/13)
Lungs	21.7%	(5/23)	61.5%	(8/13)[a]
Bones	39.1%	(9/23)	23.1%	(3/13)
Liver	17.4%	(4/23)	0.0%	(0/13)
Other	13.0%	(3/23)	7.7%	(1/13)

[a] $p < 0.05$, X^2 test.

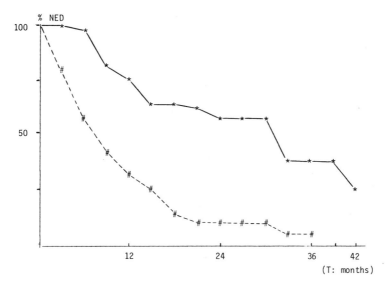

FIG. 2. Disease-free interval for historical control (70) and levamisole-treated (33) group. *—*, Levamisole; #--- #, historical control; NED.

The treated group shows a median time of 31 months, and at 42 months 25.9% are free of disease.

The sites and frequency of metastasis in both groups are summarized in Table 6. A similar percentage of lung metastasis is shown for the historical control (18.5%) as for the randomized control (21.7%); there exists a higher percentage for the levamisole-treated group (47.4%) ($p < 0.05$, X^2 with Yates correction). In the treated group the frequency of lung metastasis was greater during the first 30 months and decreased after that period of follow-up ($\overline{X}$: 23.2 months).

TABLE 6. *Comparison of sites of metastasis in historical control and 33 levamisole-treated patients*

Site of metastasis	Historical control		Levamisole	
Local recurrence	16.7%	(9/54)	36.8%	(7/19)[a]
Skin	16.7%	(9/54)	5.3%	(1/19)
Nodes	22.2%	(12/54)	10.5%	(2/19)
Lungs	18.5%	(10/54)	47.4%	(9/19)[b]
Bones	37.0%	(20/54)	21.1%	(4/19)
Liver	5.6%	(3/54)	5.3%	(1/19)
Other	3.7%	(2/54)	5.3%	(1/19)

[a] $p < 0.025$, X^2 test.
[b] $p < 0.05$, X^2 test.

Survival

The actuarial curves for the first two groups are shown in Fig. 3. The median survival time for the control group was 22 months and 41.5 months for the treated group ($p < 0.05$, generalized Wilcoxon test). At 30 months 78% are alive in the levamisole group and only 23.7% in the control group. At the end of the follow-up, 49.9% of the treated group compared to 19% of control patients is alive. Some of these alive patients (n = 3) in the treated group had shown local progression that was controlled by surgical excision or localized radiation and afterwards showed no further progression or metastasis.

The historical control group showed a median survival time of 22 months, and a 25% survival rate was reached at 32 months. At 42 months only 11.3% of historical control patients were alive. The treated group shows a median survival of 42 months, and survival at 48 months was 49.9% ($p < 0.01$, generalized Wilcoxon test) (Fig. 4).

Skin tests

Levamisole treatment was associated with an increase in positive test as compared with pretreatment reactivity (60 versus 83.3%) in the same group ($p < 0.01$ by the McNemar test) or with untreated controls ($p = 0.05$ Fisher's exact test). The treatment was associated with an increase in the number of strong positive reactions to 100 μg DNCB (Fig. 5), but not all the

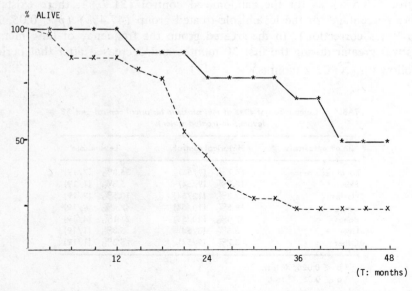

FIG. 3. Survival time for levamisole (20) and control (23) group. *—*, Levamisole; x---x, control.

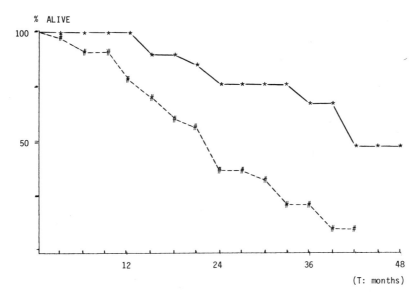

FIG. 4. Survival for historical control (70) and levamisole-treated (33) group. *—*, Levamisole; #--#, historical control.

patients increased their reactions. The treated patients could be divided into three groups—patients with negative reactions that showed no changes, patients with weak reactions, and patients with strong reactions to DNCB 100. The evolution of each group is shown in Fig. 6. The patients whose reactions decreased and reached the negative or weak groups further evolved like the

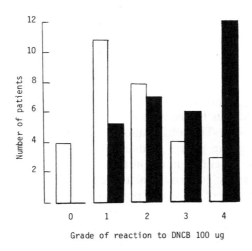

FIG. 5. Grade of reaction to DNCB before (☐) and after (■) 20 months of levamisole treatment.

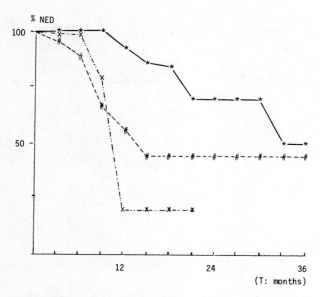

FIG. 6. Disease-free interval for levamisole-treated patients according to their skin reactivity to DNCB 100 (see text). *—*, Strong; #--- #, weak; x—··—x, negative.

low-level-of-reactions group. Patients (n = 4) whose reactions increased from negative to strong positives had a very different course. The median disease-free interval for patients with negative reactions (n = 5) with no increase or decrease from this level is 10 months, and 25% of the patients was disease free at 12 months. The patients with weak reactions (n = 10) that had fallen to this level had a median time of 13.5 months but are 45% disease free up to 42 months. The patients with strong reactions or who changed from another level to this one had 33 months of disease-free interval and are 38% disease free up to 42 months.

DISCUSSION

We oberved a significantly longer disease-free interval in levamisole-treated patients than in the control group (median 22.5 months versus 8.9 months, respectively). This observation was supported by the study of the historical control group with a median disease-free interval of 7.5 months. The great number of patients in the historical group with no further treatment after radiation therapy confirms that the clinical course of our first control group is representative of the whole population of patients without treatment. The evolution of the treated patients is statistically different from both control groups in that the levamisole treatment was associated with a better disease-free interval and survival. This observation is consistent with the finding of Chirigos et al. (4,5) and Amery et al. (14). Toxicity was negligible.

Several patients have taken more than 35 g without evidence of cumulative toxicity.

The manner of disease progression appeared to be modified by levamisole intake; patients who developed recurrence after 30 months showed local progression without other localization. Since this local recurrence can be controlled by local procedures, the patient can enter a new period with no evidence of disease, and three patients are in this condition. For the actuarial curves these patients were considered to have recurrences. The increase of pulmonary and pleural metastasis with levamisole was more evident during the first months, and had a median time of 23 months. The radiation and levamisole treatment probably had an immunomodulation effect on pulmonary tissue. This result was also present when compared with the historical control ($p < 0.05$).

Administration of levamisole was associated with an increase in reactivity to DNCB. Patients whose reactions increased to strong positive showed the best results in their clinical course. On the other hand, patients whose negative reactions to DNCB did not increase had the worst evolution. Similar results have been reported by Tripodi et al. (16), Brugmans et al. (3), and Fisher et al. (7). In four patients with negative reactions, DNCB responsiveness increased, gradually converting to weak positive and then to strongly positive over periods as long as 9 months. Only one of these has recurrent disease at 36 months.

Levamisole is effective by mouth, with no important or hazardous toxicity, and has shown to be effective in stage III breast cancer as an adjuvant to primary treatment. We do not know how levamisole affects cell-mediated immune responses, but an increase in skin test reactivity appears to correlate with the clinical responses.

SUMMARY

A clinical trial of levamisole was begun in 1972 in women with primary inoperable breast cancer (stage III). After being rendered clinically disease free by radiotherapy to the breast, supraclavicular area, and axilla, patients were allocated alternately to a control group (no further treatment) or a levamisole-treated group (150 mg orally, three times a week, every other week) and were followed up with physical examination and laboratory tests. A significant prolongation of the median disease-free interval and survival was seen in the 20 treated patients (22.5 months, 41.5 months) compared with the 23 control patients (9 months, 22 months). Before treatment no differences were found between both groups in tumoral size or hormone behavior. To confirm these results, a retrospective study of the clinical course of 70 breast cancer stage III patients irradiated from 1971 to 1974 was carried out. This historical control showed 7.5 months of median disease-free interval and 22 months median survival time.

Levamisole was associated with an increase in the percentage and intensity of delayed hypersensitivity skin reactions, and there was no major toxicity.

Our experience in breast cancer stage III led us to treat all these patients after radiation treatment because of the prolongation of clinical course and the negligible toxicity observed.

ACKNOWLEDGMENTS

We gratefully acknowledge Raquel Baldrich and Magdalena Racedo for their skillful technical assistance and Mariana Pradier for help in the preparation of this chapter.

This study has been supported in part by Cancer Research Institute, Inc.

REFERENCES

1. Bently, H. P., Hughes, E. R., and Peterson, D. A. (1974): Effect of hypophysectomy on a virus-induced T-cell leukaemia. *Nature,* 252:747.
2. Braun, W., Ishizuka, M., Yajima, Y., Webb, D., and Winchurch, R. (1971): In: *Biological Effects of Polynucleotides,* edited by R. F. Beers and W. Braun, p. 139. Springer-Verlag, New York.
3. DeJager, R., Pinsky, C., Kaufman, R., Ochoa, M., Oettgen, H. F., and Krakoff, haegen, H., Van Nimmen, L., Louwagie, A. C., and Stevens, E. (1973): Restoration of host defense mechanisms in man by levamisole. *Life Sci.,* 13:1499–1504.
4. Chirigos, M. A., Pearson, J. W., and Fuhrman, F. S. (1974): Effect of tumor load reduction on successful immunostimulation. *Proc. Am. Assoc. Cancer Res.,* 15:116.
5. Chirigos, M. A., Pearson, J. W., and Pryor, J. (1973): Augmentation of chemotherapeutically induced remission of a murine leukemia by a chemical immunoadjuvant. *Cancer Res.,* 33:2615–2618.
6. Fessell, W. J., and Forsyth, R. P. (1963): Hypothalamic role in control of globulin levels. *Arthritis Rheum.,* 6:770 (Abstr.)
7. Fischer, G. W., Oi, U. T., Ampaya, E. P., Kelley, J. L., and Bass, J. W. (1974): Enhanced host defense mechanism with Phenylimidothiazole. *Pediatr. Res.,* 8:138 (Abstr.)
8. Gehan, E. A. (1965): A generalized two samples Wilcoxon test for doubly sensored data. *Biometrika,* 52:650.
9. Goldberg, N. D., O'Dea, R. F., and Haddox, M. K. (1973): In: *Advances in Cyclic Nucleotide Research,* Vol. 3, edited by P. Greengard and G. A. Robinson, p. 209. Raven Press, New York.
10. Macris, N. T., Schiavi, R. C., Camerino, M. S., and Stein, M. (1970): Effect of hypothalamic lesion on immune processes in the guinea pig. *Am. J. Physiol.,* 219:1205–1209.
11. Renoux, G., and Renoux, M. (1974): Modulation of immune reactivity by phenylimidothiazole salts in mice immunized by sheep red blood cells. *J. Immunol.,* 113:779–790.
12. Renoux, G., and Renoux, M. (1971): Effet immunostimulant d'un imidothiazole dans l'immunisation des souris contre l'infection par Brucella abortus. *C. R. Acad. Sci.[D],* 272:349–350.
13. Rojas, A. F., Mickiewicz, E., Feierstein, J. N., Glait, H., and Olivari, A. J. (1976): Levamisole in advanced human breast cancer. *Lancet,* 1:211–215.
14. Study Group for Bronchogenic Carcinoma (1975): Immunopotentiation with Levamisole in resectable bronchogenic carcinoma: A double-blind controlled trial. *Br. Med. J.,* 3:461–464.
15. Thienpoint, D., Brugmans, J., Abadi, K., and Tanamal, S. (1969): Evaluation of

tetramisole in the treatment of nematode infections in man. *Am. J. Trop. Med. Hyg.,* 18:520–525.

16. Tripodi, D., Parks, L. C., and Brugmans, J. (1973): Drug-induced restoration of cutaneous delayed hypersensitivity in anergic patients with cancer. *N. Engl. J. Med.,* 289:354–357.

Question and Answer Session

Dr. Spitler: As I understand it, in your randomized trial, initially 24 patients were entered in each group. You reported results on 20 in the levamisole and 23 in the control, which means there were four lost in the levamisole group, and one lost in the control group. Why were they lost and if they were included in your analysis of the data, would it change your results?

Question: Perhaps I can try to answer the question. As I remember the data from the publication on the same study in the *Lancet,* it was stated that most of these patients just failed to come back.

Dr. Fudenberg: You state that patients were rendered "clinically free of disease by radiotherapy." What do you mean by "clinically free"?

Dr Olivari: The examination comprised a physical examination and liver and bone scans.

Dr. Salmon: The abstract refers to alternate allocation of patients into treatment groups, but your slides referred to a randomized allocation. Was it truly randomized or were they alternate patients?

Dr. Olivari: They were alternate patients.

Immunotherapy of Cancer: Present Status of
Trials in Man, edited by W. D. Terry and D. Windhorst.
Raven Press, New York © 1978.

Corynebacterium Parvum as Adjuvant to Combination Chemotherapy in Patients with Advanced Breast Cancer: Preliminary Results of a Prospective Randomized Trial

Carl M. Pinsky, Robert L. DeJager, Robert E. Wittes, Peter P. Wong, Richard J. Kaufman, Valerie Miké, John A. Hansen, Herbert F. Oettgen, and Irwin H. Krakoff

Memorial Sloan-Kettering Cancer Center, New York, New York 10021

We have recently reported (3) on the combination of cyclophosphamide, doxorubicin hydrochloride (Adriamycin®), methotrexate, and 5-fluorouracil (CAMF) in patients with advanced breast cancer. Initial response rate (complete and partial) was 65%. The patients were randomized to CAMF alone or CAMF plus *Corynebacterium parvum* (*C. parvum*). At the time of the previous report, there were no differences in response rate yet apparent. We report here that although response rate continues to be similar, response duration and survival appear to be longer in the group that receives CAMF plus *C. parvum*.

MATERIALS AND METHODS

Patients

To be eligible each patient had to have (a) histologically confirmed breast cancer, metastatic or locally recurrent, (b) prior oophorectomy or be postmenopausal, (c) measurable disease, (d) expected survival of over 4 weeks, (e) white blood cell count (WBC) > 4,000, platelets > 150,000, (f) normal electrocardiogram—absence of congestive heart failure, (g) normal serum creatinine, (h) no hormonal therapy in the past 4 weeks, no ablative surgery in the past 8 weeks unless disease was progressing, and (i) no prior cytotoxic chemotherapy.

Statistical Analysis

Eligible patients were randomly allocated to CAMF alone or CAMF + *C. parvum* after stratification by prior oophorectomy (yes or no), disease-free interval (less than, or more than, 1 year), radiation therapy (yes or no), and site of involvement (soft tissue, bone, or major organ). Response duration and survival were plotted according to the method of Kaplan and Meier (9) and tests for significance of difference carried out according to the method of Gehan (4).

Treatment

CAMF is an intermittent cyclic regimen in which four drugs are given during the first week of every 4-week cycle. CAMF consists of doxorubicin hydrochloride 40 mg/m² i.v. on day 1, methotrexate 15 mg/m² i.v. on days 3 and 8, 5-fluorouracil 400 mg/m² i.v. on days 3 and 8 and cyclophosphamide 125 mg/m² p.o. on days 3 through 8. Doxorubicin hydrochloride is discontinued after a total dose of 450 mg/m², and CMF as described by Canellos et al. (1) is continued thereafter.

All patients randomized to chemoimmunotherapy received *C. parvum* 4 mg s.c. weekly throughout the duration of trial. This preparation is formalin-killed, washed, and supplied by Burroughs-Wellcome Co.

Initial doses were repeated, as scheduled, with the following changes—for nadir of WBC < 3,000/mm² and/or platelets < 50,000/mm³, a 50% reduction in chemotherapy dosage for the next course; for severe liver dysfunction (bilirubin > 3 mg%), a 50% reduction in doxorubicin hydrochloride dosage; for local or systemic toxicity to *C. parvum,* a reduction of dose to 1 or 2 mg weekly.

Baseline Evaluation and Follow-up

Clinical evaluation to define the extent of disease and an immunological profile were performed before and at regular intervals after entering the study as follows: blood counts weekly, liver function tests and chest X-ray monthly, and skeletal survey or bone scan and liver scan every 3 months. Tumor measurements and/or photographs of visible lesions were repeated monthly. An immunological profile was obtained prior to treatment or shortly thereafter if it could not be obtained earlier. Every patient was sensitized with 2,4-dinitrochlorobenzene (DNCB) and challenged with four common antigens [tuberculin, mumps, *Candida,* and streptokinase/streptodornase (SK/SD)]. The details have been described previously (11).

Immune parameters *in vitro* (absolute lymphocyte counts, response to the lymphocyte mitogens phytohemagglutinin, conconavalin-A, and pokeweed mitogen, and lymphocyte response to common microbial antigens) (6) were obtained in a majority of the patients. Skin tests and immune parameters were repeated at 3, 6, and 12 weeks and then every 3 months.

Criteria of Response

Complete response was taken to be disappearance of all symptoms and signs of breast cancer. *Partial response* was taken to be a 50% decrease in the product of the two largest perpendicular diameters of all lesions with recalcification of bone metastases. A *minor response* with less than 50% decrease in the size of lesions was not computed in the response rate. Moertel's criteria were used in evaluating liver disease (10); these include reduction in the sum of the measurements below the xyphoid process and each costal margin at the midclavicular line of at least 30%. The duration of response was calculated from day 1 on the protocol. An adequate trial required 1 month on treatment with evidence of drug toxicity. Treatment was continued until progression of disease occurred.

RESULTS

Clinical and Immunological Characteristics

The two groups were comparable in their clinical and immunological characteristics (Table 1). Stratification insured that the prognostic factors would be equally represented in the two groups. Immunological reactions were also

TABLE 1. *Clinical and immunological characteristics*

	CAMF	
Characteristics	Without C. parvum (23 patients)	With C. parvum (24 patients)
Median age	57	57
(range)	(36–73)	(30–75)
Oophorectomy	6	9
Radiation therapy	17	17
Disease-free interval (less than 1 year)	8	9
Predominant site of metastasis		
Soft tissue	2	5
Bone	4	5
Major organ	17	14
DNCB negative	8/18[a]	15/24
Intradermal tests (all negative)	7/21	9/24
Absolute lymphocytes (< 1,000/mm³)	5/13	13/21
Subnormal mitogen response	9/12	15/21
Subnormal antigen response	5/12	3/19
Any of above	7/9	18/19
All of above	1/9	1/19

[a] Number abnormal/number tested.

comparable. Most patients had at least one defect in delayed hypersensitivity, but few were abnormal in all tests.

Toxicity

The treatment was generally well tolerated and suitable for out-patient administration. No toxic death occurred. Total alopecia was seen in all patients, nausea and vomiting were frequent after doxorubicin hydrochloride, and mucositis was seen in about 25%. *C. parvum* injection caused local erythema, induration, and subcutaneous nodules. Rarely, local signs or fever required a decrease in the weekly dose to 1 or 2 mg. The dose-limiting toxicity of the CAMF was hematopoietic with the nadir of leukocyte and platelet depression occurring after 15 to 18 days. There was no difference in myelosuppression between the two groups, nor was there any difference in the number of patients who had dose reductions or delays in retreatment. There are no data in this study, to date, that *C. parvum* increases the bone marrow tolerance for chemotherapy.

Antitumor Effects

Sixty-seven patients were entered and 47 are presently evaluable. Similar proportions of patients achieved complete or partial response in the two arms. Of adequately treated patients, 11 of 23 or 48% responded to CAMF alone and 14 of 24 or 58% to CAMF + *C. parvum*. Responses were seen in

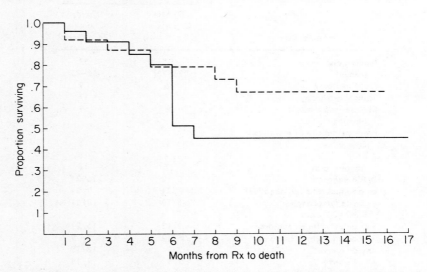

FIG. 1. The survival of the patients who received CAMF alone or CAMF plus *C. parvum* is shown in this figure. The apparent difference is not statistically significant. ————, CAMF (23 total, 13 alive); --- CAMF + *C. parvum* (24 total, 17 alive).

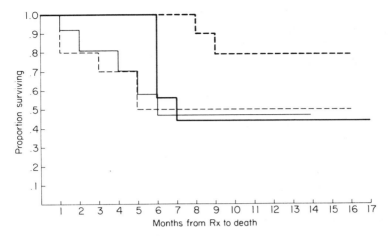

FIG. 2. The survival of patients who responded versus those who did not is compared for the two treatment arms. Although there is no difference for the nonresponders, survival is significantly longer for the responders who received CAMF plus C. parvum versus CAMF alone. Responders: ————, CAMF (11 total, 6 alive); ----, CAMF + C. parvum (14 total, 12 alive). Nonresponders: ————, CAMF (12 total, 7 alive); ---- CAMF + C. parvum (10 total; 5 alive).

patients with metastases in skin (including inflammatory carcinoma), lymph nodes, bone, pleura, lung, and liver, but not central nervous system. Only three patients had complete response, one treated with CAMF alone and two with CAMF plus *C. parvum.*

The survival curves (9) for the patients adequately treated with CAMF and CAMF plus *C. parvum* are shown in Fig. 1, indicating a difference in favor of the *C. parvum* group. This difference, however, is not statistically significant, possibly because of the small sample size and relatively short follow-up on many patients. When the data are further broken down into nonresponders versus responders, the corresponding survival curves (Fig. 2) show complete agreement in the survival experience of the two nonresponding groups but a pronounced difference between the two groups of responders. Whereas 5 of 11 patients who responded to CAMF alone have already relapsed and died, 12 of 14 patients responding to CAMF + *C. parvum* have continued their response and are still alive. Comparison of these two groups by the generalized Wilcoxon test (4) yields $p < 0.05$ (two-sided). The difference in response duration between the two groups, again, favors the *C. parvum* patients, but this difference is not statistically significant.

DISCUSSION

These preliminary results suggest that immunotherapy with *C. parvum* is effective in increasing the response duration and survival in patients with advanced breast cancer treated with chemotherapy. The data do not show evidence that *C. parvum* increases the bone marrow tolerance to chemotherapy, and preliminary data do not indicate that the group receiving *C. parvum* had increased immunological reactivity in terms of the parameters that were measured.

In this study, the response rates were lower than those previously reported by others (5,8) and ourselves (2) with similar chemotherapy programs. One possible explanation is that the proportion of patients with major organ involvement is higher in this series than it was in the others. Nonetheless, in patients with measurable breast cancer, complete responses in all studies remain infrequent and ultimate survival limited. The apparent increased duration of response and survival with the addition of *C. parvum* is a promising lead to follow. Although the number of patients in our study is small, the fact that similar findings have been reported by Israel and Edelstein (7) for *C. parvum* and Gutterman et al. (5) for Bacillus Calmette-Guerin gives greater credence to the notion that adding an immunopotentiator to partially effective chemotherapy may be of additional benefit in patients with advanced breast cancer.

SUMMARY

Sixty-seven patients with advanced carcinoma of the breast have been treated with a combination of cyclophosphamide, doxorubicin hydrochloride, methotrexate, and 5-fluorouracil, CAMF. By random assignment, half of the patients received *C. parvum* in addition to CAMF. The groups were stratified according to prior oophorectomy, disease-free interval, radiation therapy, and major site of metastasis. Of the 47 evaluable patients, 11 of 23 (48%) had complete or partial response to CAMF alone and 14 of 24 (58%) had complete or partial response to CAMF plus *C. parvum*. The toxicity and immunological responses were also similar in the two groups. On the other hand, both response duration and survival were longer in the group that received CAMF plus *C. parvum*. These results suggest that adding an immunopotentiator to partially effective chemotherapy may be of additional benefit in patients with advanced breast carcinoma.

ACKNOWLEDGMENT

The work reported here is supported by grants CA-05826, CA-08748, and contract CB-53873-S from the National Cancer Institute.

REFERENCES

1. Canellos, G. P., De Vita, V. T., Gold, G. L., Chabner, B. A., Schien, P. S., and Young, R. C. (1974): Clinical combination chemotherapy for advanced breast carcinoma. *Br. Med. J.,* 1:218–220.
2. DeJager, R., Kaufman, R., Ochoa, M., and Krakoff, I. H. (1975): Chemotherapy of

advanced breast cancer with a combination of Cytoxan, Adriamycin and 5-FU (CAF). *Proc. Am. Soc. Clin. Oncol.,* 16:273.

3. DeJager, R., Pinsky, C., Kaufman, R., Ochoa, M., Oettgen, H. F., and Krakoff, I. H. (1976): Chemotherapy of advanced breast cancer with a combination of Cyclophosphamide, Adriamycin, Methotrexate and 5-Fluorouracil (CAMF) with and without *C. parvum. Proc. Am. Soc. Clin. Oncol.,* 17:296.

4. Gehan, E. A. (1965): A generalized Wilcoxon test for comparing arbitrarily singly-censored samples. *Biometrika,* 52:203–223.

5. Gutterman, J. V., Mavligit, G. M., Burgess, M. A., Cardenas, J. O., Blumenshein, G. R., Gottlieb, J. A., McBride, Ch. M., McCredie, K. B., Bodey, G. P., Rodriguez, V., Freireich, E. J., and Hersh, E. M. (1976): Immunotherapy of breast cancer, malignant melanoma and acute leukemia with BCG: Prolongation of disease free interval and survival. *Cancer Immunol. Immunother.,* 1:99–107.

6. Hansen, J. A., Bloomfield, C. D., Dupont, B., Gajl-Peczalska, K. J., Kiszkiss, D., and Good, R. A. (1974): Lymphocyte subpopulations and immunodeficiency in lymphoproliferative malignancies. In: *Proceedings of the Eighth Leucocyte Culture Conference,* edited by K. Lindahl-Kissling and D. Osaba, pp. 119–125. Academic Press, New York.

7. Israel, L., and Edelstein, R. (1975): Nonspecific immunostimulation with *Corynebacterium parvum* in human cancer. In: *26th Annual M. D. Anderson Symposium: Immunological Aspects of Neoplasia* pp. 485–504. The Williams and Wilkins Company, Baltimore, Maryland.

8. Jones, S. E., Durie, B. G. M., and Salmon, S. E. (1975): Combination chemotherapy with adriamycin and cyclophosphamide for advanced breast cancer. *Cancer,* 36:90–97.

9. Kaplan, E. L., and Meier, P. (1958): Nonparametric estimation from incomplete observations. *J. Am. Stat. Assoc.* 53:457–481.

10. Moertel, C. G., Schutt, A. J., Hahn, R. G., and Reitemeier, R. J. (1975): Therapy of advanced colorectal cancer with a combination of 5-Fluorouracil, Methyl-1, 3-cis (2-chlorethyl)-1-nitrosourea, and Vincristine. *J. Natl. Cancer Inst.,* 54:69–72.

11. Pinsky, C. M., El Domeiri, A., Caron, A. S., Knapper, W. H., and Oettgen, H. F. (1974): Delayed hypersensitivity reactions in patients with cancer. In: *Recent Results in Cancer Research, Vol. 47,* edited by G. Mathe and R. Weiner, pp. 37–41. Springer-Verlag, Heidelberg, Berlin.

Question and Answer Session

Dr. Woodruff: Did you look at the level of antibody response to *C. parvum?* The reason I ask is that, as you know, in all animal models, subcutaneous *C. parvum* is so ineffective, even where it's highly effective when given intravenously. When you give *C. parvum* intravenously to people, you get quite markedly raised levels of antibody to the organism itself. It seems to me this is an important marker.

Dr. Pinsky: We have collected the sera but they have not yet been analyzed. There are experimental animal data suggesting the subcutaneous route may not be the best route for *C. parvum.* One of the important factors that led us to use the subcutaneous route in combination with chemotherapy was the rather striking evidence that Dr. Lucian Israel has generated by this approach. I certainly cannot disagree that other routes and other schedules should be evaluated.

Dr. Fudenberg: You stated that *C. parvum* immunotherapy prolonged remission duration. What is the evidence that *C. parvum* is acting as immunotherapy rather than perhaps by some other effect—for example, by direct killing of tumor cells?

Dr. Pinsky: We have certainly not proved in this study that the *C. parvum* is acting through an immunological mechanism, and Dr. Fudenberg's comment is well taken.

Dr. Salmon: My question relates to the adverse overall experience of this group of patients. Either these patients were in a very far advanced stage and more so than other comparable groups of patients treated in other centers, or the chemotherapy regimen itself had an increased adverse effect on the nonresponsive patients. I say this because the median survival in that group was exceedingly short.

Dr. Pinsky: I think we have some evidence that it's the patient population. There's a very high proportion of patients with major organ metastasis. About 20 fewer patients were evaluable than entered the study. Half of this difference represents patients who were too early for analysis, but the other half consisted of patients who died before they could get the first month of treatment. This was a very bad group and the early deaths occurred in both arms. There wasn't any preponderance in one arm versus the other.

Before we began this randomized trial at our center, CAMF was used and gave a 60 to 65 percent response rate. That combination, therefore, seems to be as active as CAF without methotrexate. It is certainly possible that by chance we have entered an exceedingly poor prognosis group of patients into this trial.

Dr. Salmon: We have seen comparable results in comparably staged patients, with just cytoxan and adriamycin without any immunotherapy.

Dr. Moertel: Have you looked at the particular characteristics of those patients who you have now followed out to the far end of your curves? Are they, in fact, comparable, or are there some imbalances in prognostic factors among them that might account for the apparent difference between the groups?

Dr. Pinsky: We have not specifically looked at the patients who have been followed the longest or who are at risk the longest to see if their prognostic features were different.

Immunotherapy of Cancer: Present Status of Trials in Man, edited by W. D. Terry and D. Windhorst. Raven Press, New York © 1978.

Chemoimmunotherapy of Advanced Breast Cancer with BCG

G. N. Hortobagyi, J. U. Gutterman, G. R. Blumenschein, A. Buzdar, M. A. Burgess, S. P. Richman, C. K. Tashima, M. Schwarz, and E. M. Hersh

Departments of Developmental Therapeutics and Medicine, The University of Texas System Cancer Center, M. D. Anderson Hospital and Tumor Institute, Houston, Texas 77030

Breast cancer continues to be the leading cause of cancer death among females (5,7). With the development of combination chemotherapy programs, utilizing a variety of active drugs with different modalities of action and toxicity, an encouraging increase in remission rates among patients with advanced disease has been achieved (3,6,12). The introduction of doxorubicin hydrochloride (Adriamycin®) in various combination programs has produced remission rates of 50 to 70% (11,13).

Despite this encouraging trend in remission rates, the duration of these responses has been short with a median of 5 to 10 months. The overall median survival with most of these combination chemotherapy programs has improved to approximately 10 to 15 months.

The importance of host defense mechanism in control of breast cancer and other tumors has become increasingly evident (1,2). As a result, immunotherapy is becoming increasingly important in the therapeutic strategy of the cancer patient (16). We recently demonstrated that immunotherapy with Bacillus Calmette-Guerin (BCG) prolonged chemotherapy-induced remissions and survival of patients with disseminated melanoma (15) and acute myelogenous leukemia (14). After we successfully worked out the use of intermittent chemotherapy with immunotherapy, we explored the question whether BCG immunotherapy could (a) increase remission rates, (b) prolong remission duration, and (c) prolong overall survival of patients with metastatic breast cancer who were receiving combination chemotherapy. Thus a program of chemoimmunotherapy for disseminated breast cancer was initiated combining BCG with our previous best combination chemotherapy regimen of 5-fluorouracil, doxorubicin hydrochloride, and cyclophosphamide. Our preliminary reports have been published elsewhere (13), and we report now an extension of the results for 105 patients.

MATERIALS AND METHODS

Since March, 1974, 105 evaluable patients with disseminated breast cancer have been treated with chemoimmunotherapy consisting of 5-fluorouracil 500 mg/m² i.v. on days 1 and 8 of each course, doxorubicin hydrochloride 50 mg/m² i.v. on day 1, and cyclophosphamide 500 mg/m² i.v. on day 1 (FAC). Lyophilized Tice or Pasteur strain BCG at a dose of 6×10^8 viable units was given by scarification, rotating all four proximal extremities as previously described on days 9, 13, and 17 of each course (17). Courses of chemoimmunotherapy were repeated every 21 days if hematological recovery permitted. Dose escalation or deescalation was performed in order to maintain the lowest granulocyte count between 1,000 and 2,000/mm³ and the lowest platelet count above 50,000/mm³. Documented infection and/or hemorrhage required a dose reduction of 25% regardless of change in blood count.

The results of this series were compared to those obtained in a comparable group of 44 patients treated with the same chemotherapy (FAC) immediately prior to the study between August, 1973 and March, 1974 (13).

Sixty-four patients were entered on the FAC chemotherapy study. Six patients were inevaluable since two died before the first course of therapy was completed (early death) and four patients had major protocol violations with totally inadequate doses of chemotherapy. Fifty-eight patients were eligible for response rate, which was 79% (*see below*). Only 44 were evaluable for remission duration and survival since 14 of the patients were given BCG after they achieved remissions. Thus, 44 patients were treated with FAC chemotherapy for the entire duration of therapy and serve as the chemotherapy control group.

One hundred and twenty-eight patients were entered on the FAC-BCG treatment program. Twenty-three (18%) were excluded from evaluation for the following reasons—nine of them received either no BCG or an inadequate dose schedule of BCG, five patients were lost to follow-up after their first course of chemotherapy, six patients had major chemotherapy-related protocol deviations, and three patients died before day 14 (early death) of the first course of treatment.

The total dose of doxorubicin hydrochloride was limited to 550 mg/m² on the first 44 patients and subsequently to 450 mg/m² in order to prevent doxorubicin hydrochloride-related cardiotoxicity. At the time doxorubicin hydrochloride was stopped maintenance therapy was begun consisting of the CMF regimen cyclophosphamide 500 mg/m² p.o. on day 2, methotrexate 30 mg/m² i.m. on days 1 and 8, and 5-fluorouracil, 500 mg/m² p.o. on days 1 and 8. In the chemoimmunotherapy group, BCG was continued on days 9, 13, and 17 of each 21-day maintenance course.

Criteria for eligibility for the FAC-BCG studies were as follows. There had to be evidence of progressive metastatic breast cancer with clearly measurable tumor, either by physical examination or by radiological or radioisotopic criteria. Patients with overt congestive heart failure were not eligible for this trial. Although prior chemotherapy did not exclude patients from entering the FAC or FAC-BCG program, evidence of progression with prior cyclophosphamide, doxorubicin hydrochloride, or 5-fluorouracil precluded their inclusions in the treatment programs.

The criteria of response to treatment were as follows. Complete remission was defined as the complete disappearance of all objective and subjective evidence of disease, including complete recalcification of bone lesions, and partial remission was interpreted as a 50% or greater reduction in the product of the diameter of measurable lesions, including partial recalcification of bone metastases. Patients with less than 50% reduction or less than 25% increase in tumor size for a minimum period of 2 months were considered to have stable disease. Progression or relapse was defined as a more than 25% increase in existing tumor masses or the appearance of new lesions.

Remission duration was determined from the day of achieving remission to the day of progression or relapse. Survival was measured from the start of treatment to the date of death or last follow-up examination.

The statistical methods used included the method of Kaplan and Meier for calculating and plotting remission and survival curves (20) and a generalized Wilcoxon test with a one-tailed analysis testing differences between remission and survival curves (10).

RESULTS

Pretreatment characteristics of evaluable patients in both groups are shown in Table 1. Factors known to alter the prognosis of these patients were similar in both groups and distribution of metastatic sites was comparable (Table 2).

Thirty-two of 44 patients (73%) treated with FAC and 78 of 105 (75%) treated with FAC-BCG achieved a partial or complete remission (Table 3). The proportion of partial and complete remissions was similar in both groups. The response according to metastatic sites was also similar in both treatment

TABLE 1. *Chemoimmunotherapy of advanced breast cancer, population characteristics*

Characteristics	FAC	FAC-BCG
No. of patients	44	105
Age (range)	51 (29–67)	53 (25–72)
Premenopausal	31%	23%
Postmenopausal	69%	77%
Prior hormonal therapy	79%	65%
Prior chemotherapy	7%	14%
Disease-free interval (months)	15 (0–104)	16 (0–140)

TABLE 2. *Chemoimmunotherapy of advanced breast cancer, distribution of metastatic sites*

Metastatic sites	FAC	FAC-BCG
Soft tissue	44%	33%
Lymph nodes	32%	28%
Bone	66%	61%
Lung	55%	33%
Pleura	16%	24%
Liver	20%	22%

TABLE 3. *Chemoimmunotherapy of advanced breast cancer, response rates*

Responses	FAC	FAC-BCG
Total no. patients	44	105
Complete remission	6 (14%)	20 (19%)
Partial remission	26 (59%)	58 (55.2%)
Stable	12 (27%)	21 (20%)
Progression	—	6 (6%)

groups (Table 4). The median time to partial and complete remission was 2 and 3 months, respectively. Age, menopausal status, disease-free interval, and response to prior hormonal manipulation did not influence the response to chemotherapy.

The duration of remission is shown in Fig. 1. Twenty-seven of 32 patients in the FAC group have relapsed with a median duration of 9 months. Forty-two of the 78 patients on FAC-BCG have relapsed with a median duration of 14 months. These differences are statistically significant at $p = 0.008$. The median duration of remission for FAC complete responders was 9 months and for the FAC-BCG complete responders 14 months. This was not statistically significant at $p = 0.2$. Four of 26 partial responders on the FAC program are still in remission with a median of 9 months. In contrast, 26 of 58 patients achieving partial remission on the FAC-BCG group are still in remission with a median duration of 14 months ($p = 0.07$). The duration of stability was identical for both groups.

TABLE 4. *Chemoimmunotherapy of advanced breast cancer, percent response by sites*

Metastatic sites	FAC	FAC-BCG
Breast and soft tissue	83	80
Lymph nodes	100	86
Bone	41	67
Lung	66	69
Pleura	63	76
Liver	58	61

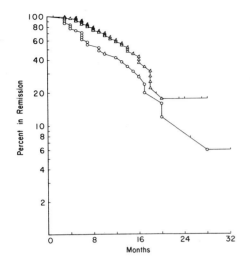

FIG. 1. Duration of remission with chemoimmuno-therapy of stage IV breast cancer. With a regimen of FAC-BCG (△) 42 of 78 have re-lapsed, and with an FAC regimen (○) 27 of 32 have relapsed. *p* = 0.008.

The most important effect of chemoimmunotherapy was prolongation of survival. Shown in Fig. 2 is the survival of the responding patients. Eleven of 32 patients in the FAC group who achieved remission are still alive with a median survival of 16 months. Fifty-one of 78 patients on FAC-BCG are still alive with a median survival of 22.5 months. These differences are statistically significant at $p = 0.004$.

At this point, survival of stable patients is superior for FAC-BCG (median, 13.5 months) compared to FAC (median, 8.8 months). These differences are suggestive ($p = 0.1$).

The survival for all patients treated with an adequate trial is shown in

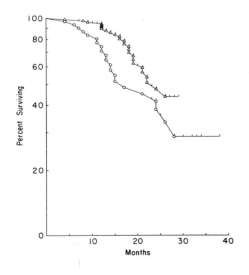

FIG. 2. Survival of responders to chemoimmuno-therapy of stage IV breast cancer. On the FAC-BCG regimen (△) 27 of 78 are dead, and on the FAC regimen (○) 21 of 32 are dead. *p* = 0.004.

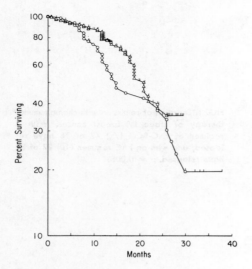

FIG. 3. Survival of all patients on chemoimmuno-therapy for stage IV breast cancer. Forty-five of 105 of the FAC-BCG group (△) have died, and 31 of 44 of the FAC group (○) have died. p = 0.02.

Fig. 3. Thirty-one of the 44 FAC-BCG patients have died with a median survival of 14.8 months. Forty-five of 105 patients on FAC-BCG have died with a median survival of 20.7 months. These differences are statistically significant at $p = 0.02$.

After progression, most of the patients in both studies were treated with second line chemotherapeutic agents such as methotrexate, vincristine, mitomycin-C, Baker's antifol, ifosphamide, and occasional hormonal manipulation. A comparative analysis of the response to secondary modalities of treatment between the two groups did not suggest any significant differences in reponses after the first relapse.

Toxicity

Treatment in both groups was well tolerated. Although nausea, vomiting, and alopecia occurred in virtually all patients, the dose-limiting toxicity was myelosuppression. Granulocytopenia was very predictable. The lowest granylocyte count was usually encountered at days 12 to 18 of each course. The recovery was prompt, and the majority of patients were able to start their courses of treatment every 21 days. Thrombocytopenia was rarely measured and was of little clinical significance. Myelosuppression was slightly cumulative, proved by the fact that by the sixth course, 50% of the patients were able to tolerate only 80% of the calculated dose.

Infectious episodes associated with granulocytopenia occurred in a small fraction of the patients in both groups, but none of these patients died as a consequence of an infectious episode. Immunotherapy did not seem to influence the degree of myelosuppression or the incidence of infectious complications.

Side effects related to BCG were mild and consisted mainly of local soreness and itching, a low-grade fever, and an ill-defined flu-like syndrome for 12 to 24 hr following most scarifications. Although a generalized rash (with a histological picture of a hypersensitivity vasculitis) was observed in three patients, no disseminated BCG disease occurred and tuberculostatic chemotherapy was not required.

Congestive heart failure, presumably secondary to doxorubicin hydrochloride-related cardiomyopathy, was observed in five patients of the FAC group and four patients of the FAC-BCG group. In all cases, digitalis and diuretic treatment achieved symptomatic control. None of the patients died as a direct consequence of the cardiotoxic effects of doxorubicin hydrochloride.

DISCUSSION

This study suggests that the prognosis of patients with advanced breast cancer treated with cyclic combination chemotherapy has been improved by the addition of immunotherapy. Remission rates have not been influenced by BCG immunotherapy, however, duration of remission has been highly significantly prolonged with FAC-CMF-BCG compared to the chemotherapy control group. However, only 20% of patients are projected to remain in remission at 20 months even with chemoimmunotherapy.

The most important therapeutic effect of BCG immunotherapy in the current study was the increase of survival among the responders. Thus, less than half the patients who achieved remission on FAC chemotherapy survived 18 months (median, 15 months). In contrast, a projected 75% of the patients achieving remission on FAC-BCG will survive more than 18 months. Thus, the 0.75 percentile is already 18 months. It is important to point out that the data with our FAC control group carried out just prior to the FAC-BCG group are nearly identical to those reported by Jones and co-workers with a similar chemotherapy combination (19) (doxorubicin hydrochloride plus cytoxan or AC). The survival of patients with partial remission (FAC, 15 months; AC, 17 months) and overall survival (median, 15 months for both studies) are identical. The allocation of 14 patients to FAC-CMF-BCG from the original 58 patients treated with FAC does not appear to have influenced the control group and thus serves as a suitable historical control.

The results, if confirmed, extend the principles established in other chemoimmunotherapy trials with BCG where remission rates were not significantly increased (except for tumor size regional to BCG scarification), but remission duration and particularly survival were significantly increased compared to chemotherapy alone (15). Similar results have been reported previously when *Corynebacterium parvum* (18) or Levamisole (23) was added to chemotherapy in breast cancer. It is hoped this preliminary report will stimulate additional trials of chemoimmunotherapy in advanced breast cancer.

Despite the encouraging results with BCG, improved modalities of immunotherapy and combination chemotherapy are needed to increase the remission rates in visceral regions as well as shift the partial remissions to complete remissions. Other immunological approaches have suggested benefit in breast cancer (22,23).

Finally, since adjuvant chemotherapy has prolonged the disease-free interval and survival in breast cancer patients with histological evidence of spread to regional lymph nodes (4,9) and adjuvant immunotherapy has been beneficial in colorectal cancer (21) and malignant melanoma (8,17), programs of combination chemotherapy and immunotherapy should be designed for patients with suspected residual microscopic disease after surgery.

Results with FAC-BCG as postoperative adjuvant therapy for breast cancer patients with positive nodes show a highly significant prolongation of the disease-free interval and survival compared to historical surgical controls (24).

ACKNOWLEDGMENTS

This work has been supported by contract N01-CB-33888 and grants 05831 and 11520 from the National Cancer Institute, Bethesda, Maryland 20014. Dr. Gutterman is the recipient of a career development award (CA-71007-2) also from the National Cancer Institute.

REFERENCES

1. Black, M. M., Kerpe, S., and Speer, F. D. (1953): Lymph node structure in patients with cancer of the breast. *Am. J. Pathol.*, 29:505–521.
2. Bloom, H. J., Richardson, W. W., and Field, J. R. (1970): Host resistance and survival in carcinoma of the breast: A study of 104 cases of medullary carcinoma in a series of 1,411 cases of breast cancer followed for 20 years. *Br. Med. J.*, 3:181–188.
3. Blumenschein, G. R., Cardenas, J. O., Freireich, E. J., and Gottlieb, J. A. (1974): FAC chemotherapy for breast cancer. *Am. Soc. Clin. Oncol.* 15:193 (Abstr. No. 839).
4. Bonadonna, G., Brusamalino, E., Valagussa, P., Rossi, A., Brugnatelli, L., Brambilla, C., De Lena, M., Tancini, G., Bajetta, E., Musumeci, T., and Vernoesi, U. (1976): Combination chemotherapy as an adjuvant treatment in operable breast cancer. *N. Engl. J. Med.*, 294:405–410.
5. *1975 Cancer Facts and Figures:* American Cancer Society, New York, New York.
6. Cannellos, G. P., Devita, V. T., Gold, G. L., Chabner, B. A., Schein, P. S., and Young, R. C. (1974): Cyclical combination chemotherapy for advanced breast carcinoma. *Br. Med. J.*, 1:218–220.
7. Cutler, S. J. (1974): Classification of extent of disease in breast cancer. *Semin. Oncol.*, 1:91–96.
8. Eilber, F. R., Morton, D. L., Holmes, E. C., Sparks, F. C., and Ramming, K. P. (1976): Immunotherapy with BCG in treatment of regional-lymph-node metastases from malignant melanoma. *N. Eng. J. Med.*, 294:240.
9. Fisher, B., Carbone, P., Economou, S. G., Frelick, R., Glass, A., Leiner, H., Redmond, C., Zelen, M., Band, P., Katrych, D., Wolmark, N., and Fisher, E. R. (1975): 1-Phenylalanine mustard (L-Pam) in the management of primary breast cancer. A report of early findings. *N. Engl. J. Med.*, 292:117–122.

10. Gehan, E. A. (1965): A generalized Wilcoxan test for comparing arbitrarily singly-censored samples. *Biometrika*, 52:203–223.
11. Gottlieb, J. A., Blumenschein, G. R., Gutterman, J. U., Freireich, E. J., and Cardenas, J. O. (1975): Adriamycin in the treatment of breast cancer. *Adriamycin Rev.*, IV:249–256.
12. Greenspan, E. M. (1966): Combination cytoxic chemotherapy in advanced disseminated breast carcinoma. *J. Mt. Sinai Hosp.*, 33:1–27.
13. Gutterman, J. U., Cardenas, J. O., Blumenschein, G. R., Hortobagyi, G., Burgess, M. A., Livingston, R. B., Mavligit, G. M., Gottlieb, J. A., Freireich, E. J., and Hersh, E. M. (1976): Chemoimmunotherapy of advanced breast cancer: Prolongation of remission and survival with BCG. *Br. Med. J.*, 2:1222–1225.
14. Gutterman, J. U., Hersh, E. M., Rodriguez, V., McCredie, K. B., Mavligit, G., Reed, R., Burgess, M. A., Smith, T., Gehan, E., Bodey, G. P., Sr., and Freireich, E. J. (1974): Prolongation of remission in myeloblastic leukemia with BCG. *Lancet*, 2:1405–1409.
15. Gutterman, J. U., Mavligit, G., Gottlieb, J. A., Burgess, M. A., McBride, C. E., Einhorn L., Freireich, E. J., and Hersh, E. M. (1974): Chemoimmunotherapy of disseminated malignant melanoma with DTIC and BCG. *N. Engl. J. Med.*, 391:592–597.
16. Gutterman, J. U., Mavligit, G. M., and Hersh, E. M. (1976): Chemoimmunotherapy of human solid tumors. *Med. Clin. North Am.*, 60:441–462.
17. Gutterman, J. U., Mavligit, G., McBride, C., Frei, E., III., Freireich, E. J., and Hersh, E. M. (1973): Active immunotherapy with B.C.G. for recurrent malignant melanoma. *Lancet*, 1:1208–1212.
18. Israel, L., and Edelstein, R., (1976): Non-specific immunostimulation with C. parvum in human cancer. In: *Immunologic Aspects of Neoplasia, 26th Symp.*, pp. 485–505. William & Wilkins, Baltimore.
19. Jones, S. E., Durie, B. G., and Salmon, S. E. (1975): Combination chemoimmunotherapy with adriamycin and cyclophosphamide for advanced breast cancer. *Cancer*, 36:90–97.
20. Kaplan, E. L., and Meier, P. (1958): Non-parametic estimation from incomplete observations. *J. Am. Stat. Assoc.*, 53:457–481.
21. Mavligit, G. M., Gutterman, J. U., Burgess, M. A., Khankhankian, M., Seibert, B. B., Speer, J. F., Jubert, A. V., Martin, R. C., McBride, C. M., Copeland, E. M., Gehan, E. A., and Hersh, E. M. (1976): Prolongation of post operative disease free interval and survival in human colorectal cancer by Bacillus Calmette Guerin (BCG) or BCG plus 5-fluorouracil. *Lancet*, 1:871–875.
22. Oettgen, H. F., Old, L. J., Farrow, J. H., Valentine, F. T., Lawrence, H. S., and Thomas, L. (1974): Effects of dialyzable transfer factor in patients with breast cancer. *Proc. Natl. Acad. Sci. USA*, 71:2319–2323.
23. Rojas, A. F., Mickiewicz, E., Feirstein, J. N., Glait, H., and Olivari, A. J. (1976): Levamisole in advanced human breast cancer. *Lancet*, 1:211–215.
24. Buzdar, A., Gutterman, J., Blumenschein, G., Tashima, C., Hortobagyi, G., Wheeler, W., Gehan, E., Freireich, E., and Hersh, E. (1977): Adjuvant chemoimmunotherapy following regional therapy in breast cancer. In: Adjuvant Therapy of Cancer, pp. 139–146. North-Holland, Amsterdam.

Question and Answer Session

Question: Some people have encountered increased leukopenia with BCG and MER. Dr. Hortobagyi, you have not seen any increased leukopenia. Just how common is this finding and is it known why it occurs?

Dr. Hortobagyi: We have not seen any difference in myelosuppression in those patients treated with chemotherapy alone or chemotherapy and immunotherapy with either BCG or MER. Similarly, we have not seen any influence on the incidence of infections, minor or major. As far as toxicity with MER, we administer MER between courses of chemotherapy. I think the main reason we encountered toxicity was because we were using a rather high dose at the beginning, and second, because we probably used the wrong route, as Dr. Weiss has told us since then.

Dr. Weiss: As Dr. Hortobagyi indicated, it really isn't surprising that a granuloma-inducing material should produce severe toxicity when injected subcutaneously. On the other hand, most animal studies indicate that schedules that cause such toxicity need not be used to have an immunostimulating or therapeutic effect.

It might, in fact, be because most patients only receive one or two treatments of MER and then have to be stopped that MER seemed to be as good as repeated administration of BCG. I want to reemphasize the evidence that, generally, undertreatment is more effective than overtreatment in immunotherapy in animal systems. That has to be borne in mind in planning and evaluating clinical trials.

Also, it might be worthwhile to consider adjusting dosage to individual cases according to reactions to the stimulant itself, rather than adhering to a predetermined absolute dose. There is some biological meaning to the extensiveness of the local reaction.

Dr. Salmon: Dr. Hortobagyi, you have about twice the percentage of patients with prior chemotherapy in the FAC-BCG arm (7 percent in FAC versus 15 percent in FAC-BCG) which could adversely affect the overall result of the chemoimmunotherapy arm. Have you analyzed those studies deleting the previously treated patients, because in most of the prior studies previous chemotherapy had an adverse influence?

Dr. Hortobagyi: I have not looked at it that way, since, as Dr. Fisher expressed earlier, this is a disease that is very heterogeneous, and numbers are very important. If we exclude more patients from our chemotherapy-alone group, we would be analyzing a very small number of patients.

Also, patients who had progressed on prior 5-FU, adriamycin, or Cytoxan were excluded from this study. Patients who had been exposed to any of the three agents but showed no evidence of progression were included.

DISCUSSION: IMMUNOTHERAPY OF BREAST CANCER

Question: Dr. Olivari, if a dose of 4,000 rads is given in the treatment of breast cancer, as a central axis dose, the variation in delivered dose could be up to 30 to 40 percent between patients. Unless there is computerized treatment planning, the variation in dose delivered could produce a "treatment effect" if, by chance, higher dosage was given to the patients who received levamisole. Did you use computerized treatment planning in the distribution of dose for these patients?

Dr. Olivari: We have not used computer planned treatment.

Question: Then it would be a central axis dose. Based on the contour of the patients, random results could be obtained. I think that is a difficulty we should watch for in the future.

Question: Drs. Moertel and Engstrom have given examples of increased leukopenia when the chemotherapy came immediately after their BCG, and this is consistent with our work on animal models using *C. parvum,* where, when cell cycle-specific drugs are given immediately after *C. parvum,* there is marked hematologic toxicity. When such agents are given immediately before *C. parvum,* there is less toxicity. This does not appear to be true for cell-cycle-nonspecific drugs, where toxicity is not altered by *C. parvum.* Presumably an agent that induces cells into more rapid proliferation will increase the sensitivity of those cells to a cell cycle-specific drug. Dr. Pinsky, in your study, was the total dose of chemotherapy equivalent in the two groups, or was there a variation in the total amount of chemotherapy for these two groups?

Dr. Pinsky: There was absolutely no difference in hematologic toxicity between the two groups. In experimental animals *C. parvum* can stimulate the bone marrow. However, if it is given in combination with chemotherapy, animal data suggest *C. parvum* could increase the hematologic toxicity. Maybe we were doing both at the same time and coming out with no difference.

Also, there are no statistically significant differences between the amount of drugs given to the two groups. However, the responders who got CAMF plus *C. parvum* eventually received less drug even though that difference was not statistically significant.

Dr. Frei: Combination chemotherapy for advanced breast cancer is moderately effective. There is a 60 to 70 percent objective response rate, a 20 percent complete response rate, and the responders survive longer than the nonresponders. Further, there is no question that the skill in using that treatment is very important to getting good results.

In any program that adds something like BCG, the patient will be seen at frequent intervals at a center where there is considerable expertise in administering chemotherapy. Patients receiving chemotherapy alone may be treated much more frequently in their home community. Factors leading to optimal chemotherapy may therefore apply to the patients receiving BCG, but not to those receiving chemotherapy alone.

I think the differences you've shown are the kinds of differences an expert chemotherapist and a less expert chemotherapist would achieve using exactly the same program. Have Dr. Pinsky and Dr. Hortobagyi analyzed their data from this point of view?

Dr. Pinsky: It might be a good thing to look at. Once we could be fairly sure about the types of reactions patients were going to have, these patients were trained to vaccinate themselves with *C. parvum*. In that situation patients receiving *C. parvum* were not seen more often than the patients who were receiving only chemotherapy.

Dr. Frei: I would like to suggest that both speakers determine how often patients received chemotherapy at Sloan-Kettering or M. D. Anderson and how often they received it from the referring physician. If there is a significant difference between the chemoimmunotherapy and the chemotherapy groups for this variable, I would be concerned.

Dr. Hortobagyi: Most of the patients at M. D. Anderson are taught to administer BCG themselves and they do it at home. A large number of them are from out of state, so they come back every third or every fourth course of chemotherapy. However, your point is valid. I will have to look at that.

Dr. Fisher: The purpose of clinical research is to apply scientific methodology to clinical problems. Any good experiment leads to another experiment. Have any of these investigators learned anything which suggests to them what the next step should be?

Dr. Hortobagyi: I think we have learned that, in patients with advanced disease, we can expect to make only modest advances with what we have available. We are talking about prolonging remission or survival by a few months, which really is not as dramatic as we would like it to be.

I believe that immunotherapy is adding something to chemotherapy and the place we should be applying our information is in the adjuvant situation, where we would be facing a minimal residual disease, and where we would have the chance of contributing in a major way to the welfare and to the survival of these patients.

Dr. Fisher: In the adjuvant situation, one can have a cleaner design, a more controlled situation.

Dr. Moertel: Dr. Fisher, would you be willing to have an immunotherapy-alone arm on your next breast cancer surgical adjuvant program?

Dr. Fisher: There are many factors to be considered. One of the important considerations to which I have addressed myself before has to do with closing doors which can't be reopened. If, for example, the first adjuvant chemotherapy for breast cancer was seven drugs that demonstrated success in 100 percent of patients, you would never be able to go back and try six drugs or five drugs or four drugs, and so on, because ethically you might be putting those patients to an inappropriate risk. When you ask me categorical questions, however, I can't give you categorical answers.

Dr. Holland: In looking at historical controls, as Dr. Hortobagyi has, it probably is important to know whether the patients developed metastatic cancer after having been operated on with no nodes in the axilla or with five or 10 nodes in the axilla. I have never seen them stratified this way. Has anyone looked at the effect of nodal status at the time of operation on the time to death, following the first demonstration of metastatic cancer?

If, in fact, the historical control had in it many people who had had four to 10 nodes at the time of operation, and the present series, because of change in medical practice over time, has in it many women who have no nodes and then develop metastatic cancer, the virulence of those tumors in those two situations might be different.

Dr. Fisher: In 1958 we did a large clinical trial, and we have a life table of the patients followed for 10 years. We started another cilincal trial in 1971, and the life table analysis is exactly the same. So one might say, "Well, this is good support for historical controls."

However, in subsets of patients, there are differences; in the 1- to 3-node groups, the difference is in one direction, and in the 4-plus node group it is in the other direction, and so they cancel out. I think this could lead you down the primrose path if you used the controls from the previous study.

Dr. Pinsky: We stratified for disease-free interval, since this seems to be a general reflection of the biologic aggressiveness of the tumor. In designing our trial we took into account a great many possible variables and leads from not only previous animal data but also from experimental clinical data including Phase I trials of optimal dose, route and schedule of administration.

To respond to Dr. Fisher's question, our study is still early, but it looks as if it will give us some leads.

Dr. Fisher: All of the investigations that have been reported here are very important. They are important in that they provide a little bit of information which in the sum total will give us reason to do or not do certain things. It is important to remember that all studies need confirmation.

Dr. Salmon: I want to respond to Dr. Fisher's question also. I will limit it just to BCG, MER, and *C. parvum,* because we haven't had enough information on levamisole to make a comment. We have learned that these agents do not increase the complete or partial response rate of any of the basic treatment regimens that have been given.

We have also learned that with basic treatment regimens that show objective response and improve remission duration or survival, the immunotherapeutic agents may appear to further improve remission duration or survival.

It isn't clear whether this effect is directly immunotherapeutic or may be an effect on the improvement of patient care.

We could say that at the very least immunotherapy has improved patient care in those trials, and it may also have had an immunotherapeutic effect.

Dr. Woodruff: It seems to me enormously important there should be a study of an immunotherapy arm as the sole adjuvant for surgery in operable breast cancer. I say that partly because I have a certain theory about immunotherapy, but more because I think our clinical tasks should be designed to answer questions, rather than to try and hit some sort of therapeutic jackpot in one shot.

Now, I accept that in the United States it may be impossible or too late at this stage to introduce that arm. There are many other parts of the world, including Britain, where an enormous number of women with operable breast cancer, rightly or wrongly, do not get adjuvant chemotherapy. While such a population exists, it is still not too late. If the patients are not going to get their adjuvant chemotherapy anyway, then I see no objection to not giving it to them in a particular trial.

I would make a plea that something of the sort should be set up. I think it's a door that might close and close very suddenly and we might miss something important.

Immunotherapy of Cancer: Present Status of
Trials in Man, **edited by** W. D. Terry **and** D. Windhorst
Raven Press, New York © 1978.

Concluding Remarks

William D. Terry

Division of Cancer Biology and Diagnosis, National Cancer Institute,
Bethesda, Maryland 20014

When we originally planned the format of the conference on which this volume is based, we hoped that the participants would be willing to engage in free discussion in an attempt to evaluate the work presented. They have done just that, and we are all very much the beneficiaries of this free and open discussion. This was a serious attempt to evaluate the best of the present studies of clinical immunotherapy and to achieve a realistic sense of our accomplishments and our failures, so that we might have a firm foundation for future efforts.

What are the take-home lessons from this review? Many of the studies have yielded negative results. There have been many examples of seemingly similar studies where some of the results have been positive and some of the results have been negative, and there are many examples of what appear to be random empiric approaches to what is a very complex biologic problem.

However, negative results are not only predictable but they are absolutely anticipated when you initiate clinical applications in a field of this complexity. Positive trials that appear to be contradicted by apparently comparable negative trials are also predictable for what is the very early phase of an attempt to harness the power of a system as complex and as poorly understood as the immune system, and to apply it to a problem of the truly awesome dimensions of clinical cancer.

We have many legacies from the development of chemotherapy when a similar pattern occurred. Some of them are quite beneficial. I have been exceedingly impressed with the quality of both the design and the implementation of most of the trials that are presented in this volume, and a comparable quality would probably not have been experienced in a chemotherapy volume 15 to 20 years ago. We have learned much from our chemotherapy colleagues. However, they have also left us with some major problems. For example, much attention has been paid to the comparative strengths and weaknesses of randomized and historically controlled trials. Although this discussion has been in the context of immunotherapy trials, this is not a specific problem of immunotherapy, but rather a general problem of all clinical experimental medicine. The issue we must address is not whether randomized studies are better than historically controlled studies, but whether it is possible to achieve a definition of the circumstances in which one or the other is the appropriate study design.

As an example of the potential value of trials using historical controls, we have the instance of osteogenic sarcoma. These studies appear to have provided one of the major advances in chemotherapy within the last few years, and these trials are all based on historical controls. Historical controls have been considered appropriate in this disease because the number of patients is small and the natural history of the disease is considered to be well established and predictable. We included a section on sarcoma in this volume because some questions had been raised about the validity of the historical controls. Some observations at the Mayo Clinic suggesting that disease-free interval was becoming longer with surgery alone. If this were universally true, it would make the historically controlled trial inevaluable. To investigate this issue, we asked other institutions to come up with comparable information. The data were acquired, evaluated, and discussed. I believe most people now are reassured about the validity of those controls, at least as regards the specific questions that were raised.

This is the way that we must proceed. We should not abolish the use of historical controls in planning studies, as long as the necessary stringent requirements for the use of such controls can be met. We also cannot reject studies simply because they have been historically controlled. Rather, if we wish to question the results of such studies, we must find the flaws in the historical controls. What we want and what we need in the entire field of clinical investigation is rational critique and not emotional rejection.

Where do we go from here?

I would say that there is no question that clinical immunotherapy is here to stay and the future is reasonably bright. For the immediate future it will be important to carefully consider the lesson that we should derive from the chapters of McKneally and Yamamura. In both experimental animals and humans, the most successful results to date have been in studies where adjuvants are introduced into the region of the tumor. Additional studies of clinical immunotherapy must take this into account. Most of the material presented is the result of studies in which this approach has *not* been pursued.

If our knowledge of the immune system and of the relationship between the immune system and an evolving tumor were to be frozen at the present level, I would be much more pessimistic. We might then be condemned to carry out an endless series of empiric studies that would be largely fruitless. Fortunately, our knowledge in these areas is rapidly expanding. There is new information every day about the nature of cell surfaces, about the nature of weak antigens, about what constitutes the grounds for establishing a stronger immune response against weak antigens, information about specific and non-specific suppressor cells and factors. And all of this information is being very rapidly applied to tumor immunology and tumor immunotherapy.

These basic developments, which represent work in progress right now, will be translated into animal experimentation and into the clinic over the next several years. I'm sure that the level of success will be considerably different within five years.

As we await this new information, we must consolidate the data that we have at this time. It is important that there be confirmation of each of the apparently positive studies, in order that we can build a firm foundation on which future clinical immunotherapy can be built.

Subject Index

AAFC, *see* Anhydroarabinosylfluorocytosine
Abscess formation, intradermal
immunotherapy and, 99
Acral lengtigenous melanoma (ALM),
1, 4
Actinomycin D, chemotherapy of soft
tissue sarcoma and, 248
Acturial life table method, *see* Life
table analysis
Acute lymphoblastic leukemia
BCG-induced remissions in, 27
immunotherapy vs. chemotherapy as
maintenance treatment of,
471–480, 481, 493–495, 496
Acute lymphocytic (lymphatic, lymphoid) leukemia
chemotherapy in, 441–450
chemotherapy followed by active
immunotherapy in, 451–466,
468–469, 473f
in children, *see* Childhood acute
lymphocytic leukemia
cures for, 443–445
immunotherapy for, 383–389, 390–
391, 410, 452–466, 468–469,
529–538
model of leukemic cell kinetics in,
441–442, 443f
multiplicity of types of, new protocols and, 463–464
Acute myeloblastic leukemia, BCG
immunotherapy in, 365–372
Acute mylocytic (myelogenous)
leukemia, manifestations and
prognostic features of, 307–313.
See also Acute myelocytic
leukemia chemotherapy; Acute
myelocytic leukemia immunotherapy
Acute myelocytic (myelogenous)
leukemia chemoimmunotherapy
with MER, 405–411, 412–413, 529
with Poly I:Poly C acid, 423–430,
431

with VCN-treated cells vs. chemotherapy, 437–352, 353
Acute myelocytic (myelogenous)
leukemia chemotherapy
with daunorubicin and cytosine
arabinoside, 316
survival and, 319t
Acute myelocytic (myelogenous)
leukemia immunotherapy
and antigens, 435–438
with BCG, 375–380, 381, 431,
432t, 433–440
with BCG by intraveous route,
393–402, 404
with BCG and leukemia cells,
315–324, 326–327
with viral oncolysate, 355–361,
362–363
Acute myeloid leukemia immunotherapy, with BCG and irradiated allogeneic blast cells,
341–345, 346
Acute nonlymphatic leukemia
immunotherapy, survival and
remission duration and, 328–
337, 339
Acute nonlymphoblastic leukemia
chemoimmunotherapy, with
Pseudomonas aeruginosa
vaccine, 415–422
ADR, *see* Doxorubicin hydrochloride
Adriamycin, *see* Doxorubicin hydrochloride
Age of patients
with acute myelocytic leukemia
and immunotherapy trials, 316,
349
incidence and, 307–308
and MER-induced remissions,
409t, 410
prognosis and, 309
BCG vaccination and, 28
in breast cancer levamisole trial,
636t
with childhood osteogenic sarcoma,